BIOLOGICAL WARFARE PATHOGEN PERSPECTIVES

PHILLIP YUAN PEI JEN Ph.D.
WILLIAM E. HOUSTON Ph.D.
AMANDA DUFFUS Ph.D.
MUSTAPHA DUROJAIYE Ph.D.

CONTRIBUTORS

DONNA JEN M.Ed.
WYATT T. CRAMBLET
RON WALTERS M.A.
JEREMY RICHARDS Ph.D
AMANDA C. ASHLEY
JIN H. SEO
ABBY M. ANDREWS
KAITLIN A. BLOODWORTH
ANDREW ODEGAARD
CHRISTOPHER B. CAMANTIGUE
PHILLIP R. GREGORY
TARA A. RIGGS

Front cover: filamentous Ebola Virus Particles taken with colorized scanning electron micrograph (25,000x magnification) budding from a chronically infected VERO E6 cell. The photomicrograph was taken by National Institute of Allergy and Infectious Diseases (NIAID) and is licenced to be reproduced under Creative Commons Attribution 2.0

Back cover: Scanning electron micrograph of *Yersinia pestis*, which causes bubonic plague, on proventricular spines of a *Xenopsylla cheopis* flea. The photomicrograph was taken by National Institute of Allergy and Infectious Diseases (NIAID) and is licenced to be reproduced under Creative Commons Attribution 2.0

BIOLOGICAL WARFARE PATHOGEN PERSPECTIVES

ISBN: 0692441212
ISBN13: 978-0692441213

Library of Congress Control Number: 2015908117
CreateSpace Independent Publishing Platform
North Charleston, South Carolina

"There are numerous books on the topic of microbiology, as well as books on biological warfare agents. However, there has not been a book designated to combine the two topics until now. Biological Warfare, Pathogen perspective is a clear and concise reference text book that combines the fundamentals of applied microbiology with a topic that is front and center of the security of the United States – biological warfare agents. This text is carefully researched, referenced and up to date with all the known and potential anti-personnel and anti-agriculture biological agents. The text is specifically designed for university courses in applied microbiology intended for future medical professionals and first responders in an effort to aid in the better understanding of biological warfare agents, their symptoms and potential treatments available. In addition, this text also includes information in regards to the methods of protection and decontamination as individuals are exposed to these agents."

Dr. William C. Patrick, III

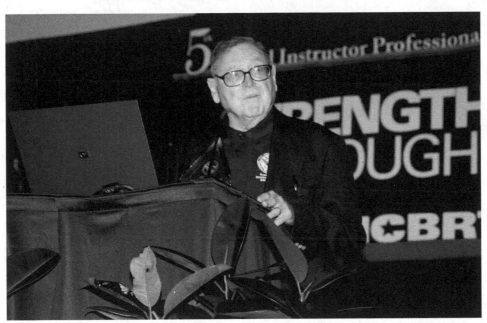

July 24, 1926 – October 1, 2010

This book is dedicated to the memory of Dr. William (Bill) Patrick III, a friend and mentor

William C. (Bill) Patrick III is a leading expert nationally and internationally on the subject of biological warfare and agents that are used in this effort. He has over 50 years of experience in the field that was foremost in the United States military retaliatory efforts in the 1950s and 1960s. Mr. Patrick served as Chief of the Products Development Division, Biological Warfare Laboratories in the US offensive program for seven years before the termination of this program in 1969 by President Richard Nixon of the United States. He holds five US patents pertaining to biological process and equipment. Mr. Patrick has authored 16 articles in the scientific literature as well as 98 major in-house Department of the Army Publications. He has performed contractual services for the Defense Intelligent Agencies, CIA, FBI and the US secret Service. Mr. Patrick has appeared on all of the major TV networks as well as Canadian Broadcasting, the BBC, History Channel and Discovery Channel in discussion of the potential use of biological agents in warfare or smaller incidences such as bio-terrorism. He has been awarded the CIA meritorious Citation and the Order of Military Medical Merit.

TABLE OF CONTENTS

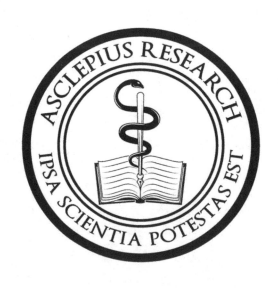

Throughout the history of man, cultural, societal and technological developments have been closely linked with conflicts. From the Bronze Age to the Digital Revolution, advancements in technology have provided advantages for one group of people to rise above others. These advantages have permitted the technologically superior participant in warfare to minimize their losses, while simultaneously inflicting devastation upon their opponents. With the imaginations of weapon designers as their only limitations, all things biotic and abiotic were considered in order to create more efficient methods of delivering death and destruction.

At first, weapons were developed to kill individuals or groups of combatants during open conflict. Slowly, as time progressed, weapons were developed to kill indiscriminately and provide the maximum amount of damage to the morale and the infrastructure of other nations. Put simply, these weapons are designed to create terror and induce submission. Presently, these weapons of mass terror and destruction include chemical, nuclear, and biological weaponry.

Biological weapons can be created from any virus, living organism or biochemical toxin found in nature that can be harnessed and "weaponized". Biological weapons are odorless and tasteless. They are designed to maim or kill at random in unsuspecting populations, animals or vegetation. Currently there are no efficient and reproducible detection and identification methods to recognize biological agents and toxins; these weapons can be disseminated with little or no prior warning. Once these agents are unleashed, the only indication of their deployment is the sheer number of casualties with similar symptoms that suddenly appear at local clinics or hospitals.[1]

Many of these biological weapons are intended to multiply and/or kill individuals from within, whether they are human or animal. These agents are capable of modifying the host's cellular functions to suit their lifecycle and, in turn, cause massive internal damage to the infected organism. Furthermore, many of these weapons are designed to proliferate in the body, causing systemic infections and/or to produce metabolic byproducts/bio-toxins, which can bring about necrosis and/or apoptosis of the host cells.

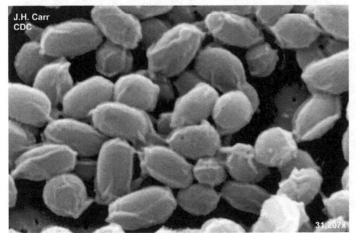

Figure I-1-1: Scanning electron micrograph (SEM) of *Bacillus anthracis* endospores

In experienced hands, biological weapons can be cheaply produced and manufactured in mass quantities with commercially available equipment. Additionally, biological weapons have a long shelf life and can be stored for long periods of time without a reduction in their devastating potential. For instance, it has been estimated that anthrax endospores can be stored for over 5 years with little or no loss of their deadly potency (Figure I-1.1).[2]

Even though the lethality of biological agents is well known, the methods of dissemination for these weapons have always posed an engineering problem for designers. Environmental factors, such as inversion, humidity, wind speed and direction, as well as landscape, population densities, etc. are all variables that have to be determined and calculated into the equation by the weapon designers in order to maximize casualties.[5] Unfortunately, due to the infinite faculties of man to provide unique solutions to problems, most of these engineering issues have been resolved by weapon designers of various nations. Nonetheless, it is fortunate for average citizens that the solutions for most of these engineering issues are still presently out of reach of would be terrorists. Even so, biological weapons, also referred to as the "poor man's nuclear weapon", when used, can provide devastating effects, both in human lives and in psychological trauma, which inevitably result after such an attack.[3, 4]

References

1. Emergency Response to Domestic Biological Incidents. Testing and Administration. Louisiana State University. National Center for Biomedical Research and Training. Module 2. A Background for Bioterrorism: Biological Events and What to Expect When One Occurs. pp. 2-3
2. Bioterrorism and Emerging Infections Education. Anthrax. University of Alabama at Birmingham. Website: http://www. bioterrorism.cme.uab.edu/CategoryA.Anthrax/Anthrax. pdf
3. National Studies Board, National Research Council. Post-Cold War Conflict Deterrence. Washington D.C.: National Academies Press, 1997. pp. 111
4. Porteus L. Weapons of Mass Destruction Handbook. June 20, 2006. Retrieved May 12, 2006, from Fox News. Web site: http:// www.foxnews.com/story/0,2933,76887, 00.html

Photo bibliography

Figure I1-2: Scanning electron micrograph of *Bacillus anthracis* endospores at 31,207X magnification. Photo was taken by Janice Haney Carr and released in 2002 by The Center for Disease Control and Prevention. Public domain photo

Researchers can date the use of biological agents as far back as 400 BC to the realm of a group of nomadic pastoralists dominating the present day areas of Iran and southwestern Russia, called Scythians. Historical records indicate that during battle, the Scythian archers would poison their arrows by dipping them in decomposing corpses and/or a mixture of blood and manure in order to inflict additional damage to their enemies. Evidence of using necrotizing tissues to spread disease during warfare persists throughout history. For example, Greeks, Persians and Romans used the decomposing carcasses of animals to contaminate wells or other water sources of their enemies.[1,2]

During the naval battle of the Eurymedon in 184 BC, Hannibal, the Carthaginian leader, ordered earthen pots filled with snakes to be hurled onto the decks of Pergamene ships. The earthen pots shattered upon impact releasing snakes among the sailors of the enemy ships. As expected, panic and chaos spread among the enemy sailors, allowing the Carthaginians to exploit the situation and achieve victory in battle.[3]

In 1346, during the Battle of Caffa (present day Feodossia), a Genoese town on the Crimean coast, the bodies of Tartar (Mongol) soldiers who had succumbed to the bubonic plague were catapulted over the city walls, so that death and disease would spread into the city's Christian population. It has been theorized by numerous historians that when some Genoese merchants escaped the besieged city, they became unwitting carriers of the disease and subsequently spread the bubonic plague throughout Europe (Figure I-2-1).[3,4]

During the Great Northern War of 1710, it has been reported that Russia utilized the same method as reported at the Battle of Caffa to instigate a plague epidemic among the Swedish soldiers.[5] Another instance of biological warfare can be found at Fort Carillon, a strategic location on Lake Champlain that protected the portage to Lake George during the French and Indian War (1754-1767). In July 1758, the British General James Abercromby led an army of approximately 16,000 British and Colonial troops against a small French force of 3,200, along with their Native American allies at Fort Carillon. During the first battle of Fort Carillon, the French and their allies were victorious, managing to inflict heavy casualties on the British forces. This debacle led to the removal of Abercromby from command. In June 1763, General Jeffery Amherst assumed command and resumed the battle. In an effort to weaken the fort's defenses, he approved the plan to offer smallpox infested blankets as a feigned gesture of friendship to the natives who had no immunity to this disease. The tactic worked; smallpox began to spread throughout the native's population, as well as within the fort. With its defenses weakened, the British finally succeeded in removing the French from Fort Carillon, renamed it Fort Ticonderoga, and set herself on the path of total victory in Canada.[3,6,7]

During World War I, Germany developed an ambitious biological warfare program, specifically targeting the agriculture and livestock of the Allies. The German Army developed anthrax, glanders, cholera, and ergot for use as biological weapons. The German biological weapons program is best described as a program of sabotage. They infected mules, cattle and horses with glanders and anthrax in allied nations such as Argentina and the United States, but never attempted to use this newly developed technology as a form of anti-human weaponry.[8,9] Nonetheless,

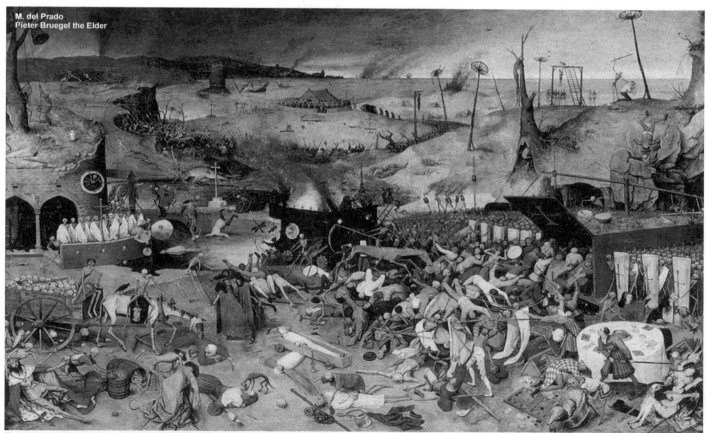

M. del Prado
Pieter Bruegel the Elder

Figure I-2-1: The painting Triumph of Death reflects the death and destruction of the Bubonic Plague. Note the dying king at the bottom left corner of the artwork which denotes the indiscriminant nature of the disease the mere speculation of a potential biological attack can cause panic among the populous. For example, the Spanish Influenza outbreak of 1918, which killed millions around the world, was falsely rumored to be a direct result of the German World War I biological warfare program. These rumors described how the Germans tainted Bayer aspirin medication with the influenza virus and subsequently sold them to the Spaniards.[10]

In an effort to address the rumors and concerns of biological, as well as, chemical warfare used during WWI, the 1925 Geneva Protocol for the Prohibition of Use in War of Asphyxiating, Poisonous or other Gases and Bacteriological Methods of Warfare was drafted. Developed by the League of Nations, the protocol addressed only the methods of warfare, but had no verification mechanism for the nations involved. Moreover, the convention did not address the issues of research and production of chemical and biological weapons.

Although well intentioned, the convention produced few tangible results. Many signatory states of the protocol refused to abandon their stockpile of chemical and biological agents and the research that accompanied them. These signatory states also reserved the right to respond to a chemical and biological attack in kind. As a glaring example of the ineffectiveness of the protocol, signatories such as Belgium, Canada, France, Great Britain, Italy, the Netherlands, Poland and the Soviet Union initiated basic research of biological warfare between World War I and II. Most notably, the United States did not ratify this 1925 Geneva protocol until 1975 under the administration of President Gerald Ford.[3, 11]

Between 1932 and the end of WWII, the Japanese actively pursued offensive biological weapon research. Under the command of Lieutenant General Shiro Ishii (Figure I-2-2), the secret biological and chemical warfare research facility, infamously known as Unit 731, was established in 1936 at the city of Pingfan, Beiyinhe, Manchuria.[3, 12]

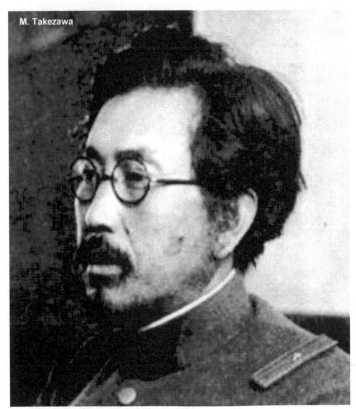

Figure I-2-2: Lieutenant General Shiro Ishii

Unit 731 consisted of approximately 150 buildings in Pingfan, 5 satellite camps and a staff of more than 3000 scientists (Figure I-2-4). A secondary research facility was also established in 1939, known as Unit Ei 1644, located in Nanking, China under the command of Lieutenant Colonel Masuda. Additionally, a third biological and chemical research facility known as Unit 100 (independent of Unit 731), under the command of Major Wakamatsu Yujiro, was also established in the city of Mokotan, Changchun, Manchuria.[3, 12]

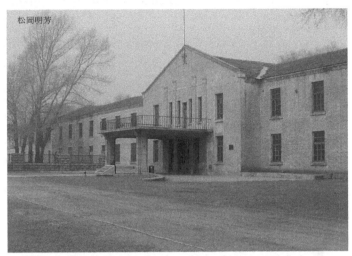

Figure I-2-3: A building on the site of the Harbin bioweapon facility of Unit 731

These secret biological research facilities carried out brutal experiments on Chinese civilians, and prisoners of war of various nationalities (e.g. Korean, Chinese, Mongolian, Soviet, American, British, Canadian, and Australian). They were cruel and deliberate in their methodologies, offering little or no consideration to their human experimental subjects, who they considered to be "untermensch" or subhuman.[3, 12]

At the height of its production, Unit 731 was producing 660 pounds of pure plague bacteria (*Yersinia pestis*) per month, 1400 pounds of anthrax (*Bacillus anthracis*), 2200 pounds of cholera vibrions (*Vibrio cholerae*), 2000 pounds of typhoid (*Salmonella typhi*), paratyphoid (*Salmonella paratyphi*), and dysentery (*Shigella dysenteriae*) combined. It is estimated that the Japanese forces exposed approximately 3000 victims to various biological agents (e.g. plague, anthrax, syphilis, etc.) in an attempt to develop the weaponized versions and to study the devastating effects of these diseases. Experiments involving porcelain bombs filled with plague infected fleas were also developed and dropped on Chinese populations with mixed results. For example, a plague attack on the Chinese city of Changteh in 1941, reportedly led to approximately 10,000 civilian casualties. However, this "field trial" also led to 1700 deaths among the Japanese occupation forces. Due to the mounting casualties among Japanese forces, the "field trials" were terminated in 1942.[13, 14] The final analysis showed that the Japanese forces lacked training and were unprepared to deal with biological weapons, even if they were they were the ones who initiated the dissemination.

During the final months of WWII, General Ishii personally planned an operation code-named "Cherry Blossoms at Night," which called for Kamikaze pilots and their specially designed planes to be transported to the west coast of the United States by submarine and spread plague contaminated fleas over the city of San Diego. Fortunately, the plan never materialized. Japan surrendered a month before the operation's September 1945 attack date.[12]

Although it is known that German medical research teams infected concentration camp prisoners with hepatitis A, *Rickettsia prowazekii* (epidemic typhus) and malaria (*Plasmodium* spp.), the German offensive biological warfare program falls short when compared to those sponsored by Japan and the Allied Nations. It has been alleged that Hitler issued specific orders prohibiting the development of biological weapons due to his own devastating experience with chemical weapons used during WWI.[1, 15] On the other hand, it is believed that the Soviets used biological weapons against the Germans during WWII. In 1942, prior to the battle of Stalingrad, a large outbreak of tularemia (*Francisella tularensis*) occurred, infecting thousands of Soviet and German soldiers alike. It has been reported that 70% of the victims had the pneumonic form of the disease, which was practically unheard of in the Soviet Union at that time. This sudden appearance of nonindigenous pneumonic form of tularemia indicates an intentional release of the agent.[13]

Back in the United States information regarding biological weapon capabilities of the Axis reached the White House. Concerned that the United States was lagging behind in biological weapons research, President Roosevelt threatened openly that the United States would retaliate with chemical weapons if faced with biological warfare. Although in principle, Roosevelt was against the use of chemical or biological weaponry, he approved the research and production of biological weapons by authorizing the War Department to establish the War Research Service in 1942.[16] By 1944, in conjunction with Great Britain and Canada, quantities of anthrax and botulinum toxins (*Clostridium botulinum*) were stockpiled. Fortunately, none of these biological weapons were ever used in battle. Nonetheless, extensive testing of explosive munitions designed to aerosolize and disperse *B. anthracis* spores as an antipersonnel weapon was conducted on Gruinard Island near the coast of Scotland in 1942. The most infamous of these stockpiles was the anthrax-laced cattle cakes that were jointly developed with Great Britain. These cattle cakes were designed to be dropped via aircraft into Axis controlled Europe in an effort to destroy the cattle industry of Germany, thereby starving the Germans of one of their important food supplies. In addition, considerable work was done in producing biological weapons that target vegetation. Plans were developed to decimate Japan's rice crops towards the end of the war although they were never implemented.[3, 17, 18]

After World War II, the United States continued its research on various offensive biological weapons, mainly at the research facilities located at Fort Detrick, Maryland; Pine Bluff, Arkansas; Edgewood, Maryland and Dugway, Utah (Figure I-2-4). The Korean War, which began in June 1950, gave additional justification for the continuation of the United States biological warfare program, especially since the Soviet Union's entry into the Korean conflict was feared. Though the Soviets remained in the background during the Korean War, in 1956 Marshal Georgy Konstantinovich Zhukov, Minister of Defense of the Soviet Union, declared that chemical and biological weapons would be used for mass destruction in future wars.[19]

In 1951 and 1954 anticrop bombs and the first antipersonnel biological weapons using *Brucella suis* were produced in the US. Within 26 years, a total of 7 antipersonnel and 3 anticrop agents were mass produced and stockpiled (please see Table 1 for more information). Fortunately, none of these biological weapons were ever used in conflicts.[3, 20]

Between 1949 and 1968, harmless organisms such as *Bacillus globigii*, *Serratia marcescens* and particulates of zinc cadmium sulfide (commonly used to study chemical and biological weapon

dispersal) were released in various geographical locations of the United States to demonstrate the vulnerability of American cities to biological and chemical attacks. For example, experiments with non-pathologic organisms were conducted at Washington National Airport. These experiments were supervised by federal personnel dressed as travelers dosing bacteria throughout the airport through a specially designed sprayer contained within a briefcase. Subsequently, the microorganisms travelling through the interior atmosphere of the airport were captured through traps that were placed throughout the facility and their rates of travel, as well as distance, were measured. Similar experiments were also conducted in the New York Subway system through light bulbs filled with harmless bacteria. After the light bulbs were purposefully broken, the bacteria were found to have spread throughout the subway system within 20 minutes.[5]

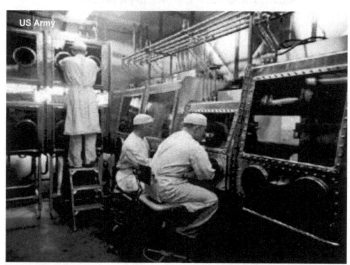

Figure I-2-4: Research personnel working with Class III cabinets at the U.S. Biological Warfare Laboratories Camp Detrick, Maryland

Table 1: Biological warfare agents produced by the United States[3]

Agents	Lethality
Bacillus anthracis	Lethal
Botulinum toxin	Lethal
Brucella suis	Incapacitant
Coxiella burnetii	Incapacitant
Fracisella tularensis	Lethal
Staphylococcal enterotoxin B	Incapacitant
Venezuelan equine encephalitis virus	Incapacitant
Rice blast	-
Rye stem rust	-
Wheat stem rust	-

◻ Targets human
▨ Targets crops

In September 1950, the first large scale aerosol vulnerability test was conducted in the San Francisco Bay area with *B. globigii* and *S. marcescens* that were conjugated with fluorescent particles.[3, 5, 21, 22] Open-air tests with anticrop agents such as rice blast, rye stem rust and wheat rust were conducted by the Department of Agriculture. Bacterial agents such as *Coxiella burnetii* and *Francisella tularensis* were released by the United States military at the Dugway Proving Ground, Eglin Air Force Base and various remote Pacific islands to examine the infectability and viability of the pathogens on animal models.[3, 22] Controversial studies to examine the susceptibility of African Americans to *Aspergillus fumigatus* were conducted on uninformed workers at Norfolk Supply Center in Virginia, using crates contaminated with *Aspergillus* spores. Additionally, light bulbs filled with *Bacillus subtilis var niger* were intentionally dropped and released in the New York Subway system (both in the ventilation and on the tracks), as well as, at the Pentagon to examine the dispersal patterns of the simulant. Furthermore, in 1956, researchers at Fort Detrick began using volunteer human test subjects in experiments. For example, biological munitions were detonated along the side of human test subjects within a hollow one million liter, spherical, metallic, aerosolization chamber known as the "eight ball." Please examine Figure I-2-5 for more information.

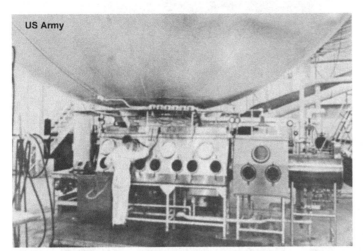

Figure I-2-5: "Eight Ball" located at Camp Detrick, Maryland

Within the "eight ball", volunteers were subjected to aerosolized pathogens such as *Francisella tularensis* and *Coxiella burnetii*, to evaluate the efficacy of vaccines, prophylaxis and therapy. These experiments were part of a congressionally approved program referred to as "Operation Whitecoat," and the primary volunteers were active-duty soldiers with conscientious objector status.[3, 11, 23, 24]

During the Nixon Administration, US policy towards biological weapon research and usage drastically changed. On November 25, 1969, during a visit to Fort Detrick, President Nixon renounced the development, production, stockpiling, and use of biological agents during war.

On April 10, 1972, the Convention on the Prohibition of the Development, Production and Stockpiling of Bacteriological (Biological) and Toxic Weapons and on their Destruction (BWC) was signed by 103 nations which included the United States, Soviet Union, United Kingdom, France, South Africa, China and Iraq. This was the first multilateral disarmament treaty banning the production of all biological weapons, with exceptions for medical research purposes. The treaty also banned any transfer of technology or expertise of biological warfare to other countries, as well as, requiring all signatories to destroy stockpiles, delivery systems and production equipment within nine months of ratifying the treaty. Although the treaty was well intentioned, there were no effective means of verification or enforcement. Therefore, the Soviet Union, as well as Iraq, and many other nations continued the research and development of biological weapons, albeit in secrecy (Figure I-2-6).[24, 25]

In response to the presidential decry and BWC, the United States Army immediately began altering the course of the biological warfare program from an offensive to defensive focus. In 1969, the United States Army Medical Research Institute of Infectious Diseases (USAMRIID) was established. USAMRIID's purpose is dedicated to developing medical defensive countermeasures to biological warfare agents (Figure I-2-7). In addition, by May 1972, all of the anti-personnel agents had been destroyed, and the production facilities at Pine Bluff were converted into a research facility. Finally, by February 1973, all of the stockpiled

anti-crop agents were also destroyed.[3, 22]

In contrast to the United States, the Soviet Union began increasing its biological warfare efforts after becoming a signatory of the BWC. The Soviet biological warfare industry comprised many institutions at approximately 52 sites under different ministries. Collectively, they were known as the Biopreparat. The Biopreparat carried out extensive offensive research, development and production under the guise of legitimate biological or medical research.[13]

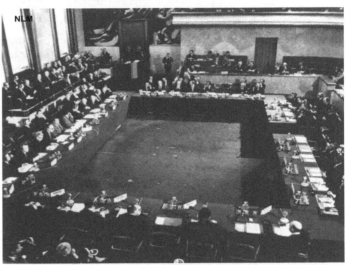

Figure I-2-6: The 1969 Conference on the Committee on Disarmament at the Palais des Nations in Geneva negotiated and led to the Convention on the Prohibition of the Development, Production and Stockpiling of Bacteriological (Biological) and Toxin Weapons and on their Destruction

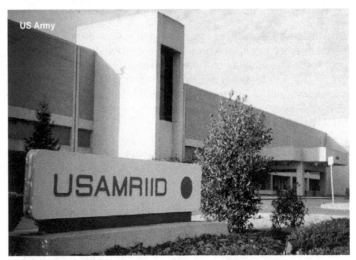

Figure I-2-7: Dan Crozier Building, USAMRIID, Fort Detrick, MD

Between 1975-1981, it is alleged that the Soviet Union supplied T-2 mycotoxin to the Lao People's Liberation Army and the Vietnamese to be used against Hmong villagers and resistance forces.[1, 26, 27, 28, 29] Between 1979-1981, the Soviets were again accused of supplying mycotoxin to the Vietnamese to use against the Khmer Rouge forces in Tuol Chrey, Kampuchea (Cambodia). Both alleged Laos and Kampuchea mycotoxin attacks have been described by eye witnesses as "yellow rain" which consists of a shower of sticky yellow liquid, clouds of dust/powder, or mists.[1, 28, 29, 30, 31]

In Afghanistan, between 1979 to 1981, the Soviet Union and their Afghan allies were accused of using mycotoxin against the Mujahidin guerrillas.[27, 28, 32] These accusations and evidence of the use of "yellow rain" by the Soviets were presented by Secretary of State Alexander M. Haig Jr. to the United States Congress in 1982, in a report titled Chemical Warfare in Southeast Asia and Afghanistan. Nonetheless, there are those in the scientific community who have challenged the accusations and stated that the "yellow rain" was nothing more than the fecal matter of honeybees dropped during their "cleansing flights." [28, 33, 34]

Unconfirmed reports have implicated the use of mycotoxin during the Egyptian attacks against Yemeni Royalists, while Iraq has been accused of using the same biological agent during the 1983-1984 Iran-Iraq War.[28, 29, 35]

The first confirmed case of the utilization of weaponized biological agents occurred in a rather unlikely place, Africa. In 1978, South African, Rhodesian security and Special Forces unleashed anthrax spores along with cholera onto the poor, black, civilian populations in Rhodesia (today's Zimbabwe). The logic was quite simple, "kill the black man's cattle, and food for the Rhodesian guerrillas dies with them." It is estimated that hundreds died from this attack but no one knows for certain the exact cost of the "Dirty War" in human terms.[36]

Between March 30th and April 3[rd,]1979, the exact date is still disputed by experts, an accidental release of anthrax from a weapons facility in Sverdlovsk, USSR, killed an estimated 66 to 105 people. The accident was caused by human error, where a filter for free floating spores was removed for cleaning but never returned, leaving the spores to flow freely out of the factory. After the accident occurred, the Soviet government claimed these deaths were due to contaminated meat, and maintained this position until Russian President Boris Yeltsin finally admitted the accident in Komsomolskaya, Pravda, on May 27, 1993 (Figure I-2-8).[13, 37, 38]

During the 1980-1990's, the miserable failure of the BWC was very apparent to experts and politicians in-the-know in all NATO countries. The inability of the world nations to verify and enforce the treaty made the international contract insignificant. This ineffectiveness of the treaty was shown to the world when the United States led the United Nation's forces in removing Iraq from Kuwait (January 16, 1991).

The allied forces knew that throughout the 1980's Iraq had actively, although covertly, pursued a biological program at Salman Pak, Al-Hakam, Taji, and Fudaliya under a government organization called Technical Research Centre. Under the guidance of Dr. Rihab Taha, also infamously known as "Dr. Germ," Iraq developed a broad spectrum of offensive biological agents which included aflatoxins, anthrax, botulinum toxin, camel pox, cholera, gas gangrene, hemorrhagic conjunctivitis virus, mycotoxins, plague, ricin, rotavirus, salmonella, smallpox, staphylcoccal enterotoxin and wheat rust.[39, 40]

After the victory of Desert Storm in March 1991, Iraq agreed to a ceasefire, which stipulated the termination of all research and production of biological weapons and other forms of weapons of mass destruction (UN Security Council Resolution 687). Furthermore, the resolution allowed UN inspectors, which includes United Nations Special Commission (UNSCOM) and International Atomic Energy Agency (IAEA), to "locate and destroy whatever documentation, hardware and software that Saddam possessed" and the ability for the United States to enforce the resolution if the agreement was ever breached.[41] After the cease fire, evidence was found by UNSCOM that Iraq had produced 4000 gallons of botulinum toxin, 1800 gallons of anthrax, 530 gallons of aflatoxin (Aspergillus spp.) and ricin (Ricinus communis), 90 gallons of gas

gangrene (Clostridium perfringens) and undisclosed amounts of smallpox (variola) and other viral pathogens (Figure I-2-9).[42]

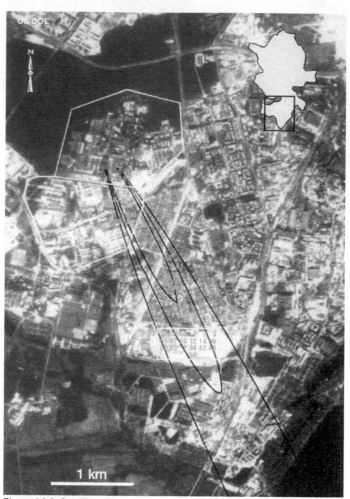

Figure I-2-8: Satellite photo shows a plume spreading out over Sverdlovsk and the locations of 64 people who died over the next 42 days. The total death toll from the accidental Anthrax release is estimated at 66-105 people

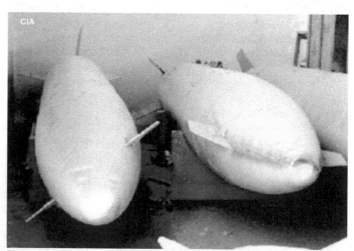

Figure I-2-9: Russian made drop tanks also known as Al-Asad are modified in Iraq for biological or chemical weapon delivery system for the Iraqi regime

The implosion of the Soviet Union in 1991 reshaped future geopolitics. The demise of this once mighty empire left an international power vacuum. No longer were weaker nation states falling in-line with the politics of superpowers from whom they were seeking economic and military support. More and more nations began striking out on their own initiatives, following their own manifest destinies.

Back in the United States both politicians and citizens were lured into a sense of false security after the "The Evil Empire" disappeared from the geopolitical scene.[43] In the 1990's, the Clinton Administration initiated a series of military cuts that reduced the U.S. standing military by an estimated 700,000 personnel. A report written by Jason Morrow in National Policy Analysis (1999) stated that the burden of this reduction, which resulted in an approximate 45% cut in personnel and budget, was made in the US Air Force and Army. The US Navy, on the other hand, faced elimination of numerous combat vessels and was forced to underman their operational ships (an approximate 36% reduction in personnel and budget). Unfortunately, the military cuts were made in haste and thoroughly underestimated the volatility of the geopolitical situation.[44]

During the 8 years of Clinton Administration, numerous new regional conflicts occurred, while unresolved disputes reappeared. During the 1990's operational commitments to Kosovo, Bosnia, Somalia and Iraq jumped by approximately 300% which further strained the US military.[44] To no small effect, these reductions and overextensions of the United States armed forces demonstrated a sign of weakness to various nations. For instance, Iraq, who signed UN Resolution 687, and agreed to the terms of the cease fire during Desert Storm, began a series of organized obstructions and/or outright intimidations to impede UN weapons inspection teams (United Nations Special Commission - UNSCOM). These active obstructions by Iraq resulted in some military actions but mainly harsh words through further UN Resolutions such as 707 (August 1991), 715 (October 1991), 949 (October 1994), 1051 (March 1996), 1060 (June 1996), 1115 (June 1997), 1134 (October 1997), 1154 (March 1998), 1194 (September 1998), 1205 (November 1998), and 1284 (December 1999).[45] Before the inspectors were finally expelled from Iraq by Saddam Hussein's regime, UNSCOM concluded that Iraq had actively maintained their biological warfare program (Figure I-2-10).[46, 47]

Sensing the weakness exhibited by the United States, terrorist attacks rose steadily in both frequency and aggressiveness during the 1990's against US targets domestic and abroad. Although these attacks were conventional in nature, they foreshadowed what was to shroud the United States in the near future. For example: On February 26, 1993, Islamic terrorists with suspected Al-Qaida connections successfully attacked the World Trade Center which killed 6 people and injured approximately 1000 individuals (Figure I-2-11).[48]

On April 14,1993, Iraqi agents attempted to assassinate Former President G.H.W. Bush during a visit to Kuwait. This resulted in President Clinton authorizing United States Navy ships to launch 23 Tomahawk missiles against the headquarters of the Iraqi Intelligence Service.[49]

On November 13, 1995, Islamic terrorists with suspected Al-Qaida connection successfully attacked the United States National Guard Training Center located in Riyadh, Saudi Arabia which killed six people (five of the individuals killed were Americans) and injuring 60 others. It is interesting to note that Riyadh, Saudi Arabia was the place of birth for Al-Qaida leader Osama Bin Laden.[50]

On June 25, 1996, the Khobar Towers located in Dhahran, Saudi Arabia were bombed by Al-Qaida killing 23 American soldiers and wounding more than 300 civilians (Figure I-2-12).[51]

The Islamic terrorist belonging to Al-Qaida attacked the United States embassies located in Nairobi, Kenya, and Dar-es-Salem,

Tanzania on August 7, 1998, which resulted in 223 people killed and approximately 4000 individuals wounded (Figure I-2-13).[52]

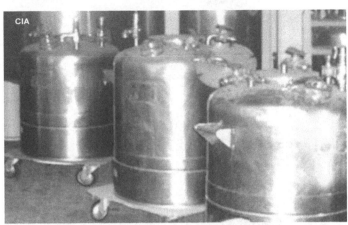

Figure I-2-10: Iraqi made 1m³ 800 liters stainless steel mobile tanks designed to transport bulk agents or used for fermentation purposes (e.g. biological agents). UNSCOM identified the remains of only two of these tanks in 1990 while the remaining 18 were never found

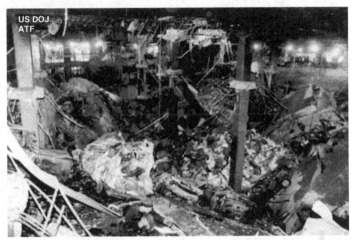

Figure I-2-11: Aftermath of World Trade Center bombing in February 25, 1993

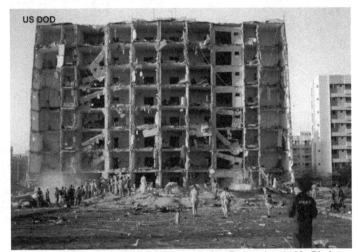

Figure I-2-12: Aftermath of the bombin at Khobar Towers located in Dhahran. Saudi Arabia on June 25, 1996

On October 12th, 2000, while harbored and refueling in the Yemeni port of Aden, United States destroyer USS Cole (DDG 67) was attacked by Islamic Terrorists belonging to Al-Qaida. The terrorists used a small dingy packed with explosives to severely damage the US warship, as well as, killed 17 sailors and injured 39 others (Figure I-2-14).[53]

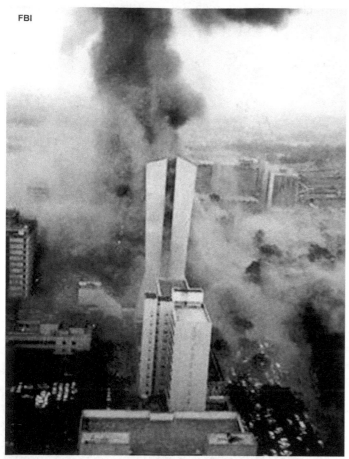

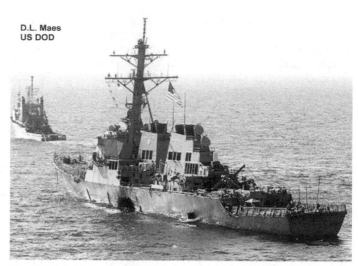

Figure I-2-14: Aftermath of USS Cole bombing in October 12, 2000

Unfortunately, these attacks received little or no attention from the administration and from the citizens of the United States. These terrorist actions led by Al-Qaida were relegated as criminal acts and isolated incidents rather than a foreshadowing sign of what was to come.

The highly contested presidential election in 2000 demonstrated to the world the volatility of America's political situation. Islamic Terrorist groups such as Al-Qaida, an international terrorist group, established by Osama Bin Laden and Muhammad Atef in 1989 "was dedicated to opposing non-Islamic governments with force and violence" selected the subsequent year for their first massive attack on US soil.[54]

Figure I-2-13: The aftermath of the 1998 embassy bombing in Nairobi, Kenya

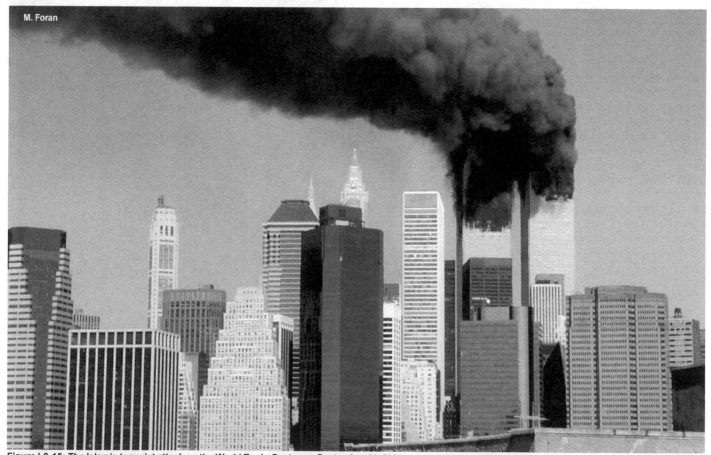

Figure I-2-15: The Islamic terrorist attack on the World Trade Center on September 11, 2001, resulted in some 2750 deaths, as well as, an additional 400 fatalities of New York City's police officers and fire fighters who rushed to the scene of the attack. An additional 184 deaths resulted during the attack on pentagon, while 40 more perished in Pennsylvania where the hijacked plane crashed after the passengers attempted to retake the plane

Al-Qaida attacks of September 11, 2001 can be identified as the date that changed the face of warfare forever. No longer was the focus of the United States directly at other regional or world powers, now the United States must deal with secretive forces without uniforms, rules of engagement and/or restricted by political or national boundaries (Figure I-2-15).

After the 9/11 attacks, one thing was made clear to the majority of the United States population and politicians, mere words and documents would not suffice against an aggressor that is intent on the destruction of the United States and other western civilizations. As the smoldering ruins of the World Trade Center loomed in the landscape of New York City, the national policy of the United States changed from police actions to an aggressive offensive engagement. "We must act and prevent the next attack before it happens by taking the war to the enemy."[55]

Operation "Enduring Freedom" was launched in October of 2001 against the Taliban and Al-Qaida in Afghanistan, thereby marking the beginning of the War on Terrorism. Subsequently, on March 20, 2003, after another UN resolution (UN resolution 1441) was ignored, the United States launched Operation "Iraqi Freedom" to address a 'clear and present danger' to the United States. Understanding, that on numerous occasions Saddam utilized WMDs' during battle with Iran and on Iraqi citizens (Figure I-2-16) and that an active "hide and seek" program was in place to hinder and/or intimidate UN inspectors which led to eleven subsequent UN Resolutions after resolution 687, it was assumed that WMDs' were actively being produced and concealed by Saddam's regime.

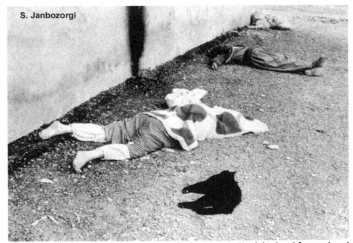

Figure I-2-16: The aftermath of a chemical weapon attack by Iraqi forces loyal to Saddam Hussein. Chemical weapons used include the Tabun, Sarin, VX, as well as mustard gas. This attack occurred in March 16, 1988 at Halabja, a Kurdish town in northern Iraq, that killed 3,200-5,000, and injured around 7,000-10,000 people

Unfortunately, after the successful invasion and the subsequent inspections, the Iraq Survey Group headed by Charles Duelfer reported that "no significant" amounts of weapons of mass destruction (WMD) had been found.[56, 57, 58, 59] Nonetheless, the shift in political attitude, increased diligence and more focused attention in national security after 9/11 resulted in thwarting 19 publically known attacks against the United States. Although these attacks were conventional in nature, it still demonstrates the perilous nature that our citizens are in when faced with an enemy that is not limited by any rules of engagement and is willing to sacrifice their lives for religious ideals.[60]

The 2008 elections marked a return to the pre-9/11 footing as war weary Americans elected Barack Hussein Obama as the 44th president of the United States. Viewing that the "cowboy diplomacy" of the Bush Administration as one of the main causes of turmoil around the world, the Obama Administration stated that open dialogue with all nations and groups, including those states that sponsor terrorism, without any preconditions would bring peace to our time.[61, 62] Mr. Obama's proclamation not only captured the attention of the majority of the people in the United States but also secured him The Nobel Peace Prize on October 9, 2009, approximately nine months after he took office. The Nobel Committee stated "only very rarely has a person to the same extent as Obama captured the world's attention and given its people hope for a better future. His diplomacy is founded in the concept that those who are to lead the world must do so on the basis of values and attitudes that are shared by the majority of the world's population."[63] Unfortunately, to those that view violence as a manner by which to achieve their goals, this new direction of the US foreign policy would only be taken as a sign of weakness which they could exploit. For example, On June 1, 2009, an American named Abdulhakim Mujahid Muhammad (born Carlos Leon Bledsoe), killed Private William Long and wounded Private Quinton Ezeagwula during a drive by shooting at a Little Rock Arkansas US military recruiting office. After his capture, Muhammad claimed that the attack was a "jihadi attack" and that he is affiliated with Al-Qaida in the Arabian Peninsula. Nonetheless, Muhammad was charged with capital murder while no terrorism charges were ever filed.[64, 65]

US Army Major Nidal Malik Hasan, a US Army psychiatrist managed to kill 12 and wound 31 others at Fort Hood Texas on November 5, 2009. Subsequent to the attack, a series of emails connecting Hasan to Anwar al Awlaki, an American imam with direct ties to Al-Qaida, came to light. Although terrorism connections were made between Hasan and Al-Qaida, he was charged and later convicted of 13 counts of murder and 32 counts of attempted murder in an act of "workplace violence". No terrorism charges were ever filed (Figure I-2-17).[66, 67, 68, 69]

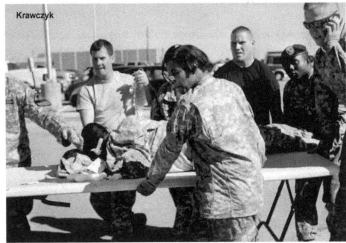

Figure I-2-17: First responders use a table as a stretcher to transport a wounded US Soldier to an awaiting ambulance at Fort Hood, Texas

On December 25, 2009, Umar Farouk Abdulmutallab, an Al-Qaida trained terrorist with direct ties to Anwar al Awlaki, was captured by fellow passengers in an attempt to ignite explosives during Northwest/Delta flight 253 from Amsterdam to Detroit. Even though Abdulmutallab was on a watch list by the U.S. National Counterterrorism Center, he was allowed to purchase a one-way ticket and board the flight bound for the United States. He was apprehended with a six-inch packet of PETN high explosives sewn into his underwear. Abdulmutallab, also known as the "underwear bomber", was charged and later convicted on

October 12, 2011 of conspiracy to commit an "act of terrorism transcending national boundaries, attempted murder within the special aircraft jurisdiction of the United States, willfully placing a destructive device on an aircraft, and attempted use of a weapon of mass destruction".[70,71,72,73]

Faisal Shahzad, a Pakistani-American citizen was arrested on May 1, 2010 for the attempted car bombing of New York Time Square. The car bombing attempt was foiled when a T-shirt vendor alerted the police that smoke was rising from the back of a parked vehicle. Apparently, the car bomb failed to detonate. Shahzad was captured at John F. Kennedy Airport on board Emirate Flight 202 as he attempted to escape to Dubai (United Arab Emirates) in route to Islamabad, Pakistan. During his trial, the unrepentant Faisal stated, "brace yourself because the war of the Muslims has just begun...the defeat of the U.S. is imminent." Faisal Shahzad pleaded guilty to 10 terror related charges and was sentenced to life in Federal prison without parole on October 5, 2010 (Figure I-2-18).[74, 75]

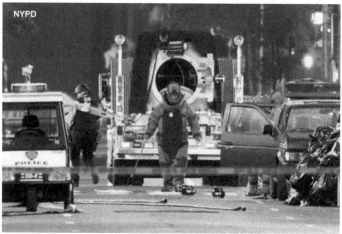

Figure I-2-18: NYPD bomb squad defusing the car bomb left by Faisal Shahzad in Time Square, New York

Mohamed Osman Mohamud, a Somali-American, attempted to detonate a car bomb during a Christmas tree lighting ceremony in Portland, Oregon on November 26, 2010. Fortunately, the bomb materials provided to Mohamud were only mock explosives provided by the FBI in a sting operation. Mohamud was charged with attempted terrorist act and sentenced to 30 years imprisonment.[76]

On September 11, 2012, Ansar al-Sharia, a Libyan militant/ terrorist group (the exact terminology is still being debated by the United States Congress and the Executive Branch), launched an assault at United States Consulate located in Benghazi, Libya which resulted in killing five Americans including US ambassador to Libya, Christopher Stevens. Presently, the exact details of what transpired during this assault are the subject of numerous congressional investigations.[77, 78]

On April 15, 2013, two homemade explosive devices were detonated near the finish line of the Boston Marathon, killing three and injuring 264. The perpetrators of the bombing were Dzhokar Tsarnaev and Tamerlan Tsarnaev, two brothers of Chechen decent. Tamerlan Tsarnaev was killed during a police shootout, while his brother Dzhokar was captured alive after an extensive manhunt. Although radicalized in their opinions against American views and policies, neither brother was directly connected to any known terrorist groups (Figure I-2-19).[79, 80, 81]

With the exception of the assault in the US consulate in Libya,

many of attempts at terroristic acts between the years of 2009 and 2014 were perpetrated by individuals or small groups responding to calls of jihad towards the citizens of the United States and her interests. Nonetheless, one particular group that managed to gain international infamy arose during this period may prove to be a serious threat to the United States. Islamic State of Iraq and the Levant (ISIL), also known as the Islamic State of Iraq and Syria (ISIS) or The Islamic State was founded by Abu Musab al-Zarqawi, a Jordanian jihadist and the leader of Al-Qaida in Iraq. It is interesting to note that it was al-Zarqawi's presence in Iraq that provided the link between Saddam Hussein and Al-Qaida.

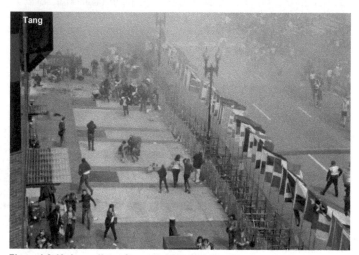

Figure I-2-19: Immediate aftermath of the Boston Marathon Bombing

Soon after the US led invasion of Iraq, al-Zarqawi established Jama'at al-Tawhid w'al-Jihad (the Party of Monotheism and Jihad) the precursor to the present day ISIL. Although al-Zarqawi shared many similar views with Osama Bin Laden, his actions proved to be much more radical. For example, al-Zarqawi's hatred was not only directed toward the United States, Israel, Western culture, and other religions, but also towards the majority Shiite population of Iraq, whom he deemed as heretics. Although this view of Sunni Muslims as the true believer of Islam was shared by Osama Bin Laden and the rank and file of Al-Qaida alike, al-Zarqawi's hatred went a step further. Instead of targeting US and coalition forces in Iraq, he directed his malevolence towards Shiite populations by bombing targets in their neighborhoods and towns. The most notorious of these attacks was detonating a massive car bomb outside of Imam Ali Shrine in Najaf, the holiest place of worship for Shiites in Iraq. This attack claimed the life of the Shiite's top cleric Ayatollah Mohammad Baqir al-Hakim, as well as, the lives of 124 others.[82] These ferocious attacks not only gained international fame for al-Zarqawi, but also the ire of Osama Bin Laden. For instance, in July 2005, Bin Laden's second in command, Ayman al-Zawahiri, wrote a letter rebuking al-Zarqawi for his drastic methods. However, the letter went unheaded.[82, 83, 84]

The drastic measures taken by Al-Qaida in Iraq eventually went too far. By 2006, al-Zarqawi began to see himself as the Emir and Caliph. He began demanding that Sharia Law be followed strictly by all Muslims under his control. Anyone who resisted his decree, no matter what status in the community they held, was summarily executed. Soon, many of the locals, Shiite and Sunni population alike, turned against al-Zarqawi and started to work with the US led coalition forces to destroy Al-Qaida in Iraq. In what was known as the "Awakening" campaign, the loose alliance of Sunni and Shiite Muslims was accompanied by a surge of US troops in Iraq. This loose coalition led to the successful elimination of al-Zarqawi by a US airstrike on his hideout just north of Baghdad.[83, 85, 86]

With the death of al-Zarqawi, Al-Qaida in Iraq floundered and its influence dissipated. Briefly, Iraq experienced a period of peace. However, as the last of the US led coalition forces withdrew from Iraq, the old animosity and open conflict between the Shiite and Sunni Muslims flared once more, which led to the resurgence of Al-Qaida in Iraq. In 2011, Al-Qaida in Iraq was led by Abu Bakr al-Baghdadi and his ranks began to swell with Iraqi Sunni Muslims. It was approximately at this time when a rebranding occurred; Al-Qaida in Iraq was renamed the Islamic State of Iraq, or ISI. Unlike the al-Zarqawi led Al-Qaida, whose ranks were filled with foreign Islamic fighters, ISI was filled by ethnically Sunni Muslim ex-Iraqi military soldiers and officers (Saddam Hussein was a Sunni Muslim and he populated his army with people of the same origin). This influx of ex-military soldiers provided the discipline and quality of a professional army rather than a militant outfit. Nonetheless, once again, the Shiite and Sunni Muslims were at war in Iraq. [83, 85]

As the civil war raged in Syria in 2011, ISI entered the fray against this Shiite led government. President Bashar al-Assad, along with most of his military commanders are Alawites, a Shiite sub-sect, therefore a natural enemy of ISI. In March 2013, ISI conquered the Syrian city of Raqqa and by January 2014, took control of Fallujah, Ramadi, and numerous smaller towns near the Turkish and Syrian borders. [83, 85] Unlike previous terrorist groups, ISI is well funded and superbly led by military tacticians and not by religious leaders.[89] Back in the United States, the laissez-faire view on the resurgence of Al-Qaida in Iraq or now known as ISI is prevalent in the political landscape. For example, during an interview with David Remnick on January 7, 2014, President Obama referred to ISI as a Junior Varsity team and not a particular serious threat.[88] It was about this time when ISI rebranded itself once more and began calling themselves ISIL (ISIS or simply the Islamic State). In June 2014, ISIL captured the city of Mosul in Iraq and suddenly became the topic of conversation around the world, as well as, in the United States. Rapidly, this previously known 'junior varsity' team is threatening to take over the entire nations of Iraq and Syria.[83, 85, 89] Presently, a US led bombing campaign targeting ISIL in Iraq is in progress, although no US ground troops or "boots on the ground" other than a few advisors have been provided. In the opinion of many military strategists, including former Defense Secretary Robert Gates, the current actions being taken are insufficient against a well-organized terrorist group.[90, 91]

Recently, a few frightening developments have been reported by various news agencies around the world but seemed to be missed by most US based news agencies. A laptop computer belonging to ISIL was captured by a moderate Syrian rebel group located in northern Syria. The files on the computer showed that ISIL have ambitions to obtain and use biological weapons, such as the bubonic plague, in terrorist actions against its enemies which include the United States. The 19 page document stored on the computer states: "The advantage of biological weapons is that they do not cost a lot of money, while the human casualties can be huge."[92] The second under reported development was submitted in letter from the Iraqi government to the United Nations stating that they have lost control of the Muthanna State Establishment, a former chemical warfare agent factory operated by Saddam Hussein's regime, located near Baghdad, to ISIL. This development indicates that ISIL may be in possession of weapons of mass destruction. This frightening admission is supported by the last major report released in 2004 by United Nation inspectors in Iraq. The report states that Bunker 13 of

Muthanna State Establishment contained 2,500 sarin-filled 122 mm chemical rockets and approximately 180 tons of sodium cyanide. This finding was further supported by an investigation by The New York Times indicating that hidden caches of chemical weaponry was discovered by US forces between 2004 and 2011. When questioned, the U.S. Defense Department spokesman, Rear Admiral John Kirby, stated: "whatever material was kept there is pretty old and not likely to be able to be accessed or used against anyone right now".[93, 94]

Unfortunately for the citizens of the United States, as well as, concerned individuals around the world, the ambition and capabilities of ISIL are presently unclear. Most information available with regards to this terrorist group are made by individuals with distinct political affiliations that may cloud the facts. What is certain is ISIL's hatred towards the United States, Israel and the West. Being a well-funded terrorist organization, it is certain that their political and territorial expansion must be immediately halted and reversed in Syria and Iraq. If ISIL is left alone and allowed to mature, it will eventually turn its attention to the United States and her allies.

References

1. Eitzen E.M., Takafuji E.T. Historical Overview of Biological Warfare. Medical Aspects of Biological Warfare. Chapter 18. Washington D.C.: The Surgeon General United States Army Medical Department Medical Center and School Borden Institute. 2007. pp. 415-423
2. Jone D.E. Poison Arrows. North American Indian Hunting and Warfare. Austin: University of Texas Press. 2007. pp. XII
3. Martin J.W., Christopher G.W., Eitzen E.M. History of Biological Weapons: From Poisoned Darts to Intentional Epidemics. Aspects of Biological Warfare. Chapter 1. Washington D.C.: The Surgeon General United States Army Medical Department Medical Center and School Borden Institute. 2007. pp. 1-20
4. Ziegler P. The Black Death. New York: The John Day Company, 1969. pp 15
5. Emergency Response to Domestic Biological Incidents. Testing and Administration. Louisiana State University. National Center for Biomedical Research and Training. Module 2. A Background for Bioterrorism: Biological Events and What to Expect When One Occurs. pp. 2-4 – 2-15
6. Popuard J.A., Miller L.A. History of Biological Warfare: Catapults to Capsomeres. Annals of New York Academy of Sciences, 1992. 666: pp 9-20
7. Daniels A. Germs against Man. National Review, December 3, 2001. Vol. 53, Issue 23. pp 23
8. Malloy C. A History of Biological and Chemical Warfare and Terrorism. Journal of Public Health Management Practice. 6: 2000. pp 32
9. Hugh-Jones M. Wickham Steed and the German Biological Warfare Research. Intelligence and National Security, 1992. 7: pp. 379-402
10. Gernhart G. A. Forgotten Enemy: PHS's Fight Against the 1918 Influenza Pandemic. Public Health Reports, 1999. 114: pp. 559-561
11. Christopher G. W., Cieslak T. J., Pavlin J. A., Eitzen Jr E. M. Biological Warfare. A Historical Perspective. JAMA. 278: August 6, 1997. pp 412-417
12. Mangold T., Goldberg J. Plague Wars: The terrifying reality of biological warfare. New York: Macmillan Publishers, 1999. pp. 15; 24-25
13. Alibek K. Biohazard. New York: Dell Publishing. 1999. pp. 29-31; 35-37; 42-43; 70-86; 81-82; 106; 131; 195-196; 295-300
14. Atlas R.M. Combating the Threat of Biowarfare and Bioterrorism. Defending against Biological Weapons is Critical to Global Security. BioScience, 1999. 49: pp. 465-477
15. Harris S. Japanese Biological Warfare Research on Humans: a Case Study of Microbiology and Ethics. Annals of the New York Academy of Sciences, 1992. 666: pp. 21-52
16. United States House of Representatives, Committee on Science and Astronautics. Technical information for Congress: A report to the subcommittee on science research and development. Washington, DC: Government Printing Office, 1971. pp 537
17. Guillemin J. Biological Weapons: From the Invention of State-Sponsored Programs to Contemporary Bioterrorism. New York: Columbia University Press, 2005. pp. 60-61
18. Bernstein B.J. The Birth of the US Biological-warfare Program. Scientific American, 1987. 256: pp. 116-121
19. Geissler E. Biological and Toxin Weapons Today. Oxford: Oxford University Press. 1986. pp. 1-207
20. US Department of the Army. US Army Activity in the US Biological Warfare Programs. Washing DC: U.S. Dept of the Army. February 24, 1977. Publication DTIC B193427
21. Broad B., Wolfinger K. Interviews with Biowarriors: Bill Patrick. NOVA, November 2001
22. Franz D.R., Parrott C.D., Takafuji E.T. The U.S. Biological Warfare and Biological Defense Programs. Medical Aspects of Chemical and Biological Warfare. Washington D.D.: Office of the Surgeon General Department of the Army, United States of America. 1997. pp. 425-436
23. Bacon D. Biological Warfare: an Historical Perspective. Seminars in Anesthesia, Perioperative Medicine and Pain, 2003. 22: pp. 224-229
24. Riedel S. Biological Warfare and Bioterrorism: a Historical Review. Baylor University Medical Center Proceedings, 2004. 17: pp. 400-406
25. Convention on the Prohibition of the Development, Production, and Stockpiling of Bacteriological (Biological) and Toxin Weapons and their Destruction. Entered into Force: March 26, 1975. Revised June 27, 2009. Retrieved May 11, 2006, Web site: http://www.nti.org/ere search/official_docs/inventory/pdfs/btwc.pdf
26. Mirocha C.J. Hazards of Scientific Investigation: Analysis of Samples Implicated in Biological Warfare. Journal of Toxicology-Toxin Reviews. 1982. 1: pp. 199-203
27. Rosen R.T., Rosen J.D. Presence of Four Fusarium mycotoxin and Synthetic Material in "Yellow Rain": Evidence for the Use of Chemical Weapons in Laos. Biomedical Mass Spectrometry, 1982. 9: pp. 443-450
28. Wannemacher R.W., Weiner S.L. Trichothecene Mycotoxins. Medical Aspects of Chemical and Biological Warfare. Chapter 34. Washington D.C.: Office of the Surgeon General Department of the Army, United States of America. 1997. pp. 655-676

29. Smart J.K. The U.S. Biological Warfare and Biological Defense Programs. Medical Aspects of Chemical and Biological Warfare. Chapter 2. Washington D.C.: Office of the Surgeon General Department of the Army, United States of America. 1997. pp. 9-86
30. Tucker J.B. The "Yellow Rain" Controversy: Lessons for Arms Control Compliance. The Nonproliferation Review, 2001. pp. 25-42
31. Ember L.R. Yellow Rain. Chemical and Engineering News, 1984. 62: pp. 8-34
32. Agarwal R., Shukla S.K., Dharmani S., Gandhi A. Biological Warfare – an Emerging Threat. Journal of Association of Physicians of India, 2004. 52: pp. 733-738
33. Haig Jr A.M. Chemical Warfare in Southeast Asia and Afghanistan. Report to the Congress from Secretary of State. Washington D.C.: United States Department of State, Bureau of Public Affairs, Office of Public Communication, Editorial Division. March 22, 1982. pp. 31
34. Robinson J., Guillemin J., Meselson M. Yellow Rain: The Story Collapses. Foreign Policy, 1987. 68: pp. 101–117
35. Ember L.R., Sorenson W.G., Lewis D.M. Charges of Toxic Arms Use by Iraq Escalate. Chemical and Engineering News, 1984. 62: pp. 16-18
36. Mangold T., Goldberg J. Plague Wars: The terrifying reality of biological warfare. New York: Macmillan Publishers, 1999. pp. 214
37. Alibek K. Biohazard. New York: Dell Publishing. 1999. pp. 70-86
38. Sidell F.R., Franz D.R. Overview: Defense Against the Effects of Chemical and Biological Warfare Agents. Medical Aspects of Chemical and Biological Warfare. Chapter 1. Washington D.C.: Office of the Surgeon General Department of the Army, United States of America. 1997. pp. 1-7
39. Mangold T., Goldberg J. Plague Wars: The terrifying reality of biological warfare. New York: Macmillan Publishers, 1999. pp. 287
40. Zilinskas R.A. Iraq's Biological Weapons: the Past as Future? The Journal of the American Medical Association, 1997. 278: pp. 418-424
41. Mangold T., Goldberg J. Plague Wars: The terrifying reality of biological warfare. New York: Macmillan Publishers, 1999. pp. 291
42. Mangold T., Goldberg J. Plague Wars: The terrifying reality of biological warfare. New York: Macmillan Publishers, 1999. pp. 294
43. Reagan, R.W. Remarks at the Annual Convention of the National Association of Evangelicals. Delivered 8 March1983, Orlando Fort Lauderdale, 1983
44. Morrow J. Greater Intervention and Military Cutbacks are a Deadly Combination. The National Center for Public Policy Research. Washington DC, 1999. pp. 249
45. UN Security Council resolutions relating to Iraq. Retrieved May 11, 2006 from United States Department of the State web site. November 8, 2002. Web site: http://www.state.gov/p/nea/rls/01fs/14906.htm
46. United Nations Security Council, "Report of Executive Chairman of the Activities of the Special Commission Established by the Secretary-General Pursuant to Paragraph to Paragraph 9 (b) (i) of Security Council Resolution 687 (1991), S/1998/920, (6 Oct. 1998), Retrieved January 2, 2007. Web Site: http://www.un.org/ Depts/unscom/sres98-920.htm
47. Iraq: The UNSCOM Experience. Stockholm International Peace Research Institute Fact Sheet. October 1998. Retrieved January 2, 2007. Web site: http://books.sipri.org/product_info? c_product_id=217#
48. Miller J., Stephen E., William B. Germs: Biological Weapons and America's Secret War. New York: Touchstone, 2002. pp. 137
49. von Drehle D., Smith J. U.S. Strikes Iraq for Plot to Kill Bush. Washington Post June 27, 1993. pp. A01
50. The Associated Press. At Least 10 Americans Killed in Saudi Terror Attack. Fox News. Revised May 13, 2003. Retrieved January 20, 2010. Website: http://www.foxnews.com/story/0,2933,86681 ,00.html
51. Shenon P. 23 U.S. Troops Die in Truck Bombing in Saudi Base. New York Times. Revised June 26, 1996. Retrieved January 27, 2010. Website: http://partners.nytimes.com/library/world/africa/ 062696binladen.html
52. "Al-Qaeda International." Testimony of J. T. Caruso, Acting Assistant Director, Counter Terrorism Division, FBI Before the Subcommittee on International Operations and Terrorism, CommitteeonForeignRelations, UnitedStatesSenate. RevisedDecember18, 2001. Retrieved January 26, 2010. Website: http://www.fbi.gov/congress/congress01/caruso121801.htm
Whitlock C. Probe of USS Cole Bombing Unravels. Plotters Freed in Yemen; U.S. Efforts Frustrated. The Washington Post, May 4, 2008. pp. A01
53. Hunting Bin Laden. Revised September 2001. Retrieved December 12 2006 from Frontline, Co-Production with New York Times and Rain Media. Web site: http://www.pbs.org/wgbh/pages/frontline/ shows/binladen/
54. Bush G.W. President Bush's weekly radio address. October 13, 2001
55. Duelfer Report: Comprehensive Report of the Special Advisor to the DCI on Iraq's WMD. October 6, 2004. Retrieved May 11, 2006. Web Site: http://www.lib.umich. edu/govdocs/duelfer.html
56. Terrill W.A. Chemical Weapons in the Gulf War. Strategic Review, 1986, pp. 53.
57. Ekeus R. Iraq's Real Weapons Threat. Washington DC. Washington Post. June 29, 2003. pp. B07
58. Gellman B. A Futile Game of Hide and Seek: Ritter, UNSCOM Foiled by Saddam's Concealment Strategy. Washington DC. Washington Post, October 11, 1998. pp. A01
59. Carafano J.J. U.S. Thwarts 19 Terrorist Attacks Against America Since 9/11. Backgrounder. The Heritage Foundation. November 13, 2007. No. 2085. pp. 1-8
60. Kristof ND. Rejoin the World. New York Times. Published November 1, 2008. Retrieved Octover 18, 2014. Website: http://www.nytimes.com/2008/11/02/opinion/02kristof.html?_r=0
61. Obama, B.H. Remarks by the President on a New Beginning. Cairo University. Cairo, Egypt. The White House, Office of the Press Secretary. Revised June 4, 2009. Retrieved January 29, 2010. Website: http://www. whitehouse.gov/the_press_office/Remarks-by-the-Preside nt-at-Cairo-University-6-04-09/
62. The Nobel Peace Prize for 2009 to President Barack Obama - Press Release. Nobelprize.org. Nobel Media AB 2014. Released October 9, 2009. Retrieved October 18, 2014. Website: http://www.nobelprize.org/nobel_prizes/pe ace/laureates/2009/press.html
63. Thomas P., Esppsito R., Date J. Recruiter Shooting Suspect Had Ties to Extremist Locations. Investigators Probing Attack to Determine Whether Shooting Suspect Acted Alone. ABC News. Revised June 3, 2009. Retrieved January 29, 2010. Website: http://abcnews.go.com/Politics/story?id=7732467
64. Dao J. Man Claims Terror Ties in Little Rock Shooting. New York Times. Published January 21, 2010. Retrieved October 18, 2014. Website: http://www.nytimes.com/20 10/01/22/us/22littlerock.html
65. Williams P., Guthrie S., Foster S., Jones K., Seidman J., Dedman B., Johnson A. Gunman kills 12, wounds 31 at Fort Hood. Army psychiatrist identified as attacker is captured alive, general says. NBC News and msnbc.com revised November 5, 2009. Retrieved October 17, 2014. Website: http://www.nbcnews.com/id/33678801/ ns/us_ne ws-crime_and_courts/t/gunman-kills-wounds-forthood/#.V E F1lzt0xZQ
66. Compoy A., Sanders P., Gold R. Hash Browns, Then 4 Minutes of Chaos. Role of Texas Shooter's Muslim Faith Is Examined; Policewoman Hailed as Hero. Revised November 9, 2009. Wall Street Journal Online. Retrieved January 29, 2010. Website: http://online.wsj.com/ article/SB125750297355533413.html
67. Carter CJ. Nidal Hasan convicted in Fort Hood shootings; jurors can decide death. CNN. Updated August 23, 2013. Retrieved October 18, 2014. Website: http://www.cnn.com/2013/08/23/ justice/nidal-hasan-court-martial-friday/
68. Chumley CK. Nidal Hasan's Fort Hood trial starts; 'workplace violence' classification denies Purple Hearts. Released August 6, 2013. Retrieved October 18, 2014. Website: http://www.washingtontimes.com/news/2013/ aug/6/nidal-hasans-fort-hood-trial-starts-workplace-viol/
69. Whittell G., Fresco A. I'm the first of many, warns airline 'bomber' Umar Farouk Abdulmutallab. Times Online. Revised December 19, 2009. Retrieved January 29, 2010. Website: http://www.timesonline .co.uk/tol/news/world/us_and_americas/article6969645.ece
70. Meeks JG, Goldsmith S. Terror Suspect Umar Farouk Abdulmutallab Faces 20 years, $250,000 Fine for Attack on Flight 253. Daily News. Published: Saturday, December 26, 2009. Retrieved October 18, 2014. Website: http://www.nydailynews.com/news/national/terr or-suspect-umar-farouk-abdulmutallab-faces-20-years-25 0-000-fine-attack-flight-253-article-1.435763
71. Finn P. Al-Awlaki directed Christmas 'underwear bomber' plot, Justice Department memo says. The Washington Post. Published February 10, 2012. Retrieved October 18, 2014. Website: http://www.washingtonpost.com/world/ national-security/al-awlaki-directed-christmas-underwear-bomber-plot-justice-department-me mo-says/2012/02/10/gIQArDOt4Q_story.html
72. Office of the Attorney General. Umar Farouk Abdulmutallab Sentenced to Life in Prison for Attempted Bombing of Flight 253 on Christmas Day 2009. Department of Justice, Office of Public Affairs. Released February 16, 2012. Retrieved October 18, 2014. Website: http://www.justice.gov/opa/pr/umar-farouk-abdulmutallab-sentenced-life-prison-attempted-bombing-flight-253-christmas-day
73. Katersky A, Esposito R. Faisal Shahzad: "War with Muslims has Just Begun." ABC News. Published Oct. 5, 2010. Retrieved October 18 2014. Website: http://abcnews.go.com/Blotter/times-square-bomber-faisal -shahzad-sentenced-life/story?id=11802740
74. Associated Press. New York City Police Find Car Bomb in Times Square. Published May 01, 2010. Retrieved October 18, 2014. Website: http://www.foxnews.com/us/ 2010/05/01/new-york-city-police-close-times-square-investigation/
75. Associated Press. Oregon: 30-Year Sentence in Bomb Plot. Published October 1, 2014 . Retreived October 18, 2014. Website: http://www.nytimes.com/2014/10/02/us /oregon-30-year-sentence-in-bomb-plot-.html
76. Irshaid F. Profile Libya's Ansar-al-sharia. BBC. Published June 13, 2014. Retrieved October 18, 2014. Website: http ://www.bbc.com/news/world-africa-27732589
77. Committee on Armed Services. Majority Interim Report: Benghazi Investigation Update. Released February 2014. Retrieved October 18, 2014. Website: http://armedservices.house.gov/index. cfm/files/serve?File_id=C4E16543-8F99-430C-BEBA-0045A6433426
78. Associated Press. A Look at the Bombing at the Boston Marathon Finish Line, Investigation into New Suspects. Published May 1 2013. Retrieved October 17 2014. Website: http://www.foxnews.com/us/2013/05/01/look-at-bombing-at-boston-marathon-finish-line-investigation-into-new-suspects/
79. Jerry Markon J, Horwitz S, Johnson J. Dzhokhar Tsarnaev charged with using 'weapon of mass destruction'. The Washington Post. Published April 22, 2013. Retrieved October 18, 2014. Website: http://www.washingtonpost.com/national/alleged-bombers -aunt-tamerlan-tsarnaev-was-religious-but-not-radical/2013/04/22/ca8f32 14-ab5c-11e2-a198-99893f10d6dd_story .html
80. CNN Library. Boston Marathon Terror Attack Fast Facts. CNN Library. Published September 26, 2014. Retrieved October 18, 2014. Website: http://www.cnn.com/2013/06/03/us/boston-marathon-terror-attack-fast-facts/
81. Wedeman B. Najaf bombing kills Shiite leader, followers say. Iraqi officials: At least 125 dead, 142 wounded. CNN. Published August 30, 2003. Retrieved October 19, 2014. Website: http://edition.cnn.com/2003/WORLD/meast/08/ 29/sprj.irq.najaf/
82. Ghoshaug B. ISIS: A Short History. The terrorist group's evolution from fervid fantasy to death cult. The Atlantic. Published August 14, 2014. Retrieved October 19, 2014. Website: http://www.theatlantic.com/international/archive/ 2014/08/isis-a-short-history/376030/
83. al-Zawahiri A. English Translation of Ayman al-Zawahiri's letter to Abu Musab al-Zarqawi. The Weekly Standard. Published October 12, 2005. Retrieved, October 18, 2014. Website: http://www.weeklystandard.com/Content/Public/Articles/000/000/006/203gpuul.asp
84. Byman DL. The History of Al-Qaida. Brookings Institute. Published September 1, 2011. Retrieved October 18, 2014. Website: http://www.brookings.edu/research/opin ions/2011/09/01-al-qaeda-history-byman
85. Knickmeyer E, Finer J. Insurgent Leader Al-Zarqawi Killed in Iraq. The Washington Post. Published June 8, 2006. Retrieved October 18, 2014. Website: http://www.washingtonpost.com/wp-dyn/content/article/2006/06/08/AR20060 60800114.html
86. Logan J. Last U.S. troops leave Iraq, ending war. Reuters. Published December 18, 2011. Retrieved October 18, 2104. Website: http://www.reuters.com/article/2011/12/18/us-iraqwithdrawal-idUSTRE7BH03320111218
87. Kessler G. Spinning Obama's reference to Islamic State as a 'JV' team. The Washington Post. Published September 3, 2014. Retrieved October 19, 2014. Website: http://www.washingtonpost.com/blogs/fact-checker/wp/2014/09/03/ spinning-obamas-reference-to-isis-as-a-jv-team/
88. Syria Iraq: The Islamic Satte Militant Group. BBC. Updated August 2, 2014. Retrieved October 19, 2014. Website: http://www.bbc.com/news/world-middle-east-24179084
89. Frizell S. President Obama Explains Why The U.S. Is Bombing ISIS. Time. Published August 9, 2014. Retrieved October 19, 2014. Website: http://time.com/3095598 /obama-iraq-isis/
90. Kaplan R. Obama Says it Again: No Ground Troops in Iraq. Published September 17, 2014. Retrieved October 19, 2014. CBS News Website: http://www.cbsnews .com/news/obama-says-it-again-no-ground-troops-in-iraq
91. Doornbos H., Moussa J. Found: The Islamic State's Terror Laptop of Doom. Foreign Policy. Published August 28, 2014. Retrieved October 19, 2014.Website:http://www.foreignpolicy.com/articles/2014/08/28/found_the_islamic_state_terror_laptop_of_doom_bubonic_plague_weapons_of_mass_destruction_exclusive
92. Thornhill T. Has ISIS looted chemical weapons from former Iraqi nerve agent factory that US failed to destroy? UN told 2,500 rockets containing deadly Sarin are in the hands of the jihadists. Mail Online. Published: October, 15 2014. Retrieved October 19, 2014. Website: http://www.dailymail.co.uk/news/article-2793731/will-rusting-chemical-weapons-cache-ignored-americans-fall-isis-hands-iraq-claims-2-500-rockets-containing-deadly-sarin-hands-terrorists.html#ixzz3GbofXeET
93. Iraq tells U.N. 'terrorist groups' seized former chemical weapons depot. Reuters. Published July 8, 2014. Retrieved October 19, 2014. Website: http://www.reuters. com/article/2014/07/08/us-iraq-security-chemicalweapons -idUSKBN0FD26K20140708

Photo Bibliography

Figure I-2-1: The painting Triumph of death reflects the death and destruction of the Bubonic Plague. Note the dying king in the left corner of the artwork which denotes the indiscriminant nature of the disease. Painting by Pieter Bruegel the Elder in 1526 and housed in Museo del Prado. Public domain photo

Figure I-2-2: Lieutenant General Shiro Ishii, commander of Unit 731 located in Beiyinhe, Manchuria. This photograph was taken by Masao Takezawa in 1932. Public domain photo

Figure I-2-3: A building on the site of the Harbin bioweapon facility of Unit 731. This photograph taken by 松岡明芳 on November, 2008. This file is licensed under the Creative Commons Attribution-Share Alike 3.0 Unported license

Figure I-2-4: Workers working with Class III cabinets at the U.S. Biological Warfare Laboratories, Camp Detrick, Maryland. Photo was taken by United States Army in the 1940s. Public domain photo

Figure I-2-5: "Eight Ball" located at Camp Detrick.[1] Photo was taken by United States Army, Fort Detrick, Maryland in the 1940s. Public domain photo

Figure I-2-6: The 1969 Conference on the Committee on Disarmament at work at the Palais des Nations at Geneva negotiated and led to the Convention on the Prohibition of the Development, Production and Stockpiling of Bacteriological (Biological) and Toxin Weapons and on their Destruction. Photo was taken by an unknown author in 1969 and released by Joshua Lederberg of the United States National Library of Medicine in April 25, 2005. Public domain photo

Figure I-2-7: Dan Crozier Building, USAMRIID, Fort Detrick, MD. Photo was taken by The United States Army, USAMRIID in September 19, 2008. Public domain photo

Figure I-2-8: Satellite photo shows a plume spreading out over Sverdlovsk and the locations of 64 people who died over the next 42 days. The total death toll from the accidental Anthrax release is estimated at 66-105 people. Photo was taken and released by the United States Department of Energy. Public domain photo

Figure I-2-9: Russian made (Al-Asad) drop tanks which are modified for biological or chemical weapon delivery system. Photo was taken and released by the Central Intelligence Agency. Public domain photo

Figure I2-10: Iraqi made 1m3 800 liters stainless steel mobile tanks that are designed to transport bulk agents or used for fermentation purposes (i.e. biological warfare agents). UNSCOM identified the remains of only two of these tanks in 1990 but 18 were never found. Photo was taken and released by the Central Intelligence Agency. Public domain photo

Figure I2-11: Aftermath of World Trade Center bombing in February 25. 1993. Photo was taken and released by Bureau of Alcohol, Tobacco, Firearms and Explosives. Public domain photo

Figure I2-12: Aftermath of Khobar Towers bombing in June 25. 1996. Photo was taken and released by Department of Defense. Public domain photo

Figure I2-13: The Islamic terrorist attack on the United States Embassies located in Nairobi, Kenya, on August 7, 1998. Photo was taken and released by Federal Bureau of Investigation. Public domain photo

Figure I2-14: Aftermath of USS Cole bombing in October 12, 2000. USS *Cole* (DDG 67) is towed away from the port city of Aden, Yemen on October 29, 2000. Photo was taken by Sgt. Don L. Maes and released by the Department of Defense. Public domain photo

Figure I2-15: Attack on the World Trade Center September 11, 2001. Photo was copyrighted ©, taken and released by Michael Foran. Printed with permission

Figure I2-16: The aftermath of a chemical weapon attack by Iraqi forces loyal to Saddam Hussein. Chemical weapons used include the Tabun, Sarin, VX, as well as mustard gas. This attack occurred in March 16, 1988 at Halabja, a Kurdish town in northern Iraq, that killed 3,200-5,000, and injured around 7,000-10,000 people. Photograph was taken by Sayeed Janbozorgi who later died in 2002 due to injuries sustain from the poison gases. This photograph is published under GFDL license

Figure I-2-17: First responders use a table as a stretcher to transport a wounded US Soldier to an awaiting ambulance at Fort Hood, Texas. Photo was taken by Sgt. Jason R. Krawczyk, US Army. Public Domain photo

Figure I-2-18: NYPD bomb squad defusing the car bomb left by Faisal Shahzad in Time Square, New York. Photo was taken and released by NYPD. Public domain photo

Figure I-2-19: Immediate aftermath of the Boston Marathon Bombing. Photo taken and released by Aaron Tang and the permission for reproduction was granted under Creative Common Attribution 2.0 license

Biological terrorism is defined as the use of biological agents by a political or religious group that is not a recognized extension of a government or a state to achieve a political or ideological objective.[1] The use of biological weapons as a form of terror attack is not just a fanciful theory, but a rude reality in recent history. For example, in September and October of 1984, 751 people were intentionally infected with *Salmonella typhimurium* by the followers of the Bhagwan Shree Rajneesh (Figure I-3-1).[2]

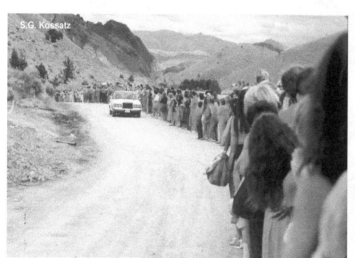

Figure I-3-1: Follower of Rajneeshee cult greet the Bhagwan at the Dalles, Oregon

The Rajneeshee cult was founded by an Indian mystic named Osho, formally known as Chandra Mohan Jain in the 1960's and they built a community known as Rajneeshpuram between the towns of Antelope and The Dalles in Wasco County, Oregon. Within a short time after establishment, the cult came into conflict with the local population and the Wasco county government over development and land practices. In an attempt to gain control of the local city government, the cult brought in thousands of homeless people from cities around the country under their "Share a Home" program, counting on their votes during the next election, as well as, plotting to sicken the local population to prevent them from voting.

The first incident of the cult using biological agents occurred on August 29, 1984, when two Wasco County commissioners were sickened by *S. typhimurium* laced water during their visit to the compound. Trial runs of disseminating biological agents were attempted prior to the November election through the contamination of the local water system and through supermarket foods but were unsuccessful. Finally, between September and October of 1984, cult members continued their trial run by contaminating foods at local restaurants by pouring *S. typhimurium* into vegetables, dressing at salad bars and coffee creamers. Subsequently, 751 people of the Wasco County developed enteritis and approximately 45 individuals were hospitalized. Since this event occurred before the establishment of 24 hour news channels, it did not attract a lot of public attention. Nonetheless, this event did attract the attention of law enforcement agencies such as the FBI and on the 28th of October 1985, Bhagwan was arrested on a thirty-five-count indictment, mainly on his conspiracy to evade immigration laws. In 1986, two members of the cult were charged and sentenced to 20 years in prison for their part in the biological terrorism event but only served 4 years of their sentence (Figure I-3-2).[1, 2, 3, 4, 5]

On March 19, 1995, a Japanese sect of the Aum Shinrikyo cult, founded and led by Shoko Asahara released sarin gas in the Tokyo subway system resulting in 12 deaths and approximately 6,000 intoxicated victims. Before their final act of releasing chemical weapons, the cult experimented, developed and attempted to disseminate biological weapons within Japan (Figure I-3-3).

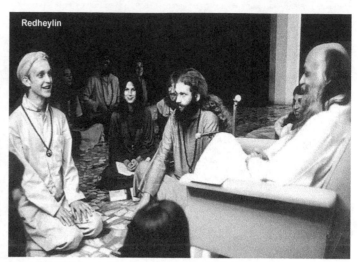

Figure I-3-2: Bhagwan Shree Rajneesh talks to disciple in 1977

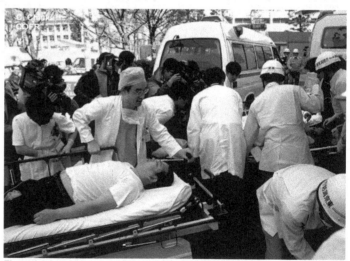

Figure I-3-3: Tokyo subway riders being cared for by emergency workers after the Sarin gas attack

The cult, with its nearly 300 million dollars in assets per year, built sophisticated laboratories and production facilities to grow *Bacillus anthracis*, *Clostridium botulinum* and *Coxiella burnetii*.[5, 6] In addition, they sent a team of their members to Zaire, in the midst of an Ebola epidemic, to acquire samples for cultivation into a biological weapon. Attempts have been made to disseminate the biological weapons they produced. For example, in April 1990, the cult made nine unsuccessful attacks (three with anthrax and six with botulinum toxin) on the Japanese Parliament, business districts in central Tokyo and Yokahama, Yosuka United States Naval Base, and Nairita International Airport. In June 1993, the cult targeted the wedding of the Crown Price of Japan by spraying botulinum toxin through the vehicle's exhaust. Later that same month, the cult installed and used a large industrial sprayer to disseminate anthrax microbes in central Tokyo (Figure I-3-4). On March 15, 1995, the cult planted three brief cases filled with botulinum toxin and released them in the Tokyo subway system. Fortunately, none of the biological attacks were successful. These failures can mainly be attributed to ineffective sprayers and the virulence of the strains of the microbes they used. Frustrated by their failed efforts, the cult finally chose chemical weapons and successfully accomplished their goals.[1, 5]

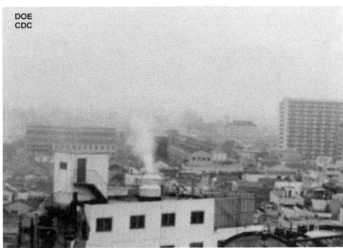

Figure I-3-4: Aum Shinrikyo cult installed and used a large industrial sprayer to disseminate anthrax microbes in central Tokyo

In 1995, members of Minnesota militia group were convicted of possession of ricin, which they had produced themselves for use in retaliation against local law enforcement officials, U.S. marshals, and IRS agents. The Minnesota Patriot Council, as they were known, was an antigovernment (anti-taxation) group that has also attempted to acquire Yersinia pestis from the American Type Culture Collection and had conducted experiments with the Sterne strain of B. anthracis.[1, 7]

In October 2001, anthrax was delivered by mail to US media and government offices. It is suspected that at least five letters (of which four have been recovered) and as many as seven anthrax tainted letters were sent in two mailings (September 18, 2001 and October 9, 2001). The first letter arrived at American Media in Boca Raton, Florida on October 4, 2001 which caused the death of one employee through inhalational anthrax - the first death from inhalational anthrax in 20 years. The remaining letters were sent to ABC News, CBS News, NBC News, New York Post, Senators Tom Daschle of South Dakota and Patrick Leahy of Vermont. These anthrax contaminated letters infected approximately 68 people; 11 people contracted inhalational form of the disease which resulted in five deaths. This attack resulted in significant disruption at the Hart United States Senate Building and the United States Postal Services. In addition, millions of dollars were spent on environmental deconta-mination (Figure I-3-5).[1, 8]

The origin of the anthrax in these letters is still unknown, however, recent accounts in the American news media point to a scientist at the US Army Medical Research Institute of Infectious Diseases (USAMRID) at Ft. Detrick, MD. Dr. Bruce Ivins, a microbiologist at the Institute, committed suicide in July 2008 before he could be charged with participating in the development and delivery of the letters containing anthrax spores. Since, he committed suicide, we may never know the true story of this incident that caused much chaos in September and October 2001.[9, 10]

In December 2002, six terrorist suspects were arrested in Manchester, England after the police raided their apartment. Apparently, their rented dwelling was serving as a "ricin

laboratory." [11] On the 5th of January, 2003, British authorities raided and arrested six suspected terrorists from Algeria and other northern African countries in their North London apartment. The British authorities believed they were using their residence as a factory for producing ricin. It was reported that at least one of these seven men had attended an Al-Qaida training camp in Afghanistan, while the others had received their training in Chechnya and the Pankisi Gorge region in the country of Georgia.[12]

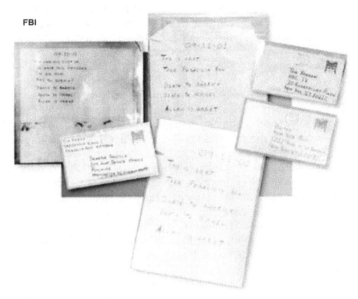

Figure I-3-5: Anthrax laced letters

United States forces, operating in Kurdish-controlled regions of Northern Iraq in 2003, seized a camp operated by Islamic militant group Ansar al-Islam, which has ties to Al-Qaida. Various pieces of equipment and materials were discovered, indicating the terrorists were working/experimenting with chemical weapons as well as ricin.[13] In October 2003, ricin was discovered in a South Carolina postal facility and on February 3, 2004, three US Senate office buildings were closed after ricin was found in a mailroom that served Senate Majority Leader Bill Frist's office, forcing the decontamination of 16 employees and the shutdown of several government buildings.[14, 15, 16, 17, 18]

On February 29th, 2008, Reuters reported that ricin was found in a Las Vegas hotel room. Roger von Bergendorff was later charged with producing and possessing a biological weapon, although it is believed that he has no direct connection to any terrorism groups.[19]

The most recent evidence that terrorist groups are attempting to develop WMDs was reported in the Washington Times in January, 2009. The report states that an Al-Qaida affiliate, located in the mountains of Tizi Ouzou Province, in Eastern Algeria, was shut down after 40 operatives were killed due to botched experiments with Yersinia pestis.[20]

TERRORISM AND WMD

In 2004, it was reported by the Central Intelligence Agency (CIA) that the threat of insurgent and terrorist groups using nonconventional materials such as chemical, biological, radiological and nuclear (CBRN) materials to achieve their political aims are significant (Please examine Table 1 for more information).[21] CIA suspected that approximately 33 designated terrorist groups and insurgents worldwide had revealed an interest in CBRN materials. Intelligence reports had indicated that many of the insurgent and terrorist groups had pursued chemical and biological (CB) programs, however, with varying degrees of success. These programs included planning or preparation to use commercially available chemicals in small-scale attacks using improvised means.[21]

It is suspected that most insurgent and terrorist groups are interested in simple chemicals or biological organisms that could be used for contamination of food and water, to create contact poisons, or for use in conjunction with conventional weapons (e.g. coating ammunition, using modified mortar rounds, or developing improvised chemical devices). It is believed that these tactics will not result in large numbers of casualties; nonetheless, these efforts may serve as a foundation for more ambitious efforts.[21]

Based on available data, the CIA have identified agents such as anthrax, botulin toxin, ricin, cyanides, mustard gas, and nerve agents (e.g. sarin) as among the most likely to be pursued or used by terrorists in the near future. It is also believed that insurgent and terrorist groups are now capable of organizing attacks using crude radiological dispersion devices (RDDs), which are likely to cause few casualties beyond those caused by any conventional explosives however, the lingering physiological effects may be substantial. While it is believed that most insurgent and terrorist groups have shown little interest in acquiring nuclear weapons or producing their own improvised nuclear devices, Al-Qaida on the other hand had taken steps to acquire such a capability.[21]

Al-Qaeda had publicly stated its interest in conducting unconventional attacks against the United States and is receiving support from sympathetic radical Islamic groups around the world. In 1998, Osama Bin Laden publicly declared that acquiring unconventional weapons was "a religious duty." The Leaders of the September 11th attacks Mohammad Atta (Figure I-3-6) and Zacharias Moussaoui expressed an interest in crop dusters. According to FBI assessment, it is possible that they were seeking ways of distributing chemical or biological weapons.[22]

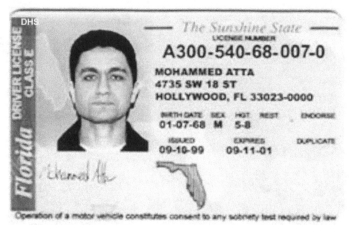

Figure I-3-6: Mohammad Atta, an Egyptian hijacker and one of the leaders of the September 11 attacks. Atta was the hijacker-pilot of American Airlines Flight 11, which crashed the plane into the North Tower of the World Trade Center

In 2003, an extremist cleric known to support Al-Qaida issued a fatwa, a religious justification, for the use of weapons of mass destruction against the United States.[21] Analysis of an Al-Qaeda

Table 1: List of terrorist actions from 1999-2004[21]

Terrorist Groups	Country	Date	Event
The Liberation Tigers of Tamil Eelam (LTTE)	Sri Lanka	1990	LTTE attacked a northern Sri Lankan Armed Forces base with chlorine gas, injuring more than 60 military Personnel
The Kurdistan Peoples' Congress (KHK)	Switzerland	1999	KHK threatened to detonate a bomb containing toxic gas inside an International Labor Organization Building in Geneva
Fuerzas Armadas Revolucionarias de Colombia (FARC)	Columbia	2001	Colombian authorities suspected that 3 members of Provisional Irish Republican Army (PIRA) that were arrested in Bogota may have provided assistance to FARC in handling chemical materials that were used in an attack that killed four policemen
Salafist Group for Call and Combat (GSPC)	USA Italy	2002	Eleven members of the GSPC were arrested. Two of the 11 GSPC members were convicted of brokering arms, explosives, and chemical weapons
Mujahidin associated with Al-Qaeda	UK	2003	Several groups of mujahidin with Al-Qaeda connections had attempted to carry out attacks in Europe with ricin
Students' Islamic Movement of India (SIMI)	India	2003	Raids on terrorist training centers of SIMI recovered potassium cyanide and sulfuric acid
Fuerzas Armadas Revolucionarias de Colombia	Columbia	2003	It is believed that FARC was using bullets and explosives soaked in chemical agents to attack Columbian government forces
Jemaah Islamiya (JI)	Philippines	2003	During raids on JI safe houses Philippine authorities recovered manuals written in Indonesian detailing procedures for making and disseminating CB agents
Ejército de Liberación Nacional (ELN)	Columbia	2004	The Colombian press reported that Colombian soldiers had seized 122 cartridges laced with cyanide
Chechen Republic	Chechnya	2004	During a raid on a Chechen base, a vial containing 200 grams of fabricated chemical poison was recovered. The actual contents of the recovered vial have not been confirmed
Chechen terrorist network*	France	2004	Six individuals were arrested and charged with terrorist activities in France. Investigators believe that they were preparing for acts of terrorism against Russian interests in Paris, and were recruiting Islamic volunteers. One of the arrested individual named Imam Shelai Benshelali attempted to make botulinum and ricin
Lashkar-e-Jhangvi (LJ)	Pakistan	2004	Pakistani authorities investigated the reports of LJ had conspired to poison food and water with sodium nitrate to Shia congregations
Revolutionary People's Liberation Party–Front (DHKP-C)	Turkey	2004	Turkish authorities captured two members of the DHKP-C and recovered 175 grams of cyanide
Fatah-Tanzim	Israel	2004	Palestinian cell member was arrested for planning to incorporate HIV-infected blood into an explosive belt and detonate it in Tel Aviv during the Passover holiday

*Chechen terrorist network includes Islamic International Peacekeeping Brigade (IIPB), Special Purpose Islamic Regiment (SPIR), Riyadus-Salikhin Reconnaissance, and Sabotage Battalion of Chechen Martyrs

documents and footage captured during Operation Enduring Freedom in Afghanistan indicated the Islamic terrorist group was suspected in experimenting with biological weapons such as anthrax, as well as, chemical weapons such as mustard agent, sarin, and VX.[23, 24, 25] In addition, further analysis of the captured documents revealed that Al-Qaeda was engaged in rudimentary nuclear research. It is believed that foreign experts such as Bashir al-Din Mahmood, a Pakistani nuclear engineer, may have provided support. According to the testimony of Jamal Ahmad Fadl, a government witness during the 2001 trial of the bombings of the American Embassies in Tanzania and Kenya, Al-Qaeda had been actively seeking nuclear material since the early 1990s. Fadl stated during his testimony that Al-Qaeda had pursued the sale of enriched uranium in Sudan however the effort was believed to be a scam perpetrated on the terrorist group since there were no credible evidence that uranium was actually acquired.[21, 26] Information released in 2003 revealed that Al-Qaeda was providing details in the construction of a cyanide-based weapon that could produce a lethal dose of this poisonous gas in an enclosed area. The plans for this chemical based weapon could be easily accessed by any would-be terrorists and could be easily constructed from readily available items and required little or no actual training to assemble and deploy.[26]

The purpose of this book is to broaden the reader's understanding of biological agents and the potential for biological terrorism. Its' objective is to offer first responders (e.g. emergency medical teams, nurses, doctors, police and fire fighters etc.) a basic understanding of virology, bacteriology and the common biological warfare/terrorism agents available. In addition, this book will discuss the methodologies of how to detect a potential biological threat and the materials and techniques needed to contend with a potential biohazard situation.

With the ever increasing uncertainty of our times, the chance of terrorist using biological agents against civilian populations escalates with each passing day. Unfortunately, it is no longer the question of if we are going to be attacked but when.

References

1. Martin J.W., Christopher G.W., Eitzen E.M. History of Biological Weapons: From Poisoned Darts to Intentional Epidemics. Aspects of Biological Warfare. Chapter 1. Washington D.C.: The Surgeon General United States Army Medical Department Medical Center and School Borden Institute. 2007. pp. 1-20
2. Miller J., Stephen E., William B. Germs: Biological Weapons and America's Secret War. New York: Touchstone, 2002. pp. 15-33; 151-164
3. FitzGerald F. A Reporter at Large. I-Rajneeshpuram. The New Yorker, September 22, 1986. pp. 46-47
4. Torok T.J., Tauxe R.V., Wise R.P., Livengood J.R., Sokolow R., Mauvais S., Birkness K.A., Skeels M.R., Horan J.M., Foster L.R. A Large Community Outbreak of Salmonellosis Caused by Intentional Contamination of Restaurant Salad Bars. The Journal of American Medical Association, 1997. 278: pp. 389-395
5. Riedel S. Biological Warfare and Bioterrorism: a Historical Review. Baylor University Medical Center Proceedings, 2004. 17: pp. 400-406
6. Miller J., Stephen E., William B. Germs: Biological Weapons and America's Secret War. New York: Touchstone, 2002. pp. 151-164
7. Tucker J.B. Historical Trends Related to Bioterrorism: an Empirical Analysis. Emerging Infectious Diseases, 1999. 5: pp. 498-504
8. Cymet T.C., Kerkvliet G.J. What is the True Number of Victims of the Postal Anthrax Attack of 2001? Journal of the American Osteopathic Association, 2004. 104: pp. 452
9. Edward L. Analyzing the Anthrax Attacks: The first 3 years. Racine, Wisconsin: Edward G. Lake, 2005. pp. 54-92
10. Vergano D. Anthrax Case Not Closed: Panel Reviews Bruce Ivins, Mail Probe. USA Today. Revised August 3, 2009. Retrieved January 24, 2010. Website: http://www.usatoday.com/tech/science/ 2009-08-03-anthrax-ivins_N .htm
11. Carter H., Ward D, Hopkins N. Murder suspect 'is senior player' in ricin plot network. The Guardian (London), January 16, 2003
12. Bale J., Bhattacharjee A. Croddy E., Pilch R. Ricin Found in London: An al-Qa'ida Connection? Center for Nonproliferation Studies, Chemical and Biological Weapons Nonproliferation Program. Update February 29, 2008. Website: http://cns.miis.edu/pubs/reports/ricin.htm
13. Cameron C. and The Associated Press. New Evidence May Link Northern Iraq Militants to Al-Qaida. Fox News. Revised April 3, 2003. Retrieved January 29, 2003. Website: http://www.foxnews.com/ story/0,2933,83047,0 0.html
14. Weil M. Suspicious Powder Found in Frist Office: 6 of 8 Tests Positive for Lethal Toxin Ricin. The New York Times, Tuesday, February 3, 2004; Page A01
15. Smart J.K. The U.S. Biological Warfare and Biological Defense Programs. Medical Aspects of Chemical and Biological Warfare. Chapter 2. Washington D.C.: Office of the Surgeon General Department of the Army, United States of America. 1997. pp. 9-86
16. Eitzen E.M., Takafuji E.T. Historical Overview of Biological Warfare. Medical Aspects of Biological Warfare. Chapter 18. Washington D.C.: The Surgeon General United States Army Medical Department Medical Center and School Borden Institute. 2007. pp. 415-423
17. Kifner J. Man is Arrested in a Case Involving Deadly Poison. New York Times. 23 December, 1995. pp. A-7
18. Goodman P.S. Seized Poison Set Off Few Alarms. Anchorage Daily News. 4 January, 1996. B-1
19. Mylchreest I. Man critical in Las Vegas after poison ricin found. February 29, 2008, from Reuter. Web site: http://www.reuters.com/article/topNews/idUSN2915050420080229?feedType=RSS&feedName=topNews
20. Lake E. Al-Qaida Bungles Arms Experiment. The Washington Times. Revised January 20, 2009. Retrieved January 29, 2009. Website: http://www.washingtontimes. com/news/2009/jan/19/al-qaeda-bungles-arms-experime nt/
21. Tenet G.J. Attachment A. Unclassified Report to Congress on the Acquisition of Technology Relating to Weapons of Mass Destruction and Advanced Conventional Munitions. Released December 2003. Retrieved September 2012. Website: https://www.cia.gov/library/reports/archived-reports-1/721report_ju ly_dec2003 .pdf
22. Hijacker Visited Crop-Duster Airfield. September 24, 2001. American Broadcasting Company (ABC News) Retrieved September 13, 2012. Website: http://abcnews.go.com/US/story?id=92436&page=1&singlePage=true#top
23. Robertson N. Disturbing Scenes of Death Show Capability with Chemical Gas. Cable News Network (CNN), Released in August 19, 2002. Retrieved September 13, 2012. Website: http://articles.cnn.com/2002-08-19/us/terror.tape.chemical_1_chemical-weapons-nerve-agent-al-qa eda-tapes?_s=PM:US
24. Kosal M.E. Near Term Threats of Chemical Weapons Terrorism. Strategic Insights, Volume V, Issue 6. Released in July 2006. Retrieved September 13, 2012. Website: http://www.nps.edu/Academics/centers/ccc/publications/OnlineJournal/2006/Jul/kosalJul06.html#references
25. Joscelyn T. Al-Qaida's anthrax scientist. The Long War Journal (LWJ). Released in December 12, 2008. Retrieved September 13, 2012. Website: http://www.longwarjournal.org/archives/2008/12/al_qaedas_anthrax_sc.php#ixzz26LzMKQVN
26. Cordesman A.H. Problem of Risk Assessment Chapter 1. Washington D.C. The Challenge of Biological Terrorism. Center for Strategic and International Studies. 2005. pp. 34

Photo Bibliography

Figure I3-1: Follower of Rajneeshee cult greet the Bhagwan at The Dalles, Oregon. Photo was copyrighted© and taken by 2003 Samvado Gunnar Kossatz. Printed with permission
Figure I-3-2: Bhagwan Shree Rajneesh talks to disciple in 1977. Photo was taken by Redheylin and released in November 30, 2009. Public domain photo
Figure I-3-3: Tokyo subway riders being cared for by emergency workers after the Sarin gas attack. Photo was taken by Chikumo Chiaki and released by Council on Foreign Relations. Public domain photo
Figure I-3-4: Aum Shinrikyo cult installed and used a large industrial sprayer to disseminate anthrax microbes in central Tokyo. Photo Taken by Department of Environment, Koto-ward Japan and released by CDC. Public domain photo
Figure I-3-5: Anthrax laced letters. Photo was taken and released by the Federal Bureau of Investigation (FBI). Public domain photo
Figure I-3-6: Mohammad Atta, an Egyptian hijacker and one of the leaders of the September 11 attacks. Atta was the hijacker-pilot of American Airlines Flight 11, which crashed the plane into the North Tower of the World Trade Center. Photo was released by the Department of Homeland Security. Public domain photo

There are numerous infectious agents in nature and many have deadly consequences. However, not all infectious agents can be successfully made into biological weapons. In order for a virus, bacterium, or toxin (from bacteria or fungi) to be made into a weapon, scientists must select the biological agents that are capable of most if not all of the following seven criteria. ① The biological agent must be highly infectious, only requiring a minuscule amount of organisms or toxin to cause the desired effect. ② The potential biological weapon must be capable of being transmitted through casual contact, if it is an infectious agent, as well as, ③ possess the capability to be easily cultivated from a small starter culture, produced in large quantities cheaply and with minimum expertise. ④ The agent must be able to be processed down to miniscule sizes (1-5 μm in particle size) and be disseminated as an aerosol. ⑤ The agent must have the capability to be stored for long periods of time and ⑥ possess natural resistance to environmental conditions, thereby allowing it to remain infectious for the desired period of time. Finally, ⑦ the biological agent must have the ability to resist conventional treatments (e.g. antibiotics, antibodies, pharmaceutical drugs, etc.).[1]

With these initial requirements, the number of biological organisms and viruses capable of becoming weapons quickly narrows. With the possibilities of potential terrorist groups using biological weapons, a final criterion must be added. The biological weapon of choice must have the ability to create mass panic, resulting in substantial social unrest and disruption, even if the maximum casualty rate of the weapon is low.[1]

Presently, the biological agents able to be weaponized have been categorized based on their potential risk. For example, the agents that have the highest potential are assigned to Category A, while the agents with the lowest level of threat are classified as Category C. Please examine Table 1 for more information.

With the advances in biotechnology during the past two decades, most biological agents capable of being weaponized are now relatively easy and inexpensive to cultivate in mass quantities within a short period of time. In general, biological weapons do not require large factories to be manufactured and can be made in small laboratories with off-the-shelf commercial and scientific equipment. For example, seed stocks for possible biological weapons can be obtained either from the natural environment or culture collections located at the Center for Disease Control and Prevention (CDC, Atlanta), State Research Center of Virology and Biotechnology located at Koltsovo, Russia or from similar agencies in numerous other countries. Information with regards to biological agent production is widely available in published scientific literature, since these technologies have applications within the pharmaceutical, food, cosmetic, and pesticide industries. Put simply, the availability of seed stock and information can be perverted and used in biological weapon production. Moreover, large scale production of biological agents can be accomplished in dual-use facilities. For example, pharmaceutical manufacturing plants could easily be converted into bio-weapons production facilities. The equipment required for manufacturing can be purchased legally via the internet or catalogues from sources both within the United States and from international providers.[3]

Out of seven countries listed by the United States in 2001 as

Table 1: Categories of potential biological threats

Category	Biological Agent	Disease Caused	Type
A	Variola Major	Smallpox	Lethal
	Bacillus anthracis	Anthrax	Lethal
	Yersinia pestis	Plague	Lethal
	Clostridium botulinum	Botulism	Lethal
	Francisella tularensis	Tularemia	Lethal
	Manchupo Virus	Bolivian hemorrhagic fever	Lethal
	Marburg Virus	Viral Hemorrhagic Fever	Lethal
	Ebola Virus	Viral Hemorrhagic Fever	Lethal
	Junin virus	Viral Hemorrhagic Fever	Lethal
	Lassa Fever Virus	Viral Hemorrhagic Fever	Lethal
	Rift Valley Fever Virus	Viral Hemorrhagic Fever	Lethal
B	Coxiella burnetii	Q Fever	Incapacitant
	Brucella spp.	Brucellosis	Incapacitant
	Burkholderia mallei	Glanders	Lethal
	Burkholderia pseudomallei	Melioidosis	Lethal
	Alphaviruses	Encephalitis	Lethal
	Rickettsia prowazekii	Typhus Fever	Lethal
	Ricin	Toxin	Lethal
	Staphylococcal enterotoxin B	Toxin	Incapacitant
	Chlamydia psittaci	Toxin	Incapacitant
	Salmonella	Food Poisoning	Incapacitant
	Escherichia coli	Food poisoning	Incapacitant
	Vibrio cholerae	Cholera	Lethal
C	Dengue Fever Virus	Viral Hemorrhagic Fever	Lethal
	Chickungunya Virus	Chickungunya fever	Incapacitant
	Congo-Crimean Hemorrhagic Fever Virus	Viral Hemorrhagic Fever	Lethal
	Monkeypox	Monkeypox	Lethal
	Nipah virus	Viral encephalitis	Lethal
	Hantavirus	Viral Hemorrhagic Fever	Lethal

sponsoring international terrorism (Cuba, Iran, Iraq, Libya, North Korea, Sudan and Syria), two nations have already been eliminated as a threat. These two nations are Iraq and Libya. This leaves five possible countries that have developed or possess the potential to developed offensive biological weapons (Table 2).[4] Nonetheless, it is the engineering and not the biological aspect of biological weaponry that provides most of the challenges for any would be biological weapons manufacturer.

There are two glaring problems associated with engineering biological weapons. The first difficulty is the containment of the biological agent prior to delivery, thereby not contaminating the workers at various stages of production. Careful handling and manufacturing techniques are necessary in order to ensure mishaps do not happen. The effort of safety in the workplace is made simpler as the equipment to construct a safe containment system is readily available for purchase on the open market

(Figure 1-1-1).

As for any biological weapon, its isolation, manipulation and small scale production require a minimum of Level 3 biohazard protocol laboratory. Establishment of a Level 3 laboratory can be done at moderate cost and labor. A task easily accomplished by any would-be terrorist and/or third world country seeking to produce WMDs. Please examine Table 3 for information in regards to various protocols of biosafety levels and Table 4 for the information about these laboratories located in the United States.

The second engineering difficulty is ensuring the safe transport and efficient delivery of the biological agent, either through open warfare or a terrorist act. In other words, biological agents must be effectively contained until the designated time and place for release. For example, biological agents must be protected from

Table 2: Examples of countries and their biological weapons program [5, 6, 7]

Countries	Biological Programs	Biological Agents Available
Algeria	Actively researching biological weapons	Unknown
Canada	Bio- weapons program initiated in 1941 and ended in 1947	Anthrax, brucellosis, rocky mountain spotted fever, plague, tularemia, typhoid, yellow fever, dysentery, rinderpest, botulinum toxin & ricin
China	Possible offensive biological weapon program	Unknown
Cuba	Possible offensive biological weapon program	Unknown
Egypt	Possible offensive biological weapon program	Unknown
France	Bio-weapon program was initiated in 1921 and Ended in 1926. The program was reinstated between 1935-1940	Anthrax, salmonella, cholera, rinderpest, botulinum toxin ricin, rinderpest potato beetle
Germany	Bio-weapon program was initiated 1915 and ended in 1918. The program was reinstated in 1940 and ended in 1945	Glanders, anthrax, foot & mouth disease, plague, rinderpest, typhus, yellow fever, potato beetle & potato blight
India	Possible offensive bio-weapon program	Unknown
Iran	Possible offensive bio-weapon program	Anthrax, foot & mouth disease, botulinum toxin & mycotoxins
Iraq	Previous active biological weapon program	Anthrax, botulinum toxin, ricin, aflatoxin, wheat cover smut weaponized; brucellosis, hemorrhagic conjunctivitis virus, rotavirus, camel pox, plague & gas gangrene toxin researched
Israel	Possible offensive biological weapon program	Unknown
Japan	Biological weapon program was initiated in 1931 and ended in 1945	Anthrax, plague, glanders, typhoid, cholera, dysentery, typhoid, paratyphoid , gas gangrene, influenza, tetanus, tuberculosis, tularemia, salmonella, typhus, glanders & tetrodotoxin
Libya	None	None
North Korea	Offensive biological weapon program	Anthrax, plague, yellow fever, typhoid, cholera, tuberculosis, typhus, smallpox & botulinum toxin weaponized
Pakistan	Possible offensive biological weapon program	Unknown
Soviet Union	Biological weapon program initiated in 1926 and presumably ended in 1992	Smallpox, plague, tularemia, glanders, Venezuelan equine encephalitis, anthrax, Q fever, Marburg, Ebola, Bolivian hemorrhagic fever, Argentinean hemorrhagic fever, Lassa fever, Japanese encephalitis, Russian spring-summer encephalitis, brucellosis, Machupo virus, yellow fever, typhus, melioidosis, psittacosis, rinderpest, African swine fever virus, wheat stem rust & rice blast
South Africa	Biological weapons program initiated in 1981 and ended 1993	Anthrax, cholera, plague, salmonella, gas gangrene, ricin & botulinum toxin
South Korea	Possible offensive biological weapon program	Unknown
Sudan	Possible offensive biological weapon program	Unknown
Syria	Possible offensive biological weapon program	Anthrax, botulinum toxin & ricin
Taiwan ROC	Possible offensive biological weapon program	Unknown
United Kingdom	Biological weapon program initiated in 1936 and ended in 1956	Anthrax, plague, typhoid & botulinum toxin
United States	Offensive biological weapon program initiated in 1943 and ended in 1969	Venezuelan equine encephalitis, Q fever, tularemia, anthrax, wheat rust, rice blast weaponized; brucellosis, smallpox, Eastern & Western equine encephalitis, Argentinean hemorrhagic fever, Korean hemorrhagic fever, Bolivian hemorrhagic fever, Lassa fever, glanders, melioidodis, plague, yellow fever, psittacosis, typhus, dengue fever, Rift Valley fever, Chikungunya virus, potato blight, rinderpest, Newcastle disease, fowl plague, staph enterotoxin B, botulinum toxin & ricin

Table 3: Biological Laboratory Protocols[7, 8, 9]

Biosafety Levels	Description
BSL-1	BSL-1 is the least secure and is generally designed to deal with agents that are known to pose no threat to the general population. Laboratories designed at level one are commonly found in most college and high school laboratories and do not have special containment equipment
BSL-2	BSL-2 is generally found in hospitals and certain university laboratories and deals with diagnostic quantities of biological agents. At this level of protocol, some containment equipment is used and the laboratory is generally located within areas of the building that are away from the general population
BSL-3	BSL-3 protocol generally involves exotic agents that may pose a threat to the general population. The level 3 laboratory is placed away from the general population and any manipulations of biological agents are performed within biological safety cabinets and/or personnel wearing biological protective suits. The air flow within the Level 3 laboratories is carefully controlled and High Efficiency Particulate Air filter (HEPTA filter) is used to filter all exhaust before being released into the atmosphere. HEPA filters are designed to filter out all particles that are 0.3 microns or larger in size limiting any possible contamination towards the general population
BSL-4	BSL-4 is designed to work with highly infectious and dangerous biological agents. Within the United States, there are 12 Level 4 laboratories (see Table 4) and they are found at various locations around the nation. These facilities are designed to be completely separate from any other facilities within these complexes and away from any potential contamination of the general population. These laboratories are constructed in isolation from the external environment which prevents any accidental contamination of insects and animals. A dedicated non-recirculation ventilation system is designed to make certain that any potentially hazardous biological agents are not accidentally released into the atmosphere. Within the confines of the laboratories, all work is confined to Class III or Class II biological safety cabinets and all personnel are required to wear a one piece, positive pressure, biological protection suit supported by a self-sustaining life support system

ultraviolet (UV) radiation (i.e. sunlight). UV radiation contains germicidal wavelengths at ~2,537 Angstroms or ~254 nm that cause the pyrimidine nucleotides (e.g. thymine) of the DNA molecule to dimerize, producing an error in the genetic strand. If enough errors accumulate within a microorganism or virus, the result will be the impediment of any further DNA replication and thereby neutralizing the biological warfare agent.

The previously mentioned technical difficulties can be managed by the careful design of the containment unit of which many are available on the open market. What cannot be controlled is associated with nature during the time of release. For example, the unpredictability of wind patterns may greatly affect the dispersal of the biological agent. If the wind is too strong, the agent may be carried too far away from the intended target. Inversely, if there is little or no wind during release, the biological agent may not be completely dispersed in the target area. Rain and other precipitation may also be a factor that could render a biological agent ineffective, where it may wash away the biological agent before it is allowed to spread in the target area. Please see Table 5 for examples and comparison of biological agents and their potential effects on a theoretical population.

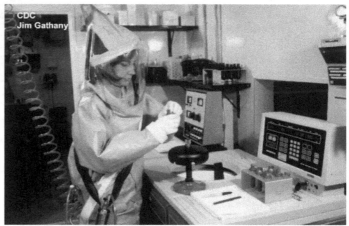

Figure 1.1-1: A CDC scientist working in a BSL-4. She is shielded from the pathogens by a protective suit with helmet and mask. The biological protective suit and equipment are readily available on the commercial market

On the opposite spectrum of the issues associated with biological weapons are the roles of the health professionals in dealing with an intentional release of a biological weapon. Unlike an overt

Table 4: BSL-4 Laboratories in the United States

Institution	Location	Name	Operational Status
Center for Disease Control and Prevention	Atlanta, Ga	CDC Special Pathogens Branch, Emerging Infectious Diseases Laboratory	Opened in 1988 and new facility operational in 2005
The United States Army Medical Research Institute for Infectious Diseases	Fort Detrick, MD	USAMRIID	Opened in 1969 and new facilities completed in 2012
Southwest Foundation for Biomedical Research	San Antonio, TX	BSL-4 Laboratory, Department of Virology and Immunology	Operational
University of Texas	Galveston, TX	Center for Biodefense and Emerging Infectious Disease	Operational
Georgia State University	Atlanta, GA	Center for Biotechnology and Drug Design	Operational
Virginia Commonwealth University	Richmond, VA	Virginia Division of Consolidated Laboratory Services (DCLS)	Operational
Department of Homeland Security	Ft. Detrick, MD	National Biodefense Analysis and Countermeasures Center (NBACC)	Operational
National Institute of Allergy and Infectious Diseases	Hamilton, MT	Rocky Mountain Laboratory Integrated Research Facility	Operational
National Institute of Allergy & Infectious Diseases	Galveston, TX	Galveston National Biocontainment Laboratory (University of Texas)	Operational
National Institute of Allergy and Infectious Diseases and Boston University	Boston, MA	BU National Center for Emerging Infectious Diseases and Biodefense	Operational
National Bio- and Agro-Defense Facility	Manhattan, KS	Department of Homeland Security	Under construction (estimated completion 2017)
National Institute of Allergy and Infectious Diseases	Ft. Detrick, MD	NIAID Integrated Research Facility at Fort Detrick	Operational

Table 5: Example and comparison for biological agent and their predicted casualty rates[2]

Biological Agent	Downwind Reach (km)	Approximate # of Dead	Approximate # of Incapacitat
B. anthracis	>20	95,000	125,000
F. tularensis	>20	30,000	125,000
R. prowazekii	5	19,000	85,000
Tick-Borne Encephalitis virus	1	9,500	35,000
Brucella spp.	10	500	125,000
C. burnetii	>20	150	125,000
Rift Valley Fever virus	1	400	35,000

attack using conventional explosives or chemical weapons, biological agents are covert in nature. It is most likely that the realization that a biological attack has taken place will occur only after scores of individuals with similar symptoms arrive at the emergency room within a narrow time frame seeking treatment.

As an example, if an intentional release of smallpox has taken place, patients will not start to arrive at their local clinician's office or the emergency room until 7 to 17 days after the initial release of the agent. This delay of onset is due to the incubation period of the disease, where no symptoms initially identifiable to the pathogen may appear.

When the patients finally arrive at their local medical facilities, they will display symptoms of an ordinary viral infection. These nonspecific symptoms will include fever, malaise, headache, body pains, fatigue and nausea. Most often the clinicians will advise the patients to obtain some over-the-counter flu medications and bedrest as treatment.

During the next four days, also known as the prodome phase of the disease, the smallpox infection becomes highly contagious. Patients will most definitely have had contact with other individuals either at home, work or during their travels. These casual contacts can possibly spread the infections to unknown numbers of other unsuspecting individuals.

After four days, the papular rash will appear. Patients will most likely revisit their local medical facilities. Often, the physician will be unfamiliar with the symptoms and signs of the condition and presume that it is an allergic response to food, fabric or stress, etc., in addition to their initial viral infection. The clinician will almost certainly send the patients home with topical creams to treat the rash and advise them to continue taking their over-the-counter medication.

Soon after, the rash will become pustules and as the patient lay dying numerous other patients will begin to appear at the medical facility with similar symptoms. It is most likely that at this time the clinician will finally reach the correct diagnosis (Figure 1.1-2).

The treatment of an intentional release of a biological agent is no different than dealing with a natural outbreak of a communicable disease. A clinician is responsible for the early diagnosis (recognition of unusual clinical syndromes and directing the appropriate tests) of the communicable agent and identifying

those that have been exposed to the infection. This, as indicated in the previous paragraphs, is a difficult task especially when the clinician is not familiar with the specific symptoms of the disease.

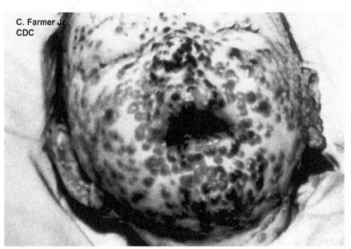

Figure 1.1-2: A photograph of an one year old child suffering from smallpox

Nonetheless, once the infection is diagnosed, the clinician should immediately proceed in implementing the treatment plan for the disease and isolate the patient from the general public, especially if the disease is contagious. Once a quarantine of the infected individuals is implemented, the clinician then needs to communicate with various federal or state health agencies in order to coordinate responses to the outbreak (Figure 1-1-3).[1] Please also examine Chapter 5.1, Disease Surveillance and Preparedness and Chapter 5.2, Federal Quarantine Powers for more information.

Similarly for the investigators of outbreaks, early recognition of an intentional biological attack is difficult. The investigators will need to recognize certain epidemiological clues that are left by an outbreak and subsequently advise the correct course of action for first responders. For example, the investigators will first be required to recognize the presence of a large and severe epidemic with an unusual route of exposure. If possible, these investigators will need to recognize the unusual geographical appearance of the disease, as well as, the potential absence of normal reservoir or vectors for the disease. For instance, most biological agents are endemic diseases of the tropical regions, so if an Ebola outbreak occurred in Chicago, IL, it would be

Table 6: Summary of diagnostic methods, tissue required and approximate time for the identification of Dengue fever[10]

Diagnostic Methods	Time	Specimens Required for Analysis	Ave. Time of Collection Post-symptom Onset
Viral isolation & serotype ID	~1-2 w	Whole blood, serum, tissue	Approximately 1-5 days
Nucleic acid detection	~1-2 d	Tissue, whole blood, serum, plasma	Approximately 1-5 days
Antigen detection	<1 d	Tissue, serum	Approximately 1-6 days
IgM ELISA	~1-2 d	Serum, plasma whole blood	Greater than (>) 5 days
IgM/IgG rapid test	~15-30 min	Serum, plasma whole blood	Greater than (>) 5 days
IgG (paired sera) ELISA	<7 d	Serum, plasma whole blood	Greater than (>) 5 days
IgG (paired sera) neutralization	<7 d	Serum, plasma whole blood	Greater than (>) 5 days

safe for the investigators to assume that the disease is most likely intentionally set or accidentally released. Nonetheless, if the disease is endemic to the particular region, investigators should recognize if there is unusual seasonality for the appearance of the disease. Additionally, another potential sign of an intentional release are the sudden appearance of multiple or simultaneous appearances of two of more different epidemics, especially when one or both of the outbreaks are zoonotic. Lastly, if it is discovered that the strain of the biological agent is unexpectedly resistant to antibacterial or general antiviral treatments, it is an additional clue that may lead investigators to determine the potential origin of the outbreak.

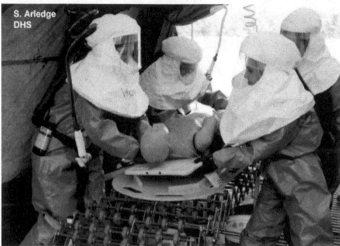

Figure 1.1-3: Healthcare workers decontaminating a simulated victim during an exercise at the Center for Domestic Preparedness (CDP) at Anniston, AL

Unfortunately, it is impossible to save every individual who has been exposed to a biological attack. There is a high probability that the few individuals who were initial infected could be unintentionally sacrificed when the physician struggles to determine the specific biological agent that caused their ailment especially when the individuals display nonspecific symptoms. In addition, unavoidable delays in diagnosis will occur when the physician is waiting for lab results to confirm the diagnosis (Table 6).

Nonetheless, once the diagnosis is made, these individuals that are initially infected will allow physicians to properly treat the individuals that are subsequently exposed to the pathogen. This fact is particular apparent especially when the physician is not familiar with the symptoms of the biological agent in question. Therefore, it is essential to properly diagnose the disease as soon as possible before the fatalities of the "initially infected" increases to an unacceptable level.

References

1. Kortepeter M.G., Parker G.W. Potential Biological Weapons Threats. Emerging Infectious Diseases, 1999. 5: pp. 523-527
2. Bellamy R.J., Freedman A.R. Bioterrorism. Quarterly Journal of Medicine, 2001. 94: pp. 227-234
3. Weapons of Mass Destruction (WMD) Biological Warfare Agent Production. GlobalSecurity.org. Retrieved May 23, 2007. Web Site: http://www.globalsecurity.org/wmd/_intro/bio_production.htm
4. Sullivan M.P. Cuba and the State Sponsors of Terrorism List. Congressional Research Service Report for Congress. Congressional Research Service, 2005. Order Code RL32251. pp. 1-13
5. Cole L.A. The Specter of Biological Weapons. Scientific American, 1996. 275: pp. 60-65
6. Nova online. Global Guide to Biological Weapons. November 2001. Retrieved July 23 2008. Web Site: http://www.pbs.org/wgbh/nova/bioterror/glob_nf.html
7. Parker H.S. Agricultural Bioterrorism: A Federal Strategy to Meet the Threat. Institute for National Strategic Studies. National Defense University. Washington D.C.: United States Government Printing Office. 2002. pp. 8-9
8. Chosewood L.C., Wilson D.E. Editors. Biosafety in Microbiological and Biomedical Laboratories (BMBL) 5th Edition. U.S. Department of Health and Human Services, Centers for Disease Control and Prevention and National Institutes of Health. Washington D.C.: U. S. Government Printing Office. 2007. pp. 1-422Gerberding J.L., Hughes J.M., Koplan

J.P.. Bioterrorism Preparedness and Response: Clinicians and Public Health Agencies as Essential Partners. American Journal of Medicine, 2002. 287: pp. 898
9. Dengue Information Center. MP Biomedicals Asia Pacific Pte Ltd. Website: http://www.mpdengueinfo.com/dengue-diagnostic.html

Photo Bibliography

Figure 1.1-1: A CDC scientist working in a BSL-4. She is shielded from the pathogens by a positive pressure protective suit with helmet and mask. The suit and equipment are readily available on the commercial market. Photo was taken in 2002 by Jim Gathany and released by the CDC. Public domain photo

Figure 1.1-2: A photograph of an one year old child suffering from smallpox. This photograph was taken by Dr. Charles Farmer Jr. in 1962 in Cardiff, Wales during an epidemic and released by CDC. Public domain photo

Figure 1.1-3: Healthcare workers decontaminating a simulated victim during an exercise at the Center for Domestic Preparedness (CDP) in Anniston, Alabama. These healthcare workers were attending the Hospital Emergency Response Training (HERT) for Mass Casualty Incidents course hosted by Federal Emergency Management Agency (FEMA). Photo was taken by Shannon Arledge (date unknown) for FEMA and the Department of Homeland Security. Public domain photo

Chikungunya Virus (CHIKV) is a potential bio-weapon listed as a Category C biological threat by the Centers for Disease Control and Prevention (CDC). Although CHIKV was not successfully weaponized by American scientists due to difficulties growing the virus in laboratory conditions, as well as, its instability in an aerosol form (the virus tends to form clumps when aerosolized), it possesses the possibility that other nations or groups may have successfully weaponized this virus.

CHIKV, also known as Buggy Creek Virus, is believed to have originated in Africa, where it maintained a sylvatic cycle involving wild primates and forest dwelling mosquitoes such as *Aedes furcifer*, *A. luteocephalus* and *A. taylori*. In humans, CHIKV is the etiologic agent of Chikungunya fever (CHIKF), which is transmitted naturally from the bites of Culicine mosquitoes (e.g. *A. aegypti* or *A. albopictus*) within urban areas (Figure 1.2-1).

It is believed that the word chikungunya is derived from Swahili, meaning "that which bends up," describing the painful contorted posture of patients suffering from the disease.[1, 2, 3] In the past, outbreaks of a type of fever with arthritic symptoms and rash were outwardly similar to CHIKV infection have been reported as early as 1824. Nonetheless, the actual Chikungunya virion was isolated in 1953 by M.C. Robinson at the Makonde Plateau, located between Tanzania and Mozambique, and has since been reported in sporadic outbreaks since that time in Sub-Saharan Africa, islands in the Indian Ocean, Southeast Asia and India (Figure 1.2-2).[4, 5, 6, 7, 8]

CHIKV belongs to the genus Alphavirus in Group IV of the family *Togaviridae*. CHIKV is approximately 70 nm in diameter and possesses an icosahedral nucleocapsid (capsid (C) protein measure 36 kDa) with T=4 symmetry surrounded by a host cell-derived envelope, containing glycoprotein spikes. The spikes are comprised of 240 heterodimers of E1 (52 kDa) and E2 (62 kDa) envelope glycoproteins arranged in 80 trimers. The Envelope 1

(E1) glycoproteins lie parallel to the viral lipid envelope, while the envelope 2 (E2) glycoproteins form the spikes (Figure 1.2-3).[9, 10]

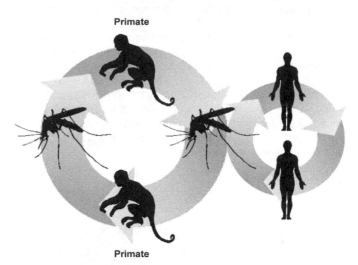

Primate

Primate

Figure 1.2-1: Sylvatic cycle of African lineage CHIKV

CHIKV possesses a positive (messenger) sense, linear, single-stranded RNA genome. The complete genome of CHIKV was determined to be 11,805 nucleotides (11.8 kb) in length (excluding the 5' cap nucleotide, an I-poly A tract and the 3' poly A tail). The viral genome comprises two long open reading frames that encode the non-structural (2474 amino acids) and structural polyproteins (1244 amino acids) (Figure 1.2-4).[11]

Presently, there are over 80 strains of CHIKV nucleotide sequences that have been isolated and characterized. These strains are grouped into four CHIKV lineages: Southeastern African, West African, Central African and Asian.[11, 12, 13, 14, 15] Unfortunately, detailed information is not available with regards

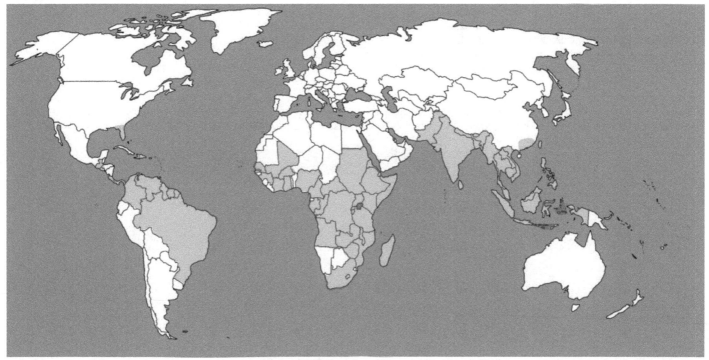

Figure 1.2-2: Distribution of Chikungunya fever (CHIKF)

to the pathophysiology of CHIKV due to a lack of suitable small animal models. Nonetheless, it is believed that the primary replication of CHIKV occurs in the fibroblast cells of connective tissues found in the connective tissue of the joints, skin and skeletal muscles. This observation was supported after muscle biopsies were taken from CHIKF patients during the acute and chronic phases of the infection, which demonstrated atrophy and necrosis of scattered muscle fibers, as well as, collagenosis, with a limited number of infiltrating inflammatory cells. However, in a 2007 study the researchers reported that viral antigens were found exclusively inside skeletal muscle progenitor cells, designed as satellite cells, and not directly found in mature skeletal muscle fibers. Regardless of the site of replication for CHIKV, which remains to be elucidated, it is believed that the concentrated numbers of nociceptors available in the muscles and at joints may account for the characteristic arthritic pains that patients experience during CHIKF.[16, 17, 18]

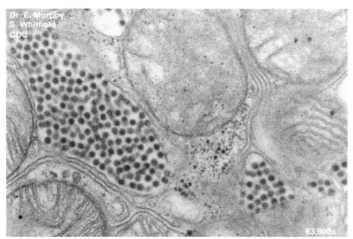

Figure 1.2-3: Transmission electron micrograph (TEM) of Alphaviruses (in red) infecting the salivary gland that had been extracted from a mosquito

Unlike other alphaviruses, CHIKV does not infect human primary monocytes, T and B lymphocytes, immature or mature monocyte derived dendritic cells. Nonetheless, CHIKV replicates in various human adherent cells, including epithelial and endothelial cells, fibroblasts, and human primary macrophages (e.g. CD14, CD4 and CCR5 macrophage lineage). It has been reported that CHIKV infection severity is critically dependent on the age of the host (where the elderly are more severely affected) and the functionality of type-1 (interferon) IFN signaling pathway.[19, 20, 21]

After inoculation, CHIKV attaches to the host receptor through E2 glycoproteins (spikes) while the E1 glycoproteins drive the virus/host cell fusion process. Unfortunately, the exact type of host cellular receptor is presently not known mainly due to its broad cell tropisms.

After the viral attachment, the E1 induces an acid-triggered membrane fusion in endosomes, thereby causing the virion to be endocytized (via clathrin-mediated pathways) into the host cell, while E2 suppresses the membrane fusion until the low pH of the endosomal compartment promotes the necessary conformational changes of the viral envelope glycoproteins thereby allowing viral fusion. [20, 21, 22, 23, 24] Subsequently, the nucleocapsid is released into the cytoplasm, followed by uncoating and the release of the viral RNA genome. The positive sense viral RNA is very similar to cellular messenger RNA, containing a 5' methylguanylate cap structure and 3' polyadenylate sequence. The process of replication and translation of the viral genome occurs after the release of the positive-sense RNA into the host cytoplasm. First the nonstructural viral proteins (nsP1-4) are coded directly via the 5' two-thirds of the positive-sense genome serving as the messenger RNA.

The functions of the nonstructural (ns) proteins are not well understood. Evidence indicates that nsP-1 serves as a guanine-7-methyltransferase and guanyltransferase for capping both genomic and subgenomic viral RNA strands. Other evidence has shown that this protein participates in the binding of the replicated complexes to the host membrane. Nonstructural (ns) P-2 serves both as a helicase (N-terminal) and a protease (C-terminus), processing nonstructural proteins. It is believed that the nsP-3 serves as a subgenomic promoter and affects the cytopathology of some host cells, while nsP-4 serves as a DNA-dependent RNA polymerase for both positive and negative RNA strand synthesis.[9]

The translation of ns proteins is followed by the replication of the positive-sense viral RNA into a negative sense complimentary ssRNA that serves as a template. This ssRNA subsequently creates a subgenomic RNA molecule (26S RNA) that constitutes the 3' one-third of the viral genome and is subsequently translated into three structural proteins (CP, E1 and E2).[9, 17, 25] It has been reported that viral RNA replication, transcription and translation are confined to the cytoplasmic surfaces of an endosome-derived vesicle called cytopathic vacuoles type I (CPVI), which are closely related to the membranes of the host endoplasmic reticulum (Figure 1.2-4).[23]

Once the viral structural proteins are translated, E1 and E2 are post-translationally modified in the endoplasmic reticulum and Golgi apparatus of the host cell before being transported to the plasma membrane, where the two proteins maintain a close association with one another, forming a trimeric heterodimer

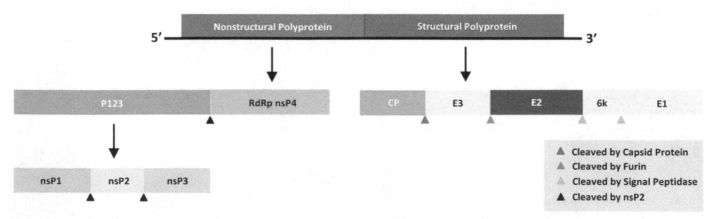

Figure 1.2-4: CHIKV genome is composed of monopartite, linear, single-stranded, positive-sense RNA genome of 11-12 kb

spike structure.

It is known that CHIKV replication and protein translation is accompanied by the inhibition of host cell functions, such as synthesis of proteins, RNA and DNA, although the exact mechanism is poorly understood and requires further elucidation.[9, 24, 26, 27, 28]

The assembly of CHIKV, similar to other *Alphaviruses*, begins with nucleocapsid assembly in the cytoplasm. Based upon experiments of other *Alphaviruses*, it is believed that the putative coiled-coil α-helix of the CP is utilized for core assembly while the N-terminus region of CP is essential for RNA-binding and packaging of the viral progeny. Again, based upon assumptions formulated from experiments of other *Alphaviruses*, it is believed that CP forms RNA-bound dimmers, while its lateral interactions with other CP units create the icosahedral shell of the virus. Once the capsid is assembled, the complex diffuse freely to the plasma membrane of the host cell.[29, 30]

The CHIKV virion is released from the host cell via budding. It is believed that during this process that CHIKV acquire a lipid bilayer envelope containing the virus-encoded glycoprotein spikes which are composed of trimeric heterodimer of E1–E2. Unfortunately, the final stages of the CHIKV replication cycle have not been investigated and require further elucidation (Figure 1.2-5).[29, 31]

SYMPTOMS

Fatalities resulting from Chikungunya fever are usually rare and in most cases the disease is self-limiting.[31] CHIKV epidemics are generally characterized by explosive outbreaks followed by several years of absence. It is believed that environmental conditions play a large part in natural outbreaks where the susceptibility of humans to the virus (in terms of health, living conditions etc.) and the populations of the mosquito vector, among others play a role.[33]

The incubation period of CHIKV is in the range of 3 to 12 (average 3 to 7) days, while the acute illness persists approximately for 3 to 5 days; patients generally recover from viral infection in 5 to 7 days. CHIKV is indiscriminant in its infections. It affects all age groups, sexes and it has been documented that pregnant women can transmit the disease transplacentally to their fetus. The time of greatest risk of CHIKV transmission from mother to fetus appears to be during birth. These cases of vertical transmission are rarely serious and newborns generally recover quickly without sequelae.[25, 34, 35, 36]

A clinical triad of fever, rashes and arthralgia is generally suggestive of CHIKF. Symptoms of this infection involve the rapid onset of fever, which may associate with rigor, could reach 39° to 40.6°C (102° to 105°F). This fever may persist for approximately two days before it suddenly subsides. In some patients, the fever demonstrates a biphasic pattern (saddle-back fever).[25, 36, 37, 38]

Patients suffering from the biphasic pattern of fever will experience a sudden onset of fever for 4 to 6 days followed by a afebrile period of a few days and then a sudden return of the fever for an additional two days.[16, 25, 35] Febrile convulsions in children infected by the virus have also been reported.[39]

Arthralgia and myalgia (general myalgia or back and shoulder pains) are the most pronounced symptoms which are observed in over 70% of CHIKV infections. Patients experiencing arthralgia will display either single or multiple (polyarticular) joint pains that may last for the duration of the infection or in some cases the pains and stiffness persisted for a year or more causing serious social and economic impacts. The arthralgias, which are generally accompanied by swelling due to accumulation of fluids, tend to affect the smaller joints of the hands, wrists, ankles and feet (the peripheral small joints) with less involvement of the larger joints. The joint pain is extreme in its severity and is known to completely immobilize many patients.[16, 25, 36, 37] Other symptoms include headache, chills, rigor, nausea, vomiting and fatigue, which may last a few days to several weeks, or even months. Insomnia (generally resulting from arthritic pains) and photophobia (excessive sensitivity to light) are also indications of the disease which may last for approximately one week. In addition, patients also suffer from conjunctival suffusion (redness of the eyes), conjunctivitis (inflammation of the conjunctiva) and cervical or generalized lymphadenopathy (swelling of the lymph nodes).[16, 25, 37]

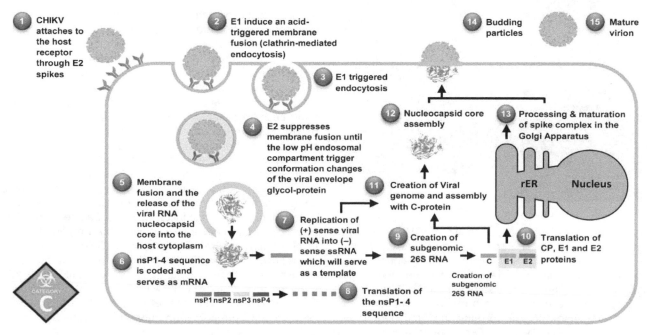

Figure 1.2-5: Diagrammatic process of CHIKV infection within an eukaryotic cell

Physical manifestations of the viral infection may include petechial rash, caused by minor hemorrhage of capillaries and arterioles, as well as, maculopapular rash surfacing as minor inflammatory bumps that do not contain pus. Both rashes are generally located along the limbs of patients, but at times they may be found along the torso. Redness or inflammation of the skin surrounding the nose (nasal blotchy erythema), as well as, freckle-like pigmentation appearing over the mid-facial area and linear (flagellate) pigmentation on face and extremities are also a common signs of the disease.[16, 25, 36, 38]

Other symptoms include white streaking and reticulate patterning of the skin (lichenoid eruption) and hyperpigmentation (patches of darker skin) in the areas of the body generally exposed to the sun (photo-distributed areas), as well as, gingival hemorrhages, commonly seen in children. Numerous aphthous-like sores may be found on the scrotum, crural (thigh or leg) areas and axilla (arm pit). In children, multiple ecchymotic spots are commonly seen, while vesiculobullous lesions are found on infants. Fluid retention resulting from a compromised lymphatic system (lympoedema), as well as, subungual hemorrhage, photo and acral urticaria are also common.[16, 36, 38]

Table 1: An overview of the clinical symptoms of CHIKF

Symptoms	+	++	+++
Fever			■
Rashes			■
Arthralgia			■
Swellings			■
Myalgia			■
Chills			■
Headache			■
Rigors			■
Nausea			■
Vomiting			■
Fatigue			■
Petechial rash			■
Maculopapular rash			■
Insomnia		■	
Photophobia		■	
Conjunctival suffusion		■	
Conjunctivitis		■	
Lymphadenopathy		■	
Nasal blotchy erythema		■	
Facial pigmentation		■	
Flagellate pigmentation		■	
lichenoid eruption		■	
Hyperpigmentation		■	
Gingival hemorrhages		■	
Aphthous-like sores		■	
Encephalitis	■		
Myelopathy	■		
Neuropathy	■		
Hematemesis	■		
Melaena	■		
Myeloneuropathy	■		
Myopathy	■		

+ Rare ++ Common +++ Frequent

Neurological manifestations as a result of CHIKV infection are extremely rare. The neurological syndromes observed include encephalitis, myelopathy, neuropathy, myeloneuropathy and myopathy. It remains unclear whether the neurological manifestations are due to persistence of the CHIKV or an inappropriate immune response. In a report by Chandak et al. (2009), the prognoses of patients suffering from neurological manifestations are generally good. Out of 49 patients examined with neurological syndromes, only three deaths were reported as a result of systemic complications while the remaining patients recovered with supportive therapy and/or corticosteroids.[40] In addition, infrequent documentation of hemorrhagic manifestations have also been reported. As reported by Sarkar et al. (1965), symptoms such as hematemesis and melaena have appeared during CHIKV infections in Southeast Asia.[38] Please examine Table 1 for an outline of CHIKV symptoms.

DETECTION

Basically, there are three main laboratory tests used to diagnose CHIKV infection: virus isolation (culture), serological tests for the demonstration of virus-specific antibodies and genomic detection by polymerase chain reaction (PCR) based methods (e.g. reverse transcriptase-PCR and quantitative-PCR). The most definitive test for CHIKV detection is virus isolation, since it shows the presence of viable virions. Presently, the isolation of the virus is done using the blood of viremic patients or infected tissues. It has been reported that the isolation of CHIKV is comparatively more simple to other viruses due to the highly cytopathic and fast-growing (high titers) nature of the virus.[21] CHIKV is known to replicate in various cultured cell lines such as C6/36, nonhuman viz, Vero, chick embryo fibroblast-like cells, BHK21, L929 and Hep-2 cells, HeLa and MRC5 cell lines.[41]

Other diagnostic tests available for CHIKV infection are based on serological and PCR techniques in order to differentiate between infections with similar symptoms such as Dengue.[42] Serodiagnostic methods are generally designed to detect CHIKV specific IgM and IgG antibodies found in human sera by using immunohistochemical techniques.[9, 20, 43] Enzyme linked immunosorbent assay (ELISA) can also be used to detect CHIKV.[9, 34, 42] Sergon et al. (2008), tested 288 sera samples from residents of Lamu (Kenya) during an outbreak of the disease in 2004 for IgM and IgG antibodies to CHIKV. The researchers reported that IgM antibodies to CHIKV were detected in 18% of the individuals tested (53/288), while IgG antibodies were detected in 72% (206/288) and IgM and/or IgG antibodies were present in 75% (215/288) of the individuals tested.[44] In addition, hemaglutination inhibition assays cab also be used to detect anti-CHIKV antibodies.[16, 20, 44]

It is important to note that virus isolation and culture are sensitive methodologies that are time consuming and must be performed under BSL-3 biosafety conditions. Additionally, the degree of success of culturing the virus is dependent on the freshness of tissue used. These factors includes the time of collection, transportation, maintenance of cold or proper freezing methods, storage and processing of samples. Therefore, virus isolation and culture are generally used for virus identification at the beginning of an epidemic. Serological methods are reliable but are not appropriate in early stages of infection. These methods are only useful after an antibody response which is detectable approximately 5 to 6 days after clinical onset. PCR analysis on the other hand, is an appropriate diagnostic tool at an early stage of infection, even while the patient is viremic.[45] For example, reverse transcription-PCR test has been developed to quickly and efficiently identify CHIKV.[46] As reported by Chahar et al. (2009), positive identification of CHIKV through reverse transcription-PCR was developed by targeting partial nucleotide sequences of the E1 gene (294 bp) of CHIKV.[47] In addition, real-time reverse transcriptase-PCR methodologies, have been developed for the detection of CHIKV, which allows the initial genome concentration to be quantified and the viral load to be accurately determined.[45, 48]

TREATMENT

Interferons (IFNs) are essential for the innate immunity to protect against CHIKV. In cell cultures, CHIKV retains full sensitivity towards both type I and II IFNs, suggesting at innate immunity responds to the virus and is responsible for the rapid decline of viremia observed during an acute infection. Presently, it is not known which IFN-induced proteins mediate the inhibition of CHIKV, but ISG15 is a strong candidate, which has recently been shown to be an antiviral molecule against another alphavirus, Sindbis virus (SINV), in mouse models.[21, 49, 50]

Currently, there is no CHIKV vaccine available to the public; however, recent scientific publications have shown some promise in the development of such a vaccine. Based on an article written by Edelman et al. (2000), a serially passaged, plaque purified, live Chikungunya vaccine was tested on 73 healthy adult volunteers, of whom 59 were immunized with the vaccine and 14 were given placebo (tissue culture fluid) to act as controls. Out of the 59 volunteers who were vaccinated, 98% of them (57 volunteers) developed CHIKV neutralizing antibodies by the 28th day, post immunization.[51]

Other experimental vaccines are also being tested in animal models which have shown promise. For example, Weger-Lucarelli et al. (2014) experimented with Modified Vaccinia Ankara (MVA) virus expressing CHIKV E2 and E3 glycoproteins. Once administered, this experimental vaccine protected the mouse model against viremia when challenged with CHIKV.[52]

Given that vaccines to CHIKV are still in the experimental/testing phase, clinicians will need to rely on the traditional manner of treatment for the disease. In view of the fact that this disease is generally non-life threatening and self-limiting, clinicians generally apply supportive therapies and direct treatments for the symptoms, such as pain and fever etc. Clinicians are advised to provide plenty of fluids for their patients and careful application of paracetamol (aceta-minophen), ibuprofen, or non-steroidal anti-inflammatory drugs (NSAIDS) such as indomethacin for symptom relief. Aspirin (acetylsalicylic acid) should be avoided due to the reports of mild hemorrhagic manifestations in patients who have received it for treatment. Some clinicians have suggested the usage of chloroquine phosphate for treating arthropathy. In an effort to prevent secondary infections; broad spectrum antibiotics may also be judiciously administered.[9, 16, 53, 54]

Clinicians are advised against indiscriminate use of corticosteroids, non-steroid based anti-inflammatory medications and various antibiotics. Excess use of these medications may cause additional symptoms or conditions such as nausea, vomiting, gastritis, thrombocytopenia and gastrointestinal bleeding.[36]

DIFFERENTIAL DIAGNOSIS

It is important to stress that CHIKV infections closely resemble other infections and can be misdiagnosed if care is not taken. For example, both CHIKV and Dengue fever demonstrate similar patterns of rash; however, clinicians need to distinguish the severe hemorrhagic symptoms that accompany Dengue, which do not appear in patients infected with CHIKV (Table 2). In addition, CHIKV infected individuals do not display retro-orbital

Table 4: Differential diagnosis of CHIKF with selected viral infections that share some similar symptoms. Note: O'nyong-nyong Fever (ONNF), West Nile Fever (WNF), Hepatitis A (HAV), Hepatitis B (HBV)

Symptoms	CHIKF	ONNF	WNF	Sindbis	Rubella	Parvovirus	HAV	HBV
Fever	●	●	●	●	●	●	●	●
Rashes	●	●	●	●	●	●	●	
Arthralgia	●	●	●	●	●	●		●
Swellings	●	●	●			●		
Myalgia	●	●	●	●			●	
Chills	●	●	●	●				
Headache	●	●	●	●		●	●	●
Rigors	●							
Fatigue	●	●	●			●	●	
Insomnia	●							
Photophobia	●	●						
Nausea	●	●	●	●			●	●
Vomiting	●	●	●	●			●	●
Petechial rash	●	●	●	●				
Maculopapular rash		●		●				
Conjunctival suffusion	●							
Conjunctivitis	●				●			
Lymphadenopathy	●	●	●		●			
Nasal blotchy erythema	●							
Facial pigmentation	●							
Flagellate pigmentation	●							
Lichenoid eruption	●	●						
Hyperpigmentation	●							
Gingival hemorrhages	●	●						
Aphthous-like sores	●							
Encephalitis	●		●					
Myelopathy	●							
Neuropathy	●							
Hematemesis	●	●						
Melaena	●	●						
Myeloneuropathy	●							
Myopathy	●							

pain which is a characteristic symptom of dengue.[55, 56]

Table 2: comparison of nonspecific symptoms observed in early stages Dengue hemorrhagic fever (DHF) and Chikungunya fever (CHIKF)[57]

Symptoms	DHF (%)	CHIKVF (%)
Injected pharynx	96.8	90.3
Vomiting	57.9	59.4
Constipation	53.5	40.0
Abdominal pain	50.0	31.6
Headache	44.6	68.4
General lymphadenopathy	40.5	30.8
Conjunctival injection	32.8	55.6
Cough	21.5	23.3
Rhinitis	12.8	6.5
Maculopapular rash	12.1	59.4
Myalgia/arthralgia	12.0	40.0
Enanthema	8.3	11.1
Abdominal reflex	6.7	0.0
Diarrhea	67.4	15.6
Palpable spleen	6.3	3.1
Coma	3.0	0.0

Table 3: Differential diagnosis of late stages of DHF/DSS and CHIKVF[57]

Symptoms	DHF (%)	CHIKVF (%)
Fever lasting 2-4 days	23.6	62.5
Fever lasting 5-6 days	59.0	31.2
Fever lasting >7 days	17.4	6.3
Positive Tourniquet test	83.9	77.4
Scattered Petechiae	46.5	31.3
Confluent Petechial rash	10.1	0.0
Epistaxis	18.9	12.5
Gum bleeding	1.5	0.0
Melena/hematemesis	11.8	0.0
Hepatomegaly	90.0	75.0
Shock	35.2	0.0

Patients suffering from Dengue hemorrhagic fever generally recover within six or seven days and are immune to the particular serotype of dengue virus that caused the infection. Nonetheless, if the patient is subsequently infected by another serotype of dengue fever viruses, the individual may develop DHF, which may lead to dengue shock syndrome (DSS).[59] The development of thrombocytopenia with concurrent hemo-concentration differences or hypotension, as well as shock, generally rule out a diagnosis of CHIKVF. These developments also rule out the diagnosis of bacterial endotoxin shock and meningococcemia (Table 3).[57]

Other common viral infections that demonstrate similarities in the representation of symptoms are O'nyong-nyong, West Nile, Sindbis, rubella, parvovirus, hepatitis A and B, mumps, as well as non-viral infections, such as disseminated gonococcal infection and rheumatoid arthritis (Table 4). Therefore, laboratory analysis is essential to differentiate CHIKV from other infections.[58]

References

1. Arias D. Chikungunya Fever has Reached United States via Global Travelers. Public Health, 2007. pp. 20
2. Brooks G.F., Butel J.S., Morse S.A. Human Arboviral Infections. Medical Microbiology. 23rd Edition. Singapore: McGraw Hill. 2004. pp. 514-524
3. Vanlandingham D.L., Hong C., Klingler K., Tsetsarkin K., McElroy K.L., Powers A.M., Lehane M.J., Higgs S. Differential Inactivities of O'nyong-nyong and Chikungunya Virus Isolates in Anopheles gambiae and Aedes aegypti Mosquitoes. American Journal of Tropical Medicine and Hygiene, 2005. 72: pp. 616-621
4. Robinson M. An Epidemic of Virus Disease in Southern Province, Tanganyika Territory, in 1952-53; I. Clinical Features. Transactions of the Royal Society of Tropical Medicine and Hygiene, 1955. 49: 28-32
5. Pastorino B., Muyembe-Tamfum J.J., Bessaud M., Tock F., Tolou H., Durand J.P., Peyrefitte C.N. Epidemic Resurgence of Chikungunya Virus in Democratic Republic of the Congo: Identification of a New Central African Strain. Journal of Medical Virology, 2004. 74: pp. 277-282
6. Lam S.K., Chua K.B., Hooi P.S. Chikungunya Infection: Emerging Disease in Malaysia. The Southeast Asian Journal of Tropical Medicine and Public Health, 2001. 32: pp. 447-

451
7. Shah K.V., Gibbs C.J.J., Banerjee G. Virological Investigation of the Epidemic of Haemorrhagic Fever in Calcutta: Isolation of Three Strains of Chikungunya Virus. Indian Journal of Medical Research, 1964. 52: pp. 676-683
8. Chikungunya Fever, a Re-emerging Disease in Asia. World Health Organization. Regional Office for South East Asia. Retrieved May 23, 2007. Website: http://www.searo.who.int/en/Section10 /Section2246.htm
9. Guerrant R.L., Walker D.H., Weller P.F. Tropical Infectious Diseases – Principles, Pathogens & Practice. Volume 1. Philadelphia: Churchill Livingstone Elsevier. 2006. pp. 831-833
10. Mavalankar D., Shastri P., Raman P. Chikungunya Epidemic in India: a Major Public-health Disaster. The Lancet Infectious Diseases, 2007. 7: pp. 306-307
11. Khan A.H., Morita K., Parquet M.C., Hasebe F., Mathenge E.G.M., Igarashi A. Complete Nucleotide Sequence of Chikungunya Virus and Evidence for an Internal Polyadenylation Site. Journal of General Virology, 2002. 83: 3075-3084
12. Vanlandingham D.L., Tsetsarkin K., Hong C., Klingler K., McElroy K. Development and Characterization of a Double Subgenomic Chikungunya Virus Infectious Clone to Express Heterologous Genes in Aedes aegypti Mosquitoes. Insect Biochemistry and Molecular Biology, 2005. 35: pp. 1162–1170
13. Schuffenecker I., Iteman I., Michault A., Murri S., Frangeul L., Vaney M.C., Lavenir R., Pardigon N., Reynes J.M., Pettinelli F., Biscornet L., Diancourt L., Michel S., Duquerroy S., Guigon G., Frenkiel M.P., Bréhin A.C., Cubito N., Desprès P., Kunst F., Rey F.A., Zeller H., Brisse S. Genome Microevolution of Chikungunya Viruses Causing the Indian Ocean Outbreak. Public Library of Science (PLoS) Medicine, 2006. 3: pp. e263
14. Parola P., De Lamballerie X., Jourdan J., Rovery C., Vaillant V., Minodier P., Brouqui P., Flahault A., Raoult D., Charrel R.N. Novel Chikungunya Virus Variant in Travelers Returning from Indian Ocean Islands. Emerging Infectious Diseases, 2006. 12: pp. 1493–1498
15. Volk S.M., Chen R., Tsetsarkin K.A., Adams A.P., Garcia T.I., Sall A.A., Nasar F., Schuh A.J., Holmes E.C., Higgs S., Maharaj P.D., Brault A.C., Weaver S.C. Genome-Scale Phylogenetic Analyses of Chikungunya Virus Reveal Independent Emergences of Recent Epidemics and Various Evolutionary Rates. Journal of Virology, 2010. 13: pp. 6497-6504
16. Lahariya C., Pradhan S.K. Emergence of Chikungunya Virus in Indian Subcontinent after 32 Years: a Review. The Journal of Vector Borne Diseases, 2006. 43: pp. 151-160
17. Couderc T., Chrétien F., Schilte C., Disson O., Brigitte M., Guivel-Benhassine F., Touret Y., Barau G., Cavet N., Schuffenecker I., Desprès P., Arenzana-Seisdedos F., Michault A., Albert M.L., Lecuit M. A mouse Model for Chikungunya: Young Age and Inefficient Type-I Interferon Signaling are Risk Factors for Severe Disease. Public Library of Science (PLoS) Pathogens, 2008. 4: pp. e29
18. Ozden S., Huerre M., Riviere J-P., Coffey L.L., Afonso P.V., Mouly V., de Monredon J., Roger J-C., El Amrani M., Yvin J-L., Jaffar M-C., Frenkiel M-P., Sourisseau M., Schwartz O., Butler-Browne G., Desprès P., Gessain A., Ceccaldi P-E. Human Muscle Satellite Cells as Targets of Chikungunya Virus Infection. Public Library of Science (PLoS) ONE, 2007. 2: e527
19. Ozden S., Huerre M., Riviere J.P., Coffey L.L., Afonso P.V., Mouly V., de Monredon J., Roger J.C., El Amrani M., Yvin J.L., Jaffar M.C., Frenkiel M.P., Sourisseau M., Schwartz O., Butler-Browne G., Despres P., Gessain A., Ceccaldi P.E. Human Muscle Satellite Cells as Targets of Chikungunya Virus Infection. Public Library of Science (PLoS) ONE, 2007. 2: e527
20. Ziegler S.A., Lu L., Travassos da Rosa A.P.A., Xiao S-Y., Tesh R.B. An Animal Model for Studying the Pathogenesis of Chikungunya Virus Infection. American Journal of Tropical Medicine and Hygiene, 2008. 79: pp. 133-139
21. Sourisseau M., Schilte C., Casartelli N., Trouillet C., Guivel-Benhassine F., Dominika Rudnicka D., Sol-Foulon N., Le Roux K., Prevost M-C, Fsihi H., Frenkiel M-P., Blanchet F., Afonso P.V., Ceccaldi P-E., Ozden S., Gessain A., Schuffenecker I., Verhasselt B., Zamborlini A., Saïb A., Rey F.A., Arenzana-Seisdedos F., Desprès P., Michault A., Albert M.L., Schwartz O. Characterization of Reemerging Chikungunya Virus. Public Library of Science (PLoS) Pathogens, 2007. 3: pp. e89
22. Johnston R.E., Peters C. Alphaviruses Associated Primarily with Fever and Polyarthritis. Third Edition. New York: Raven Press. 1996. pp. 843-898
23. Kielian M., Rey F.A. Virus Membrane-fusion Proteins: More Than One Way to Make a Hairpin. Nature Reviews Microbiology, 2006. 4: pp. 67-76
24. Garoff H., Sjöberg M., Cheng R.H. Budding of Alphaviruses. Virus Research, 2004. 106: pp. 103-116
25. Yadav J.S. A Special Issue on Chikungunya. Envis News Letter, 2006. 3: pp. 1-12
26. Sourisseau M., Schilte C., Casartelli N., Trouillet C., Guivel-Benhassine F., Rudnicka D., Sol-Foulon N., Le Roux K., Prevost M-C., Fsihi H., Frenkiel M-P., Blanchet F., Afonso P.V., Ceccaldi P-E., Ozden S., Gessain A., Schuffenecker I., Verhasselt B., Zamborlini A., Saïb A., Rey F.A., Arenzana-Seisdedos F., Desprès P., Michault A., Albert M.L., Schwartz O. Characterization of Reemerging Chikungunya Virus, 2007. 3: pp. e89
27. Anthony R.P., Brown D.T. Protein-protein Interactions in an Alphavirus Membrane. The Journal of Virology, 1991. 65: pp. 1187-1194
28. Paredes A.M., Brown D.T., Rothnahel R., Chiu W., Schoepp R.J., Johnston R.E., Prasad B.V. Three-dimensional Structure of a Membrane-containing Virus. Proceedings of the National Academy of Science United States of America, 1993. 90: pp. 9095-9099
29. Solignat M., Gay B., Higgs S., Briant L., Devaux C. _Replication cycle of Chikungunya: A re-emerging arbovirus. Virology, 2009. 25: pp. 183–197
30. Perera R., Owen K.E., Tellinghuisen T.L., Gorbalenya A.E., Kuhn R.J. Alphavirus Nucleocapsid Protein Contains a Putative Coiled Coil Alpha-Helix Important for Core Assembly. Journal of Virology, 2001. 75: pp. 1–10
31. Ekström M., Liljeström P., Garoff H. Membrane Protein Lateral Interactions Control Semliki Forest Virus Budding. European Molecular Biology Organization (EMBO) Journal, 1994. 1: pp. 1058-1064
32. Sarkar J.K., Chatterjee S.N., Chakravarty S.K. Haemorrhagic Fever in Calcutta: Some Epidemiological Observations. Indian Journal of Medical Research, 1964; 52: pp. 651–659
33. Lahariya C., Pradhan S.K. Emergence of Chikungunya Virus in Indian Subcontinent after 32 Years: a Review. Journal of Vector Borne Diseases, 2006. 43: pp. 151-160
34. Robillard P.Y., Boumahni B., Gerardin P., Michault A., Fourmaintraux A., Schuffeneccker I., Carbonnier M., Djémili S., Choker G., Roge-Wolter M., Barau G. Vertical Maternal Fetal Transmission of the Chikungunya Virus. Ten Cases among 84 Pregnant Women. La Nouvelle Presse Médicale, 2006. 35: pp. 785-788
35. Sam I.C., AbuBakar S. Chikungunya Virus Infection. The Medical Journal of Malaysia, 2006. 61: pp. 264-269
36. Guerrant R.L., Walker D.H., Weller P.F. Tropical Infectious Diseases – Principles, Pathogens & Practice. Volume 1. Philadelphia: Churchill Livingstone Elsevier. 2006. pp. 836
37. Mohan A. Chikungunya Fever: Clinical Manifestation & Management. Indian Journal of Medical Research, 2006. 124: pp. 471-474
38. Sakar J.K., Chatterjee S.N., Chakravarti S.K. Chikungunya Virus Infection with Hemorrhagic Manifestations. Indian Journal of Medical research, 1965. 53: pp. 921
39. Sebastian M.R., Lodha R., Kabra S.K. Chikungunya Infection in Children. Indian Journal

of Pediatrics, 2009. 76: pp. 185-189

40. Chandak N.H., Kshyap R.S., Kabra D., Karandikar P., Sha S.S., Morey S.H., Purohit H.J., Taori G.M., Daginawala H.F. Neurological Complications of *Chikungunya Virus* Infection. Neurology India, 2009. 57: pp. 177-180

41. Parida M.M., Santhosh S.R., Dash P.K., Lakshmana Rao P.V. Rapid and Real-time Assay for Detection and Quantification of Chikungunya Virus. Future Virology, 2008. 3: pp. 179-192

42. Johnston R.E., Peters C.J. Alphaviruses Associated Primarily with Fever and Polyarthritis. Fields Virology. Philadelphia: Lippincott-Raven Publishers. 1996. pp. 843–98

43. Mohan A. Chikungunya Fever Strikes in Andhra Pradesh. The National Medical Journal of India, 2006. 19: pp. 240

44. Sergon K., Njuguna C., Kalani R., Ofula V., Onyango C., Konongoi L.S., Bedno S., Burke H., Dumilla A.M., Konde J., Njenga M.K., Sang R., Breiman R F. Seroprevalence of *Chikungunya Virus* (CHIKV) Infection on Lamu Island, Kenya, October 2004. American Journal of Tropical Medicine and Hygiene, 2008. 78: pp. 333–337

45. Bustin S.A., Mueller R. Real-time Reverse Transcription PCR (qRTPCR) and its Potential use in Clinical Diagnosis. Clinical Science, 2005. 109: pp.365–379

46. Couderc T., Khandoudi N., Grandadam M., Visse C., Gangneux N., Bagot S., Prost J-F, Lecuit M. Prophylaxis and Therapy for *Chikungunya Virus* Infection. The Journal of Infectious Diseases, 2009. 200: pp. 516–523

47. Chahar H.S., Bharaj P., Dar L., Randeep G., Kabra S.K., Broor S. Co-infections with *Chikungunya Virus* and Dengue Virus in Delhi, India. Emerging Infectious Diseases, 2009. 15: pp. 1077-1080

48. Laurent P., Le Roux K., Grivard P., Bertil G., Naze F., Picard M., Staikowsky F., Barau G., Schuffenecker I., Michault A. Development of a Sensitive Real-Time Reverse Transcriptase PCR Assay with an Internal Control to Detect and Quantify Chikungunya Virus. Clinical Chemistry, 2007. 53: pp. 1408–1414

49. Sheng T., Kwan-Gett C., Kemp C., Kovarik C. Infectious and Tropical Diseases, a Handbook for Primary Care. St. Louis: Elsevier Mosby. 2006. pp. 140.

50. Lenschow D.J., Lai C., Frias-Staheli N., Giannakopoulos N.V., Lutz A., Wolff T., Osiak A., Levine B., Schmidt R.E., García-Sastre A., Leib D.A., Pekosz A., Knobeloch K-P., Horak I., Virgin IV H.W. IFN-stimulated Gene 15 Functions as a Critical Antiviral Molecule Against Influenza, Herpes, and Sindbis Viruses. Proceedings of the National Academy of Science United States of America, 2007. 104: pp. 1371-1376

51. Edelman R., Tacket C.O., Wasserman S.S., Bodison S.A., Perry J.G., Mangiaffico J.A. Phase II Safety and Immunogenicity Study of Live *Chikungunya Virus* Vaccine. American Journal of Tropical Medicine and Hygiene, 2000. 62: pp. 681-685

52. Weger-Lucarelli J., Chu H., Aliota, M.T., Partidos C.D., Osorio J.E. A Novel MVA Vectored *Chikungunya Virus* Vaccine Elicits Protective Immunity in Mice. Public Library of Science (PloS) Neglected Tropical Diseases, 2014. 8: pp 1-14

53. Brighton S.W. Chloroquine Phosphate Treatment of Chronic Chikungunya Arthritis. An Open Pilot Study. South African Medical Journal, 1984. 66: pp. 217-218

54. Powers A.M., Logue C.H. Changing Patterns of *Chikungunya Virus*: Re-emergence of a Zoonotic Arbovirus. Journal of General Virology, 2007. 88: pp. 2363-2377

55. Jadhav M., Namboodripad M., Carman R.H., Carey D.E., Myers R.M. Chikungunya Disease in Infants and Children in Vellore: a Report of Clinical and Haematological Features of Virologically Proved Cases. Indian Journal of Medical Research, 1965. 53: pp. 764-776

56. Myers R.M., Carey D.E., Concurrent Isolation from Patient of Two Arbo Viruses, Chikungunya and Dengue Type 2. Science, 1967. 157: pp. 1307-1308

57. Nimmannitya S., Halstead S., Cohen S.B. Margiotta M.R. *Dengue* and *Chikungunya virus* infection in man in Thailand. American Journal of Tropical Medicine and Hygiene, 1960. 18: pp. 954-971

58. Hasebe F., Parquet M.C., Pandy B.D., Mathenge E.G.M., Morita K., Balasubramaniam V., Saat Z., Yusop A., Sinniah M., Natkunam S., Igarashi A.. Combined Detection and Genotyping of *Chikungunya Virus* by a Specific Reverse Transcription-polymerase Chain Reaction. Journal of Medical Virology, 2002. 67: 370-374

59. World Health Organization. Dengue Haemorrhagic Fever – Diagnosis, Treatment, Prevention and Control 2nd Edition. WHO Library Cataloging in Publication Data, 1997. pp. 13

Photo Bibliography

Figure 1.2-2: Transmission electron micrograph (TEM) of *Togaviridae* virus family and the genus *Alphavirus* (Eastern Equine Encephalitis virus) infecting the salivary gland that had been extracted from a mosquito Photo was taken by Dr. Fred Murphy and Sylvia Whitfield of the CDC in 1968. This TEM is magnified at 83,900x Public domain photo

Figure 1.2-3: Computer-generated model of the surface of an alphavirus derived by cryoelectron microscopy. Graphic was designed and released by the CDC in 2007. Public domain photo

Figure 1.2-4: Genomic protein graphics produced and released by the National Institute of Health (NIH). Public domain photo

Crimean-Congo Hemorrhagic Fever virus (CCHFV) belongs to the family *Bunyaviridae* and is a member of the genus *Nairovirus*. This virus is the caustic agent of Congo-Crimean Hemorrhagic Fever (CCHF) (Figure 1.2-1).[1]

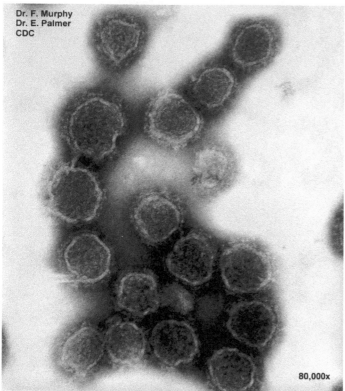

Dr. F. Murphy
Dr. E. Palmer
CDC

80,000x

Figure 1.3-1: Negatively-stained transmission electron micrograph (TEM) of numerous virions in the family *Bunyaviridae*

CCHFV is a tick-borne virus that causes endemic infections in approximately 30 nations of Africa, Asia, Southeastern Europe and the Middle East (Figure 1.2-2).[2, 3, 4, 5] CCHF is believed to be an ancient disease with its first description dated as early as 12th century from southwestern Russia, in what is today Tadzhikistan.[6] The first well documented case of CCHF occurred in the Crimean Peninsula (Russia) in mid-1944 after an outbreak of hemorrhagic fever in agricultural workers of the region. Nonetheless, the virion was not isolated until 1956 in Zaïre (presently known as The Democratic Republic of Congo).[7]

Typically, CCHFV is a zoonosis, which can be transmitted from wild animals to domestic animals and on some occasions to humans. CCHFV is transmitted to humans either through the bite of an infected tick, contact with contaminated blood, tissue or through aerosolized virus via the respiratory tract. The majority of naturally transmitted infections in humans involve workers in agriculture, the livestock industry, veterinary practice and other related fields.[8, 9] Livestock and animal ticks *Hyalomma dermacentor, H. amblyomma* and *H. rhipicephalus*, as well as, approximately 28 other species of ticks, and one species of biting midge (*Culicoides* spp.) serve as vectors and are the reservoir of CCHFV.[10] The initial transmission of this disease to humans involves direct contact of humans with infected animal blood. The subsequent human to human transmission involves direct contact with infected blood and bodily fluids (Figure 1.3-3).[11]

CCHFV has been successfully cultured and aerosolized in small quantities and is a potential biological weapon/ terrorism threat. Nonetheless, mass production of CCHFV has not been successful, thereby excluding it from being categorized as a Category A or B mass casualty weapon.[9]

CCHFV is a spherical, enveloped virus that is approximately 90 nm in diameter. The genome of the CCHFV consists of a tripartite (three parts), single stranded, negative-sense RNA, with highly conserved complementary nucleotide sequences 5'-UCUCAAAGA and 3'AGAGUUUCU at the segment ends. It has been reported that the intrastrand base pair interaction between these terminal nucleotides develops a non-covalently closed circular RNA providing the functional promoter region for

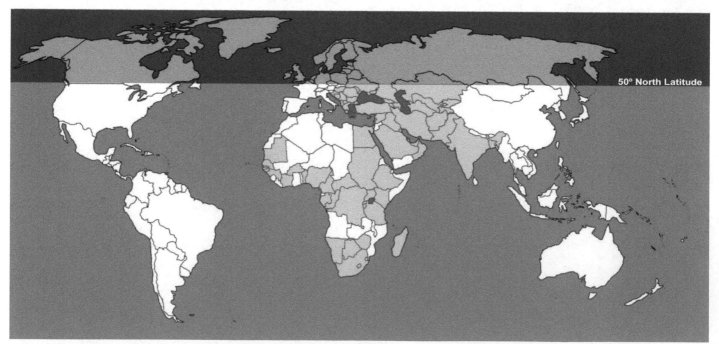

50° North Latitude

Figure 1.3-2: Distribution of Crimean-Congo hemorrhagic fever. Please note that the 50° north latitude is the limit for the distribution of *Hyalomma* ticks

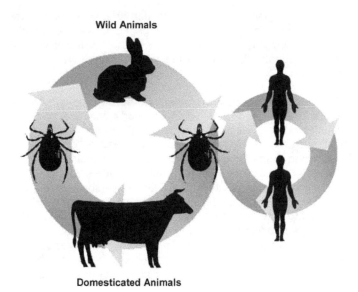

Wild Animals

Domesticated Animals

Figure 1.3-3: Sylvatic cycle of Crimean-Congo hemorrhagic virus

the interaction of the viral polymerase and genome segments.[12, 13, 14, 15]

The three genome segments of CCHFV are divided into large, medium and small segments. The large (L) genome segment encodes the RNA-dependent RNA polymerase (RDRP), or the L protein. The medium (M) genome segment encodes the glycoproteins G_N and G_C. The small (S) genome segment encodes the nucleoprotein (NP) (Figure 1.3-4).[16, 17, 18]

The glycoproteins G_N and G_C are inserted into the lipid envelope of CCHFV during assembly as spike like structures and the induction of neutralizing antibodies by the hosts' immune system.[16]. A recent report indicated that G_C is the candidate essential for gaining entry into the host cell, while the surface protein molecule nucleolin, is proposed to be a possible CCHFV entry factor.[19] It is believed that the virus enters the host cell via receptor mediated clathrin-dependent endocytosis. After gaining entry, the internalized clathrin-coated vesicles fuse with lysosomes and subsequently an acid-triggered process permits for the necessary conformational changes of the virus, allowing

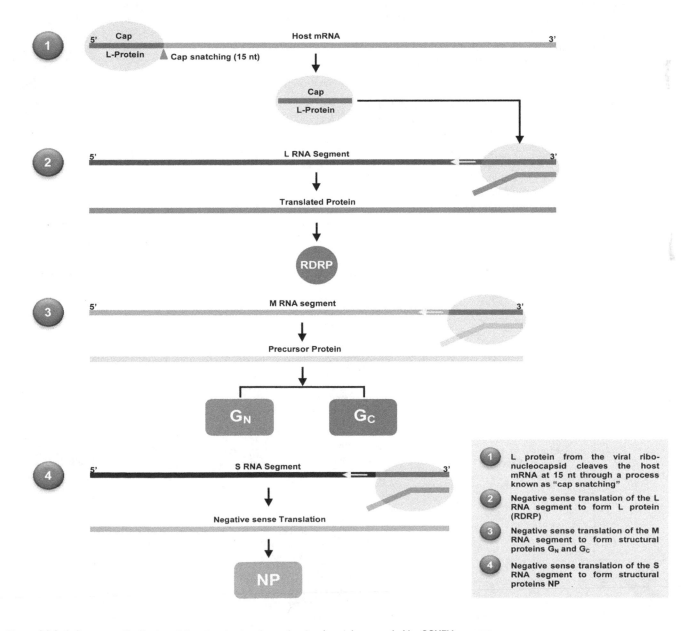

Figure 1.3-3: A diagrammatic display of the structural and nonstructural proteins encoded by CCHFV genome

it to escape.[19, 20, 21]

The cytoplasm of the host cell is dense and does not permit efficient long range diffusion of the virus. Therefore, the intracellular movement of the virus requires the recruitment of the host cellular cytoskeletal transport machinery. It has been reported that the intracellular transport of the virus to the cellular sites for viral transcription and replication is mediated by microtubule or actin filaments and their associated motor proteins (e.g. kinesin, dynein-dynactin) although the exact mechanism presently remains unknown.[22]

Initial replication of CCHFV is believed to be similar to other viruses of the *Bunyaviridae*. It is thought that the replication of the tri-segmented negative sense RNA strands of the CCHKV into positive sense complimentary strands via the L protein occurs within the cytoplasm of the host cell.[20] This explanation is supported by the isolation of only positive sense RNA within the initial 6 hours after infection.[22] Nonetheless, the exact manner by which the replication occurs requires further elucidation

CCHFV, like other Bunyaviridae, possesses a unique "cap stealing" strategy. Experimental evidence has shown that the L protein is responsible for cleaving host cellular mRNA at 15 nucleotides (nt) from their 5' ends and utilizing the cut segment as spliced leader RNA cap to prime the transcription of the nonpolyadenylated mRNA on the three viral (large, medium and small) RNA segments.

It has been reported that the termination of the transcription is completed when the availability of the hairpin loops on the viral RNA template are reached. Hairpin loops are formed when two regions of the same strand possess complementary nucleotide sequence and form a double helix that ends in an unpaired loop (Figure 1.3-5). However, it is uncertain how the CCHFV changes from transcription of mRNA transcripts into full-length complementary positive sense RNA transcription.[23, 24]

During replication, viral structural protein NP is directed to the perinuclear region, the space between the inner and outer nuclear membranes, where it is engaged in viral assembly. Viral assembly has been reported to be host cell cytoskeletal actin-dependent, while independent from any virally encoded glycoproteins.[25]

CCHFV utilizes the host endoplasmic reticulum to synthesize glycoprotein G_N and G_C.[26] Recent reports indicate that the presence of G_N is essential to promote the correct folding of G_C. Additionally, G_N serves as a chaperone molecule for G_C during its transport to the Golgi apparatus. [22, 23, 27, 28] Once the virion is assembled, the mature virus particles bud into vesicles and are transported via the intact host cellular micro-tubule network to the cell surface and are released via the secretory pathway.[24] It is important to note that some research has indicated that CCHFV matures by budding through the endoplasmic reticulum into the cytoplasmic vesicles formed from the Golgi membranes. The assembly and budding of the virus seems to be defined by the retention of the G_N and C_C at the Golgi apparatus (Figure 1.3-6).[23]

The pathogenesis of CCHFV is complex and not well described. Presently, the limited knowledge of pathogenesis is primarily based upon descriptions of autopsied tissues thereby restricting our understanding to the terminal stages of the disease.[29]

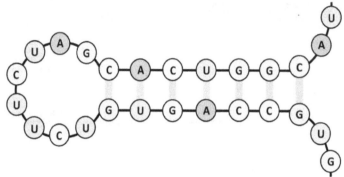

Figure 1.3-5: An example of a "hairpin loop" that serves as a termination site of CCHFV transcription on the RNA template

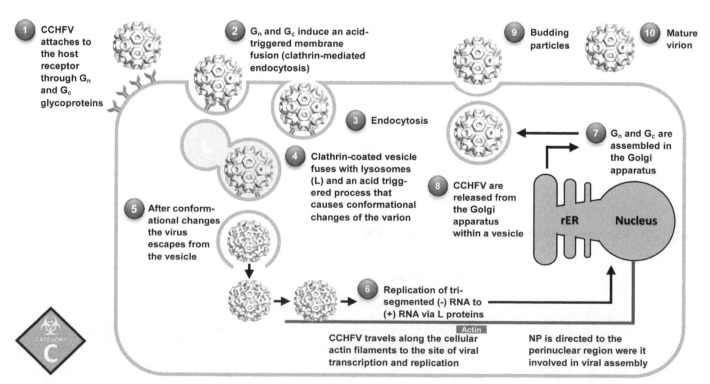

Figure 1.3-6: Diagrammatic process of CCHFV infection within an eukaryotic cell

It is believed that the main targets of CCHFV are mononuclear phagocytes, vascular endothelial cells and hepatocytes. CCHFV infection of the liver is generally accompanied by parenchymal necrosis of that organ (Figure 1.3-7 and 1.3-8).

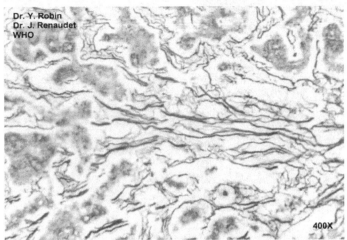

Figure 1.3-7: A Wilder's reticulin-stained photo-micrograph demonstrates the cytoarchitectural changes found in a liver tissue specimen extracted from a Congo/Crimean hemorrhagic fever patient. This micrograph depicts a thickening and disassociation or the fibers of the reticular network

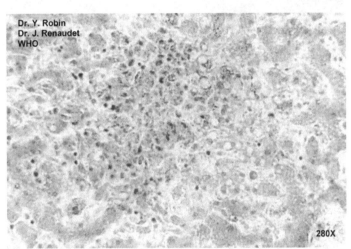

Figure 1.3-8: Photomicrograph demonstrates the coagulation necrosis of hepatocytes with an associated perifocal inflammatory reaction in a liver tissue specimen extracted from a Congo/Crimean hemorrhagic fever patient. In addition several cells can be seen to be undergoing fatty degeneration. The slide was prepared with hematoxylin-eosin (H&E) stain

Viral antigens and RNA are present within cells (e.g. Kupffer cells and endothelial cells) lining the hepatic sinusoids. Additionally, viral antigens and RNA were found in the endothelial cells and lymphoreticular cells of the spleen and are assumed to be responsible for the depletion of lymphoid cells within the splenic tissue of infected individuals. Presently, it is presumed that the presence of CCHFV within mononuclear phagocytes and vascular endothelial cells is indicative of the phagocytic and immunologic activities of these cells related to viral clearance, or it may be supporting the replication and shedding of the virus back into circulatory system. For example, the absence of necrosis in infected mononuclear phagocytes and the depletion of splenic lymphoid tissue may protect the virus from phagocytosis and suppress the immune response, thereby allowing CCHFV to replicate and spread within the host.[8]

CCHFV infection of mononuclear phagocytes and endothelial cells may play a role in the pathogenesis of CCHF by inducing the secretion of cytokines and other inflammatory mediators.[8]

For example, it has been reported that inappropriately activated T helper 1 (CD4 Th1) lymphocytes produce tumor necrosis factor-alpha (TNF-α) and interferon gamma (IFN-γ). This increased secretion of TNF-α and IFN-γ promote macrophage co-activation and the subsequent over secretion of interleukin-1 (IL-1) and IL-6 by the phagocyte. In addition, the vascular endothelium is also directly affected (infected or damaged) by CCHFV and responds by secreting cytokines that stimulate the production of vasodilators, platelet aggregation factors and the activation of coagulant proteins, believed to contribute to the development of disseminated intravascular coagulation and multi-organ failure.[30]

SYMPTOMS

CCHFV is an indiscriminant killer with a mortality rate of approximately 50%, ranging typically between 25-75%, with most deaths occurring 5-14 days after the onset of illness.[31] Research has indicated that there are 4 clinical phases of the CCHF: (1) incubation, (2) pre-hemorrhagic, (3) hemorrhagic and (4) convalescence.[7]

The incubation period of CCHFV within a human host is highly dependent on the route of exposure. For example, the incubation period for the disease after a direct tick bite is generally around 2-7 days, but when infection is due to a direct contact with infected blood, tissue fluid, or a biological weapons attack, the incubation period for the virus is approximately 10 to14 days.[10, 32, 33]

The onset of the symptoms of CCHF is sudden. During the pre-hemorrhagic phase the symptoms of infection include flu-like conditions including sudden onset of fevers (~38°C or 101°F), that last 5 to 20 days. The initial fever will be followed by chills, myalgia, arthralgia, general weakness, neck pains and stiffness, severe headaches, dizziness, conjunctivitis, jaundice, eye pains and photophobia. Occasionally, nausea, vomiting, diarrhea, sore throat and pains in the epigastria and lumbar regions have been reported during the early stage of infection.[16, 33, 34] Neuropsychiatric changes were also observed, patients developed altered consciousness progressing to aggressive behaviors and subsequent unconsciousness.[33] In addition, cardiovascular changes, such as bradycardia and low blood pressure have also been noted.[10] The pre-hemorrhagic phase of the disease may be biphasic with fever lasting 2-3 days before the disease proceeds into remission (afebrile) for several days. The afebrile period is followed by the return of fever along with epistaxis, petechiae, purpura and thrombocytopenia.[16, 33, 36]

The hemorrhagic phase of the infection may last 3 to 10 days, where hemorrhages often begin with blood leakages at the inoculation site(s) (site of initial exposure). Blood loss at inoculation site(s) may become quite profuse.[16] During this time, petechial hemorrhages can be found in and around the mouth, throat and skin, which may slowly spread to ecchymoses or hemorrhages covering a larger area of the epidermis (Figure 1.3-9, 1.3-10 and 1.3-11).

During the later stages of the hemorrhagic phase, other hemorrhages may also appear. For example, hematuria, hematemesis, hemoptysis, melaena (black stools resulting from bleeding of the upper gastrointestinal tract), epistaxis, bloody gums, cytopenia (e.g. leukopenia and thrombo-cytopenia), and bloody otorrhea (inflammation of the middle ear) are frequently observed in patients. Additionally, consumptive coagulopathy (blood throughout the patient's body begins to coagulate) resulting from sepsis, may also be observed in patients.[8, 10]

Hemorrhages are a result of numerous small blood clots caused by the virus replicating throughout the body, which is clinically known as disseminated intravascular coagulation. Wherever one of these clots is found, a small section of tissue downstream will die from lack of nutrients and oxygen. The human body will attempt to compensate for the formation of the clots by secreting substantial amounts of plasmin designed to dissolve fibrin clots. As a result, massive uncontrollable bleeding occurs throughout the body.[37]

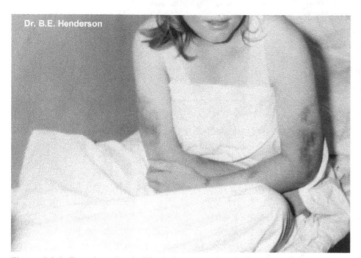

Figure 1.3-9: Female patient with ecchymoses located on her arms

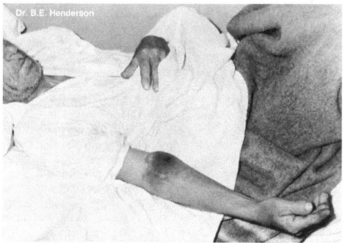

Figure 1.3-10: Male patient with ecchymoses located on his right antibrachial region

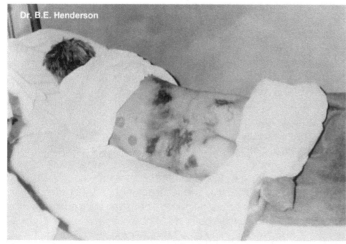

Figure 1.3-11: Male patient with consumptive coagulopathy

Table 1: An overview of the clinical symptoms of CCHF

Symptoms	+	++	+++
Fevers			■
Chills			■
Myalgia			■
Arthralgia			■
Neck pains			■
Stiffness			■
General weakness			■
Severe headaches			■
Confusion			■
Dizziness			■
Dryness of the mouth			■
Sweating			■
Conjunctivitis			■
Jaundice			■
Eye pains			■
Photophobia			■
Nausea & vomiting			■
Diarrhea			■
Sore throat			■
Pains epigastria region			■
Pains lumbar region			■
Altered consciousness		■	
Aggressive behavior		■	
Unconsciousness		■	
Epistaxis		■	
Petechiae		■	
Purpura		■	
Thrombocytopenia		■	
Venipuncture bleeding		■	
Petechial hemorrhages		■	
Ecchymoses		■	
Hematuria		■	
Hematemesis		■	
Hemoptysis		■	
Melaena		■	
Epistaxis		■	
Bloody gums		■	
Leukopenia		■	
Thrombocytopenia		■	
Leukopenia		■	
Bloody otorrhea		■	
Con. coagulopathy		■	
Insomnia		■	
Depression		■	
Lethargy		■	
Sudden mood swings		■	
Hepatitis	■		
Hepatomegaly	■		
Splenomegaly	■		
Tachycardia	■		
Lymphadenopathy	■		
Shock	■		
Liver failure	■		
Kidney failure	■		
Pulmonary failure	■		
Cerebral hemorrhage	■		
Anemia	■		
Dehydration	■		
Myocardial infarction	■		
Pulmonary edema	■		
Pleural effusion	■		
Hair loss	■		
Bradycardia	■		
Low blood pressure	■		

+ Rare ++ Common +++ Frequent

In addition to the hemorrhagic manifestations, patients may also experience insomnia, depression, lethargy, and sudden mood swings. Hepatitis may occur in some patients, it may result in jaundice and hepatomegaly. Physical manifestation of the disease such as splenomegaly, tachycardia, and lymphadeno-pathy may also be detected. In approximately 30% of severe cases, patients may experience shock accompanied by liver failure, kidney failure, pulmonary failure cerebral hemorrhage (e.g. encephalopathy), anemia, dehydration, diarrhea, myocardial infarction, pulmonary edema and pleural effusion which may lead to death.[8, 10, 16, 33]

Patients that survive the hemorrhagic manifestations of CCHFV will proceed into a convalescent phase, which generally begins approximately 15 to 20 days after the initial onset of symptoms. During this phase, the fever will subside, as well as the hemorrhagic symptoms. The convalescent phase is characterized by general weakness, weak pulse, tachycardia, confusion, asthenia, alopecia and neuralgias. In addition, other symptoms such as sweating, dryness of the mouth, nausea, poor appetite, labored breathing and memory loss have also been reported. Patients may also experience possible hair loss and dizziness. It has been estimated that recovery from CCHF typically requires 2-4 weeks.[10, 16, 33, 36, 38] Please examine Table 1 for an overview of the clinical signs of CCHF.

DETECTION

Early diagnosis of CCHF is essential, both for the outcome of the patient and to prevent further transmission of disease. Presently, accurate detection of CCHFV requires BSL 4 facilities. The virus can be isolated via inoculation of infected blood or bodily fluids into newborn mice (intracerebrally), Vero cells or other susceptible cell lines (e.g. LLC-MK2, BHK-21, and SW-13). Intracerebrally inoculation of infected serum into new borne mice is considered to be the more sensitive methodology, however, using cell cultures is far simpler and provides more rapid results. Cell culture generally detect high concentrations of virus and is most effective during the first five days of illness. Once the virus is isolated, it can be identified using CCHFV-specific antibodies through direct immunofluorescence.[39, 40, 41] Although effective, viral isolation and subsequent identification is time consuming and it may take days before any results are available.[10, 16]

Enzyme linked immunoassay (ELISA) can be used to detect CCHFV specific IgG and IgM antibodies in infected human serum samples approximately seven days after the onset of disease.[32, 42, 43] Although less sensitive in comparison to classic virus isolation methods, the assay is a valuable tool when used in severe CCHF cases due to the higher viral titer and prolonged viremia. ELISAs could be employed to detect the CCHFV specific antibodies in patient's serum within 5 to 6 hours.[44] A new, more sensitive, methodology involving recombinant nucleoprotein -based IgG and IgM ELISA for serological diagnosis of CCHFV infections has been developed.[45] However, in 30% of patients with fatal infection, the levels of antibodies are so low that ELISA may not be able to detect.[12] Put simply, the levels of these antibodies titers are directly linked to the likelihood of survival of patients. For those patients that have low CCHFV antibodies, the virus can be isolated from blood or tissues within the first five days of infection and grown in cell cultures by applying immunofluorescence (EIA) to directly detect viral antigen.[46]

Molecular-based diagnostic assays, such as the reverse transcription-polymerase chain reaction (RT-PCR), can provide a useful complement to serological diagnosis of CCHFV. RT-PCR is designed to detect RNA specific to CCHFV, thereby making this diagnostic tool highly specific without the need for specialized biological containment laboratory facilities. In addition, RT-PCR may allow a presumptive diagnosis to be reported within 8 hours of receiving the first specimen, in comparison with other described methodologies which may take days. However, due to the genetic variability of the CCHFV, there are no single sets of primers that can be used to detect all variants. Therefore, most reverse transcriptase-PCR assays are designed to detect a specific variant. Additional improvements of reverse transcriptase-PCR are the development of automated real-time assays. The real-time reverse transcriptase-PCR assay has many advantages over conventional RT-PCR methods. These advantages include lower contamination rates, higher sensitivity, and greater specificity, as well as, providing rapid results in minutes instead of hours.[10, 47, 48, 49]

TREATMENT

Early diagnosis of CCHF is essential for the survival of infected individuals. However, at present, there are no specific antiviral therapies and vaccines that have been approved by the Food and Drug Administration for the treatment of CCHF. Nonetheless, a mouse brain, formalin-inactivated CCHF vaccine was developed and approved for use in the Soviet Union and Bulgaria during the 1970's. Recently, a study has shown that the Bulgarian vaccine elicited cellular and humoral response to CCHFV. Nonetheless, the study also reported that the amount of neutralizing antibody titers formed, even after repeated vaccination, was low.[50, 51]

The suggested treatment for CCHF consists mainly of supportive therapies, which involve the careful management of a patient's hematological imbalances as well as their fluid and electrolyte intake.[16] Various treatment methodologies have been devised, however their effectiveness remains to be determined. For example, intravenous injection of fresh platelets (3×10^{11} apheresis platelet suspension), plasma and erythrocytes can also be administered and have been reported to be effective although this treatment's success has not been replicated.[8, 30, 33]

Some experimental treatment methods have been devised and are presently in the testing phase with regards to their usefulness. For example, intravenous and oral treatment with the broad spectrum antiviral agent ribavirin, coupled with corticosteroids, has shown some promise when clinical trials were performed, but to this date no controlled studies have been performed to confirm its effectiveness.[11, 30, 34] The suggested doses for ribavirin are 30 mg/kg of body weight for the initial dose followed by 16 mg/kg every 6 hours for 4 days and finally 8 mg/kg every 8 hours for the remaining 6 days of treatment.[52] In an effort to prevent secondary infections, broad spectrum antibiotics (combinations such as cloxacillin, chloramphenicol and tobramycin) can also be administered.[16, 53]

Immunotherapy is another treatment that has been reported to show some promise. The specific immunoglobulin CCHF-venin isolated from donors was prepared using a combined enthanol-polyethyleneglycol fractionation method with ion-exchange purification and was intravenously introduced into patients suffering from CCHF. As reported by Vassilenko et al. (1989), seven patients with severe CCHF received immunotherapy, resulting in the recovery of all patients treated.[54] It has been reported that CCHF immune serum (hyperimmune serum) administered intravenously in a dose of 250 ml over 1 to 2 hours on successive days has shown to be successful. However, the evidence of immunotherapy's effectiveness is based upon clinical improvement and the studies did not include placebo control patients.[16, 54, 55, 56]

Table 2: Differential diagnosis of CCHF with other bacterial and viral infections that share similar symptoms. Note: Rocky Mountain spotted fever (RMSF), Leptospirosis (Weils Syndrome - WS), Borreliosis (Lyme Disease – LD), Hantavirus hemorrhagic fever (HFRS), Lassa fever (LF), Ebola hemorrhagic fever (EHF), Marburg hemorrhagic fever (MHF), Dengue hemorrhagic fever (DHF)

Symptoms	CCHF	RMSF	WS	LD	HFRS	LF	EHF	MHF	DHF
Fevers	■	■	■		■	■	■	■	■
Chills	■	■	■	■	■	■	■	■	■
Myalgia	■	■	■		■	■	■	■	■
Arthralgia	■	■	■	■	■		■		■
Stiffness	■				■				
General weakness	■		■		■		■	■	
Severe headaches	■	■	■	■	■	■	■	■	
Confusion						■	■		
Sweating	■								
Dizziness	■	■	■	■					
Insomnia	■								
Lethargy	■						■		■
Sudden mood swings	■								
Jaundice			■	■				■	
Nausea	■	■	■	■	■		■		
Vomiting	■	■	■	■	■	■	■	■	■
Diarrhea	■	■					■		■
Sore throat	■								
Conjunctivitis	■	■				■	■		
Photophobia	■	■			■			■	■
Pains in the epigastria region	■		■	■					
Pains in the lumbar region	■								
Aggressive behavior	■								
Epistaxis						■		■	
Petechiae	■	■	■			■		■	■
Purpura	■		■				■		
Thrombocytopenia	■	■		■				■	
Venipuncture bleeding	■						■		
Petechial hemorrhages	■				■		■		
Ecchymoses	■			■			■		
Hematuria	■		■					■	■
Hematemesis	■					■		■	■
Hemoptysis	■					■	■	■	■
Melaena	■						■	■	■
Epistaxis	■						■	■	■
Bloody gums	■					■	■	■	■
Leukopenia	■						■		
Thrombocytopenia	■				■		■		■
Bloody otorrhea	■					■			
Consumptive coagulopathy	■	■	■				■		
Hepatitis	■		■						
Hepatomegaly	■		■	■		■			
Splenomegaly	■			■	■				
Tachycardia	■					■			■
Lymphadenopathy	■		■	■					
Shock	■					■	■	■	
Liver failure	■		■				■	■	
Kidney failure	■				■		■		
Pulmonary failure	■					■			
Cerebral hemorrhage	■	■							
Anemia	■		■						
Dehydration	■	■							
Myocardial infarction	■	■							
Pulmonary edema	■	■	■						
Pleural effusion	■					■			
Bradycardia	■				■				■
Low blood pressure	■								

DIFFERENTIAL DIAGNOSIS

It is essential to obtain an early diagnosis of CCHF in order to prevent the further spread of the disease, as well as the benefit of the patient. Nonetheless, CCHF could be mistaken for other infections therefore care must be employed during the examination of the patient. For example, careful documentation of clinical symptoms, patient history (including travels to endemic areas), insect bites (e.g. tick) and/or exposure to tissue, blood of humans and/or livestock could provide the first indicators of CCHF. Differential diagnosis of early CCHF symptoms should include rickettsiosis which could be caused by tick-borne typhus (Rocky Mountain spotted fever - RMSF) and African tick bite fever (ATBF), leptospirosis, and borreliosis (relapsing fever). In addition, other infections, such as meningococcal infections, Hantavirus hemorrhagic fever, Lassa fever, malaria, Ebola, Marburg, Yellow fever, Kyasanur Forest disease, dengue fever, Omsk hemorrhagic fever should also be placed under consideration (Table 2).[7, 8]

References

1. Fisher-Hoch S.P., McCormick J.B., Swanepoel R., Van Middlekoop A., Harvey S., Kustner H.G. Risk of Human Infections with Crimean-Congo Hemorrhagic Fever Virus in a South African Rural Community. American Journal of Tropical Medicine and Hygiene, 1992. 47: pp. 337-345
2. Yashina L., Petrova I., Seregin S., Vysbemirskii O., Lvov D., Aristova V., Kuhn J., Morzunov S., Gutorov V., Kuzina I., Tyunnikov G., Netesov S., Petrov V. Genetic Variability of Crimean-Congo Haemorrhagic Fever Virus in Russia and Central Asia. Journal of General Virology, 2003. 84: pp. 1199 - 1206
3. Simpson D.I., Knight E.M., Courtois G., Williams M.C., Weinbren M.P., Kibukamusoke J.W. Congo virus: A Hitherto Undescribed Virus Occurring in Africa. I. Human Isolations - Clinical Notes. East African Medical Journal, 1967. 44: pp. 86-92
4. Hassanein K.M., el-Azazy O.M., Yousef H.M. Detection of Crimean-Congo Haemorrhagic Fever Virus Antibodies in Humans and Imported Livestock in Saudi Arabia. Transactions of the Royal Society of Tropical Medicine and Hygiene, 1997. 91: pp. 536-537
5. Drosten C., Minnak D., Emmerich P., Schmitz H., Reinicke T. Crimean-Congo Hemorrhagic Fever in Kosovo. Journal of Clinical Microbiology, 2002. 40: pp. 1122–1123
6. Gear J.H.S. Crimean-Congo Hemorrhagic Fever. Handbook of Viral and Rickettsial Hemorrhagic Fevers. Boca Raton: Chemical and Rubber Company (CRC) Press. 1988. pp. 121-129
7. Whitehouse C.A. Crimean-Congo Hemorrhagic Fever. Antiviral Research, 2004. 64: pp. 145 - 160
8. Guerrant R.L., Walker D.H., Weller P.F. Tropical Infectious Diseases – Principles, Pathogens & Practice. Volume 1. Philadelphia: Churchill Livingstone Elsevier. 2006. pp. 756-761
9. Schwarz T.F., Nitschko H., Jager G., Nsanze H., Longson M., Pugh R.N., Abraham A.K. Crimean-Congo haemorrhagic fever in Oman. Lancet, 1995. 346: pp. 1230
10. The Center for Food Security & Public Health. Iowa State University. Crimean-Congo Hemorrhagic Fever. Revised August 20, 2009. Retrieved December 24, 2009. Website: http://www.cfsph.iastate.edu/Factsheets /pdfs/crimean_congo_hemorrhagic_fever.pdf
11. Morikawa S., Qing T., Xinqin Z., Saijo M., Kurane I. Genetic Diversity of the M RNA Segment among Crimean-Congo Hemorrhagic Fever Virus Isolates in China. Virology, 2002. 296: pp. 159 – 164
12. Suleiman M.N., Muscat-Baron J.M., Harries J.R., Satti A.G., Platt G.S., Bowen E.T., Simpson D.I. Congo/Crimean haemorrhagic fever in Dubai: an outbreak at the Rashid Hospital. Lancet, 1980. 2: pp. 939-941
13. Clerex-van Haaster C.M., Clerex J.P., Ushijima H., Akashi H., Fuller F., Bishop D.H. The 3' Terminal RNA Sequences of *Bunyaviruses* and *Nairoviruses* (*Bunyaviridae*): Evidence of End Sequence Generic Differences within the Virus Family. Journal of General Virology, 1982. 61: pp. 289–292
14. Elliott R.M., Schmaljohn C.S., Collett M.S. *Bunyaviridae* Genome Structure and Gene Expression. Current Topics in Microbiology and Immunology, 1991. 169: pp. 91–141
15. Flick R., Elgh F., Pettersson R.F. Mutational Analysis of the Uukuniemi Virus (*Bunyaviridae* Family) Promoter Reveals Two Elements of Functional Importance. Journal of Virology, 2002. 76: pp. 289-292
16. Flick R., Whitehouse C.A. Crimean-Congo Hemorrhagic Fever Virus. Current Molecular Medicine, 2005. 5: pp. 753-760
17. Kinsella E., Martin S.G., Grolla A., Czub M., Feldmann H., Flick R. Sequence Determination of the Crimean-Congo Hemorrhagic Fever Virus L Segment. Virology, 2004. 321: pp. 23-28
18. Honig J.E., Osborne J.C., Nichol S.T. Crimean-Congo Hemorrhagic Fever Virus Genome L RNA Segment and Encoded Protein. Virology, 2004. 321: pp. 29–35
19. Xiao X., Feng Y., Zhu Z., Dimitrov D.S.Identification of a putative Crimean-Congo hemorrhagic fever virus entry factor. Biochemical and Biophysical Research Communications. 2011. 411: pp. 253-258
20. Simon M., Johansson C., Mirazimi A. Crimean-Congo Hemorrhagic Fever Virus Entry and Replication is Clathrin-, pH – and Cholesterol-dependent. Journal of General Virology, 2009. 90: pp. 210-215
21. Marsh M., Helenius A. Virus Entry: Open Sesame. Cell, 2006. 124: pp. 729–740
22. Simon M., Johansson C., Lundkvist A., Mirazimi A. Microtubule-Dependent and Microtubule-Independent Steps in Crimean–Congo Hemorrhagic Fever Virus Replication Cycle. Virology, 2009. 385: pp. 313–322
23. Schmaljohn C.S., Nichol S.T. Bunyaviridae. Fields Virology - 5th Edition. Philadelphia: Lippincott Williams and Wilkins, 2007. pp. 1741- 1789
24. Garcin D., Lezzi M, Dobbs M., Elliott R.M., Schmaljohn C., Kang C.Y., Kolakofsky D. The 5' ends of Hantaan Virus (*Bunyaviridae*) RNAs Suggest a Prime-and-Realign Mechanism for the Initiation of RNA Synthesis. The Journal of Virology, 1995. 69: pp. 5754–5762
25. Kraus A.A., Mirazimi A. Molecular Biology and Pathogenesis of Crimean–Congo Hemorrhagic Fever Virus. Future Virology, 2010. 5, pp. 469-479
26. Andersson I., Simon M., Lundkvist A., Nilsson M., Holmström A., Elgh F., Mirazimi A. Role of Actin Filaments in Targeting of Crimean Congo Hemorrhagic Fever Virus Nucleocapsid Protein to Perinuclear Regions of Mammalian Cells. Journal of Medical Virology, 2004. 72: pp. 83–93
27. Haferkamp S., Fernando L., Schwarz T.F., Geldmann H., Flick R. Intracellular Localization of Crimean-Congo Hemorrhagic Fever (CCHF) Virus Glycoproteins. Virology Journal, 2005. 2: pp. 42
28. Shi X., van Mierlo J.T., French A., Elliott R.M. Visualizing the replication cycle of *bunyamwera orthobunyavirus* expressing fluorescent protein-tagged GC glycoprotein. The Journal of Virology, 2012. 84: pp. 8460–8469.
29. Bertolotti-Ciarlet A., Smith J., Strecker K., Paragas J., Altamura L.A., McFalls J.M., Frias-Staheli N., Garcia-Sastre A., Schmaljohn C.S., Doms R.W. Cellular Localization and Antigenic Characterization of Crimean-Congo Hemorrhagic Fever Virus Glycoproteins. Journal of Viology, 2005. 79: pp. 6152-6261
30. Burt F.J., Swanepoel R., Shieh W-J., Smith J.F., Leman P.A., Greer P.W., Coffield L.M., Rollin P.E., Ksiazek T.G., Peters C.J., Zaki S.R. Immunohistochemical and in situ Localization of Crimean-Congo Hemorrhagic Fever (CCHF) Virus in Human Tissues and Implications for CCHF Pathogenesis. Archives of Pathology and Laboratory Medicine, 1997. 121: pp. 839-846
31. Duru F., Fişgin T. Hematological Aspects of Crimean-Congo Hemorrhagic Fever. Turkish Journal of Hematology, 2009. 26: 161-166
32. Schwarz T.F., Nsanze H., Ameen A.M. Clinical Features of Crimean-Congo Haemorrhagic Fever in the United Arab Emirates. Infection, 1997. 25: pp. 364-367
33. Van Eeden P.J., van Eeden S.F., Joubert J.R., King J.B., van de Wal B.W., Michell W.L. A Nosocomial Outbreak of Crimean-Congo Haemorrhagic Fever at Tygerberg Hospital. Part II. Management of Patients. South African Medical Journal, 1985. 68: pp. 718-721
34. Tavana A.M., Tavakkoli H.R. Review on Crimean-Congo Haemorrhagic Fever in the World. International Journal of Virology, 2008. 4: pp. 26-29
35. Jabbaria A., Besharat S., Abbasi A., Moradi A., Kalavik K. Crimean-Congo Hemorrhagic Fever: Case Series from a Medical Center in Goldstan Province, Northeast of Iran. Indian Journal of Medical Science, 2004. 60: pp. 327-329
36. Swanepoel R., Gill D.E., Shepherd A.J., Leman P.A., Mynhardt J.H., Harvey S. The Clinical Pathology of Crimean-Congo Hemorrhagic Fever. Reviews of infectious diseases, 1989. 11: pp. S794-S800
37. Drönder Ergönül. Crimean-Congo Haemorrhagic Fever The Lancet Infectious Diseases, 2006. 6: pp. 203-214
38. Peters C.J., Olshaker M. Virus Hunter. Thirty Years of Battling Hot Viruses around the World. New York: Anchor Books. 1997. pp. 218-219
39. Hoogstral J. The Epidemiology of Tick-borne Crimean-Congo Haemorrhagic Fever in Asia, Europe and Africa. Journal of Medical Entomology, 1979. 15: pp. 307-314
40. Zeller H. Crimean-Congo Hemorrhagic Fever. Laboratory Diagnosis of Crimean-Congo Hemorrhagic Fever. Dordrecht: Springer Netherlands. 2007. pp. 233-243
41. Bertolotti-Ciarlet A., Smith J., Strecker K., Paragas J., Altamura L.A., McFalls J.M., Frias-Stäheli N., García-Sastre A., Schmaljohn C.S., Doms R.W. Cellular Localization and Antigenic Characterization of Crimean-Congo Hemorrhagic Fever Virus Glycoproteins. The Journal of Virology, 2005. 79: pp. 6152–6161
42. Saijo M., Qing T., Niikura M., Maeda A., Ikegami T., Sakai K., Prehaud C., Kurane I., Morikawa S. Immunofluorescence Technique Using HeLa Cells Expressing Recombinant Nucleoprotein for Detection of Immunoglobulin G Antibodies to Crimean-Congo Hemorrhagic Fever Virus. Journal of Clinical Microbiology, 2002. 40: pp. 372–375
43. Bryan J.P., Iqbal M., Ksiazek T.G., Ahmed A., Duncan J.F., Awan B., Krieg R.E., Riaz M., Leduc J.W., Nabi S., Qureshi M.S., Malik I.A., Legters L.J. Prevalence of Sand Fly Fever, West Nile, Crimean-Congo Hemorrhagic Fever and Leptospirosis antibodies in Pakistani Military Personnel. Military Medicine, 1996. 161: pp. 149-153
44. Chinikar S., Mazaheri V., Mirahmadi R., Nabeth P., Daron M.F., Salehi P., Hosseini N., Bouloy M., Mirazimi A., Lundkvist A., Nilsson M., Mehrabi-Tavana A. A Serological Survey in Suspected Human Patients of Crimean-Congo Hemorrhagic Fever in Iran by Determination of IgM-Specific ELISA Method during 2000-2004. Archives of Iranian Medicine, 2005. 8: pp. 52-55
45. Donets M.A., Rezapkin G.V., Ivanov A.P., Tkachenko E.A. Immunosorbent Assays for Diagnosis of Crimean-Congo Hemorrhagic Fever (CCHF). The American Journal of Tropical Medicine and Hygiene, 1982. 31: pp. 156-162
46. Masayuki M., Tang Q., Bawudong S., Han L., Zhang G.Y., Muer A., Dong T., Akihiko M., Ichiro K., Shigeru M. Recombinant Nucleoprotein-based Serological Diagnosis of Crimean-Congo Hemorrhagic Fever Virus Infections. Journal of Medical Virology, 2005. 75: pp. 295-299
47. Logan T.M., Linthicum K.J., Moulton J.R., Ksiazek T.G. Antigen-capture Enzyme-linked Immunosorbent Assay for Detection and Quantification of Crimean-Congo Haemorrhagic Fever virus in the Tick, Hyalomma truncatum. Journal of Virological Methods, 1993. 42: pp. 33-44
48. Karti S.S., Odabasi Z., Korten V., Yilmaz M., Sonmez M., Caylan R., Akdogan E., Eren N., Koksal I., Ovali E., Erickson B.R., Vincent M.J., Nichol S.T., Comer J.A., Rollin P.E., Ksiazek T.G. Crimean-Congo Hemorrhagic Fever in Turkey. Emerging Infectious Disease, 2004. 10: pp. 1379-1384
49. Drosten C., Gottig S., Schilling S., Asper M., Panning M., Schmitz H., Gunther S. Rapid detection and quantification of RNA of Ebola and Marburg viruses, Lassa Virus, Crimean-Congo Hemorrhagic Fever Virus, Rift Valley Fever Virus, Dengue Virus, and Yellow Fever Virus by Real-Time Reverse Transcription-PCR. Journal of Clinical Microbiology, 2002. 40: pp. 2323 - 2330
50. Bente D.A., Forrester N.L., Watts D.M., McAuley A.J., Whitehouse C.A., Bray M. Crimean-Congo hemorrhagic fever: History, epidemiology, pathogenesis, clinical syndrome and genetic diversity. Antiviral Research, 2013. 100: pp. 159–189
51. Mousavi-Jazi M., Karlberg H., Papa A., Christova I., Mirazimi A. Healthy individuals' immune response to the Bulgarian Crimean–Congo hemorrhagic fever virus vaccine. Vaccine, 2012. 30: pp. 6225–6229.
52. Whitehouse, C. A. Crimean-Congo Hemorrhagic Fever. Antiviral Research, 2004. 64: pp. 145-160
53. Huggins J.W. Prospects for Treatment of Viral Hemorrhagic Fevers with Ribavirin, a Broad-Spectrum Antiviral Drug. Reviews of Infectious Diseases, 1989. 11: S750-S761
54. Gear J.H.S., Thomson P.D., Ledger J., Berkowitz F.E. Congo-Crimean Haemorrhagic Fever in South Africa: Report of a Fatal Case in Transvaal. South African Medical Journal, 1982. 62: pp. 576-580
55. Vassilenko S.M., Vassilev T.L., Bozadjiev L.G., Bineva I.L., Kazarov G.Z. Specific Intravenous Immunoglobulin for Crimean-Congo Haemorrhagic Fever. Lancet, 1990. 8692: pp. 791 – 792
56. Vassilev T., Valchev V., Kazarov G., Razsukanova L., Vitanov. A Reference Preparation for Human Immunoglobulin against Crimean/Congo Hemorrhagic Fever. Journal of the International Association of Biological Standardization, 1991. 19: pp. 57

Photo Bibliography

Figure 1.3-1: Negatively-stained transmission electron micrograph (TEM) of numerous California encephalitis virus virions in the family *Bunyaviridae*. Photo was taken at 80,000x magnification by Dr. Fred Murphy and Dr. Erskine Palmer of the CDC in 1975. Public domain photo

Figure 1.3-6: Virus graphics is produced by Los Alamos National Laboratory and National Institute of Allergy and Infectious Diseases. Public domain photo

Figure 1.3-6: Genomic protein graphics produced and released by the National Institute of Health (NIH). Public domain photo

Figure 1.3-7: Under Wilder's reticulin-stained photomicrograph demonstrates the cytoarchitectural changes found in a liver tissue specimen extracted from a Congo/Crimean hemorrhagic fever patient. This micrograph depicts a thickening and disassociation or the fibers of the reticular network. Photo was taken in 1980 by Dr. Yves Robin and Dr. Jean Renaudet, Arbovirus Laboratory at the Pasteur Institute in Dakar, Senegal of the World Health Organization. Public domain photo

Figure 1.3-8: Hematoxylin-eosin-stained (H&E) photomicro-graph demonstrates the coagulation necrosis of hepatocytes with an associated perifocal inflammatory reaction in a liver tissue specimen extracted from a Congo/Crimean hemorrhagic fever patient. In addition several cells can be seen to be undergoing fatty degeneration. Photo was taken in 1980 by Dr. Yves Robin and

Dr. Jean Renaudet, Arbovirus Laboratory at the Pasteur Institute in Dakar, Senegal of the World Health Organization. Public domain photo

Figure 1.3-9: Female patient with Crimean-Congo hemorrhagic fever. Note the ecchymoses located on her arms. Photo was taken by Dr. B.E. Henderson of the CDC in 1969. Public domain photo

Figure 1.3-10: Male patient with Crimean-Congo hemorrhagic fever. Note the ecchymoses located on the right antibrachial region. Photo was taken by Dr. B.E. Henderson of the CDC in 1969. Public domain photo

Figure 1.3-11: Male patient with Crimean-Congo hemorrhagic fever. Note the consumptive coagulopathy. Photo was taken by Dr. B.E. Henderson of the CDC in 1969. Public domain photo

The Dengue fever virus belongs to the genus *Flavivirus* in the family *Flaviviridae*. Dengue fever virus is a small positive-sense, single stranded RNA, enveloped virus possessing a polyhedral capsid. The word dengue is generally thought to be derived from the Swahili word "Ki-denga pepo" which describes a cramp-like seizure that is caused by an evil spirit.

There are four closely related but antigenically distinct serotypes of dengue fever viruses (DENV 1 to 4) with the main reservoir being humans (Figure 1.4-1).[1]

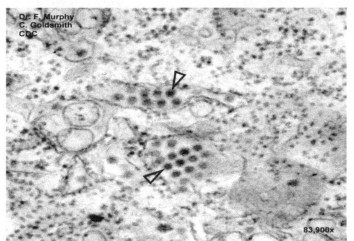

Figure 1.4-1: Transmission electron micrograph (TEM) of Dengue virus (round particles indicated by blue arrows) in hepatocytes of the human liver

Each serotype of Dengue fever virus is capable of producing a wide spectrum of clinical manifestations ranging from a self-limiting febrile illness known as Dengue fever (DF) to the more severe Dengue hemorrhagic fever (DHF).[2] Please examine Figure 1.4-2 for information regarding the various manifestations of Dengue virus infection.

DHF is characterized by hemorrhage, thrombocytopenia, as well as, hypovolemia where plasma has leaked into the interstitial space. It has been reported that patients suffering from hypovolemia may also deteriorate into circulatory collapse.

DHF is categorized into 4 grades: from less severe, grade 1, to most severe, grade 4. Patients suffering from DHF grades 3 and 4 may exhibit signs of plasma leakage so severe that shock occurs. This extremely serious condition is also referred to as dengue shock syndrome (DSS) (Table 1).[2, 3]

Table 1: Grading of Severity for DHF

Grade	Symptoms
Grade 1	Fever accompanied by non-specific symptoms. Hemorrhagic manifestations only appear after a tourniquet test and/or easy bruising
Grade 2	Along with symptoms of Grade 1 with additional symptoms of spontaneous bleeding via the skin
Grade 3	Circulatory failure with a rapid, weak pulse and narrowing of pressure of hypotension with defervescence
Grade 4	Profound shock with barely detectable blood pressure

DENV serotypes 1 to 4 are responsible for epidemics and pandemics that have occurred in approximately 100 countries throughout recent history.[4] In nature, the virus is transmitted to humans via a mosquito vector such as *Aedes aegypti* and to a lesser extent, *Ae. albopictus, Ae. polynesiensis*, and *Ae. scutellaris*. At present, the sylvatic cycle of dengue transmission to human infection is unknown (Figure 1.4-3).

Historical reports of Dengue-like symptoms date back to the Chin, Tang and Northern Sung Dynasties in China, later reports of similar outbreaks are found in Panama in 1699, while the first actual case report of the disease occurred in 1779-1780 involving epidemics occurring almost simultaneously in Africa, Asia and North America.[5, 6, 7, 8]

In 1789, Dr. Benjamin Rush (1745-1813), in his effort to name and describe the symptoms of the disease, coined the term "breakbone fever."[9] Soon after World War II, a pandemic of DF broke out of its previously set geographical boundaries and spread around the world. It is assumed that technological improvements in air and sea transportation allowed the virus and its vector, the mosquito, to spread rapidly, with the assistance of human population (Figure 1.4-4).

Presently, it is estimated that 50 to 100 million cases of dengue fever occur annually and approximately 500,000 cases develop into life-threatening DHF or DSS. Among the patients that developed DHF and DSS, an estimated 2.5% of the cases are fatal, while 95% occur in children under the age of 15.[10]

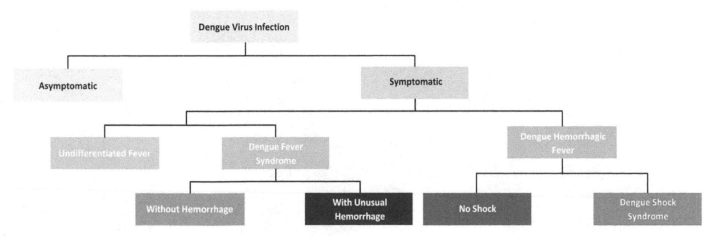

Figure 1.4-2: Diagrammatic displays of various manifestations of DENV Infection

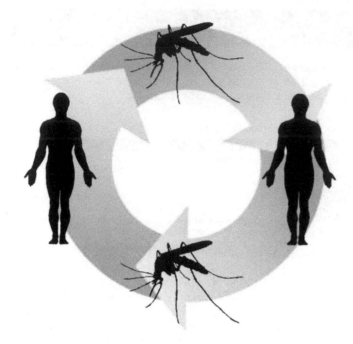

Figure 1.4-3: Transmission cycle of Dengue Fever virus. The viruses are efficiently transmitted between mosquitoes and humans without the need for an enzootic amplification host. Nonetheless, at present the sylvatic cycle of dengue transmission to human infection is unknown

The RNA genome of DENV (serotypes 1 to 4) consists of a single open reading frame, which is translated as a single, long polyprotein, cleaved by viral and host proteases to yield the 10 viral proteins. The viral proteins produced consist of structural proteins, such as the capsid (C), membrane (prM) and envelope (E) proteins, as well as, seven non-structural proteins NS1, NS2A, NS2B, NS3, NS4A, NS4B and NS5.[11]

DENV (serotypes 1 to 4) is introduced cutaneously, after a mosquito blood meal. It is commonly accepted that the replication of virus begins when the DENV viron infects a permissive host cell of the mononuclear lineage, such as dendritic cells, monocytes and/or macrophages, although other cells such as lymphocytes, endothelial cells, hepatocytes, neuronal cells and cells of the bone marrow have been shown to be susceptible to viral propagation in vitro. Viremia is generally detected 6-8 hours preceding the onset of symptoms.[10, 12, 13, 14, 15]

DENV gains entry into susceptible host cells via clatherin-mediated endocytosis.[16] Clathrin-mediated endocytosis involves internalization of the DENV viron through a clathrin-coated cellular membrane pit and buds into the cytosol via an early endosome to late endosome and a lysosome.[16, 17, 18] Various host cell receptors have been proposed to contribute DENV entry into the host cell. These receptors include heparin-sulfate, CD14, heat shock proteins 70 and 90 (HSP 70, HSP 90), GRP78/BiP, 37-kDa/67-kDa high affinity laminin receptor, liver/lymph node-specific ICAM-3-grabbing nonintegrin and dendritic cell-specific ICAN-3 grabbing nonintegrin (DC-SIGN).[19, 20, 21, 22, 23, 24, 25, 26, 27, 28]

Out of all the potential cell membrane receptors, DC-SIGN has been reported to be able to mediate infections in all four serotypes of DENV. In addition, the propensity of ectopic expression of DC-SIGN renders many other cell lines infectable by DENV.[29, 30] Research has demonstrated that DENV viral E glycoprotein, organized in 90 homodimers on the surface of the virion, binds to DC-SIGN through the addition of high-mannose glycans to residue N67 and thus gains entry to the host cell.[28, 29] Other research has proposed that the receptor-mediated endocytosis of DENV involves two or more receptors, such as a DC-SIGN that initially captures and increases the local concentration of the virus at the cell surface while a second high affinity receptor (presently unknown) mediates internalization of the virion.[31]

The E glycoprotein of DENV is comprised of three domains. Domain 1 is a centrally located β barrel which is a large beta-sheet that twists to create a closed structure where the first strand is hydrogen bonded to the last strand. Domain 2 contains

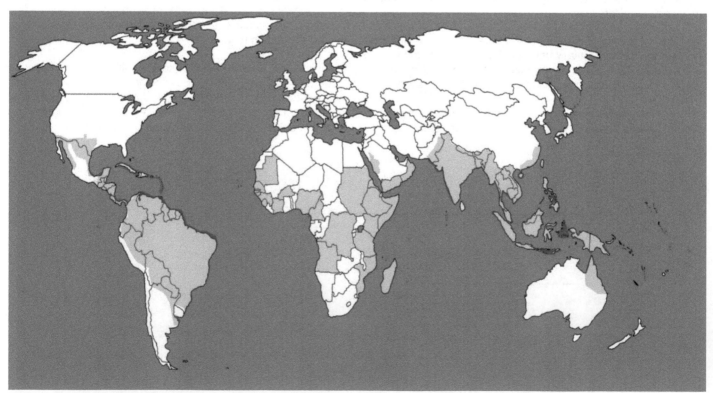

Figure 1.4-4: Areas that are in risk of Dengue and Dengue Hemorrhagic Fever

a dimerization region and the fusion peptide while Domain 3 is responsible for receptor binding. In the mature DENV virion, the E proteins exist as homodimers where domain 2 is inaccessible.

Once endocytized into the host cell, the low pH of the endosomes causes the E protein to undergo trimerization, thereby exposing the fusion peptide of domain 2, mediating endosomal fusion with viral capsid and the subsequent release of the viral genome into the cytoplasm of the host cell.[32, 33, 34, 35]

Once the DENV genome gains entry into the cytoplasm, the positive sense viral RNA genome immediately undergoes translation to generate viral RNA replicase enzyme that initiates the infection. The translation of the DENV genome is initiated when the small ribosomal subunit locates the initiation codon. The DENV genome, like the genome of other positive sense viruses, is similar in structure to host cellular mRNA. The DENV genome possesses a 5' type 1, 7-methyl guanosine cap, 5' untranslated region, a single open reading frame, and a 3' untranslated region. The only notable exception is that the DENV genome does not possess a polyadenylated (poly-A) tail. It is presumed that with the absence of a poly-A tail, DENV does not use the same mechanism for translation as cellular mRNAs, although the exact mechanisms remain to be elucidated. Nonetheless, translation and replication of positive sense RNA viruses occur in association with the membrane structures of the host cell's rough endoplasmic reticulum (rER) (Figure 1.4-5).[14]

It has been reported that both co- and post-translational cleaving during the formation of the DENV polyprotein is completed through a combination of signal peptidases, viral serine proteases (NS2B and NS3 forms a cofactor that forms NS2B-NS3 protease complex) and various host cellular proteases.[14, 36] For example, DENV nonstructural proteins NS2A-NS2B, NS2B-NS3, NS3-NS4A, and NS4B-NS5 are cleaved by the NS2B-NS3 protease complex. The cleavage between NS4A-NS4B, as well as, structural proteins C and prM, involves both the protease complex and the host cell endoplasmic reticulum (ER) signalase. The cleavage of prM-E involves host enzymes, furin-like Golgi protease and ER signalase, while the cleavage between E-NS1 and NS1-NS2A requires only ER signalase.[36, 37, 38, 39]

NS1 (~48 kDa) is a glycoprotein that can be detected in the cytoplasm and the plasma membrane of infected cells. This glycoprotein is also secreted in a soluble form (sNS1) that is found in the circulatory system of patients where the amounts detected correlates with increased severity of DENV infection. It has been reported that the immuno-recognition of NS1 located on the plasma membrane of infected cells serves an important part of the mechanism that triggers vascular leakage during severe DENV infection. Furthermore, it is believed that the interactions between NS1 and NS4A are responsible for RNA-dependent RNA polymerase (RdRP) function during replication. Nonetheless, the exact manner by which NS1 becomes associated with the plasma membrane or the exact nature of its function (s) remains to be elucidated.[40, 41, 42, 43]

As mentioned previously, NS2B (~14 kDa) has been reported to form a stable complex with NS3 to act as a cofactor for NS2B-3 serine protease to form the NS2B-NS3 protease complex. This protease complex has been shown to mediate cleavage activities at various junctions of structural and nonstructural proteins.[36, 37, 38]

NS3 (70kDa) has been reported to be a multifunctional protein. NS3 possesses 5'-terminal RNA triphosphatase (RTPase) activity where it has been suggested to perform dephosphorylation of the 5'-end of the viral RNA genome prior to the addition of the 5'-cap. In addition, at the C terminal, NS3 also possesses a coupled nucleoside 5'-triphospha-tase (NTPase) activity that provides the necessary energy for RNA unwinding actions of the helicase.[40, 41]

NS4B (~27 kDa) has been reported to interact with NS3 and NS5A and plays a role in viral RNA replication where it presumably induces morphological changes in the ER membrane. Nonetheless, its exact function remains unknown.[40]

Little is known about the individual protein functions of NS2A (~22 kDa), NS4A (~16 kDa) and NS4B although they are

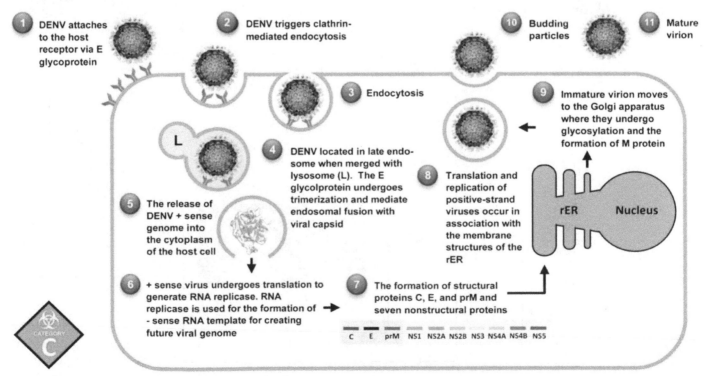

Figure 1.4-5: Diagrammatic process of DENV infection within a host cell

believed to contribute to the inhibition of the interferon alpha/beta response of the infected host cell. Through the examination of another flavivirus, Kunjin virus, NS2As are localized to the sites of RNA synthesis and may coordinate the shift between RNA packaging and RNA replication. During reverse genetic and localization studies with DENV replicons, NS4A and NS4B have been demonstrated to be necessary for DENV replication. Experimental evidence showed that NS4B modulates DENV replication via an interaction with helicase domain of NS3 while NS4A appears to play a role in the induction of host cellular membrane alterations that may serve as a scaffold to anchor the viral replication complex.[40]

NS5 (103 kDa) is the largest of the DENV nonstructural proteins that possesses RdRp activities in its C terminal domain and in its N terminal, (guanine-N7) - methyltransferase and nucleoside-2'-O methyltransferase activities that are required for sequential methylation of 5' end cap structure of the flavivirus RNA.[44] Please examine Figure 1.4-6 for a summary of DENV nonstructural proteins and their function.

After the DENV positive-sense genome has undergone the translation process, the virus switches to the production of viral RNA, which involves the formation of a negative-sense strand template for the generation of viral genomic RNA (positive-sense) strands.[45, 46]

The addition of the RNA cap is a critical process for the DENV genome. This RNA cap allows the viral RNA to be efficiently translated by the cellular translational machinery, as well as, providing protection from the exonucleases of host cells during forthcoming infections. DENV genomic RNA is modified at the 5' end to generate a type 1 cap structure (me^7-GpppA-me^2) through the enzymatic actions of RNA triphosphatase (RTPase) which is found within the helicase domain of NS3 and guanylyltransferase (Gtase), 2'-O methyl-transferase (2'-OMTase) and N7-methyltransferase (Guanine-N7-Mtase) which are located on the N-terminal capping enzyme domain of NS5. Please note that the C-terminal domain of the NS5 functions as the DENV RNA dependent RNA polymerase.[47]

Finally, the immature virus particles move to the Golgi apparatus where they undergo glycosylation. During the latter part of the maturation process, the DENV prM is processed to form M proteins through the enzymatic actions of furin within the trans-Golgi compartment. The formation of the M proteins marks the generation of matured DENV virion, which is subsequently released via secretory vesicle.[14, 45, 46]

In individuals infected with DF, both innate and adaptive immune responses play a role in combating the viral infection. For example, elevated levels of interferon-gamma (IFN-γ), tumor necrotic factor alpha (TNF-α), soluble tumor necrotic factor receptors (sTNFRs), soluble interleukin-2 receptors, CD4, CD8, interleukin-8 and interleukin-2 are released by activated T-lymphocytes which have a positive correlation with the severity of the disease.[48, 49, 50] Cytokines, such as TNF-α, interleukin-1β (IL-1β) and interleukin-6 (IL-6), have been associated with both

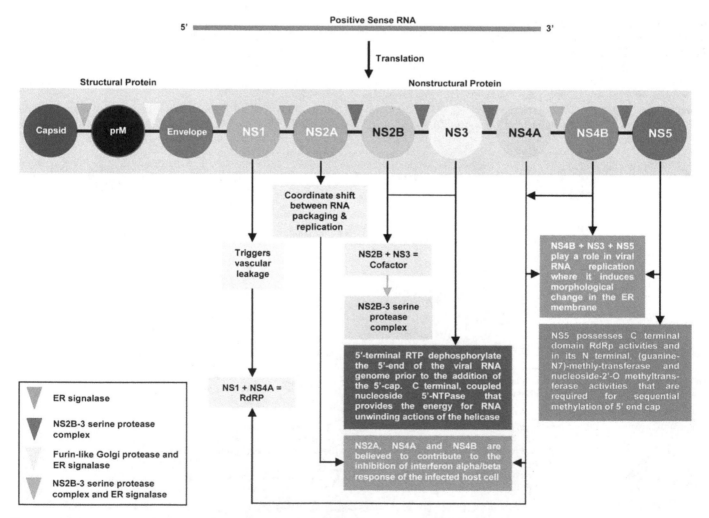

Figure 1.4-6: Protein products of DENV. A summary of structural and nonstructural proteins and their functions

coagulation and fibrinolysis activation. It has been shown that this activation is more pronounced in patients with the severe clinical manifestations of DHF and DSS.[10, 51, 52, 53, 54]

Reports have shown that some inflammatory mediators, such as IL-1β, IFN-γ, interleukin-4 (IL-4), IL-6, interleukin-13 (IL-13), interleukin-7 (IL-7) and granulocyte-monocyte colony-stimulating factor (GM-CSF) were significantly increased in patients with severe dengue infection, when compared to those found in individuals suffering from the mild form of the disease. Additionally, IL-1β, IL-8, chemokine (C-C motif) ligand 5 (RANTES), sTNFRs, TNF-α and monocyte chemoattractant protein type 1 (MCP-1), as well as, complement activation may cause plasma leakage and were also associated with thrombocytopenia leading to shock and bleeding in the severe form of the disease.[50, 55, 56, 57, 58] Increased MCP-1 and GM-CSF levels correlated with hypotension in DHF patients. In contrast, levels of macrophage inflammatory protein (MIP-1β), which is produced by human monocytes, dendritic cells, NK cells and lymphocytes, increased in patients with mild dengue.[10, 51]

Alibek (1999) reported that the Biopreparat of the Soviet Union had conducted research to genetically alter Dengue Fever Virus in an effort to heighten its infectivity, whereby paving the way for the development of pathogens capable of overcoming potential vaccines.[59] Nonetheless, recent experiments have shown that this virus is not transmissible in small-particle aerosol form, therefore, it is not considered to be a primary threat as a biological weapon.[60, 61]

SYMPTOMS

Symptoms of the dengue fever are dependent on the age of the victim. Infants and children often develop an undifferentiated febrile disease coupled with maculopapular rash, while older children and adults may either develop a mild febrile symptom or the classic incapacitating disease.[62]

On average, dengue fever (DF) infections in older children and adults last approximately 6-7 days, with a 5-10 day incubation period. The initial symptoms of DF is a sudden onset of high fever (~40°C or ~104°F) which generally lasts 2-7 days. The fever is followed by an afebrile period that varies with the patient and then an additional 1-2 days of high fever. The second period of high fever is also accompanied by severe headaches, myalgia (aches in the lumbar, legs and joints), fatigue, arthralgia, lymphoedema, retro-orbital pains on eye movement, conjunctival injection, macular hemorrhages, as well as, red petechial rash that generally appears on the lower limbs and chest, although in some cases, the rash spreads thorough out the body.[63, 64] In addition, clinicians often observe that the patient's pulse is slow in comparison to the temperature exhibited.

Photophobia accompanied by puffy eye lids, as well as, enlarged lymph nodes are also common.[65] Other symptoms include nausea, vomiting, loss of appetite, abdominal pains, chills and diarrhea, with marked signs of gastritis. Bouts of extreme exhaustion and bradycardia are commonly seen in patients that display the symptoms described above and may last for months after initial onset of the disease.[66, 67]

Laboratory indications including leucopenia, thrombocytopenia and mild elevations in serum hepatic transaminases concentrations are commonly observed, while in some cases non-hemoconcentration bleeding, such as epistaxis, gingival bleeding, gastrointestinal bleeding, hematuria and menorrhagia are reported (Table 2).[68, 69]

Transplacental infections of the fetus in pregnant women do occur on rare occasions, but it is believed that the protective antibodies developed by the mother do provide the fetus with sufficient immune protection on most occasions, at least until birth.[69] It has been reported that children born to dengue-immune mothers have a great risk of developing DHF. This high proportion of children suffering from DHF is believed to be caused by a condition known as antibody-dependent enhancement (ADE).[70, 71, 72]

Table 2: An overview of the clinical symptoms of DF

Symptoms	+	++	+++
Biphasic high fever			■
Severe headaches			■
Myalgia			■
Fatigue			■
Arthralgia			■
Lymphedema			■
Retro-orbital pains			■
Red petechial rash			■
Maculopapular rash			■
Conjunctival injection		■	
Photophobia		■	
Enlarged lymph nodes		■	
Nausea		■	
Vomiting		■	
Loss of appetite		■	
Abdominal pains		■	
Chills		■	
Diarrhea		■	
Extreme exhaustion		■	
Bradycardia		■	
Leucopenia		■	
Thrombocytopenia		■	
Epistaxis	■		
Gingival bleeding	■		
Gastrointestinal bleeding	■		
Hematuria	■		
Menorrhagia	■		

+ Rare ++ Common +++ Frequent

It is known that the maternal anti-dengue antibodies can cross the placenta and protect the infants from dengue infection at birth, however, with time, the maternal antibody concentration will steadily decrease until about the third month postnatal when the infant will start producing their own antibodies. If this infant is subsequently (secondarily) infected with dengue viruses of a different serotype, the pre-existing non-neutralizing heterotypic antibodies to different dengue serotype that was acquired from the mother will actually enhance the entry and replication of the virus in macrophages in the phenomenon of ADE, which leads to a more serious form the disease.[71, 72] Please examine Table 3 for more information in regards to the symptoms of DHF.

As stated previously, in some cases patients suffering from DF develop much milder symptoms, where with the exception of fever, no other symptoms appear. In these rare occurrences the patients are generally misdiagnosed as having the flu or another similar viral infection. Due to this misdiagnosis, these patients are not isolated form the general population thereby allowing the possibility of transmitting the infection, through mosquito bites or by contaminated blood, to others.[6] Nonetheless, the fatality rate of DF is calculated to be less than 1%. Patients suffering from DF generally recover within six or seven days and are immune to the particular serotype of dengue virus that caused the infection. However, if the patient is subsequently infected by another serotype of DENV, the individual may develop a second, more deadly type of infection, known as Dengue Hemorrhagic Fever (DHF).[73]

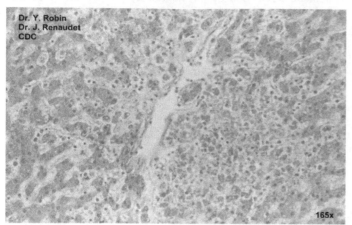

Figure 1.4-7: Hematoxylin-eosin-stained (H&E) photomicro-graph shows the cytoarchitectural changes found in a liver tissue specimen extracted from a Dengue hemorrhagic fever patient in Thailand. This particular view reveals mid-lobular necrosis, with accompanying acidophilic degeneration, and moderate hypertrophy of Kupffer cells

DHF occurs when the DF patients are subsequently infected by another serotype of dengue fever virus. The initial symptoms includes sudden onset of high fever (~40°C, ~104°F), headaches (although less severe in comparison with people suffering from DF), hemorrhagic phenomena associated with easy bruising and bleeding at venipuncture sites. Hepatomegaly is also a frequent symptom of DHF. Histological examination of liver biopsy samples typically shows acidophilic degeneration and necrosis (Figure 1.4-7). Soon after the onset of initial symptoms, patients generally experience circulatory failure which last 2 to 7 days. During this time, patients may become either lethargic or restless. They may also exhibit a rapid but weak pulse, hypotension, displaying signs of acute abdominal pain, possessing cold extremities, as well as, suffering from oliguria.[71, 73]

The critical stage of DHF occurs at the end of febrile stage, when the patient will experience defervescence (a rapid drop in core temperature). This afebrile stage will last approximately 24 hours as the patients' temperature gradually increases to normal range. During this time, patients will generally develop signs of hemo-concentration and petechiae rash, lesions appearing purple in coloration, as well as, ecchymosis (subcutaneous purpura larger than one centimeter in diameter).[74]

During the 24 hours after defervescence the disease is marked by hemorrhagic manifestations and thrombocytopenia (<100,000/

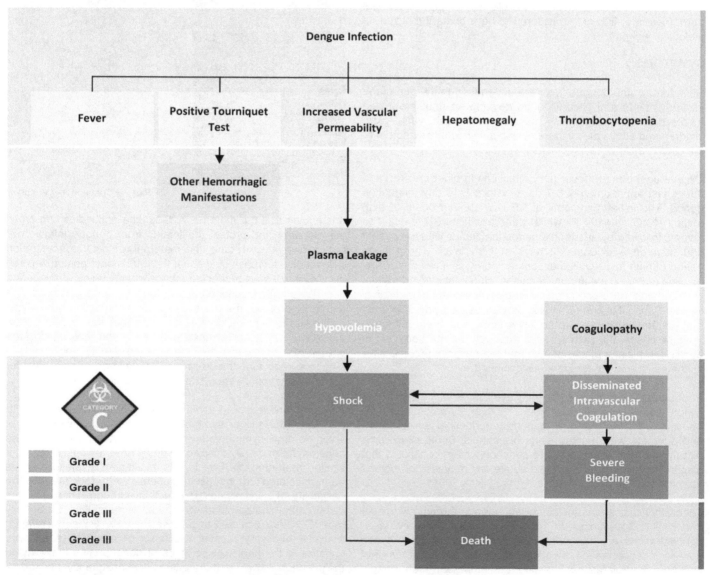

Figure 1.4-9: Diagrammatic display of various manifestation of DHF and DSS

mm³). The capillaries of the patients will become highly permeable (vascular permeability) and the skin of patents is easily bruised. Additionally, patients will suffer from nose and gums bleed, as well as, showing signs of internal bleeding (Figure 1.4-8). The signs of internal bleeding include a rise in hematocrit which may lead to bleeding diathesis or disseminated intravascular coagulation (DIC). It has been reported that patients will also demonstrate low serum total protein level and low albumin concentration.[75, 76]

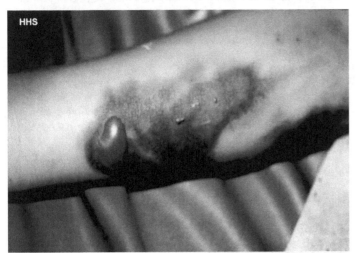

Figure 1.4-8: A patient suffering from Dengue Hemorrhagic Fever demonstrates a large subcutaneous hemorrhage on the arm

Table 3: An overview of the clinical symptoms of DHF

Symptoms	+	++	+++
High fever			■
Headaches			■
Easy bruising			■
Venipuncture			■
Hepatomegaly			■
Circulatory failures			■
Lethargic			■
Restless			■
Rapid but weak pulse			■
Hypotension			■
Acute abdominal pain			■
Cold extremities			■
Oliguria			■
Defervescence			■
Hemo-concentration			■
Petechiae rash			■
Ecchymosis			■
Thrombocytopenia			■
Rise in hematocrit			■
Bleeding diathesis		■	
Intravascular coagulation		■	
Epistaxis		■	
Gastrointestinal hemorrhages		■	
Hematuria		■	
Pleural effusions	■		
Pneumonitis	■		
Hemoptysis	■		
Pulmonary hemorrhages	■		
Acute respiratory distress	■		
Shock	■		

+ Rare ++ Common +++ Frequent

Other symptoms include epistaxis, gastro-intestinal hemorrhages and hematuria. Rare cases of pleural effusions, pneumonitis, hemoptysis, pulmonary hemorrhages and shock have been described.[75, 76] A single case of a DHF patient developing pulmonary hemorrhages and subsequently acute respiratory distress syndrome (ARDS) was reported by Setlik et al. (2004).[65] It has been estimated that the mortality rates associated with DHF are estimated to be 10% to 30% (Table 3).[73]

Despite hospitalization and intensive supportive health management, approximately 20-30% of the DHF cases develop Dengue shock syndrome (DSS) which leads to multisystem failures and death.[77] If the correct treatments are not administered at this stage, patients will proceed into shock where their pulse and blood pressure become barely detectable. Patients generally expire within 12 to 24 hours after proceeding into DSS. The mortality rates for DSS varies from 10% to 30%.[78] Please examine Figure 1.4-9 for an overview of various manifestations of DHF and DSS.

It has been reported by Kalayanarooj et al. (2007) that the severity of DHF seems to be directly linked to the ABO blood type of the individual. In their study, they have shown that individuals with blood type AB will suffer the most severe case of DHF. Presently, the exact manner of this correlation has yet to be further elucidated.[79]

DETECTION

The detection of DF is generally made clinically by assessing various physical and physiological conditions described in the previous section. Similarly, the detection of DHF is also made through clinical assessments while other examinations can be employed to detect the hemorrhagic tendencies of this disease.

For example, the tourniquet test is used to demonstrate the easy bruising of DHF patients. In addition, patients demonstrating bleeding at venipuncture sites can also be used to indicate possible DHF infections.[79] Further examinations for signs of thrombocytopenia and changes in the hematocrit levels can also reveal DHF infections. For example, an examination of blood platelet and hematocrit levels could be performed between the third and eighth day of the infection. If the blood platelet count drops below 100,000 per mm³ and the patient's blood demonstrates a rise in the hematocrit levels (demonstrating plasma leakage) it is highly possible that the individual is affected by the disease. White blood cell counts vary between leucopenia and leukocytosis during the early stages of infection. Nonetheless, nearing the end of the febrile phase, a sudden drop in leukocyte count (especially the numbers of neutrophils) is almost always observed. However, immediately before the onset of shock, a sudden onset of lymphocytosis, with the presence of atypical lymphocytes, is similarly almost always observed. At the initial stage of shock, assay for coagulation factors will show a marked reduction of fibrinogen, prothrombin, factor VII, factor XII, and antithrombin III. In severe cases of shock, liver dysfunction is followed by a notable drop in vitamin K dependent factors V, VII, IX and X which of course marks the impairment of platelet functions.[80, 81] Please examine Table 1 for more information in regards to the different grades of severity of DHF and Figure 1.4-10 for more information regarding the reduction of coagulation factors during initial stages of shock and severe shock.

Unfortunately, the initial onset of Dengue virus infection is similar to flu-like conditions, where symptoms may vary from patient to patient. Therefore, the clinical diagnosis methods for the disease are rather time consuming, making early detection of the disease nearly impossible because they are seldom fully employed.

In recent years, various detection methods have been made available in an effort to accurately detect DF and DHF in order to commence the appropriate series of treatments. For example, antibodies such as IgM, IgG and hemagglutination-inhibiting antibodies can be detected through antibody-capture enzyme-linked immunesorbent assay (MAC-ELISA). It has been reported that 50% of patients will suffer from primary dengue fever symptoms while the remaining 50% of the patients will display signs of anti-dengue antibodies within 2-3 days after defervescence.[82]

Diagnostic tests based on the detection of DENV Non Structural Protein 1 (NS1) antigen and IgM Capture ELISA assays are presently commercially available (e.g. Panbio Dengue Early NS1 and IgM Capture ELISA assays). However, a recent study completed in eight Indonesia cities demonstrated a relatively low sensitivity of detection for DENV. It is postulated by the researchers that the low sensitivity of NS1 antigen detection is not related to the genetic diversity of the NS1. Instead, it is believed that the performance of the antigen test was directly influenced by the "infection status of patients and geographical origin of samples."[83]

Other detection methods for detecting DENV utilizes reverse transcription-polymerase chain reaction (RT-PCR) have been successfully developed to detect the RNA genome of the DENV.[84] For example, the CDC Real Time RT-PCR assay have been shown to detect DENV in most cases during the first 5 days of the infection. This RT-PCR DENV assay has since been distributed to most domestic and international health agencies.[84, 85, 86]

Presently, experiments involving monoclonal antibodies designed to detect dengue E and NS-1 proteins are being performed, but are still unavailable outside of experimental laboratories. These methods involve in situ hybridization and/or immunocytochemistry, they are theoretically more sensitive and could dramatically change the detection methods of this disease.[87, 88]

TREATMENT

There are no commercially available vaccines for treating DF and/or DHF. Nonetheless, in 2012 the results of a Phase IIB clinical trial of a DENV vaccine were published. The results demonstrated a prospect of a preventive vaccine that in immunogenic for all four DENV serotypes and protected individuals from DENV serotypes 1, 3, and 4.[89]

Presently, there are no effective antiviral medications for treating DF or DHF, therefore the basis of treatment is mainly supportive therapy. During the febrile phase of the infection, paracetamol may be cautiously used to reduce fevers over 39°C (102.2 °F). Please examine Table 4 for information regarding age and dosing.[90]

Table 4: Paracetamol dosage per age groups[90]

Age of Patient (years)	Paracetamol
Less than 1	60 mg/dose
1-3	60-120 mg/dose
3-6	120 mg/dose
6-12	240 mg/dose

Clinicians may also prescribe acetaminophen to combat fever and inflammatory symptoms, aspirin and non-steroid anti-inflammatory drugs should be avoided. Aspirin is known to

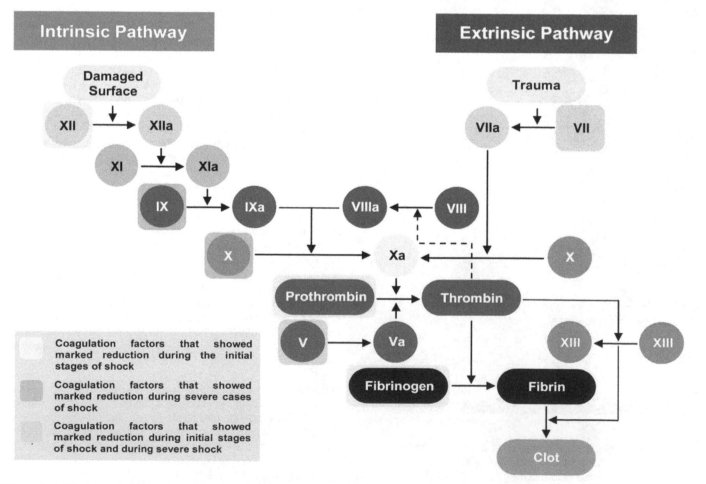

Figure 1.4-10: Diagrammatic display showing various reductions of coagulation factors during initial stages of shock and severe shock

reduce the concentration of prothrombin in plasma and acts as an anticoagulant. Therefore, it is essential that aspirin is not administered to the patients, since it may promote internal hemorrhages in patients. In addition, NSAIDS, such as non-acetylated medications and cox-2 inhibitors are also known to show similar effects as aspirin should also be avoided. In an effort to prevent secondary infections, broad spectrum antibiotics may be administered.[90]

Patients suffering an increase in hemo-concentration or loss of plasma from increase in vascular permeability will require continuous intake of fluids orally and/or intravenously to prevent dehydration. Oral intake of fruit juice is preferable to water, because it replaces both lost fluids and electrolytes of the patient. Careful observations should be made of the patient for any sign of DSS. The most important period to watch for DSS occurs on the third day, when the patient transitions from febrile to afebrile phase of the disease. Excessive loss of plasma, if uncorrected, will result in anoxia, metabolic acidosis and eventually death.[91] Judicious management of fluid replacement is required and careful monitoring of the volume and rate of plasma loss for each and every patient. Rates of fluid loss can be accessed by monitoring the changes in the hematocrit, vital signs or volume of urine output. Please examine Table 5 for calculations of intravenous infusion based upon body weight.

Table 5: Intravenous infusion of fluids for patients suffering from DHF[91]

Body Weight (Kg)	Volume of Fluids (ml) per 24 hours
10	100/kg
10-20	1000 + 50 for each kg over 10 kg
Over 20	1500 + 20 for each kg over 20 kg

Patients showing symptoms of thrombocytopenia will require platelet transfusions when the platelet count falls below 50,000 per mm^3 with signs of hemorrhage and bleeding or 20,000 per mm^3 without hemorrhage or bleeding.[79]

The mortality rate of treated DHF, as well as DSS, is approximately 3% while the mortality rate of untreated DHF and DSS is approximately 50%.[92]

DIFFERENTIAL DIAGNOSIS

The differential diagnosis during the early stage of the infection for DF may be confused with numerous other viral (e.g. flu), bacterial and parasitic infections. One of these viral infections is Chikungunya fever (CHIKVF) which is extremely difficult to clinically differentiate with DF without laboratory analysis.[92] Please examine Table 6 for a comparison between non-specific symptoms observed in DHF/DSS and CHIKVF.

Table 6: Comparison of nonspecific symptoms observed in early stages of Dengue hemorrhagic fever (DF) and Chikungunya fever (CHIKF)[93]

Symptoms	DHF (%)	CHIKVF (%)
Injected pharynx	96.8	90.3
Vomiting	57.9	59.4
Constipation	53.5	40.0
Abdominal pain	50.0	31.6
Headache	44.6	68.4
General lymphadenopathy	40.5	30.8
Conjunctival injection	32.8	55.6
Cough	21.5	23.3
Rhinitis	12.8	6.5
Maculopapular rash	12.1	59.4
Myalgia/arthralgia	12.0	40.0
Enanthema	8.3	11.1
Abdominal reflex	6.7	0.0
Diarrhea	67.4	15.6
Palpable spleen	6.3	3.1
Coma	3.0	0.0

Unfortunately, laboratory analysis may take up to four days to determine and this diagnostic delay may prove to be fatal for the patient. Because of the delay in diagnosis or misdiagnosis, these

Table 8 – An overview of the possible differential diagnosis of Dengue Fever (DF). Note: Chikungunya Virus (CHIKV), O'nyong-nyong Fever (ONNF), West Nile Fever (WNF), Parvovirus (PV), Hepatitis A (HAV), Hepatitis B (HBV)

Symptoms	DHF	CHIKV	ONNF	WNF	Sindbis	Rubella	PV	HAV	HBV
Biphasic high fever	■	■							
Chills	■	■	■	■	■				
Severe headaches	■	■	■	■	■	■	■	■	■
Myalgia	■	■	■	■	■			■	
Fatigue	■	■	■	■			■	■	■
Arthralgia	■	■	■	■	■	■	■		■
Lympoedema	■	■							
Abdominal pains	■								
Nausea	■			■	■			■	■
Vomiting	■	■	■	■	■			■	■
Diarrhea	■								
Loss of appetite	■								
Photophobia	■								
Conjunctival injection	■	■							
Retro-orbital pains	■								
Red petechial rash	■	■							
Maculopapular rash	■	■							
Enlarged lymph	■	■							
Extreme exhaustion	■	■							
Bradycardia	■								
Leucopenia	■								
Thrombocytopenia	■								
Epistaxis	■	■							
Gingival bleeding	■	■							
Gastrointestinal bleeding	■	■							
Hematuria	■								

Table 9 – An overview of the possible differential diagnosis of Dengue Hemorrhagic Fever (DHF). Note: Chikungunya Virus (CHIKV), Crimean–Congo hemorrhagic fever (CCHF), Hantavirus hemorrhagic fever (HFRS), Lassa fever (LF), Ebola hemorrhagic fever (EHF), Marburg hemorrhagic fever (MHF)

Symptoms	DHF	CHIKV	CCHF	HFRS	LF	EHF	MHF
High fever	■	■	■	■	■	■	■
Headaches	■	■	■	■	■	■	■
Easy bruising	■		■	■	■	■	■
Bleeding at puncture sites	■		■	■	■	■	■
Hepatomegaly	■				■		
Circulatory failures	■						
Lethargic	■					■	
Restless	■						
Rapid but weak pulse	■						
Hypotension	■		■				
Acute abdominal pain	■		■				
Cold extremities	■						
Oliguria	■						
Defervescence	■						
Hemo-concentration	■						
Petechiae rash	■	■			■		■
Ecchymosis	■						
Rise in hematocrit	■						
Bleeding diathesis	■	■	■	■	■	■	■
Intravascular coagulation	■		■		■	■	■
Epistaxis	■		■				
Gastrointest. hemorrhages	■						
Hematuria	■					■	
Pleural effusions	■				■		
Pneumonitis	■						

patients are not isolated which may allow their infection to be transmitted to others.[6]

Patients suffering from DF generally recover within six or seven days and are immune to the particular serotype of dengue virus that caused the infection. Nonetheless, if the patient is subsequently infected by another serotype of DENV, the individual may develop DHF which may lead to DSS.[73] The development of thrombocytopenia with concurrent hemo-concentration differences or hypotension, as well as shock, generally rule out a diagnosis of CHIKVF. These developments also rule out the diagnosis of bacterial endotoxin shock and meningococcemia (Table 7).[93] Please examine Table 8 and 9 for differential diagnosis of DF and DHF with other similar viral infections.

Table 7: Differential diagnosis of late stages of DHF/DSS and CHIKVF[93]

Symptoms	DHF (%)	CHIKVF (%)
Fever lasting 2-4 days	23.6	62.5
Fever lasting 5-6 days	59.0	31.2
Fever lasting >7 days	17.4	6.3
Positive Tourniquet test	83.9	77.4
Scattered Petechiae	46.5	31.3
Confluent Petechial rash	10.1	0.0
Epistaxis	18.9	12.5
Gum bleeding	1.5	0.0
Melena/hematemesis	11.8	0.0
Hepatomegaly	90.0	75.0
Shock	35.2	0.0

References

1. Gubler D.J. Dengue and Dengue Hemorrhagic Fever. Clinical Microbiology Reviews, 1998. 11: pp. 480-496
2. Rocco I.M., Barboas M.C., Kanomata E.H. Simultaneous Infections with Dengue 1 and 2 in a Brazilian Patient. Review of the Institute Medical Tropico at San Paulo, 1998. 40: pp. 151-154
3. World Health Organization. Department of Child and Adolescent Health and Development. Dengue, Dengue Haemorrhagic Fever and Dengue Shock Syndrome in the Context of the Integrated Management of Childhood Illness. Geneva: Switzerland. 2005. pp. 1-34
4. Guzman M.G., Kouri G. Dengue: An Update. The Lancet Infectious Disease, 2002. 2: pp. 33-42
5. Gubler D.J., Kuno G. Dengue and Dengue Hemorrhagic Fever. London, CAB International. 1997. pp. 1-22
6. Guerrant R.L., Walker D.H., Weller P.F. Tropical Infectious Diseases – Principles, Pathogens & Practice. Volume 1. Philadelphia, Churchill Livingstone Elsevier. 2006. pp. 813
7. McSherry J.A. Some Medical Aspects of the Darien Scheme: was it Dengue? Scottish Medical Journal, 1982. 27: pp. 183-184
8. Halstead S.B. Dengue Hemorrhagic Fever – a Public Health Problem and a Field for Research. Bulletin of the World Health Organization, 1980. 58: pp. 1-21
9. Rigau-Pérez J.G. The Early Use of Break-Bone Fever (Quebranta Huesos, 1771) and Dengue (1801) in Spanish. American Journal of Tropical Medicine and Hygiene, 1998. 59: pp. 272-274
10. Waidab W., Suphapeetiporn K., Thisyakorn U. Pathogenesis of Dengue Hemorrhagic Fever: From Immune to Genetics. Journal of Pediatric Infectious Diseases, 2008. 3: pp. 221-227
11. Kuhn R., Zhang W., Rossmann M., Pletnev S., Corver J., Lenches E., Jones C., Mukhopadhyay S., Chipman P., Strauss E. Structure of Dengue Virus: Implications for Flavivirus Organization, Maturation, and Fusion. Cell, 2002. 108: pp. 717-725
12. Vaughn D.W., Green S., Kalayanarooj S., Innis B.L., Nimmannitya S., Suntayakorn S., Rothman A.L., Ennis F.A., Nisalak A. Dengue in the Early Febrile Phase: Viremia and Antibody Responses. The Journal of Infectious Diseases, 1997. 176: pp. 322–330
13. Sakuntabhai A., Turbpaiboon C., Casadémont I., Chuansumrit A., Lowhnoo T., Kajaste-Rudnitski A., Kalayanarooj S.M., Tangnararatchakit K., Tangthawornchaikul N., Vasanawathana S., Chaiyaratana W., Yenchitsomanus P., Suriyaphol P., Avirutnan P., Chokephaibulkit K., Matsuda F., Yoksan S., Jacob Y., Lathrop G.M., Malasit P., Desprès P., Julier C. A Variant in the CD209 Promoter is Associated with Severity of Dengue Disease. Nature Genetics, 2005. 37: pp. 507 – 513
14. Clyde K., Kyle J.L., Harris E. Recent Advances in Deciphering Viral and Host Determinants of Dengue Virus Replication and Pathogenesis. Journal of Virology, 2006. 80: pp. 11418–11431
15. Hung S. L., Lee P. L., Chen H.W., Chen L. K., Kao C. L., King C. C. Analysis of the Steps Involved in Dengue Virus Entry into Host Cells. Virology, 1999. 257: pp. 156–167
16. Hase T., Summers P.L., Eckels K.H. 1989. Flavivirus Entry into Cultured Mosquito Cells and Human Peripheral Blood Monocytes. Archives of Virology, 1989. 104: pp. 129–143
17. Gruenberg J., van der Goot F.G. (2006) Mechanisms of Pathogen Entry through the Endosomal Compartments. Nature Review Molecular Cell Biology, 2006. 7: pp. 495–504
18. van der Schaar H.M., Rust M.J., Chen C., van der Ende-Metselaar H., Wilschut J., Zhuang X., Smit J.M. Dissecting the Cell Entry Pathway of Dengue Virus by Single-Particle Tracking in Living Cells. Public Library of Science Pathogens, 2008. 4: pp. e1000244
19. Chen Y., Maguire T., Hileman R.E., Fromm J.R., Esko J.D., Linhardt R.J., Marks R.M. Dengue Virus Infectivity Depends on Envelope Protein Binding to Target Cell Heparan Sulfate. Nature Medicine,1997. 3: pp. 866-871
20. Hilgard P., Stockert R. 2000. Heparan Sulfate Proteoglycans Initiate Dengue Virus Infection of Hepatocytes. Hepatology, 2000. 32: pp. 1069-1077
21. Germi R., Crance J.M., Garin D., Guimet J., Lortat-Jacob H., Ruigrok R.W., Zarski J.P., Drouet E. Heparan Sulfate-Mediated Binding of Infectious Dengue Virus Type 2 and Yellow Fever Virus. Virology, 2002. 292: pp.162-168
22. Chen Y. C., Wang S.Y., King C.C. Bacterial Lipopolysaccharideinhibits Dengue Virus Infection of Primary Human Monocytes/Macrophages by Blockade of Virus Entry via a CD14-Dependent Mechanism. Journal of Viology, 1999. 73: pp. 2650-2657
23. Valle J.R.D., Chavez-Salinas S., Medina F., del Angel R.M. Heat Shock Protein 90 and Heat Shock Protein 70 are Components of Dengue Virus Receptor Complex in Human Cells. Journal of Virology, 2005. 79: pp. 4557-4567
24. Jindadamrongwech S, Thepparit C., Smith D.R. Identification of GRP 78 (BiP) as a Liver Cell Expressed Receptor Element for Dengue Virus Serotype 2. Archives of Virology, 2004. 149: pp. 915-927
25. Thepparit C., Smith D.R. Serotype-Specific Entry of Dengue Virus into Liver Cells:

Identification of the 37-Kilodalton/67-Kilodalton High Affinity Laminin Receptor as a Dengue Virus Serotype 1 Receptor. Journal of Virology, 2004. 78: pp. 12647-12656
26. Navarro-Sanchez E., Altmeyer R., Amara A., Schwartz O., Fieschi F., Virelizier J.L., Arenzana-Seisdedos F., Despres P. Dendritic-Cell Specific ICAM3-Grabbing Non-Integrin is Essential for the Productive Infection of Human Dendritic Cells by Mosquito-Cell-Derived Dengue Viruses. European Molecular Biology Organization (EMBO) Report, 2003. 4: pp. 723-728
27. Tassaneetrithep B., Burgess T.H., Granelli-Piperno A., Trumpfherer C., Finke J., Sun W., Eller M.A., Pattanapanyasat K., Sarasombath S., Birx D.L., Steinman R.M., Schlesinger S., Marovich M.A. DC-SIGN (CD209) Mediates Dengue Virus Infection of Human Dendritic Cells. The Journal of Experimental Medicine, 2003. 197: pp. 823-829
28. Lozach P. Y., Burleigh L., Staropoli I., Navarro-Sanchez E., Harriague J., Virelizier J.L., Rey F.A., Despres P., Arenzana-Seisdedos F., Amara A. Dendritic Cell-Specific Intercellular Adhesion Molecule 3-Grabbing Non-Integrin (DC-SIGN) Mediated Enhancement of Dengue Virus Infection is Independent of DC-SIGN Internalization Signals. The Journal of Biological Chemistry, 2005. 280: pp. 23698-23708
29. Navarro-Sanchez E., Altmeyer R., Amara A., Schwartz O., Fieschi F., Virelizier J.L., Arenzana-Seisdedos F., Despres P. Dendritic-Cell Specific ICAM3-Grabbing Non-Integrin is Essential for the Productive Infection of Human Dendritic Cells by Mosquito-Cell-Derived Dengue Viruses. European Molecular Biology Organization (EMBO) Report, 2003. 4: pp. 723-728
30. Lozach P-Y, Burleigh L., Staropoli I., Navarro-Sanchez E., Harriague J., Virelizier J-L, Rey F.A., Després P., Arenzana-Seisdedos F., Amara A.Dendritic Cell-specific Intercellular Adhesion Molecule 3-grabbing Non-integrin (DC-SIGN)-mediated Enhancement of Dengue Virus Infection Is Independent of DC-SIGN Internalization Signals. The Journal of Biological Chemistry, 2005. 280: pp. 23698-23708
31. Pokidysheva E., Zhang Y., Battisti A.J., Bator-Kelly C.M., Chipman P.R., Xiao C.A., Gregorio G.G., Hendrickson W.A., Kuhn R.J., Rossmann M.G.. 2006. Cryo-EM Reconstruction of Dengue Virus in Complex with the Carbohydrate Recognition Domain of DC-SIGN. Cell, 2006. 124: pp. 485-493
32. Hung S. L., Lee P.L., Chen H.W., Chen L.K., Kao C.L., King C.C. Analysis of the Steps Involved in Dengue Virus Entry into Host Cells.Virology, 1999. 257: pp. 156–167
33. Lozach P. Y., Burleigh L., Staropoli I., Navarro-Sanchez E., Harriague J., Virelizier J.L., Rey F.A., Despres P., Arenzana-Seisdedos F., Amara A. Dendritic Cell-Specific Intercellular Adhesion Molecule 3-Grabbing Non-Integrin (DC-SIGN)-Mediated Enhancement of Dengue Virus Infection is Independent of DC-SIGN Internalization Signals. The Journal of Biological Chemistry, 2005. 280: pp. 23698–23708
34. Guirakhoo F., Hunt A.R., Lewis J.G., Roehrig J.T. Selection and Partial Characterization of Dengue 2 Virus Mutants that Induce Fusion at Elevated pH. Virology, 1993. 194: pp. 219–223
35. Chambers, T. J., Nestorowitz, A., Rice, C. M. Mutagenesis of the Yellow Fever Virus NS2B/3 Cleavage Site: Determinants of Cleavage Site Specificity and Effects on Polyprotein Processing and Viral Replication. Journal of Virology, 1995. 69: pp. 1600-1605
36. Lin, C., Amberg S. M., Chambers, T. J., Rice, C. M. Cleavage at a Novel Site in the NS4A Region by the Yellow Fever Virus NS2B-3 Proteinase is a Prerequisite for Processing at the Downstream 4A/4B Signalase Site. Journal of Virology, 1993. 67: pp. 2327-2335
37. Khumthong R., Angsuthanasombat C., Panyim S., Katzenmeier G. In Vitro Determination of Dengue Virus Type 2 NS2B-NS3 Protease activity with Fluorescent Peptide Substrates. Journal of Biochemistry and Molecular Biology, 2002. 35: pp. 206-212
38. Falgout B., Markoff L. Evidence that Flavivirus NS1-NS2A Cleavage Is Mediated by a Membrane-Bound Host Protease in the Endoplasmic Reticulum. Journal of Virology, 1995. 69: pp. 7232–7243
39. Miller S., Romero-Brey I., Bartenschlager R. Frontiers in Dengue Research. Norfolk, Caister Academic Press. 2010. pp. 35-38
40. Lindenbach, B. D., Rice, C. M. Trans-Complementation of Yellow Fever Virus NS1 Reveals a Role in Early RNA Replication. Journal of Virology, 1997. 71: pp. 9608–9617
41. Lindenbach, B. D., Rice, C. M. Genetic Interaction of Flavivirus Nonstructural Proteins NS1 and NS4A as a Determinant of Replicase Function. Journal of Viology, 1999. 73: pp. 4611–4621
42. Xu T., Sampath A., Chao A., Wen D., Nanao M., Chene P., Vasudevan S.G., Lescar J. Structure of the Dengue Virus Helicase/Nucleoside Triphosphatase Catalytic Domain at a Resolution of 2.4 Å. Journal of Virology, 2005. 79: pp. 10278–10288
43. Ackermann, M., Padmanabhan, R. (2001). De Novo Synthesis of RNA by the Dengue Virus RNA-dependent RNA Polymerase Exhibits Temperature Dependence at the Initiation but Not Elongation Phase. The Journal of Biological Chemistry, 2001. 276: pp. 39926-39937
44. Modis Y., Ogata S., Clements D., Harrison S.C. Structure of the Dengue Virus Envelope Protein after Membrane Fusion. Nature, 2004. 427: pp. 313–319
45. Stadler K., Allison K.L., Schalich,J., Heinz F.X. 1997. Proteolytic Activation of Tick-Borne Encephalitis Virus by Furin. Journal of Viology, 1997. 71: pp. 8475-8481
46. S.L. Alcaraz-Estrada, M. Yocupicio-Monroy, R. M. del Angel. Insights into Dengue Virus Genome Replication. Future Virology, 2010. 5: pp. 575–592
47. Henderson B.R., Saeedi B.J., Campagnola G., Geiss B.J. Analysis of RNA Binding by the Dengue Virus NS5 RNA Capping Enzyme. Public Library of Science (PLoS) One, 2011. 6: pp. e25795
48. Kurane I., Innis B.L., Nimmannitya S., Nisalak A., Meager A., Janus J., Ennis F.A. Activation of T lymphocytes in Dengue Virus Infections. High Levels of Soluble Interleukin 2 Receptor, Soluble CD4, Soluble CD8, Interleukin 2, and Interferon-gamma in Sera of Children with Dengue. The Journal of Clinical Investigation, 1991. 88: pp. 1473-1480
49. Gagnon S.J., Ennis F.A., Rothman A.L. Bystander Target Cell Lysis and Cytokine Production by Dengue Virus-Specific Human CD4+ Cytotoxic T-Lymphocyte Clones. Journal of Virology, 1999. 73: pp. 3623–3629
50. Green S., Vaughn D.W., Kalayanarooj S., Nimmannitya S., Suntaykorn S., Nisalak A., Lew R., Innis B.L., Kurane I., Rothman A.L., Ennis F.A. Early Immune Activation in Acute Dengue Illness is related to Development of Plasma Leakage and Disease Severity. The Journal of Infectious Diseases, 1999. 179: pp. 755-762
51. Bozza F.A., Cruz O.G., Zagne S.M.O., Azeredo E.L., Nogueira R.M.R., Assis E.F., Bozza P.T., Kubelka C.F. Multiplex Cytokine Profile from Dengue Patients: MIP-1beta and IFN-gamma as Predictive Factors for Severity. Biomed Central Infectious Diseases, 2008. 8: pp. 2-11
52. Suharti C., van Gorp E.C., Setiati T.E., Dolmans W.M., Djokomoeljanto R.J., Hack C.E., Ten C.H., Meer J.W. The Role of Cytokines in Activation of Coagulation and Fibrinolysis in Dengue Shock Syndrome. Thrombosis and Haemostasis, 2002. 87: pp. 42-46
53. Avila-Aguero M.L., Avila-Aguero C.R., Um S.L., Soriano-Fallas A., Canas-Coto A., Yan S.B. Systemic Host Inflammatory and Coagulation Response in the Dengue Virus Primo-Infection. Cytokine, 2004. 27: pp. 173-179.
54. Nguyen T.H., Lei H.Y., Nguyen T.L., Lin Y.S., Huang K.J., Le B.L., Lin C.F., Yeh T.M., Do Q.H., Vu T.Q., Chen L.C., Huang J.H., Lam T.M., Liu C.C., Halstead S.B. Dengue Hemorrhagic Fever in Infants: A Study of Clinical and Cytokine Profiles. The Journal of Infectious Diseases, 2004. 189: pp. 221-232
55. Bethell D.B., Flobbe K., Cao X.T., Day NP, Pham T.P., Buurman W.A., Cardosa M.J., White N.J., Kwiatkowski D. Pathophysiologic and Prognostic Role of Cytokines in Dengue Hemorrhagic Fever. The Journal of Infectious Diseases, 1998. 177: pp. 778-782
56. Avirutnan P., Malasit P., Seliger B., Bhakdi S., Hussmann M. Dengue Virus Infection of Human Endotheliual Cells Leads to Chemokine Production, Complement Activation, and Apoptosis. The Journal of Immunology, 1998. 161: pp. 6338-6346
57. Lee Y.R., Liu M.T., Lei H.Y., Liu C.C., Wu J.M., Tung Y.C., Lin Y.S., Yeh T.M., Chen S.H., Liu H.S. MCP-1, a Highly Expressed Chemokine in Dengue Haemorrhagic Fever/Dengue Shock Syndrome Patients, May Cause Permeability Change, Possibly Through Reduced Tight Junctions of Vascular Endothelium Cells. The Journal of General Virology, 2006. 87: pp. 3623-3630
58. Wang L., Chen R.F., Liu J.W., Yu H.R., Kuo H.C., Yang K.D. Implications of Dynamic Changes Among Tumor Necrosis Factor-alpha (TNF-alpha), Membrane TNF Receptor, and Soluble TNF receptor Levels in Regard to the Severity of Dengue Infection. American Journal of Tropical Medicine and Hygiene, 2007. 77: pp. 297-302
59. Alibek K. Biohazard. New York: Dell Publishing. 1999. pp. 281
60. Jahrling P.B. Viral Hemorrhagic Fevers. Medical Aspects of Chemical and Biological Warfare. Falls Church: Office of the Surgeon General, Department of the Army, United States of America. 1997. pp. 591-602
61. Peters C.J., Jahrling P.B., Khan A.S. Patients Infected with High-hazard Viruses. Achieves of Virology Supplement, 1996.11: pp. 141-168
62. World Health Organization. Dengue Haemorrhagic Fever – Diagnosis, Treatment, Prevention and Control 2nd edition. WHO Library Cataloging in Publication data, 1997. pp. 12
63. Domingues R.B., Kuster G.W., de Castro F.L., Souza V.A., Levi J.E., Pannuti C.S. Headache Features in Patients with Dengue Virus Infection. Cephalalgia, 2006. 26: pp. 879-882
64. Laude A., Chlebicki M.P., Ang B., Barkham T. Maculopathy and Dengue. Emerging Infectious Diseases, 2007. 13: pp. 347-348
65. Fernando R.L., Fernando S.E., Leong S.Y. Tropical Infectious Diseases – Epidemiology, Investigation, Diagnosis & Management. London: Greenwich Medical Media. 2001. pp. 282
66. Premaratna R., Bailey M.S., Ratnasena B.G., de Silva H.J. Dengue Fever Mimicking Acute Appendicitis. Transactiuons of the Royal Society of Tropical Medicine and Hygiene, 2007. 101: pp. 683-685
67. Lateef A., Fisher D.A., Tambyah P.A. Dengue and Relative Bradycardia. Emerging Infectious Diseases, 13: pp. 650-651
68. World Health Organization. Dengue Haemorrhagic Fever – Diagnosis, Treatment, Prevention and Control 2nd Edition. WHO Library Cataloging in Publication Data, 1997. pp. 12-13
69. Mathew A., Rothman A.L. Understanding the Contribution of Cellular Immunity to Dengue Disease Pathogenesis. Immunological Reviews, 2008. 225: pp. 300-313
70. Dale-Carroll I., Toovey S., Gompel A.V. Dengue Fever and Pregnancy – A Review and Comment. Travel Medicine and Infectious Disease, 2007. 5: pp. 183-188
71. Halstead S.B., O'Rourke E.J. Dengue Viruses and Mononuclear Phagocytes. I. Infection Enhancement by Non-neutralizing Antibody. The Journal of Experimental Medicine, 1977. 146: pp. 201-217
72. Halstead S.B. Pathogenesis of Dengue: Challenges to Molecular Biology. Science, 1988. 239: pp. 476-481
73. World Health Organization. Dengue Haemorrhagic Fever – Diagnosis, Treatment, Prevention and Control 2nd Edition. WHO Library Cataloging in Publication Data, 1997. pp. 13
74. Setlik R.F., Morgan J., Dorsey D., Horvath L., Purcell B. Pulmonary Hemorrhage Syndrom Associated with an Autochthonous Case of Dengue Hemorrhagic Fever. Southern Medical Journal, 2004. 97: pp. 688-691
75. Nelson E.R. Haemorrhagic Fever in Children in Thailand. Journal Paediatrics, 1960. 56: pp. 101-108
76. Liam C.K., Yap B.H., Lam S.K. Dengue Fever Complicated by Pulmonary Haemorrhage Manifesting as Haemoptysis. Journal of Tropical Medicine and Hygiene, 1993. 96: pp. 197-200
77. Ong A., Sandar M., Chen M.I., Sin L.Y. Fatal Dengue Hemorrhagic Fever in Adults during a Dengue Epidemic in Singapore. International Journal of Infectious Diseases, 2007. 11: pp. 263-267
78. World Health Organization. Dengue Haemorrhagic Fever – Diagnosis, Treatment, Prevention and Control 2nd edition. WHO Library Cataloging in Publication data, 1997. pp. 15
79. Kalayanarooj S., Gibbons R.V., Vaughn D., Green S., Nisalak A., Jarman R.G., Mammen M.P., Perng G.C. Blood Group AB is Associated with Increased Risk for Severe Dengue Disease in Secondary Infections. Journal of Infectious Diseases, 2007. 195: pp. 1014-1017
80. World Health Organization. Dengue Haemorrhagic Fever – Diagnosis, Treatment, Prevention and Control 2nd Edition. WHO Library Cataloging in Publication Data, 1997. pp. 16-17
81. World Health Organization. Dengue Haemorrhagic Fever – Diagnosis, Treatment, Prevention and Control 2nd Edition. WHO Library Cataloging in Publication Data, 1997. pp. 22
82. World Health Organization. Dengue Haemorrhagic Fever – Laboratory Diagnosis 2nd Edition. WHO Library Cataloging in Publication Data, 1997. pp. 34-35
83. Aryati, Trimarsanto H., Yohan B., Wardhani P., Fahri S., Sasmono R.T. Performance of commercial dengue NS1 ELISA and molecular analysis of NS1 gene of dengue viruses obtained during surveillance in Indonesia. Biomedical Central Infectious Diseases, 2013. 13: pp. 611
84. World Health Organization. Dengue Haemorrhagic Fever – Laboratory Diagnosis 2nd Edition. WHO Library Cataloging in Publication data, 1997. pp. 38-39
85. CDC DENV-1-4 Real-Time RT-PCR Assay for Detection and Serotype Identification of Dengue Virus. Revised July 12, 2013. Retrieved October 30, 2014. Website: http://www.cdc.gov/dengue/clinicalLab/realTime.html
86. He J., Kraft A.J., Fan J., Van Dyke M., Wang L., Bose M.E., Khanna M., Metallo J.A., Henrickson K.J. Simultaneous Detection of CDC Category "A" DNA and RNA Bioterrorism Agents by Use of Multiplex PCR & RT-PCR Enzyme Hybridization Assays. Virus, 2009. 1: pp. 441-459
87. Wu T.Z., Su C.C., Chen L.K., Yang H.H., Tai D.F., Peng K.C. Piezoelectric Immunochip for the Detection of Dengue Fever in Viremia Phase. Biosensors and Bioelectronics, 2005. 21, 5: pp. 689-695
88. Chen Y.C., Huang H.N., Lin C.T., Chen Y.F., King C.C., Wu H.C. Generation and Characterization of Monoclonal Antibodies against Dengue Virus Type 1 for Epitope Mapping and Serological Detection by Epitope-based peptide Antigens. Clinical and Vaccine Immunology, 2007. 14: pp. 404-411
89. Sabchareon A., Wallace D., Sirivichayakul C., Limkittikul K., Chanthavanich P., Suvannadabba S., Jiwariyavej V., Dulyachai W., Pengsaa K., Wartel T.A., Moureau A.,

Saville M., Bouckenooghe A., Viviani S., Tornieporth N.G., Lang J. Protective efficacy of the recombinant, live-attenuated, CYD tetravalent dengue vaccine in Thai schoolchildren: a randomised, controlled phase 2b trial. Lancet, 2012. 380: pp. 1559-1567

90. World Health Organization. Dengue Haemorrhagic Fever – Diagnosis, Treatment, Prevention and Control 2nd Edition. WHO Library Cataloging in Publication Data, 1997. pp. 24-25

91. World Health Organization. Dengue Haemorrhagic Fever – Diagnosis, Treatment, Prevention and Control 2nd Edition. WHO Library Cataloging in Publication Data, 1997. pp. 26

92. Halliday M.A., Segar W.E. Maintenance Need for Water in Parenteral Fluid Therapy. Pediatrics, 1957. 19: pp. 823

93. Nimmannitya S., Halstead S., Cohen S.B. Margiotta M.R. Dengue and Chikungunya virus infection in man in Thailand. American Journal of Tropical Medicine and Hygiene, 1960. 18: pp. 954-971

Photo Bibliography

Figure 1.4-1: Transmission electron micrograph (TEM) of Dengue virus (round particles) in hepatocytes. Photo was taken by Frederick Murphy and Cynthia Goldsmith at 83,000x in 2010 and released by the CDC. Public domain photo

Figure 1.4-5: Diagrammatic process of DENV infection within a host cell. The virus graphics was developed by Paredes A. M., Ferreira D., Horton M., Saad A., Tsuruta H., Johnston R., Klimstra W., Ryman K., Hernandez R., Chiu W., Brown D. T. Conformational changes in Sindbis virions resulting from exposure to low pH and interactions with cells suggest that cell penetration may occur at the cell surface in the absence of membrane fusion. Virology, 2004. 324: pp. 373-86 and released by Oak Ridge National Laboratory, Department of Energy. Public domain photo

Figure 1.4-5: Genomic protein graphics produced and released by the National Institute of Health (NIH). Public domain photo

Figure 1.4-7: Hematoxylin-eosin-stained (H&E) photomicro-graph shows the cytoarchitectural changes found in a liver tissue specimen extracted from a Dengue hemorrhagic fever patient in Thailand. This particular view reveals mid-lobular necrosis, with accompanying acidophilic degeneration, and moderate hypertrophy of Kupffer cells. The photomicrograph was taken by Dr. Yves Robin and Dr. Jean Renaudet in 1980 and released by Arbovirus Laboratory at the Pasteur Institute in Dakar, Senegal; World Health Organization and CDC. Public domain photo

Figure 1.4-8: A patient suffering from dengue hemorrhagic fever demonstrates a large subcutaneous hemorrhage on the upper arm. Photo is attributed to WHO/TDR/STI/Hatz and was released by United States Department of Health and Human Services, National Institute of Health. Public domain photo

The Ebola virus (EBOV) belongs to the genus *Ebolavirus* of the family *Filoviridae*. EBOV, along with the closely related Marburg virus, are members of the order *Mononegavirales*.[1]

EBOV is a non-segmented, single-stranded, ~19-kb, negative sense, linear RNA and enveloped virus that is specific to primates (including human). EBOV is responsible for causing Ebola Hemorrhagic Fever, also known as Ebola Virus Disease (EVD), is highly pathogenic in humans and is one of the most deadly and virulent infections known to mankind (Figure 1.5-1).[1]

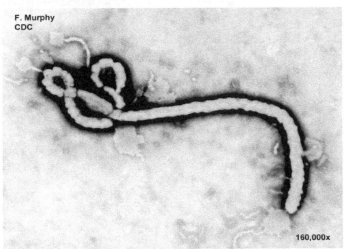

Figure 1.5-1: Colorized transmission electron micrograph (TEM) of an Ebola virus particle

Presently, there are five recognized strains of Ebola virus and they are identified and named based on the location where they were first discovered.[2] Ebola-Zaire (ZEBOV) was identified near the Ebola River Valley (Yambuku) in Zaire (presently the Democratic Republic of Congo).[3] ZEBOV strain first appeared in 1976-1977 and resulted in an 88% mortality rate among the infected patients. The second strain is called Ebola-Sudan (SEBOV) and it was discovered in 1976. Like ZEBOV, SEBOV is a severe infection and caused 53% mortality rate in patients.[4] The third strain, called Ebola-Côte d'Ivoire (CIEBOV), also known as Ebola-Ivory Coast, was found in one patient in 1994 and did not result in a fatality.[5] The fourth strain is called Ebola-Bundibugyo (BEBOV) and was identified in Bundibugyo, Uganda during an outbreak that occurred between November 2007 and February 2008. This outbreak resulted in 25% case fatality rate.[6] The fifth and final strain is called Ebola-Reston (REBOV). REBOV was identified in Reston, Virginia in imported primates (cynomolgous monkeys) from the Philippines in 1989-1990. REBOV caused severe disease in non-human primates and swine. Human infections by REBOV have only been serologically identified and no diseases or fatalities have resulted.[7, 8]

With the exception of REBOV, the remaining four strains of Ebola are responsible for causing hemorrhagic fevers in humans. In addition to genomic differences, these 4 Ebola strains differ in their rate of secondary transmission and case fatality ratios. Please examine Figure 1.5-2 and Table 1 for the chronology of Ebola out-breaks and the distribution of this disease.

Presently, the reservoir(s) and origin of the Ebola virus is unknown. Based on the available evidence, scientists believe that Ebola is a zoonotic virus, native to the African continent. Available information shows that handling primates (e.g. monkeys, chimpanzees, gorillas etc.) and forest antelopes (in the case of Ebola-Côte d'Ivoire), pigs, horses, civets and fruit bats can potentially promote the spread of the disease (Figure 1.5-3).[9, 10, 11, 12]

There is no evidence suggesting that EVD has a predilection for a particular sex or race. However, there is some evidence that EBOV preferentially infects adults rather than children under the age of 17 years. During the 1995 Democratic Republic of Congo outbreak only 27 (8.6%) out of 315 people infected were children

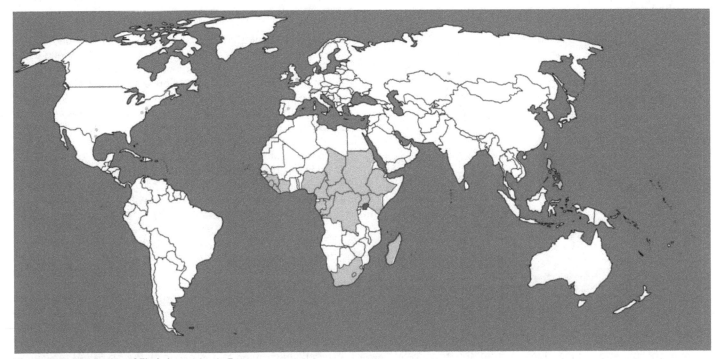

Figure 1.5-2: Distribution of Ebola hemorrhagic Fever

Table 1: Chronology of Ebola outbreaks. Please note that the indicated case and fatality rate of the 2014 Ebola infection are numbers provided by the CDC as of January 30, 2015

Year	Nation	Strain	Cases	Deaths	% of fatalities
1976	Congo (Democratic Republic of Congo)	ZEBOV	318	280	88%
1976	Sudan (Republic of the Sudan)	SEBOV	284	151	53%
1976	England (United Kingdom)	SEBOV	1	0	0%
1977	Congo (Democratic Republic of Congo)	ZEBOV	1	1	100%
1979	Sudan (Republic of the Sudan)	SEBOV	34	22	65%
1989	USA (United States of America)	REBOV	4	0	0%
1989-1990	Philippines	REBOV	3	0	0%
1990	USA (United States of America)	REBOV	0	0	0%
1992	Italy (Italian Republic)	REBOV	0	0	0%
1994	Gabon (Gabonese Republic)	ZEBOV	52	31	60%
1994	Ivory Coast (Republic of Côte d'Ivoire)	CIEBOV	1	0	0%
1995	Liberia (Republic of Liberia)	CIEBOV	1	0	0%
1995	Congo (Democratic Republic of Congo)	ZEBOV	315	250	81%
1996	Gabon (Gabonese Republic)	ZEBOV	37	21	57%
1996-1997	Gabon (Gabonese Republic)	ZEBOV	60	45	74%
1996	South Africa (Republic of South Africa)	ZEBOV	2	1	50%
1996	USA (United States of America)	REBOV	0	0	0%
1996	Philippines (Republic of the Philippines)	REBOV	0	0	0%
1996	Russia	ZEBOV	1	1	100%
2000-2001	Uganda (Republic of Uganda)	SEBOV	435	224	53%
2001-2002	Gabon (Gabonese Republic)	ZEBOV	65	53	82%
2001-2002	Congo (Democratic Republic of Congo)	ZEBOV	57	43	75%
2002-2003	Congo (Democratic Republic of Congo)	ZEBOV	143	128	89%
2003	Congo (Democratic Republic of Congo)	ZEBOV	35	29	83%
2004	Sudan (Republic of the Sudan)	SEBOV	17	7	41%
2004	Russia	ZEBOV	1	1	100%
2007	Congo (Democratic Republic of Congo)	ZEBOV	264	187	71%
2007-2008	Uganda	BEBOV	149	37	25%
2008	Philippines	REBOV	6	0	0%
2008-2009	Congo (Democratic Republic of Congo)	ZEBOV	32	15	47%
2011	Uganda	SEBOV	1	1	100%
2012	Uganda	SEBOV	11	4	36.4%
2012	Congo (Democratic Republic of Congo)	BEBOV	36	13	36.1%
2012-2013	Uganda	SEBOV	6	3	50%
2014-Present	Guinea, Liberia, Sierra Leone, Nigeria, Spain, USA	ZEBOV	22136	8833	40%

although approximately 50% of the population of DRC at that time was younger than 17 years. Definitive evidence of the age selection is presently unavailable; however, it is known that other hemorrhagic fevers selectively infect adults over children.[13]

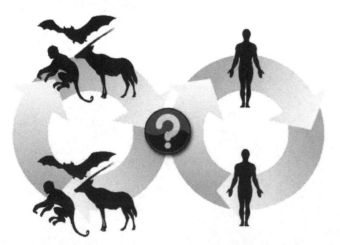

Figure 1.5-3: Possible transmission cycle of Ebola virus. The viruses are efficiently transmitted among the human population through physical contact or exchange of bodily fluids without the need for an enzootic amplification host. At present the sylvatic cycle of Ebola transmission to human is unknown

EBOV is approximately 80 nm in diameter and is surrounded by phospholipid membrane derived from the host cell. The average size of the EBOV genome is ~18.9 kb and consists of a non-segmented, linear single negative strand RNA molecule. The genome comprises ~1.1% of the total virion mass of approximately 4.0×10^6 Da. [14, 15, 16]

The primary targets of EBOV infections are mononuclear phagocytes such as macrophages, monocytes, dendritic cells, Kupffer's cells and other antigen presenting immunological cells. Additional target of EBOV infection also includes endothelial cells.[17] The exact manner of viral transcription and translation is presently unknown, mainly due to the highly infectious and dangerous nature of the virus. Nonetheless, it is believed that EBOV uses similar mechanisms of transcription, translation and replication as other negative sense RNA viruses. For example, it has been postulated that after gaining entry into the cytoplasm of the host cell, EBOV is transcribed and generates a polyadenylated sub-genomic messenger RNA (mRNA) with a characteristic gene order of 3' leader, nucleoprotein (NP), virion protein 35 (VP35), VP40, glycoprotein (GP), VP30, VP24, polymerase (L) protein and 5' trailer.[14, 15, 17] Subsequent transcription and translation will produce 7 structural polypeptides, where 4 of the polypeptides, NP, VP30, VP35 and L protein, are associated with the virus genomic RNA in a ribonucleoprotein complex associated with viral transcription and replication. VP40 and VP24 are matrix proteins that are linked to the ribonucleoprotein complex are involved in nucleocapsid formation, budding, viral assembly as well as, host range determination.[17] VP30 is assumed to be a transcription activation factor, essential for the EBOV replication cycle (Figure 1.5-4 and 1.5-5).[17, 18, 19]

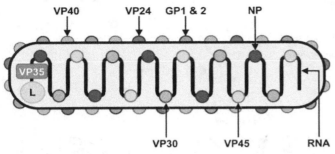

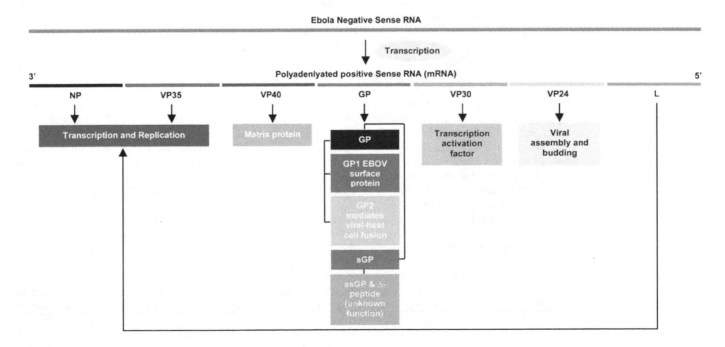

Figure 1.5-4: Internal diagram of an Ebola virus demonstrating negative (-) sense RNA genome, structural and nucleoproteins

It has been reported that 80% of the transcriptional product of the *GP* gene codes for a precursor of the nonstructural soluble glycoprotein (pre-sGP). Subsequently, pre-sGP is post-translationally cleaved through the enzymatic actions of furin or furin-like endo-protease into secretory glycoprotein (sGP), delta peptide (Δ-peptide), glycoproteins 1 and 2 (GP$_{1,2}$) transmembrane trimeric protein spikes, and a recently discovered soluble secreted glycoprotein (ssGP). Once produced, sGP, Δ-peptide and ssGP are secreted systemically within the infected individual and are detected in the blood samples of patients infected with EBOV (Figure 1.5-5).[17, 20, 21, 22, 23, 24, 25]

Presently, the exact function of sGP is unknown, nonetheless, numerous hypotheses have been proposed. Kindzelskii *et al.* (2000), have indicated that sGP deactivates neutrophils through their interactions with the neutrophilic membrane receptor CD16b (a neutrophil-specific form of Fc-γ receptor III that interacts with the Fc portion of IgG).[26] However, this concept has been challenged by other researchers who propose that sGP may serve as a 'decoy' released by EBOV during an infection. For example, sGP shares neutralizing epitope with GP$_1$, GP$_2$ trans-membrane spikes and may be released to bind with circulating neutralizing antibodies in order to distract the immune system, thereby escape detection. Additional studies have indicated that

sGP may function as a mediator in the activation of target cells, as well as, causing the increased vascular endothelial permeability which leads to hemorrhage and shock.[17, 27, 28, 29, 30, 31]

It has been suggested that Δ-peptide, may play an important role during EBOV pathogenesis and can function as mediators of endothelial dysregulation.[32, 33, 34] However, the experiments conducted by Wahl-Jensen *et. al.* (2005), have indicated that Δ-peptide is not involved in endothelial cell activation and/or reduced endothelial cell barrier functions.[35] Other studies have presented evidence that Δ-peptide is responsible for preventing super-infection of target cells and/or prevents mature virions from being trapped within the endoplasmic reticulum.[17] In summary, the exact function of Δ-peptide remains to be elucidated.

Recently, a third secreted glycoprotein known as ssGP has been discovered. ssGP is a N-glycosylated disulfide-linked homodimer that shares similar molecular weight and biochemical properties as sGP. However, at present, the precise function of ssGP remains unknown.[17, 36]

The remaining 20% of the *GP* gene are synthesized as a single polypeptide, 676 amino acids in length, where the 32 amino acids of the N-terminal act as a the signal peptide which is cleaved after translation.[14, 37] Once cleaved, the product proceeds through N-glycosylation in the endoplasmic reticulum of the host cell to form pre-GP molecules and are further processed in the Golgi apparatus to form glycosylated GP (GP0) molecules. GP0 is again cleaved by furin or furin-like endoprotease into disulfide-linked fragments GP$_1$ (surface subunit) and GP$_2$ (transmembrane subunit) which will be used as transmembrane trimeric protein spikes eventually located on the viral particle.[38, 39] GP$_1$ is responsible for receptor binding, while GP$_2$ mediates viral-host cell membrane fusion and receptor mediated endocytosis in a pH-dependent manner (Figure 1.5-5 and 1.5-6).[40, 41, 42]

It has been postulated that asialoglycoprotein receptor, folate receptor-α, integrins (e.g. β1), dendritic-cell specific intercellular adhesion molecule-grabbing nonintegrin (DC-SIGN) and liver/lymph node specific intercellular adhesion molecule-grabbing

Figure 1.5-5: Translational products of EBOV

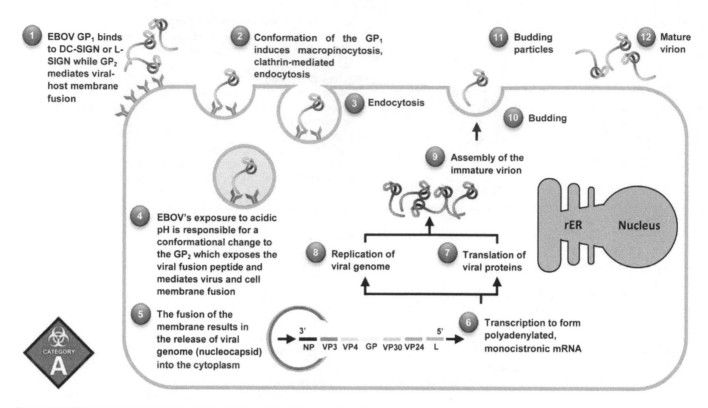

Figure 1.5-6: Diagrammatic process of EBOV infection within an eukaryotic cell

nonintegrin (L-SIGN) are some of the potential attachment sites.[15, 17, 43] Conformational changes of the EBOV GP_1 and GP_2 spikes must take place in order to allow the hydrophobic fusion domain to be inserted in the host cellular membrane. Chandran *et al.* (2005) proposed that proteolysis by two endosomal cytosine proteases, cathepsin B and cathepsin L, which are active at a low-pH, produce the conformation changes of the viral surface glycoprotein necessary to induce entry to the host cell. Cathepsin B and cathepsin L have been reported to cleave GP_1 yielding an approximately 18-kD N-terminal fragment which is further cleaved by cathepsin B. It is suggested that the subsequent cleavage of this fragment by cathepsin B initiates membrane fusion by GP_2. Research has also shown that glycoprotein-mediated infections are substantially reduced in cells that are lacking in these proteases.[44, 45]

Once the nucleocapsid, along with the negative sense RNA genome has entered into the cytoplasm of their primary targeted cells (e.g. macrophage and dendritic cells etc.), it is postulated that VP24 and VP35 play a vital role in preventing these phagocytes from reacting towards the infection. For example, it has been reported that VP24 and VP35 prevent the accumulation of signal transducer and activator 1 (STAT1) thereby blocking the activities of interferon regulatory factor-3 and -7. Additionally, VP24 is believed to be responsible for obstructing the p38 mitogen-activated protein kinase pathway, which in turn, eliminates cellular response to cytokines. VP35, on the other hand, is believed to be responsible for preventing the activation of double stranded RNA dependent protein kinase thereby blocking the production of interferons (IFN).[17, 46]

It is believed that NP, along with other EBOV proteins, triggers transcription of the viral genome. This initial transcription yield polyadenylated, momocistronic mRNAs in 3' to 5' direction from the encapsidated genomic RNA template. Viral transcription involves a process of starts (conserved start sequence) and stops (polyadenylated stop sequence) as the polymerase complex moves along the viral genome.[45]

The initial expression of transcribed viral gene (antigenomic viral positive sense RNA) leads to a buildup of viral proteins (NP, VP35, VP40, GP, VP30, VP24 and L protein). This buildup (especially of NP) is believed to trigger a switch from transcription to replication. It has been reported that NP mRNA can be detected as early as seven hours post infection and peaks around 18 hours.[47, 48, 49]

Replicated antigenomic viral positive sense RNA serves as a template to synthesize genomic negative sense RNA. After the formation of genomic negative sense RNA, it is rapidly encapsidated. It has been reported that the depletion of viral proteins leads to a switch from replication to transcription and translation. Eventually, equilibrium is reached between transcription, translation, and replication, whereby the viral particles accumulate and are directed to the plasma membrane for virion assembly and budding.[49]

Of the remaining membrane associated non-glycosylated proteins, VP-40 and VP24, it is known that VP-40 functions as a matrix protein, while VP24 is believed to be involved in viral assembly and budding, however its exact function(s) require further elucidation.[15, 45] Please examine Figure 1.5-6 for a diagrammatic process of EBOV infection and Figure 1.5-7 for a transmission electron micrograph of EBOV within a host cell.

In humans and primates, EBOV infections are associated with hypotension and problems associated with fluid distribution and coagulation, causing fulminant shock and multi-organ system failure. Viral replication, along with the dys-regulation of the immune and vascular systems, plays a major role in the development of disease. It has been demonstrated that EBOV creates a marked disruption of the parafollicular regions in the spleen and lymph nodes, as well as, the proliferation of the virus in mononuclear phagocytes.[15, 50, 51] In non-human primates, lymphopenia is believed to be the result of "bystander apoptosis", which is thought to be caused by mediators such as tumor necrosis factor (TNF)-α, fatty acid synthase ligand (Fas/Fas ligand), TNF-α-related apoptosis-inducing ligand (TRIAL) and nitric oxide (NO) released from virus-activated primary cells or by unidentified interactions between viral and host products. Nonetheless, presently there is little information regarding the role of apoptosis resulting from EBOV pathogenesis in humans, with the exception of the loss of CD8+ T cells and plasma cells.[15, 17, 51, 52]

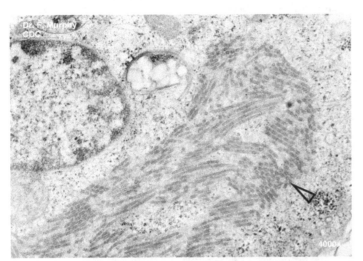

Figure 1.5-7: Transmission electron micrograph showing assembly and maturing EBOV (arrow) within the cytoplasm of a monocytic host cell

Much research has indicated that EBOV infection of monocytes and macrophages triggers the release of vast amounts of interleukin-1β (IL-1β), IL-2, IL-6, IL-8 and IL-10. Additionally, the infection also triggers the release of tumor necrosis factor - α (TNF-α), monocyte chemo-attractant protein - 1 (MCP-1), regulated upon activation normal T cell expressed and presumably secreted (RANTES), reactive oxygen species (ROS) and reactive nitrogen species (RNS). This triggered release of massive amounts of cytokines and chemokines, also referred to as the "cytokine storm", is responsible for recruiting additional phagocytes to the site(s) of infection whereby increasing the number of host cells available for additional infections.[17]

Evidence shows that there are clear differences in the expression of the types of cytokines between non-fatal and fatal EBOV infections. For example, in non-fatal ZEBOV acute hemorrhagic cases, the concentration of IL-1β, along with elevated levels of IL-6, tumor necrosis factor-α (TNFα), macrophage inflammatory protein-1α (MIP-1α) and MIP-1β during the early phase of the disease is followed by the availability of IL-1 receptor antagonist (IL-1RA) and soluble receptors for TNFα (sTNF-R) and IL-6 (sIL-6R) within the plasma of patients, towards the end of the symptomatic phase and after recovery. These are considered to indicate non-fatal infections. On the other hand, patients with normal levels of MIP-1α and MIP-1β (similar to those of endemic controls), moderate levels TNFα and IL-6 and elevated levels of IL-10, neopterin, sTNF-R and IL-1 receptor A (IL-1RA) are seen within a few days after the onset of the disease and are indicative of fatal EBOV infections.[53, 54, 55, 56, 57, 58]

While infections with EBOV lead to a moderate cytopathic effect in susceptible tissue culture cells, the exact mechanism of cellular destruction is presently unknown. It is speculated that the production and accumulation of viral proteins, as well as, substantial numbers of maturing viral particles at the plasma membrane may be involved in cellular death (Figure 1.5-8).[15] It

has also been postulated that viral proteins such as GP$_1$ and GP$_2$ may play a part in the cytopathic effect of the virus in tissue and susceptible host cells. Research has indicated that the serine-threonine-rich mucin-like domain of GP$_1$ mediated cytotoxicity in human embryonic kidney 293T cells, as well as, in human endothelial cells.[59] Additional studies have shown that GP$_2$ is involved in a phosphorylation-dependent signal cascade which caused the detachment of 293T from the tissue culture without cell death.[60]

The breakdown of the blood-tissue barrier, which is mainly controlled by endothelial cells in EBOV infected individuals, is an important part of the disease's pathogenesis. It has been reported that the endothelial cells can be affected directly by EBOV infection, leading to activation and cytopathogenic replication and/or indirectly through mediator-induced inflammatory response.[15] For example, the uncontrollable release of cytokines originating from EBOV infected mononuclear phagocytic cells, have been demonstrated to break down the endothelial barrier functions in vitro. Although the mechanism of breakdown in the endothelial barrier is presently unknown, experimental data provides evidence that changes occur in the organization of the endothelial intercellular junctions (e.g. cadherin-catenin complex) of the vascular endothelium. These alterations in the membrane permeability may explain the imbalance of fluid between the intravascular and extravascular tissue spaces in EBOV infected patients. Additionally, the breakdown of the blood-tissue barrier contributes to the rapid dissemination of infected phagocytes systemically thereby allowing the release of EBOV in various lymphoid organs (e.g. spleen, thymus etc.), liver, lungs, as well as other secondary sites for viral replications. [15, 17, 53, 54, 61, 62]

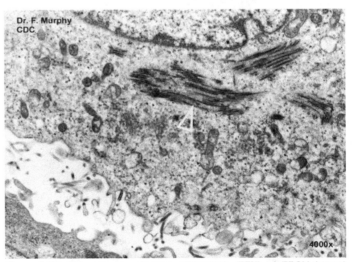

Figure 1.5-8: Transmission electron micrograph (TEM) of EBOV (arrow) within a host cell. Please note the accumulation of assembling virus and virus particle within the cytoplasm and the budding of viruses at the plasma membrane

The United States biological weapons program placed restrictions on itself to produce biological weapons that have known antibiotic treatments and vaccines. However, the former Soviet Union specifically targeted biological agents that have no known cure and produced large quantities of aerosolized form of Ebola viruses until 1992.[61, 62] As reported by Alibek, Ebola virus was classified as N2 by the Soviet Union biological weapons program and was researched and produced at the Institute of Ultra-Pure Biopreparations in Leningrad, Omutninsk, Kirov, Obolensk, outside of Moscow, the Lyubuchany Institute of Immunology in Chekhov, (near Moscow) and Vector Research and testing was located in Novosibrisk (the small town of Koltsovo) in Siberia.[63, 64]

In 1993, the Aum Shinrikyo cult unsuccessfully attempted to obtain Ebola virus in Zaire as part of their effort to create biological weapons that would be used to bring about the end of the world. Based on Ebola's potential of widespread person to person transmission, illness and death, the CDC classified Ebola as a biosafety level 4 and Category A biological weapon agent (Figure 1.5-9).[65, 66, 67]

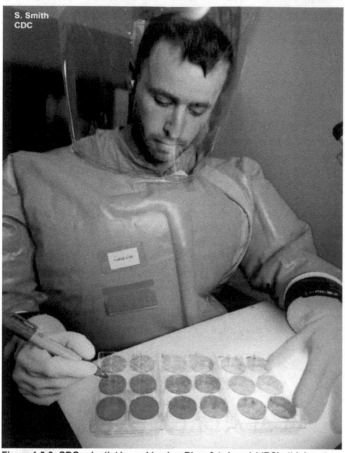

Figure 1.5-9: CDC scientist is working in a Biosafety Level 4 (BSL-4) laboratory within an air-tight, self-contained, positively-pressurized suit

SYMPTOMS

EBOV is transmitted by contact with contaminated blood, bodily fluids, fecal matter, vomit, breast milk, urine, semen, as well as organs of the infected individuals. For example, it has been reported that EBOV can persist in semen for approximately 70-90 days after infection.[68, 69, 70] Contact can be defined as direct contact with the patients, either alive or dead. Contamination is frequently seen in individuals who participate in traditional burial practices, where the body of the deceased, after succumbing to EVD, is washed and cleansed by family members. Additional evidence indicates that transmission could be spread from indirect contact via a cough or a sneeze. Evidence has shown that direct contact with the patients' linens, clothing and/or other inanimate objects that previously had interaction with the afflicted individual during the infection or just after death can also result in the transmission of the disease.[63, 68] There are frequent reports of cases of infection in individuals who do not follow proper sanitation procedures after coming into contact with an infected EVD patient. Therefore, health care workers on the site of an outbreak are most commonly exposed through close contact with patients if infection control procedures are not carefully followed.[12, 68, 69, 70]

The targets of EBOV range from mononuclear phagocytic cells, as well as, the endothelial cells of the respiratory and digestive

tracts.[69, 70, 71] EBOV is also capable of infecting hepatocytes, fibroblast cells and the parenchymal cells of the liver, spleen and lymphoid tissues respectively, causing extensive necrosis (examine Figure 1.5-10 and 1.5-11).[71, 72, 73] In addition to the exponential growth of EBOV within mononuclear phagocytic cells (e.g. monocytes, macrophages etc.) and endothelial cells, the virus can also initiate the secretion of significant concentrations of various chemokines and proinflamatory cytokines, including RANTES, monocyte chemotactic protein-1, microphage inflammatory protein-1α, tumor necrosis factor-α, interleukin-6, interleukin-8 and growth related oncogenic-α.[61, 71, 73, 74, 75] Furthermore, the Ebola virus inhibits infected cells from secreting interferon-α, an important immunomodulatory and antiviral cytokine.[76, 77, 78]

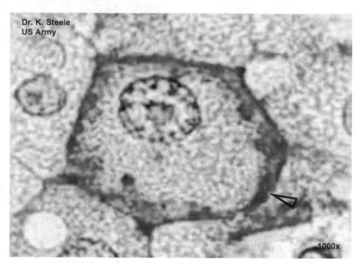

Figure 1.5-10: Photomicrograph of a formalin fixed Ebola virus in a monkey hepatocyte (arrow)

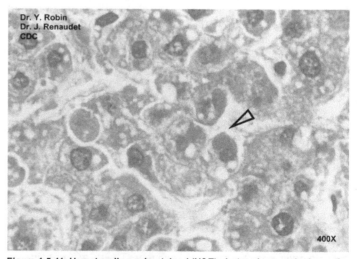

Figure 1.5-11: Hematoxylin-eosin-stained (H&E) photo-micrograph shows the cytoarchitectural changes in a liver specimen. This tissue was extracted from a patient suffering from EBOV in Zaire. Note the acidophilic necrosis leading to the formation of a Councilman hyaline body (eosinophilic globule: arrow) and cytoplasmic inclusions

Once EBOV enters the system, an incubation period of approximately 4 to 10 days (2 to 21 days stated by WHO Fact sheet N°103) occurs before the first signs of EVD are apparent.[9, 68, 79, 80] The onset of EVD is characterized by flu-like symptoms including high fever (~40°C or 104°F), chills, malaise, myalgia, arthralgia, prostration, severe fatigue, extreme asthenia, cephalalgia, disequilibrium and sore throat with odynophagia. These initial symptoms are followed by prostration, lethargy, nausea, emesis, diarrhea, exhaustion, asthenia (general muscle weakness), anorexia, and abdominal pains. A maculopapular rash, which first appears on the lateral sides of the trunk, groin and axillary spaces will quickly spread to the entire body with the exception of the face.[75] Additional symptoms may also appear, including chest pains, shortness of breath, cough, conjunctival injection, headaches, confusion and seizures.[80] Subsequently, symptoms such as purpura and hemorrhagic manifestations will appear. These hemorrhagic manifestations are generally limited to petechiae, ecchymoses, uncontrollable bleeding from venipuncture sites, epistaxis, hematuria and melena. Other symptoms such as thrombocytopenia, lymphopenia and leucopenia will also develop. Furthermore, secondary symptoms of edema, postural hypotension, hypovolemia, tachycardia and signs of impaired kidney and liver functions due to renocyte and hepatocyte necrosis are also commonly seen.[17, 71, 79, 80]

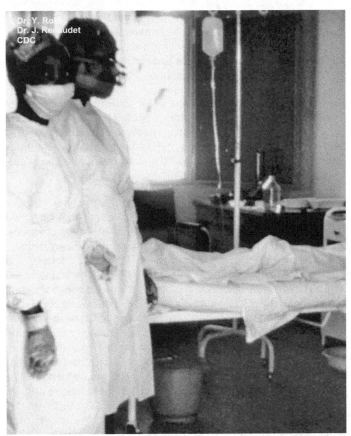

Figure 1.5-12: This 1976 photograph shows two nurses standing in front of Ebola case #3. This patient who was treated but later died at Ngaliema Hospital, in Kinshasa, Zaire

Within a few days of infection, the patient will also develop neutrophilia and an increase in aspartate aminotransferase and alanine aminotransferase concentrations. At the later stages of infection, most patients develop external hemorrhaging from orifices, such as the nose and mouth. The hemorrhaging is a result of numerous small blood clots formed throughout the body, clinically known as disseminated intravascular coagulation (DIC). Where ever these clots are found, a small section of tissue downstream will die from lack of nutrients and oxygen. The body will attempt to compensate for the formation of clots by secreting substantial amounts of plasmin and extrinsic tissue factors, secreted by lymphoid macrophage and monocytes in the blood stream. As a result, massive uncontrollable bleeding occurs throughout the body space (Figure 1.5-12).[79, 80, 81, 82, 83]

During the final stages of EVD, myocarditis and pulmonary edema are also common symptomatic developments. Terminally ill patients will suffer from shock, convulsions, and severe

metabolic disturbances, as well as, displaying an expressionless Hippocratic face. Patients will often succumb to the disease during the second week in a tachypneic, hypotensive, anuric state or more often, in a coma.[79, 80, 81, 82, 83] Please examine Table 2 for more information in regards to the symptoms of EVD.

Table 2: An overview of the clinical symptoms of EVD

Symptoms	+	++	+++
High fever & chills			■
Malaise			■
Myalgia			■
Arthralgia			■
Prostration			■
Severe fatigue			■
Cephalalgia			■
Disequilibrium			■
Sore throat (odynophagia)			■
Lethargy			■
Nausea			■
Emesis			■
Diarrhea			■
Exhaustion			■
Anorexia			■
Abdominal pain			■
Maculopapular rash			■
Chest pains			■
Shortness of breath			■
Cough			■
Conjunctival injection			■
Headaches			■
Confusion			■
Seizures			■
Purpura			■
Petechiae hemorrhage			■
Ecchymoses hemorrhage			■
Venipuncture bleeding			■
Epistaxis			■
Hematuria			■
Melena			■
External hemorrhaging			■
Thrombocytopenia			■
Lymphopenia			■
Leucopenia			■
Edema		■	
Postural hypotension		■	
Hypovolemia		■	
Tachycardia		■	
Impaired kidney functions		■	
Impaired liver functions		■	
Shock		■	
Convulsions		■	
Metabolic disturbances		■	
Anuric state		■	
Tachypneic state		■	
Hypotensive state		■	
Coma		■	

+ Rare ++ Common +++ Frequent

It is suspected that the Ebola virus can cross the placental barrier and infect the fetus. Evidence has shown that in 15 cases of pregnant women infected with EVD, almost all aborted their fetuses, while only one delivered the child at term. Unfortunately, the baby died 3 days after birth due to high fever.[84]

DETECTION

The detection of EVD is generally made clinically by assessing various physical and physiological conditions described in the previous section. Unfortunately, the symptoms of EVD are similar to those described for other hemorrhagic fevers. Therefore, laboratory methodologies are required to definitively diagnose EVD.[85]

During the acute phase of the disease, virus, viral antigen and viral RNA in serum or blood can be isolated through cell culture. For example, the most commonly used cell line for both viral propagation and isolation are the Vero cell lines (e.g. E6 clone). In addition, human adrenal carcinoma cell lines, such as MA-104 and SW13, as well as, cell cultures of monocytes, macrophages and endothelial cells have also proven to be useful in primary viral isolation.[57, 61, 86, 87, 88]

EBOV can be directly identified through electron microscopy of tissue (Figure 1.5-13) culture supernatants, blood, serum or though scanning of cell cultures for the cytopathic effect. Indirect immunofluorescence of cell cultures may also be used to identify EBOV.[79, 89, 90] Additional methods such as antigen-capture enzyme-linked immuno-sorbent assay (ELISA) can be used for the identification of Ebola antigens. Through ELISA, anti-Ebola IgM and IgG can be detected within a few days of the onset infection.[8, 89] However, if the antibodies levels are low, reverse transcriptase polymerase chain reaction (RT-PCR) can be used to detect the RNA genome of the virus. It has been reported that RT-PCR and antigen-capture diagnostic assays were very effective methodologies for detecting EBOV in patient serum, plasma, and whole blood. The RT-PCR assay can detect EBOV RNA 24 to 48 hours prior to detection by antigen capture.[91, 92] Nonetheless, definitive detection of the EVD involves the direct isolation of the Ebola virus in tissue culture coupled with serologic testing which takes time.

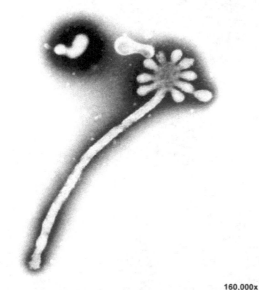

C. Humphrey
A. Sanchez
CDC

160,000x

Figure 1.5-13: Negatively-stained transmission electron micrograph (TEM) reveals some of the ultrastructural morphologic features displayed by an Ebola virion discovered from the Ivory Coast of Africa

It is known that early detection and confirmation of EVD are hampered by collecting appropriate clinical samples, the availability of suitable laboratories and/or the risks associated with transporting such a dangerous specimen to these laboratories. In addition, the availability of properly trained personnel, as well as, cultural objections to taking blood or other invasive samples may impede the infection identification process. For these reasons, scientists are attempting to develop a faster, less invasive manner for the identification of EVD.[93] For example, scientists are developing a method of identification for the Ebola

virus using saliva. At present, this method is still in the testing phase and requires more time before the proper procedures are elucidated.[94]

TREATMENT

Presently, the only available FDA approved treatment is supportive management of specific symptoms that develop as a result of EVD. The clinician needs to closely monitor the patient's pulmonary, renal and cardiac functions throughout the course of infection. Most often, in severe cases of EVD, patients are dehydrated and in need of intravenous fluids. In addition, electrolytes and nutrition will also have to be intravenously introduced, since symptoms of nausea and vomiting will complicate ingestion. It is essential that the clinician closely monitors/maintains oxygen levels as well as the blood pressure of the victim. In an effort to prevent secondary infections, broad spectrum antibiotics may also be administered. In addition, the clinician may provide patients with replacement plasma heparin before the onset of clinical shock and may consider administering corticosteroids to control inflammation.[95]

As with any type of hemorrhagic fever, intramuscular injections should be avoided due to the possibility of uncontrollable intramuscular bleeding. In addition, administering acetyl-salicylic acid (e.g. Aspirin) and non-steroid anti-inflammatory drugs for fever should always be avoided. Clinicians may prescribe aceta-minophen to combat fever and inflammatory symptoms.[96, 97]

The antiviral agent ribavirin has been used with some success in other forms of hemorrhagic fever. However, ribavirin failed in protecting primates infected with EBOV in laboratory trials. Recently, three new anti-EBOV treatments have been devised that demonstrated their effectiveness in animal models and some success in individuals infected with EVD. The first is called MB-003, which is comprised of three chimeric mouse/human monoclonal anti-EBOV antibodies: c13C6, h-13F6 and c6D8. The three monoclonal antibodies were produced in Chinese hamster ovary and in *Nicotiana benthamiana*. During experimental trials, MB-003 successfully protected rhesus macaques from lethal challenges 1 hour post infection and provided significant protection 24-48 hours post infection.[98] The second anti-EBOV agent is called ZMAb which is composed of three mouse derived monoclonal antibodies directed against EBOV GP. In animal trials, ZMab protected 2 out of 4 (50%) non-human primates from lethal EBOV challenges, administered 2 days post-infection. To improve its effectiveness, the researchers combined ZMAb with adenovirus-vectored interferon-α (Ad-IFN) and tested it against infected primates. In one experiment, ZMAb with Ad-IFN protected 3 out of 4 (75%) cynomolgus macaques from lethal EBOV challenges, administered 3 days post-infection. In a subsequent experiment, the ZMAb combination drug protected 4 out of 4 rhesus macaques (100%) from lethal EBOV challenges, administered 3 days post-infection.[99, 100] The third and final treatment also known as ZMapp was developed through various combinations of chimeric mouse/human monoclonal antibodies. The final formulation contains 3 antibodies from MB-003 and ZMAb. During experimental trials on non-human primates, the researchers administered lethal doses of EBOV to 3 groups of 6 non-human primates per group. The first group received ZMapp 3, 6 and 9 days post infection. The second group received ZMapp four, seven, and ten days post infection. The third and final group received ZMapp at five, eight and eleven days post infection. The result of the experiment showed that ZMapp was a complete success as all animals recovered.[101, 102]

During the 1995 outbreak in the Democratic Republic of Congo, human convalescent plasma was used to treat 8 patients suffering from confirmed EVD; seven out of eight patients who received this treatment recovered from the disease.[96, 97] The results from this convalescent antiserum treatment have not been confirmed through *in vitro* and *in vivo* examinations, and laboratory tests showed little or no significant neutralization of the Ebola virus by the antiserum.[17, 103]

Clinical developments and trials of Ebola vaccines have been conducted by Health Canada and the US Army Medical Research Institute of Infectious Diseases at Fort Detrick. As reported by the Medical Laboratory Observer, trials of the Ebola vaccine on macaque monkeys have shown promise, since none of the vaccinated animals contracted EVD, even after ingestion of large doses of the Ebola virus.[17, 104, 105, 106] Recent research in EBOV vaccines uses numerous different platforms for development. The first platform that successfully protected non-human primates and other animal models against lethal EBOV challenges utilized recombinant adenovirus serotype 5 (rAd5) vector expressing EBOV (serotype SEBOV and CIEBOV) GP and NP. Regardless of these promising results, rAd5 based vaccines have limited usage in human subjects where most individuals around the world possess circulating anti-rAd5 neutralizing antibodies which would eliminate the adenovirus before achieving its designed effects.[107, 108] Similar issues faced researchers when they utilized recombinant human parainfluenza virus 3 (HPIV3) that

Table 3: An overview of the differential diagnosis of EHF and other viral infections with similar symptoms. Note: Marburg hemorrhagic fever (MHF), Dengue hemorrhagic fever (DHF), Crimean-Congo hemorrhagic fever (CCHF), Lassa fever (LF), Bohemian hemorrhagic fever (Machupo virus - BHF)

Symptoms	EHF	MHF	DHF	CCHF	LF	Junin	BHF
High fever	■	■		■		■	■
Chills	■	■		■		■	
Malaise	■	■	■	■	■	■	■
Myalgia	■	■		■	■	■	■
Arthralgia	■	■		■	■		■
Prostration	■	■					■
Severe fatigue	■	■					■
Cephalalgia	■						
Disequilibrium	■						
Sore throat with odynophagia	■	■		■	■		
Prostration	■	■					
Lethargy			■	■		■	
Nausea		■		■		■	■
Emesis	■	■		■	■	■	■
Diarrhea	■	■		■	■	■	
Exhaustion		■					
Anorexia	■					■	■
Abdominal pain	■	■	■				
Maculopapular rash	■	■					
Chest pains	■	■					
Shortness of breath	■						
Cough	■				■	■	
Conjunctival injection	■			■	■		■
Headaches	■	■	■	■	■	■	■
Confusion	■						
Seizures	■				■		■
Purpura	■			■			
Petechiae hemorrhage	■	■		■		■	■
Ecchymoses hemorrhage	■	■		■			
Bleeding at puncture sites	■	■		■			
Epistaxis	■			■	■		
Hematuria	■			■		■	
Melena	■			■			
External hemorrhaging	■				■		
Thrombocytopenia	■	■	■	■			
Lymphopenia	■	■					
Leucopenia	■			■			■
Edema	■						
Postural hypotension	■	■			■		
Hypovolemia	■						
Tachycardia				■			
Impaired kidney functions	■			■			
Impaired liver functions	■			■			
Shock	■		■				■
Convulsions	■						
Severe metabolic disturbances							■
Anuric state	■					■	
Tachypneic state	■				■		
Hypotensive state	■	■	■	■	■	■	■
Coma	■						■

expressed EBOV GP and NP. Although the vaccine completely protected non-human primates and other animal models against lethal EBOV challenges, it had limited effect on human subjects. Like the rAd5, most human populations possess anti-HPIV3 neurtralizing antibodies.[17, 109] In order to circumvent this problem, Bukreyev et al. (2009) created a chimeric HPIV3 that expresses only EBOV GP as its only surface protein. The researcher reported that a single dose of the vaccine protected guinea pigs against lethal EBOV challenges. Although successful, more analysis is required to evaluate the toxicity of the vaccine in non-human primates and human test subjects.[110]

DIFFERENTIAL DIAGNOSIS

EBOV infection may be difficult to differentiate from other viral hemorrhagic fevers, such as Marburg hemorrhagic fever (MHF), Dengue hemorrhagic fever (DHF), Crimean-Congo hemorrhagic fever (CCHF), Argentine Hemorrhagic Fever (AHF), and Bolivian hemorrhagic fever (BHF). In the early stages of the disease, EBOV infection can be hard to differentiate from Lassa fever, malaria and typhoid fever.[79, 111]

A physician can discriminate EVD from Lassa fever through Lassa fever's more insidious symptoms of sore throat, pharyngitis and in later stages, facial edema. However, with the exception of mucosal bleeding, the pronounced hemorrhagic symptoms of EVD should be easily distinguished from the disseminated intravascular coagulation and massive uncontrollable bleeding that occurs throughout the body space.[79, 111]

Malaria is generally presented with anemia, jaundice, sweating, and vomiting where these symptoms do not appear in EVD. Typhoid fever may present with rash, gastrointestinal symptoms, lymphadenopathy, relative bradycardia, cough and leucopenia, which also do not appear in EVD. Again, the appearance of disseminated intravascular coagulation and massive uncontrollable bleeding will preclude the diagnosis of malaria and typhoid fever.[79, 111]

Hemorrhagic complications resulting from other VHFs are extremely difficult to differentiate from EVD. However, unlike other VHFs, EVD is marked by extreme prostration and weight loss. With the exemption of dengue virus infection, maculopapular rash have not been observed in other VHFs. Careful epidemiological investigation may show a pattern of insect mediated transmission (EBOV is transmitted from person to person). Nonetheless, the only certain diagnosis of the particular VHF that patient or patients are infected with are through laboratory testing and confirmation (Table 3).[79, 111]

AUTHOR'S NOTE

The most recent EVD outbreak began in 2013 with the first cases in December, and even though the disease frequency has diminished significantly, EVD is still exhibiting cases in June 2015, some 18 months after the beginning of the outbreak. This is the worst outbreak of EVD in history, affecting multiple countries in West Africa. Although the majority of the cases were in Guinea, Sierra Leone, and Liberia, a small number of cases were reported in Nigeria and Mali. EVD has caused significant mortality with reported case fatality rates up to 70% in isolated areas. There have been 869 confirmed health care worker infections reported in the 3 countries involved. Two imported, including one death in health care workers in the United States, attesting to the quality of health care in this country. To date (June 2, 2015) the World Health Organization has reported 27,135 confirmed cases with 11,145 deaths (attributing to the lethality and the communicable nature of EVD. Although the worst of the outbreak is over, sporadic cases of the disease are still being reported in Guinea and Sierra Leone.[112]

References

1. McCormick J.B. Ebola Virus Ecology. Journal of Infectious Diseases, 2004. 190: pp. 1893-1894
2. Kuhn J.H., Becker S., Ebihara H., Geisbert T.W., Johnson K.M., Kawaoka Y., Lipkin W.I., Negredo A.I., Netesov S.V., Nichol S.T., Palacios G., Peters C.J., Tenorio A., Volchkov V.E., Jahrling P.B. Proposal for a revised taxonomy of the family Filoviridae: classification, names of taxa and viruses, and virus abbreviations. Archives of Virology, 2010. 155: pp. 2083-2103
3. Ebola Haemorrhagic Fever in Zaire, 1976. Bulletin of the World Health Organization, 1978. 56: pp. 271-293
4. Ebola Haemorrhagic Fever in Sudan, 1976. Report of a World Health Organization/International Study Team. Bulletin of the World Health Organization, 1978. 56: pp. 247-270
5. Formenty P., Hatz C., Le Guenno B., Stoll A., Rogenmoser P., Widmer A. Human Infection Due to Ebola Virus, Subtype Côte d'Ivoire: Clinical and Biologic Presentation. The Journal of Infectious Diseases, 1999. 179: pp. S48-S53
6. Roddy P., Howard N., Van Kerkhove M.D., Lutwama J., Wamala J., Yoti Z., Colebunders R., Palma P.P., Sterk E., Jeffs B., Van Herp M., Borchert M. Clinical Manifestations and Case Management of Ebola Haemorrhagic Fever Caused by a Newly Identified Virus Strain, Bundibugyo, Uganda, 2007–2008. Public Library of Science (PLoS) One, 2012. 7: pp. e52986
7. Miranda M.E., Ksiazek T.G., Retuya T.J., Khan A.S., Sanchez A., Fulhorst C.F., Rollin P.E., Calaor A.B., Manalo D.L., Roces M.C., Dayrit M.M., Peters C.J. Epidemiology of Ebola (subtype Reston) Virus in the Philippines, 1996. Journal of Infectious Diseases, 1999. 179: pp. S115-S119
8. MacNeil A., Reed Z., Rollin P.E.Serologic Cross-Reactivity of Human IgM and IgG Antibodies to Five Species of Ebola Virus. Public Library of Science (PLoS) Neglected Tropical Diseases, 2011. 5: pp. e1175
9. Ebola Haemorrhagic Fever. World Health Organization. Revised December 2008. Retrieved February 25, 2010. Website: http://www.who.int/mediacentre/factsheets/fs103/en/
10. Wang S., Lau S., Woo P., Yuen K.Y. Bats as a Continuing Source of Emerging Infections in Humans. Reviews in Medical Virology, 2007. 17: pp. 67-91
11. Choi C.Q. Going to Bat. Scientific American, 2006. 294: pp. 24-24B
12. Ebola Haemorrhagic Fever – Fact Sheet Revised in May 2004. Weekly Epidemiological Record, 2004. 49: pp. 435-439.
13. Dowell S.F., Mukunu R., Ksiazek T.G., Khan A.S., Rollin P.E., Peters C.J. Transmission of Ebola Hemorrhagic Fever: A Study of Risk Factors in Family Mmebers, Kikwit, Democratic Republic of the Congo, 1995. The Journal of Infectious Diseases, 1999. 179: S87-S91
14. Sanchez A., Khan A.S., Zaki S.R., Nabel G.J., Ksiazek T.G., Peters C.G. 2001. Filoviridae: Marburg and Ebola Viruses. Fields Virology. Volume 1. 4th Edition. Philadelphia: Lippincott Williams and Wilkins. 2001. pp. 1279-1304
15. Feldmann H., Jones S., Klenk H-D., Schnittler H-J. Ebola Virus: From Discovery to Vaccine. Nature Reviews Immunology, 2003. 3: pp. 677-685
16. Peters, C. J., Khan A. S. Filovirus Diseases. Current Topics in Microbiology and Immunology, 1999. 235: pp. 85-95
17. Choi J.H. Croyle M.A. Emerging Targtes and Novel Approaches to Ebola Virus Prophylaxis and Treatment. BioDrugs, 2013. 27: pp. 565-583
18. Basler C.F., Wang X., Mühlberger E., Volchkov V., Paragas J., Klenk H-D., Garcia-Sastre A., Palese P. The Ebola Virus VP35 Protein Functions as a Type I IFN Antagonist. The Proceedings of the National Academy of Sciences of the United States of America, 2000. 97: pp. 12289-12294
19. Volchkov V.E., Volchkova V.A., Muhlberger E., Kolesnikova L.V., Weik M., Dolnik O., Klenk H.D. Recovery of Infectious Ebola Virus from Complementary DNA: RNA Editing of the GP Gene and Viral Cytotoxicity. Science, 2001. 291: pp. 1965-1969
20. Sanchez A., Kiley M.P., Holloway B.P., Auperin D.D. Sequence Analysis of the Ebola Virus Genome: Organization, Genetic Elements, and Comparison with the Genome of Marburg virus. Virus Research, 1993. 29: pp. 215-240
21. Volchkov V. E., Becker S., Volchkova V.A., Ternovoj V.A., Kotov A.N., Netesov S.V., Klenk H.D. GP mRNA of Ebola Virus is edited by the Ebola Virus Polymerase and by T7 and Vaccinia Virus Polymerases. Virology, 1995. 214: pp. 421-430
22. Sanchez A., Trappier S.G., Mahy B.W., Peters C.J. The Virion Glycoproteins of Ebola Viruses are Encoded in Two Reading Frames and are Expressed Through Transcriptional Editing. Proceedings of the National Academy of Sciences of the United States of America, 1996. 93: pp. 3602-3607
23. Volchkova V. A., Feldmann H., Klenk H.D., Volchkov V.E. The Nonstructural Small Glycoprotein sGP of Ebola Virus is Secreted as an Antiparallel-Orientated Homodimer. Virology, 1998. 250: pp. 408-414
24. Volchkova V. A., Klenk H.D., Volchkov V.E. 1999. Delta-Peptide is the Carboxy-Terminal Cleavage Fragment of the Nonstructural Small Glycoprotein sGP of Ebola Virus. Virology, 1999. 265: pp. 164-171
25. Sanchez A., Trappier S.G., Mahy B.W., Peters C.J., Nichol S.T. 1996. The Virion Glycoproteins of Ebola Viruses are Encoded in Two Reading Frames and are Expressed Through Transcriptional Editing. Proceedings of the National Academy of Sciences of the United States of America, 1996. 93: pp. 3602-3607
26. Kindzelskii A. L., Yang Z., Nabel G.J., Todd III R.F., Petty H.R. 2000. Ebola Virus Secretory Glycoprotein (sGP) Diminishes Fc Gamma RIIIB-to-CR3 Proximity on Neutrophils. The Journal of Immunology, 2000. 164: pp. 953-958
27. Lee J.E., Fusco M.L., Hessell A.J., Oswald W.B., Burton D.R., Saphire E.O. Structure of the Ebola Virus Glycoprotein Bound to an Antibody From a Human Survivor. Nature, 2008. 454: pp. 177-182
28. Ray R.B., Basu A., Steele R., Beyene A., McHowat J., Meyer K., Ghosh A.K., Ray R. Ebola Virus Glycoprotein-Mediated Anoikis of Primary Human Cardiac Microvascular Endothelial Cells. Virology, 2004. 321: pp.181-188
29. Ströher U., West E., Bugany H., Klenk H.D., Schnittler H.J., Feldmann H. Infection and Activation of Monocytes by Marburg and Ebola Viruses. Journal of Viology, 2001. 75: pp. 11025-11033
30. Sullivan N., Yang Z-Y., Nabel G.J. Ebola Virus Pathogenesis: Implications for Vaccines and Therapies. Journal of Virology, 2003. 77: pp. 9733-9737
31. Schnittler H. J., Feldmann H. 2003. Viral Hemorrhagic Fever—a Vascular Disease? Journal of Thrombosis and Haemostasis, 2003. 89: pp. 967-972
32. Feldmann H., Bugany H., Mahner F., Klenk H.D., Drenckhahn D., Schnittler H.J. Filovirus-Induced Endothelial Leakage Triggered by Infected Monocytes/Macrophages. Journal of Viology, 1996. 70: pp. 2208-2214

33. Feldmann H., Volchkov V.E., Volchkova V.A., Klenk H.D. The Glycoproteins of Marburg and Ebola Virus and Their Potential Roles in Pathogenesis. Archives of Virology, 1999. 15:159-169
34. Geisbert T. W., Hensley L.E., Larsen T., Young H.A., Reed D.S., Geisbert J.B., Scott D.P., Kagan E., Jahrling P.B., Davis K.J. Pathogenesis of Ebola Hemorrhagic Fever in Cynomolgus Macaques: Evidence that Dendritic Cells are Early and Sustained Targets of Infection. The Americal Journal of Pathology, 2003. 163: pp. 2347-2370
35. Wahl-Jensen V.M., Afanasieva T.A., Seebach J., Ströher U., Feldmann H., Schnittler H-J. Effects of Ebola Virus Glycoproteins on Endothelial Cell Activation and Barrier Function. Journal of Virology, 2005. 79: pp. 10442–10450
36. Mehedi M., Falzarano D., Seebach J., Hu X., Carpenter M.S., Schnittler H-J., Feldmann H. New Ebola Virus Nonstructural Glycoprotein Expressed through RNA Editing. Journal of Virology, 2011. 85: pp. 5406–5414
37. Manicassamy B., Wang J., Jiang H., Rong L. Comprehensive Analysis of Ebola Virus GP1 in Viral Entry. The Journal of Virology, 2005. 79: pp. 4793–4805
38. Volchkov V.E., Feldmann H., Volchkova V.A., Klenk H.D. Processing of the Ebola Virus Glycoprotein by the Proprotein Convertase Furin. Proceedings of the National Academy of Sciences of the United States of America, 1998. 95: pp. 5762-5767
39. Jeffers S. A., Sanders D.A., Sanchez A. Covalent Modifications of the Ebola Virus Glycoprotein. The Journal of Virology, 2002. 76: pp. 12463-1247
40. Feldmann H., Volchkov V.E., Volchkova V.A., Stroher U., Klenk H.D. Biosynthesis and Role of Filoviral Glycoproteins. Journal of General Virology, 2001. 82: pp. 2839-2848
41. Takada A., Robison C., Goto H., Sanchez A., Murti K.G., Whitt M.A., Kawaoka Y. A System for Functional Analysis of Ebola Virus Glycoprotein. Proceedings of the National Academy of Sciences of the United States of America, 1997. 94: pp. 14764-14769
42. Wool-Lewis R. J., Bates P. 1998. Characterization of Ebola Virus Entry by using Pseudotyped Viruses: Identification of Receptor-Deficient Cell Lines. The Journal of Virology, 1998. 72: pp. 3155-3160
43. Hans Z., Boshra H., Sunyer J.O., Zwiers S.H., Paragas J., Harty R.N. Biochemical and Functional Characterization of the Ebola Virus VP24 Protein: Implications for a Role in Virus Assembly and Budding. The Journal of Virology, 2003. 77: pp. 1793-1800
44. Chandran K., Sullivan N.J., Felbor U., Whelan S.P., Cunningham J.M. Endosomal Proteolysis of the Ebola Virus Glycoprotein is Necessary for Infection. Science, 2005. 308: pp. 1643-1645
45. Yoshihiro K. How Ebola Virus Infects Cells. New England Journal of Medicine, 2005. 352: pp. 2645-2646
46. Martinez O., Leung L.W., Basler C.F. The Role of Antigen-Presenting cells in Filoviral Hemorrhagic Fever: Gaps in Current Knowledge. Antiviral Research, 2012. 93: pp. 416-428
47. Baize S., Leroy E.M., Mavoungou E., Fisher-Hoch S.P. Apoptosis in Fatal Ebola Infection. Does the Virus Toll the Bell for Immune System? Apoptosis, 2000. 5: pp. 5-7
48. Sanchez A. Kiley M.P. Identification and Analysis of Ebola Virus Messenger RNA. Virology, 1987. 157: pp.414-420
49. Knipe D.M., Howley P.M. Fields Virology. Volume 1. Philadelphia: Lippincott William & Wilkins. 2007. pp. 1410-1448
50. Ryabchikova E.I., Kolesnikova L.V., Luchko S.V. An Analysis of Features of Pathogenesis in Two Animal Models of Ebola Virus Infection. The Journal of Infectious Diseases, 1999. 179: pp. S199-S202
51. Geisbert T.W., Hensley L.E., Gibb T.R., Steele K.E., Jaax N.K., Jahrling P.B. Apoptosis induced in vitro and in vivo during Infection by Ebola and Marburg Viruses. Laboratory Investigation, 2000. 80: pp. 171-186
52. Bente D., Gren J., Strong J.E., Feldmann H. Disease Modeling for Ebola and Marburg Viruses. Disease Models and Mechanisms, 2009. 2: pp. 12-17
53. Baize S., Leroy E.M., Georges A.J., Georges-Courbot M-C., Capron M., Bedjabaga I., Lansoud-Soukate J., Mavoungou E. Inflammatory Responses in Ebola Virus-Infected Patients. Clinical and Experimental Immunology, 2002. 128: pp. 163–168
54. Villinger F., Rollin P.E., Brar S.S., Chikkala N.F., Winter J., Sundstrom J.B., Zaki S.R., Swanepoel R., Ansari A.A., Peters C.J. Markedly Elevated Levels of Interferon (IFN)-gamma, IFN-alpha, Interleukin (IL)-2, IL-10, and Tumor Necrosis Factor-alpha Associated with Fatal Ebola Virus Infection. The Journal of Infectious Diseases, 1999. 179: pp. S188-S191
55. Leroy E.M., Baize S., Volchkov V.E., Fisher-Hoch S.P., Georges-Courbot M.C., Lansoud-Soukate J., Capron M., Debré P., McCormick J.B., Georges A.J. Human Asymptomatic Ebola Infection and Strong Inflammatory Response. Lancet, 2000. 355: pp. 2210-2215
56. Maruyama T., Buchmeier M.J., Parren P.W. H. I., Burton D.R., Yang Z-Y., Delgado R., Xu L., Todd R.F., Nabel E.G., Sanchez A., Nabel G.J. Ebola Virus, Neutrophils, and Antibody Specificity. Science, 1998. 282: pp. 843
57. Ströher U., West E., Bugany H., Klenk H-D., Schnittler H.J., Feldmann H. Infection and Activation of Monocytes by Marburg and Ebola Viruses. Journal of Virology, 2001. 75: pp. 11025-11033
58. Volchkov V.E., Volchkova V.A., Slenczka W., Klenk H.D., Feldmann H. Release of Viral Glycoproteins during Ebola Virus Infection. Virology, 1998. 245: pp. 110-119
59. Yang Z.Y., Duckers H.J., Sullivan N.J., Sanchez A., Nabel E.G., Nabel G.J. Identification of the Ebola Virus Glycoprotein as the Main Viral Determinant of Vascular Cell Cytotoxicity and Injury. Nature Medicine, 2000. 6: pp. 886-889
60. Chan S.Y., Ma M.C., Goldsmith M.A. Differential Induction of Cellular Detachment by Envelope Glycoproteins of Marburg and Ebola (Zaire) Viruses. The Journal of General Virology, 2000. 81: pp. 2155-2159
61. Feldmann H., Bugany H., Mahner F., Klenk H.D., Drenckhahn D., Schnittler H.J. Filovirus-induced Endothelial Leakage Triggered by Infected Monocytes/macrophages. Journal of Virology, 1996. 70: pp. 2208-2214
62. Schnittler H.J., Feldmann H. Molecular Pathogenesis of Filovirus Infections: Role of Macrophages and Endothelial Cells. Current Topics in Microbiology and Immunology, 1999. 235: pp. 175-204
63. Alibek K. Biohazard. New York: Dell Publishing. 1999. pp. 18
64. Johnson E., Jaax N., White J., Jahrling P. Lethal Experimental Infections of Rhesus Monkeys by Aerosolized Ebola virus. International Journal of Experimental Pathology, 1995. 76: pp. 227-236
65. Alibek K. Biohazard. New York: Dell Publishing. 1999. pp. 20-42
66. Maron D.F. Weaponized Ebola: Is It Really a Bioterror Threat? What would it take to hijack the virus in west Africa and turn it into a bioterror agent elsewhere? Sceintific American. Published September 25, 2014. Retrieved November 2, 2014. Website: http://www.scientificamerican.com/article/weaponized-ebola-is-it-really-a-bio terror-threat/
67. Olson K.B. Aum Shinrikyo: Once and Future Threat. Emerging Infectious Diseases, 1999. 5: pp. 513-516
68. What we know about transmission of the Ebola virus among humans. Ebola situation assessment. World Health Organization. Released 6 October 2014. Retrieved November 2, 2014. Website: http://www.who.int /mediacentre/news/ebola/06-october-2014/en/
69. Bausch D.G., Towner J.S., Dowell S.F., Kaducu F., Lukwiya M., Sanchez A., Nichol S.T., Ksiazek T.G., Rollin P.E. Assessment of the Risk of Ebola Virus Transmission from Bodily Fluids and Fomites. The Journal of Infectious Diseases, 2007. 196: pp. S142–S147
70. Francesconi P., Yoti Z., Declich S., Onek P.A., Fabiani M., Olango J., Andraghetti R., Rollin P.E., Opira C., Greco D., Salmaso S. Ebola Hemorrhagic Fever Transmission and Risk Factors of Contacts, Uganda. Emerging Infectious Diseases, 2003. 9: pp. 1430-1437
71. Bosio C.M., Aman M.J., Grogan C., Hogan R., Ruthel G., Negley D., Mohamadzadeh M., Bavari S., Schmaljohn A. Ebola and Marburg Viruses Replicate in Monocyte-derived Dendritic Cells without Inducing the Production of Cytokins and full Maturation. Journal of Infectious Diseases, 2003. 188: pp. 1630-1638
72. Mahanty S., Hutchinson K., Agarwal S., McRae M., Rollin P.E., Pulendran B. Cutting Edge: Impairment of Dendritic Cells and Adaptive Immunity by Ebola and Lassa Viruses. Journal of Immunology, 2003. 170: pp. 2797-2801
73. Bray M., Mahanty S. Ebola Hemorrhagic Fever and Septic Shock. The Journal of Infectious Diseases, 2003. 188: pp. 1613-1617
74. Stroher U., West E., Bugany H., Klenk H.D., Schnittler H.J., Feldmann H. Infection and Activation of Monocyte by Marburg and Ebola Viruses. The Journal of Virology, 2001. 75: pp. 11025-33
75. Hensley L.E., Young H.A., Jahrling P.B., Geisbert T.W. Proinflammatory Response during Ebola Virus Infection of Primate Models: Possible Involvement of Tumor Necrosis Factor Receptor Superfamily. Immunology Letters, 2002. 80: pp. 169-179
76. Gupta M., Manhanty S., Ahmed R., Rollin P. Monocyte Derived Human Macrophage and Peripheral Blood Mononuclear Cells Infected with Ebola Virus Secrete MIP-1 Alpha and TNF-alpha and Inhibit Poly-IC Induced IFN-alpha in Vitro. Virology, 2001. 284: pp. 20-25
77. Harcourt B.H., Sanchez A., Offermann M.K. Ebola Virus Selectively Inhibits Responses to Interferons, but not to Interleukin -1beta, in Endothelial Cells. The Journal of Virology, 1999. 73: pp. 3491-3496
78. Basler C.F., Wang X., Muhlberger E., Volchkov V., Paragas J., Klenk H.D., Garcia-Sastre A., Palese P. The Ebola virus VP35 Protein Functions as a Type I IFN Antagonist. Proceedings of the National Academy of Science, 2000. 97: pp. 12289-12294
79. Guerrant R.L., Walker D.H., Weller P.F. Tropical Infectious Diseases – Principles, Pathogens & Practice. Volume 1. Philadelphia: Churchill Livingstone Elsevier. 2006. pp. 784-796
80. Bente D., Gren J., Strong J.E., Feldmann H. Disease Modeling for Ebola and Marburg Viruses. Sisease Models and Mechanisms, 2009. 2: pp. 12-17
81. Bwaka M., Bonnet M.J., Calain P., Colebunders R., Roo A.D., Guimard Y., Katwiki K.R., Kibadi K., Kipasa M.A., Kuvula K.J., Mapanda B.B., Massamba M., Mupapa K.D., Muyembe-Tamfum J.J., Ndaberey E., Peters C.J., Rollin P.E., Van den Enden E. Ebola Hemorrhagic Fever in Kikwit, Democratic Republic of the Congo: Clinical Observations in 103 Patients. The Journal of Infectious Diseases, 1999. 179: pp. S1-S7
82. Peters C.J., Olshaker M. Virus Hunter. Thirty Years of Battling Hot Viruses around the World. New York: Anchor Books.1997. pp. 218-219
83. Geisbert T.W., Young H.A., Jahrling P.B., Davis K.J., Kagan E., Hensley L.E. Mechanisms Underlying Coagulation Abnormalities in Ebola Hemorrhagic Fever; Over Expression of Tissue Factor in Primate Monocytes/Macrophages is a Key Event. Journal of Infectious Diseases, 2003. 188: pp. 1618-1629
84. Kibadi M., Woliere M., Ado B.M., Mungala K., Ann D., Kivudi K., Kapay K., Matondo M., Djuma N., Robert C., Muyembe-Tamfum, J.J. Ebola Hemorrhagic Fever and Pregnancy. The Journal of Infectious Diseases, 1999. 179: pp. S11- S12
85. Peters C.J., Zaki S.R., Rollin P.E. Viral Hemorrhagic Fevers. Atlas of Infectious Diseases. Philadelphia: Churchill Livingstone. 1997. pp. 10.2-10.26
86. Shurtleff A.C., Biggins J.E., Keeney A.E., Zumbrun E.E., Bloomfield H.A., Kuehne A., Audet J.L., Alfson K.J., Griffiths A., Olinger G.G., Bavari S. Standardization of the Filovirus Plaque Assay for Use in Preclinical Studies. Viruses, 2012. 4: pp. 3511-3530
87. Feldmann H., Kiley M.P. Classification, Structure and Replication of Filoviruses. Current Topics in Microbiology and Immunology, 1999. 235: pp. 1-21
88. McCormick J.B., Bauer S.P., Elliott L.H., Webb P.A., Johnson K.M. Biologic Differences Between Strains of Ebola Virus from Zaire and Sudan. The Journal of Infectious Diseases, 1983. 147: pp. 264-267
89. Truant A.L., Regnery R.L., Kiley M.P. Development of an Immunofluorescence Focus Assay for Ebola Virus. Journal of Clinical Microbiology, 1983. 18: pp. 416-419
90. Beniac D.R., Siemens C.G., Wright C.J., Booth T.F. A Filtration Based Technique for Simultaneous SEM and TEM Sample Preparation for the Rapid Detection of Pathogens. Virus, 2014. 6: pp. 3458-3471
91. Towner J.S., Rollin P.E., Bausch D.G., Sanchez A., Crary S.M., Vincent M., Lee W.F., Spiropoulou C.F., Ksiazek T.G., Lukwiya M., Kaducu F., Downing R., Nichol S.T. Rapid Diagnosis of Ebola Hemorrhagic Fever by Reverse Transcription-PCR in an Outbreak Setting and Assessment of Patient Viral Load as a Predictor of Outcome. Journal of Virology, 2004. 78: pp. 4330-4341
92. He J., Kraft A.J., Fan J., Van Dyke M., Wang L., Bose M.E., Khanna M., Metallo J.A., Henrickson K.J. Simultaneous Detection of CDC Category "A" DNA and RNA Bioterrorism Agents by Use of Multiplex PCR & RT-PCR Enzyme Hybridization Assays. Virus, 2009. 1: pp. 441-459
93. Ksiazek T.G., West C.P., Rollin P.E., Jahrling P.B., Peters C.J. ELISA for the Detection of Antibodies to Ebola Viruses. The Journal of Infectious Diseases, 1999. 179: pp. S192-198
94. Nokes D.J., Enquselassie F., Nigatu W., Vyse A.J., Cohen B.J., Brown D.W., Cutts F.T. Has Oral Fluid the Potential to Replace Serum for the Evaluation of Population Immunity Levels? A Study of Measles, Rubella and Hepatitis B in Rural Ethiopia. Bulletin of the World Health Organization, 2001. 79: pp. 588-595
95. Formenty P., Leroy E.M., Epelboin A., Libama F., Lenzi M., Sudeck H., Yaba P., Allarangar Y., Boumandouki P., Nkounkou V.B., Drosten C., Grolla A., Feldmann H., Roth C. Detection of Ebola Virus in Oral Fluid Specimens during Outbreaks of Ebola Virus Hemorrhagic Fever in the Republic of Congo. Clinical Infectious Diseases, 2006. 42: pp. 1521-1526
96. McConnell E.A. Combating Infection. Ebola: Preparing for the Worst. Nursing, 2001. 31: pp. 30
97. Mupapa K., Massamba M., Kibadi K., Kuvula K., Bwaka A., Kipasa M., Colebunders R., Muyembe-Tamfum J.J. Treatment of Ebola Hemorrhagic Fever with Blood Transfusions from Convalescent Patients. The Journal of Infectious Diseases, 1999. 179: S18-S23
98. Olinger Jr. G.G., Pettitt J., Kim D., Working C., Bohorov O., Bratcher B., Hiatt E., Hume S.D., Johnson A.K., Morton J., Pauly M., Whaley K.J., Lear C.M., Biggins J.E., Scully C., Hensley L., Zeitlin L. Delayed treatment of Ebola virus infection with plant-derived monoclonal antibodies provides protection in rhesus macaques. Proceedings of the National Academy of Sciences of the United States of America, 2012. 109: pp. 18030–18035
99. Qiu X., Wong G., Fernando L., Audet J., Bello A., Strong J., Alimonti J.B., Kobinger G.P. mAbs and Ad-Vectored IFN-α Therapy Rescue Ebola-Infected Nonhuman Primates When Administered After the Detection of Viremia and Symptoms. Science Translational Medicine, 2013. 5: 207ra143
100. Qiu X., Audet J., Wong G., Fernando L., Bello A., Pillet S., Alimonti J.B., Kobinger G.P. Sustained protection against Ebola virus infection following treatment of infected nonhuman primates with ZMAb. Scientific Reports, 2013. 3: pp. 3365
101. Geisbert T.W. Medical Research: Ebola Therapy Protects Severely Ill Monkeys. Nature,

2014. 514: pp. 41-43

102. Qiu X., Wong G., Audet J., Bello A., Fernando L., Alimonti J.B., Fausther-Bovendo H., Wei H., Aviles J., Hiatt E., Johnson A., Morton J., Swope K., Bohorov O., Bohorova N., Goodman C., Kim D., Pauly M.H., Velasco J., Pettitt J., Olinger G.G., Whaley K., Xu B., Strong J.E., Zeitlin L., Kobinger G.P. Reversion of advanced Ebola virus disease in nonhuman primates with ZMapp. Nature, 2014. 514: pp. 47-53
103. Huggins J.W. Prospects for Treatment of Viral Hemorrhagic Fevers with Ribavirin, a Broad Spectrum Anti-viral Drug. Reviews of Infectious Diseases, 1989. 4: pp. S750-S761
104. Peters C.J., Olshaker M. Virus Hunter. Thirty Years of Battling Hot Viruses around the World. New York: Anchor Books. 1997. pp. 225
105. Potential Marburg and Ebola Vaccines. Medical Laboratory Observer, 2005. 37: pp. 8
106. Nierengarten M.B., Lutwick L.I. Vaccines for Viral Hemorrhagic Fevers: Filoviruses and Arenaviruses. Medscape Infectious Disease, 2002. 4: Retrieved July 6, 2007. Web Site: http://www.medscape.com/viewarticle/43 3535
107. Choi J.H., Schafer S.C., Zhang L., Kobinger G.P., Juelich T., Freiberg A.N., Croyle M.A. A Single Sublingual Dose of an Adenovirus-based Vaccine Protects Against Lethal Ebola Challenge in Mice and Guinea pigs. Molecular Pharmaceutics, 2012. 9: pp. 156–167.
108. Mast T.C., Kierstead L., Gupta S.B., Nikas A.A., Kallas E.G., Novitsky V., Mbewe B., Pitisuttithum P., Schechter M., Vardas E., Wolfe N.D., Aste-Amezaga M., Casimiro D.R., Coplan P., Straus W.L., Shiver J.W. International epidemiology of human pre-existing adenovirus (Ad) type-5, type-6, type-26 and type-36 neutralizing antibodies: correlates of high Ad5 titers and implications for potential HIV vaccine trials. Vaccine, 2010. 28: pp. 950–957.
109. Bukreyev A., Skiadopoulos M.H., Murphy B.R., Collins P.L. Nonsegmented negative-strand viruses as vaccine vectors. Journal of Virology, 2006. 80: pp. 10293–10306
110. Bukreyev A., Marzi A., Feldmann F., Zhang L., Yang L., Ward J.M., Dorward D.W., Pickles R.J., Murphy B.R., Feldmann H., Collins P.L. Chimeric Human Parainfluenza Virus Bearing the Ebola Virus Glycoprotein as the Sole Surface Protein is Immunogenic and Highly Protective Against Ebola Virus Challenge. Virology, 2009. 383: pp. 348–361
111. Tomori O. Ebola: Clinical Features and Public Health Issues. The Philippine Journal of Microbiology and Infectious Diseases, 1996. 25: pp. S8-S15
112. Ebola virus disease. Fact sheet N°103. World Health Organization. Released April 2015. Retrieved June 3, 2015. Website: http://www.who.int/mediacentre/factsheets/fs103/en

Photo Bibliography

Figure 1.5-1: Colorized transmission electron micrograph (TEM) of Ebola virus. This micrograph was taken at 160,000x magnification by Dr. Frederick Murphy and released by the CDC. Public domain photo

Figure 1.5-7: Transmission electron micrograph showing assembly and maturing EBOV within the cytoplasm of a monocytic host cell. The micrograph was taken at 4000x magnification by Dr. Fredrick Murphy in 1977 and released by the CDC. Public domain photo

Figure 1.5-8: Transmission electron micrograph (TEM) of EBOV within a host cell. Please note the accumulation of assembling virus and virus particle within the cytoplasm and the budding of viruses at the plasma membrane. The micrograph was taken at 4000x magnification by Dr. Fredrick Murphy in 1977 and released by the CDC. Public domain photo

Figure 1.5-9: CDC microbiologist Zachary Braden is working in a Biosafety Level 4 (BSL-4) laboratory within an air-tight, self-contained, positively-pressurized suit. Photo was taken by Dr. Scott Smith and released by the CDC. Public domain photo

Figure 1.5-10: Photomicrograph of a formalin fixed Ebola virus in monkey hepatocyte (indicated by the blue arrow). The photomicrograph was contributed by Dr. Keith Steele, US Army Medical Research Institute of Infectious Disease, Frederick, Maryland. Public domain photo

Figure 1.5-11: Hematoxylin-eosin-stained (H&E) photomicro-graph demonstrates the cytoarchitectural changes in a liver tissue specimen. This specimen was extracted from a patient suffering from EBOV in Zaire. Note the acidophilic necrosis leading to the formation of a Councilman hyaline body (eosinophilic globule) and cytoplasmic inclusions. The photomicrograph indicates that the hepatocytes are undergoing apoptosis. Photo was taken by Dr. Yves Robin and Dr. Jean Renaudet, Arbovirus Laboratory at the Pasteur Institute in Dakar, Senegal; World Health Organization and released by the CDC. Public domain photo

Figure 1.5-12: This 1976 photograph shows two nurses standing in front of Ebola case #3. This patient who was treated but later died at Ngaliema Hospital, in Kinshasa, Zaire. Photo was taken by Dr. Lyle Conrad and released by the CDC. Public domain photo

Figure 1.5-13: Negatively-stained transmission electron micrograph (TEM) revealed some of the ultrastructural morphologic features displayed by an Ebola virion discovered from the Ivory Coast of Africa. This electron micrograph was taken at 160,000x by Charles Humphrey and Anthony Sanchez and released by the CDC. Public domain photo

The hantavirus (HV) is a spherical, negative sense, enveloped, single stranded, tri-segmented (tripartite) RNA virus and belonging to the genus *Hantaviridae* of the family *Bunyavioridae*.[1] The three segments of the genome are ambisense single RNA strands composed of large, medium and small segments. Research has shown that the reverse compliment of the large RNA segment encodes the RNA-dependent RNA polymerase (L-protein 250 kD). The reverse complement of the medium RNA segment encodes a glycoprotein precursor (GPC) that cleaves to form two glycoproteins: G_1 (72 kD) and G_2 (54 kD). Finally the reverse complement of small RNA segment encodes the nucleocapsid (N) proteins (48 kD).[1, 2, 3, 4, 5]

There are approximately 43 species of HV, 23 of which have been isolated in laboratories and serotyped. Approximately 24 species are known to be capable of causing either hemorrhagic fever with renal syndrome (HFRS: Old World disease) or hantavirus pulmonary syndrome (HPS: New World disease) in humans (Table 1).[1] Presently, it is estimated that there are between 60 and 100 thousand reported cases of Hantavirus infections annually, with the bulk of the infections reported in European Russia and China (Figure 1.6-1).[6, 7]

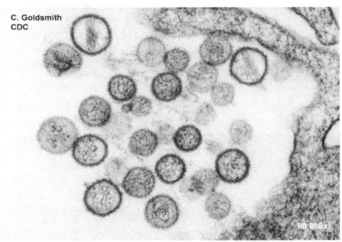

C. Goldsmith
CDC

Figure 1.6-1: Transmission electron micrograph (TEM) of numerous Hantavirus virions

It is believed that the diseases caused by HV infection has appeared under many different names throughout history. Researchers recognized that the first reported cases of hantavirus may date back nearly one thousand years in China. Other reported cases, with similarly described symptoms, have also been discovered in European and Asian historical medical literature.[8] Researchers believed that other outbreaks, which could be attributed to HFRS have been recorded between 1913-1932 in Russia, as well as, among Japanese troops in Manchuria during 1932.[9] During the Korean War (1951-1953), more than three thousand United Nations and US troops suffered from HFRS, with a mortality rate between 7 and 10%.[10,11] However, it was not until 1977 that the first species of the HV was isolated and received its name from the location where it was discovered, the Hantaan River, in Korea.[12]

HV is a zoonosis and its common reservoir are rodents belonging in the Subfamily *Muridae, Arvicolinae* or *Sigmodontinae* and are commonly found throughout all corners of the world.[1, 13] Nonetheless, it is known that one insectivore (*Suncus murinus*),

which lies outside of the *Muridae* is a vector of HV.[14]

Table 1: Serotypes of Hantavirus, its reservoir and the diseases it causes

Type of Hantavirus	Location/Serotype	Disease
Andes	S. America	HPS
Amur	E. Russia	HFRS
Anajatuba	Brazil	HPS
Araraquara	Brazil	HPS
Bayou	N. America	HPS
Bermejo	N.W. Argentina	HPS
Black Creek Canal	N. America	HPS
Bloodland Lake	N. America	-
Blue River	N. America	-
Cano Delgadito	S. America	-
Calabazo	Panama	-
Castelo dos Sonhos	Brazil	HPS
Central Plata	Uruguay	HPS
Choclo	Panama	HPS
Dobrava-Belgrade	Balkans	HFRS
El Moro Canyon	N. America	-
Hantaan	E. Asia	HFRS
Hu39694	C. Argentina	HPS
Isla Vista	N. America	-
Juquitiba	Brazil	HPS
Khabarovsk	Russia	-
Laguna Negra	S. America	HPS
Lechiguanas	C. Argentina	HPS
Limestone Canyon	S.W. US, Mexico	-
Maciel	C. Argentina	-
Maporal	Venezuela	-
Monongahela	N. America	HPS
Muleshoe	N. America	-
New York-1	N. America	HPS
Oran	NW Argentina	HPS
Pergamino	C. Argentina	-
Prospect Hill	N. America	-
Puumala	Russia, Europe	HFRS
Rio Mamore	Bolivia	-
Rio Mearim	Brazil	-
Rio Segundo	Costa Rica	-
Saaremaa	Europe	HFRS
Seoul	Worldwide	HFRS
Sin Nombre	N. America	HFRS
Thailand	S.E. Asia	HFRS
Thottapalayam	S.E. Asia	-
Topografov	Siberia	-
Tula	Russia, Slovakia & Czech	-

■ Vector unknown
□ Rodent
▨ Shrew

Traditionally, it is believed that HV and its reservoir, the murid rodents, shared a period of co-evolution. As a result, there are no known diseases identified in the rodent reservoir that are caused by HV.[15] However, current studies show clinically detectable disease can be found within the host (e.g. histological lesions of the lungs and various other organs), although no mortalities of the hosts due to the infections have been found (Figure 1.6-2).[16, 17, 18]

Experimental evidence indicates that there are no limitations as to the specific species of rodent that can be the vector of HV. To the contrary, more than one rodent species can become the reservoir for the various species of HV.[15] This occurrence is particularly problematic since the ecological distribution of HV may cross a broad range of geographical boundaries around the world.[15,19]

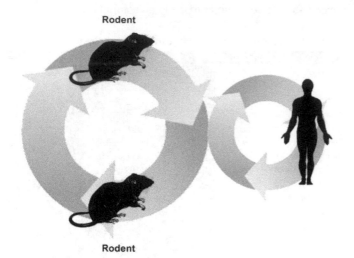

Figure 1.6-2: Sylvatic cycle of hantavirus

HV is responsible for causing hemorrhagic fever with renal syndrome (HFRS) and hantavirus pulmonary syndrome (HPS) in individuals that come in close proximity with murid rodents. HFRS is most commonly seen in Europe and East Asia, while in North and South America, HPS is the prevalent disease. For example, the Hantaan virus is responsible for HFRS in China, Russia and Korea, while the Seoul virus has worldwide distribution. To a lesser extent, Thailand virus inflicts HFRS to the population of Southeast Asia (e.g. Thailand and China).[20] In Western Europe, Russia and Scandinavia, the Puumala virus is the main source for HFRS. The Puumala virus causes a less severe case of HFRS and its infections are commonly referred to as nephrpopathia epidemica (NE).[8] Less significantly, the Saaremaa virus, a serotype of Dobrava-Belgrade virus, causes HFRS within the same geographical distribution as Puumala.[21] Lastly, the Dobrava-Belgrade virus is found to be the cause of

HFRS in the Balkans.[22]

In North America, the common agent for causing HPS is the Sin Nombre virus, which is also referred to as the Four Corners virus. Other less prevalent types can also cause HPS in North America including the New York-1 virus, Black Creek Canal virus, and the Bayou virus. In South America, there are three virus types that can cause HPS; Andes virus, Cano Delgadito and the Laguna Negra virus.[23] Please see Table 1 and Figure 1.6-3 for more information.

HV virions measure between 120-160 nm in diameter, which when inhaled, will pass successfully through the nose, and move into the terminal respiratory bronchioles and alveolar sacs, where initial infection occurs.[24] It is known that the naked HV RNA genome is non-infectious. An infectious virus, requires encapsulation of the RNA genome by nucleoprotein (NP, small RNA segment) forming the nucleocapsid core, in association with the RNA-dependent RNA polymerase (large RNA segment). The remaining viral proteins, such as G_1 and G_2 are found embedded in the phospholipid membrane, derived from the host cell.[1]

In vitro and *in vivo* experiments have demonstrated that HV infects endothelial cells and monocytic cells (Figure 1.6-4).[25, 26, 27] Although, a single report has stated that HV induced apoptosis in cultured endothelial cells.[28] Histological examinations of infected tissues have indicated that HV-infected patients did not show major endothelial cell death, nor did HV alter the permeability or tight junction structures of these cells *in vitro*.[29,30] Therefore, it is presumed that HV is capable of affecting the function of endothelial cells in a limited fashion, without causing obvious cytopathic effects, unlike other hemorrhagic fever viruses, such as filoviruses.[31]

Human beta (β) 3 integrins are cellular receptors found on endothelial cells and platelets. They are critical adhesive protein receptors that regulate vascular permeability, platelet activation and adhesion. For HV, Human β3 integrins are the targeted attachment site, as well as the site of entry into these susceptible host cells via clathrin-dependent endocytosis. It has been

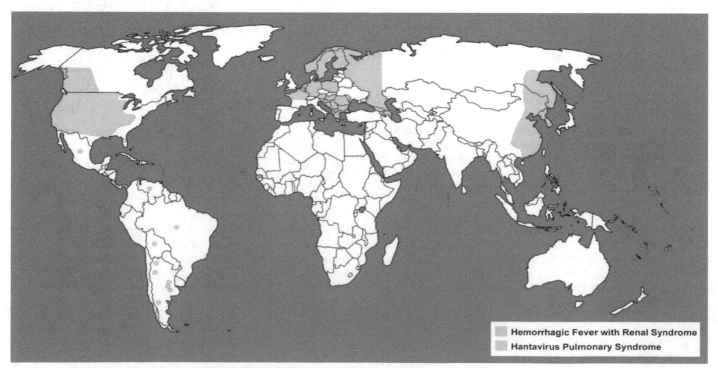

Hemorrhagic Fever with Renal Syndrome
Hantavirus Pulmonary Syndrome

Figure 1.6-3: Distribution of New world and old world Hantavirus

shown that viral proteins are co-localized in early endosome, approximately 90 minutes post-infection, while detected in the late endosome and lysosome approximately four hours post infection.[1, 32, 33, 34]

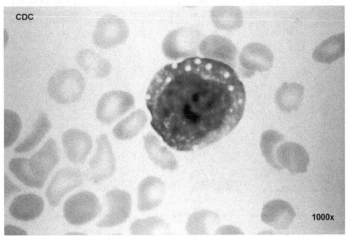

Figure 1.6-4: A photomicrograph of an atypical enlarged lymphocyte found in the blood smear from a HPS patient

Although all HV serotypes utilize β3 integrin as the site of attachment and entry into host cells, there is a divergence of HV surface glycol-proteins depending on the serotype. The use of β3 integrin by all HV species may suggest that common elements exist on the G_1 or the highly conserved G_2 surface glycoprotein that mediates attachment of the virus. Nonetheless, the variation of the G_1 and G_2 glycoproteins of HV are likely to contribute to additional interactions, which may establish pathogenic responses associated with individual viruses. Unfortunately, at present there is no research that elucidates the virion attachment protein, although, the development of antibodies that recognize HV attachment proteins while blocking integrin interactions is of particular interest, since it is likely to provide an additional point for therapeutic intervention and vaccine development.[35]

Soon after the HV virus is taken into the host cell through clathrin-dependent endocytosis, viral replication is initiated after the release of the viral ribonucleoprotein (RNP) core into the cytoplasm. Immediately, HV utilizes the RNA-dependent RNA polymerase (L protein embedded in the ribonucleoprotein core) to transcribe each of the negative sense RNA segments into viral mRNA (positive sense segments). The process of synthesizing HV mRNA requires "cap-snatching," where the virus cleaves host cellular capped mRNAs from the 5' terminus and generates capped RNA oligonucleotides that are used as primers by viral RNA-dependent RNA polymerase during transcription initiation.[1, 36] It has been reported that the N protein of Black Creek Canal, Puumala, and Seoul hantaviruses are localized in the perinuclear region (i.e. cytoplasmic region around the nucleus). Therefore, it is theorized that transcription of negative sense viral RNAs into mRNA occurs within the vicinity of that region. Nonetheless, other reports have indicated that transcription may occur within the cytoplasm.[1, 37, 38] Presently, the exact location of transcription remains unknown, however, the result of transcription is the production of functional mRNA segments, which is used either to produce more viral proteins or to transcribe negative sense viral genomes (Figure 1.6-5).[1, 39]

It has been reported that the relative amount of the mRNA synthesized is inversely proportional to the length of the viral genome. For example, the S mRNA is most abundantly synthesized while the L mRNA is the least synthesized. One proposed explanation of the amounts of viral mRNA synthesized is that this may be due to the discontinuous nature of the transcription and elongation process where the RNA-dependent RNA polymerase (L-protein) pauses and presumably prematurely terminates at specific sites along the viral genome. Therefore, it is assumed that the longer the gene, the higher the probability of the existence of pausing (early termination) sites.[1, 40]

Although the manner by which HV switches from transcription to translation is presently unknown, research has shown that the viral protein translated reflects the amount of viral mRNA that is previously synthesized. It has been reported that the N and L-protein (RNA-dependent RNA polymerase) are translated via free ribosomes, while GPC is translated on membrane

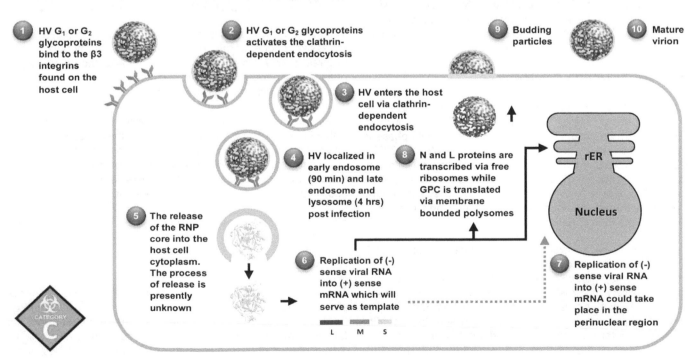

Figure 1.6.5: Diagrammatic process of HV infection within an eukaryotic cell

bounded polysomes on the rough endoplasmic reticulum (GPC is subsequently cleaved to form G_1 and G_2 glycoproteins).[1, 41]

The assembly of the virus begins as soon as sufficient amounts of viral structural proteins and negative sense genome segments have been synthesized. It is currently assumed that the assembly of the virus particle occurs in the Golgi apparatus. This is supported by the accumulation of G_1 and G_2 proteins in the Golgi.[41] After assembly, HV is sent to the Golgi cisternae where it is transferred into secretory vesicles. Subsequently, HV virions are transported (in secretory vesicles) to the plasma membrane and released via exocytosis (Figure 1.6-5).[1, 41]

HV infected patients develop cellular and humoral immune responses before or immediately after the onset of clinical symptoms leading to the speculation that these symptoms may be due to immunopathogenesis.[42] In addition to virus-specific immunity, elevated levels of tumor necrosis factor alpha (TNF-α), interleukin-6 (IL-6) and IL-10 have also been reported.[43] It is known that TNF-α increases vascular permeability by targeting two TNF-α receptors, TNF-R75 and TNF-R55, found in endothelial cells.[44,45,46] In addition, TNF-α also induces the release of cytokines and chemokins from the endothelial cells as well as up-regulates the production of enzymes such as cyclo-oxygenaseses (Cox-2) and nitric oxide synthases (NOS) although the significance of the release of the latter two enzymes requires further elucidation.[31] Presently, the HV is not considered to be a significant biological weapon threat, however in the future, improved culturing technology may promote this virus from a potential biological weapon to a serious biological weapon threat.[24]

SYMPTOMS

It is known that rodent saliva, feces and urine contain live HV. Natural transmission of this virus occurs during rodent bites or when rodent secretion and fecal matter become airborne and enter the human body through the respiratory tract, cuts in the skin, and the eyes.[47,48,49,50] There is no evidence of vector transmission of HV via arthropods and it is believed that human to human transmission of HV is highly unlikely.[51,52] Once the virus enters the body, it is believed that the incubation period ranges from one to six weeks, with an average of about two weeks before the first sign of disease can be seen.

Hemorrhagic Fever with Renal Syndrome

The course of HFRS infection is generally divided into five overlapping phases. Also, it is not uncommon for one or more of the phases to be absent. The first phase, the febrile phase is indicated by the sudden onset of a high fever (~102°F or 39°C), headaches, malaise, nausea, chills, bradycardia, myalgia (i.e. abdominal and back pain) lasting three to seven days, as well as myositis. To a lesser extent, the febrile phase may also exhibit pharynx enanthema, photophobia, albuminuria and a diffused reddening of the face (Table 2).[1, 8]

The initial phase is followed by a hypotensive phase, which lasts from a few hours to six days. This phase is marked by thrombocytopenia, petechial hemorrhages appearing on the palate and axillary skin folds, as well as, conjunctival injection, blurred vision, conjunctival hemorrhages, acute myopia (i.e. decreased visual acuity with or without pain) tachycardia, hypoxemia, hypotension, proteinuria and renal failure (Table 3).[53]

The oliguric phase generally lasts for three to seven days and is marked with hemorrhagic manifestations (i.e. severe gastrointestinal hemorrhages) becoming more prominent. In addition, during the oliguric phase, hypervolemia, oliguria or anuria may appear as additional symptoms (Table 4).[53]

Table 2: An overview of the clinical symptoms of the febrile phase of HFRS

Symptoms	Rare	Common	Frequent
High fever			■
Headaches			■
Malaise			■
Nausea			■
Chill			■
Bradycardia			■
Myalgia			■
Myositis			■
pharynx enanthema		■	
Photophobia		■	
Albuminuria		■	
Reddening of the face		■	

Table 3: An overview of the clinical symptoms of the hypotensive phase of HFRS

Symptoms	Rare	Common	Frequent
Thrombocytopenia			■
Petechial hemorrhages			■
Conjunctival injection			■
Blurred vision			■
Conjunctival hemorrhages			■
Acute myopia			■
Tachycardia			■
Hypoxemia			■
Hypotension			■
Renal failure			■
Proteinuria			■

Table 4: An overview of the clinical symptoms of the oliguric phase of HFRS

Symptoms	Rare	Common	Frequent
Hemorr. manifestations			■
Gastrointestinal hem.			■
Hypervolemia		■	
Oliguria		■	
Anuria		■	

The diuretic phase can last several weeks and is indicated by an excessive amount of urine production (polyuria) by patients (up to three to six liters of urine per day). Finally, the convalescent phase is generally prolonged, requiring weeks to months (3 weeks to 6 months) before the patient recovers.[53]

Depending upon the type of HV, mortality rates associated with HFRS can be as low as 0.1%, as in the cases of Puumala infections[50], to approximately 6-15%[6] in the cases of Hantaan infections. Deaths from HFRS generally occur during the hypotensive or oliguric phase of the disease. Patients generally succumb to shock, multi-organ hypoperfusion due to the loss of blood volume via vascular leakage during the hypotensive phase. In the course of the oliguric phase, the patient generally dies from hypervolemia, uremia and renal failure.[53]

Hantavirus Pulmonary Syndrome

The course of an HPS infection is generally divided into three phases. The initial phase, the prodromal phase, is indicated by flu-like symptoms including fever (101-104°F or 38.33-40°C), fatigue, myalgia, myositis, dizziness, nausea and gastrointestinal manifestations such as diarrhea, vomiting and weight loss (Table 5).[53] The initial phase is followed by the cardiopulmonary phase, which includes coughing and shortness of breath. This second stage of the infection will proceed rapidly. Patients will suffer from severe respiratory insufficiency caused by non-cardiogenic pulmonary edema, and hypotension, as well as, rhabdomyolysis (Figure 1.6-6).[11]

Unlike HFRS, hemorrhagic tendencies of HPS is mainly isolated in the lungs which, during the course of the second phase, patients may require assisted ventilation within 24 hours of the initial onset of respiratory symptoms. Furthermore, during the cardio-pulmonary phase, neutrophilic leukocytosis, hemoconcentration, thrombocyto-penia and circulating immunoblasts are also commonly observed (Figure 1.6-7).[8]

Table 5: An overview of the clinical symptoms of the prodromal phase of HPS

Symptoms	Rare	Common	Frequent
Fever			■
Fatigue			■
Myalgia			■
Myositis			■
Dizziness			■
Diarrhea			■
Nausea			■
Vomiting			■
Weight loss			■

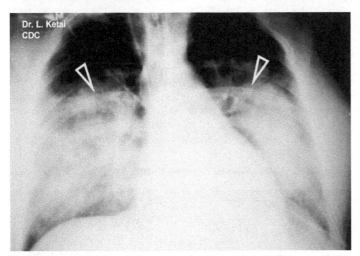

Figure 1.6-6: Chest X-ray from a patient suffering from HPS demonstrating interstitial pulmonary edema (indicated by the arrows), progressing to alveolar edema with severe bilateral involvement

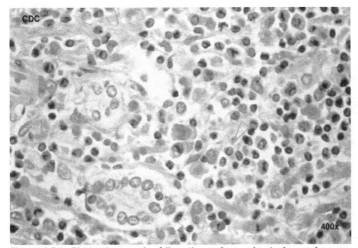

Figure 1.6-7: Photomicrograph of liver tissue from a hantavirus pulmonary syndrome (HPS) patient. Note the high concentration of immunoblasts (lymphoblasts) within the portal triads (indicated by the arrow)

Depending upon the species of Hantavirus (e.g. Sin Nombre, Bayou, Black Creek Canal, Andes, etc.), renal failure is also a common symptom. Finally, the convalescent phase is generally prolonged and may take several months before the patient returns to normal (Table 6).[53]

Table 6: An overview of the clinical symptoms of the cardiopulmonary phase of HPS

Symptoms	Rare	Common	Frequent
Coughing			■
Shortness of breath			■
Pulmonary edema			■
Hypotension			■
Rhabdomyolysis			■
Hemorrhage in the lungs			■
Neutrophilic leukocytosis		■	
Hemoconcentration		■	
Thrombocytopenia		■	
Circulat. immunoblasts		■	
Renal failure	■		

The mortality rate for patients suffering from HPS is not confirmed, but it is estimated to be 40-50%. The reason for the high mortality rate is mainly due to the fact that patients are usually admitted to the hospital when pulmonary edema occurs. Unfortunately for the patient, as well as the medical practitioner, death generally occurs within three days after the onset of pulmonary edema, leaving a very short period of time for treatment.[54] Patients generally succumb to shock, myocardial dysfunction, hypoperfusion, respiratory failure and acute renal failure during the cardiopulmonary phase. Nonetheless, many of the survivors of the disease recover rapidly and experience complete restoration of lung functions.[53]

DETECTION

Commercially available indirect immunofluore-scence assays can be used to detect anti-Hantavirus IgM and IgG.[55] Hantavirus can also be identified by IgM capturing enzyme-linked immunosorbent assay (ELISA) using infected cell lysate as antigen and an uninfected control for each unknown serum.[56] Western blot assays have been used and found to be useful as a diagnostic tool.[55, 57] Other identification methods such as antigen identification via immuno-histochemistry, recombinant immunoblot assay (RIBA), and reverse transcriptase polymerase chain reaction (RT-PCR) have also be used.[58, 59]

TREATMENT

Clinical trials of ribavirin have been shown to dramatically reduce the mortality rate of patients suffering from HFRS, if the treatment is applied in the first 5 days of the infection. However, the treatment of patients suffering from HPS with ribivirin is inconclusive and requires further clinical trials.[60] The use of α-interferon on patients suffering from HFRS has shown no effect on the course of the infection.[61] Presently, there are no known trials using α-interferon on patients suffering from HPS. It has been suggested that antiviral agents, such as tragacanthin poly-saccharides, be used in the treatment of both HFRS and HPS since they show promise in the treatment of other types of viruses in the family *Bunyavioridae*. However, there are no laboratory and clinical trials examining the potential of this compound against Hantavirus infections.[62]

Supportive management is presently the mainstay of treatment for HFRS and HPS. Maintaining the patients' intravascular volume, along with their cardiac output, is essential. This is accomplished by carefully managing fluids and electrolyte balance. If needed, external inotropic support of the patients' cardiac function may be used to maintain homeostasis. The use of acute peritoneal dialysis or hemodialysis, where wastes such as urea, potassium and excess fluids are removed after renal failure may further aid recovery. Furthermore, if consumptive coagulo-pathy occurs, heparin and platelet infusions may be lifesaving. In patients suffering from HPS, extracorporeal membrane oxygenation (ECMO) may be needed to aid in the cases where the lungs and heart are severely compromised. In an effort to prevent secondary infections broad spectrum antibiotics may also be administered.[63]

As with any type of hemorrhagic fever, intramuscular injections should be avoided due to the possibilities of uncontrollable intramuscular bleeding. In addition, administering acetylsalicylic acid (e.g. Aspirin) and non-steroid anti-inflammatory drugs should always be avoided. Clinicians should prescribe acetaminophen to combat fever and inflammatory symptoms.

Various vaccines have been developed to combat to HFRS and HPS. For example, formalin-inactivated HTNV vaccines for Hantaan and Seoul viruses have shown to prompt the production of IgG specific antibodies in 100% of the volunteers during trials and prompted the production of neutralizing antibodies in 80% of the tested individuals. This vaccine, now commercially available is called Hantavax ® (produced by the Korean Green Cross, Seoul, Korea) and is derived from virally infected rodent brain tissue.[64] However, the effects of immunization with the vaccine is very short lived [60] and the antibody titers decline rapidly within months; booster vaccines produce no subsequent increase in antibody production.[65,66] Long term studies of Hantavax ® demonstrate only a 30-50% protection rate.[67] Other formalin-inactivated HTNV vaccines have been produced and tested,

however, the results are very similar to those for Hantavax®.[68]

By using recombinant DNA technology, viral components were obtained and tested for their immunogenicity and protective potential. Viral structural proteins have shown promise for the development of vaccines in animal models such as bank voles and mice.[69,70] In 2000, a vaccinia-vectored Hantaan virus vaccine was tested with human volunteers and showed that it elicited neutralizing antibodies in 72% of the tested individuals. Nonetheless, the developmental work on recombinant DNA vaccines is still ongoing and presently there is no vaccine that has received worldwide approval.[71]

DIFFERENTIAL DIAGNOSIS

HFRS could be misdiagnosed as leptospirosis, murine or louse-borne typhus, pyelonephritis, malaria, poststrepyococcal glomerulonephritis, blood dyscrasias, glaucoma, and acute abdominal emergencies. In addition, the hemorrhagic symptoms of HFRS could be easily confused with other hemorrhagic fevers. Severe cases of HFRS may be confused with fulminant sepsis, while milder cases with fever and myalgia may lead to a misdiagnosis of influenza, hepatitis A, or streptococcal pharyngitis. The appearance of myelocytes and atypical lymphocytes that resulted from leukemoid reaction occasionally seen in HFRS may be confused with leukemia. Clinician may misinterpret the elevated hematocrit as a sign of dehydration and administer excessive fluid loads via rapid infusion of intravenous fluids, as well as unwarranted amounts of antibiotics (Table 7).[1, 55]

Diagnosis of HPS is difficult during the prodromal phase of the infection. Nonetheless, once the common signs of HPS such as dyspnea, thrombocytopenia, and an increase in the number of immature leukocytes in the peripheral blood appear, the diagnosis of HPS should be clearly made. Hypoxemia is one of

Table 7: An overview of the differential diagnosis of HFRS. Note: Leptospirosis (Lepto), Murine-borne typhus (MbT), Ebola hemorrhagic fever (EHF), Crimean-Congo Hemorrhagic Fever (CCHF), Chikungunya fever (CHIKF)

Symptoms	HFRS	Lepto	MbT	Malaria	EHF	CCHF	CHIKF
High fever	■	■	■	■	■	■	■
Chills	■	■	■	■	■	■	■
Headaches	■	■	■	■	■	■	■
Nausea	■	■	■	■	■	■	■
Malaise	■	■		■	■	■	■
Bradycardia	■					■	
Myalgia	■	■	■	■	■	■	■
Myositis	■						
Pharynx enanthema	■						
Photophobia	■	■	■				■
Albuminuria	■	■		■			
Diffused reddening of the face	■						
Thrombocytopenia	■	■		■	■	■	■
Petechial hemorrhages	■	■		■	■	■	
Conjunctival injection	■						
Blurred vision	■						
Conjunctival hemorrhages					■		
Acute myopia	■						
Tachycardia	■			■	■	■	■
Hypoxemia	■						
Hypotension	■				■	■	
Renal failure	■			■		■	
Proteinuria	■	■					
Hemorrhagic manifestations	■	■		■			
Gastrointestinal hemorrhages	■						
Hypervolemia	■						
Oliguria	■	■					
Anuria	■	■					

Table 8: An overview of the differential diagnosis of HPS. Argentine Hemorrhagic fever (AHF), Dengue fever (DF), Leptospirosis (Lepto), influenza and pneumonia (Flu/Pneu)

Symptoms	HPS	AHF	DF	Lepto	Flu/ Pneu	Tularemia
Fever	■	■		■	■	■
Fatigue	■	■			■	■
Myalgia	■	■	■	■	■	■
Myositis	■					
Dizziness	■	■	■			
Diarrhea	■	■			■	■
Vomiting	■	■	■	■		■
Weight loss	■	■				
Coughing	■			■	■	■
Shortness of breath	■			■	■	■
Pulmonary edema	■			■		
Hypotension	■	■		■		
Rhabdomyolysis	■					
Hemorrhage in the lungs	■			■		
Neutrophilic leukocytosis	■					
Hemoconcentration	■	■	■			
Thrombocytopenia	■	■	■			
Circulating immunoblasts	■					
Renal failure	■					

the early signs of this condition and could aid in diagnosis of this disease. The appearance of abdominal pain and symptoms involving gastrointestinal tract may easily be misdiagnosed with acute abdominal emergencies. Symptoms of fever and myalgia may lead to the misdiagnosis of influenza, however, the clinician should notice the absence of cough and coryza from HPS until later stages when the patient enters cardiorespiratory phase of the illness. The symmetric finding of interstitial infiltrates which progresses to pulmonary edema in patients suffering from HPS should allow the clinician to rule out pneumococcal and other pneumonias (Table 8).[1, 5]

References

1. Guerrant R.L., Walker D.H., Weller P.F. Tropical Infectious Diseases – Principles, Pathogens & Practice. Volume 1. Philadelphia: Churchill Livingstone Elsevier. 2006. pp. 763
2. Schmaljohn C.S., Jennings G.B., Hay J., Dalrymple J.M. Coding Strategy of the S Genome Segments of Hantaan Virus. Virology, 1986. 155: pp. 633-643
3. Schmaljohn C.S., Schmaljohn A.L., Dalrymple J.M. Hantaan Virus M RNA: Coding Strategy, Nucleotide Sequence, and Gene Order. Virology, 1987. 157: pp. 31-39
4. Schmaljohn C.S. Nucleotide Sequence of the L Genome Segment of Hantaan Virus. Nucleic Acids Research, 1990. 18: pp. 6728
5. Elliott, R.M. Molecular biology of the Bunyaviridae. Journal of General Virology, 1990. 71: pp. 501-522
6. Lee H.W. The Bunyaviridae. Epidemiology and Pathogenesis of Hemorrhagic Fever with Renal Syndrome. New York: Plenum Press. 1996. pp. 253-367
7. Oncul O., Atalay Y., Onem Y, Turhan V., Acar A., Uyar Y., Caglayik D.Y., Ozkan S., Gorenek L. Hantavirus Infection in Istanbul, Turkey. Emerging Infectious Disease Journal, 2011. 17: pp. 303-304
8. McCaughey C., Hart C.A. Hantaviruses. Journal of Medical Microbiology, 2000. 49: pp. 587-599
9. Casals J., Henderson B.E., Hoogstraakm G. A Review of Soviet Viral Hemorrhagic Fevers. The Journal of Infectious Diseases, 1969. 122: pp. 437-453
10. Muranyi W., Bahr U., Zeier M., van der Woude F.J. Disease of the Month Hantavirus Infection. Journal of the American Society of Nephrology, 2005. 16: pp. 3669-3679
11. Smadel J.E. Epidemic Hemorrhagic Fever. American Journal of Public Health, 1953. 43: pp. 1327-1330
12. Lee H.W., Lee P.W., Johnson K.M. Isolation of the Etiologic Agent of Korean Hemorrhagic Fever. The Journal of Infectious Diseases, 1978. 137: pp. 298–308
13. Hurtley S. Of Mice. Science, 2004. 5705: pp. 2164
14. All about Hantavirus. National Center for Infectious Diseases Special Pathogens Branch. Retrieved June 20, 2007. Website: http://www.cdc.gov/ncidod/diseases /hanta/hps/
15. Weidmann M., Schmidt P., Vackova M., Krivanec K., Munclinger P., Hufert F.T. Identification of Genetic Evidence for Dobrava Virus Spillover in Rodents by Nested Reverse Transcription (RT)-PCR and TaqMan RT-PCR. Journal of the American Society of Nephrology, 2005. 2: pp. 808-812
16. Netski D., Thran B.H., St. Jeor S.C. Sin Nombre Virus Pathogenesis in Permyscus Maniculatus. Journal of Virology, 1999. 73: pp. 585-591
17. Lyubsky S., Gavrilovskaya I., Luft B., Mackow E. Histopathology of Peromyscus Leucopus Naturally Infected with Pathogenic NY-1 Hantaviruses: Pathologic Markers of HPS Viral Infection in Mice. Laboratory Investigations, 1996. 74: pp. 627-633
18. Fulhorst C., Milazzo M., Duno G., Salas R.A. Experimental Infection of the Sigmodon Alstoni Cotton Rat with Cano Delgadito Virus, a South American Hantavirus. American Journal of Tropical Medicine and Hygiene, 2002. 1: pp. 107-111
19. Cross R.W., Waffa B., Freeman A., Riegel C., Moses L.M., Bennett A., Safronetz D., Fischer E.R., Feldmann H., Voss T.G., Bausch D.G.Old World hantaviruses in rodents in New Orleans, Louisiana. The American Journal of Tropical Medicine and Hygiene, 2014. 90: pp. 897-901
20. Hantavirus. Studies conducted in Thailand, Finland and the People's Republic of China have updated our knowledge about hantavirus. Hospital Business Week, 2007; March 4: pp. 1085.
21. Sjölander B., Golovljova K.I., Vasilenko V., Plyusnin A., Lundkvist Å. Serological Divergence of Dobrava and Saaremaa Hantaviruses: Evidence for Two Distinct Serotypes. Epidemiology and Infection, 2002. 128: pp. 99-103
22. Klempa B., Tkachenko E.A., Dzagurova T.K., Yunicheva Y.V., Morozov V.G., Okulova N.M., Slyusareva G.P., Smirnov A., Kruger D.H. Hemorrhagic Fever with Renal Syndrome Caused by 2 Lineages of Dobrava Hantavirus, Russia. Emerging Infectious Diseases, 2008. 14: pp. 617-625
23. Monroe M.C., Morzunov S.P., Johnson A.M., Bowen M.D., Artsob H., Yates T., Peters C.J., Rollin P.E., Ksiazek T.G., Nichol S.T. Genetic Diversity and Distribution of Peromyscus-Borne Hantaviruses in North America. Emerging Infectious Diseases, 1999. 1: pp. 75-86
24. Lundkvist A., Niklasson B. Hemorrhagic Fever with Renal Syndrome and other Hantavirus Infections. Reviews in Medical Virology, 1994. 4: pp. 177-184
25. Pensiero M.N., Sharefikin J.B., Dieffenbah C.W., Hay J. Hantaan Virus Infection of Human Endothelial Cells. Journal of Virology, 1992. 66: pp. 5929-5936
26. Raftery M.J., Kraus A.A., Ulrich R., Kruger D.H., Schonrich G. Hantavirus Infection of Dendritic Cells. Journal of Virology, 2002. 76: pp. 10724-10733
27. Yanagihara R., Silverman D.J. Experimental Infection of Human Vascular Endothelial Cells by Pathogenic and Nonpathogenic Hantavirus. Archives of Virology, 1990. 111: pp. 281-286
28. Kang J.I., Park S.H., Lee P.W., Ahn B.Y. Apoptosis is Induced by Hantavirus in Cultured Cells. Virology, 1999. 264: pp. 99-105
29. Nolte K.B. Feddersen R.M., Foucar K., Zaki S.R., Koster F.T., Madar D., Merlin T.L., McFeeley P.J., Umland E.T., Zumwalt R.E. Hantavirus Pulmonary Syndrome in the United States: A Pathological Description of a Disease Caused by a New Agent. Human Pathology, 1995. 26: pp. 110-120
30. Zaki S.R., Greer P.W., Coffiold L.M., Goldsmith C.S., Nolte K.B., Foucar K., Feddersen R.M., Zumwalt R.E., Miller G.L., Khan A.S., Rollin P.E., Ksiazek T.G., Nicole S.T., Mahy B.W.J., Peters C.J. Hantavirus Pulmonary Syndrome. Pathogenesis of an Emerging Infectious Disease. American Journal of Pathology, 1995. 146: pp. 552-579
31. Niikura M., Maeda A., Ikegami T., Saijo M., Kurane I., Morikawa S. Modification of Endothelial Cell Function by Hantaan Virus Infection: Prolong Hyper-permeability Induced by TNF-alpha of Hantaan Virus-infected Endothelial Cell Monolayers. Archives of Virology, 2004. 149: pp. 1279-1292
32. Jin, M., Park, J., Lee, S., Park, B., Shin, J., Song, K.J., Ahn, T.I., Hwang, S.Y., Ahn, B.Y., Ahn, K. Hantaan Virus Enters Cells by Clathrin-Dependent Receptor-Mediated Endocytosis. Virology, 2002. 294: pp. 60-69
33. Gavrilovskaya I., Brown E., Ginsberg M., Mackow E. Cellular Entry of Hantaviruses which Cause Hemorrhagic Fever with Renal Syndrome is Mediated by B3 Integrins. Journal of Virology, 1999. 73: pp. 3951-3959
34. Gavrilovskaya I., Shepley M., Shaw R., Ginsberg M., Mackow E. B2 Integrins Mediate the Cellular Entry of Hantaviruses that Cause Respiratory Failure. The Proceedings of the National Academy of Science United States of America, 1998. 95: pp. 7074-7079
35. Mackow E.R., Gavrilovskaya I.N. Cellular Receptors and Hantavirus Pathogenesis. Current Topics in Microbiology and Immunology, 2001. 256: pp. 91-115
36. Mir M.A., Hjelle B., Ye C., Panganiban A.T. Cap snatching Revised: Viral storage of cellular 5' mRNA caps in P bodies. The proceedings of the National Academy of Science United States of America, 2008. 105: pp. 19294-19299
37. Ravkov, E.V. & Compans, R.W. Hantavirus Nucleocapsid Protein is Expressed as a Membrane-Associated Protein in the Perinuclear Region. Journal of Virology, 2001. 75: pp. 1808-1815
38. Kariwa, H., Tanabe, H., Mizutani, T., Kon, Y., Lokugamage, K., Lokugamage, N., Iwasa, M.A., Hagiya, T., Araki, K., Yoshimatsu, K., Arikawa, J., & Takashima, I. Synthesis of Seoul Virus RNA and Structural Proteins in Cultured Cells. Archives of Virology, 2003. 148: pp. 1671-1685
39. Hutchinson K.L., Peters C.J., Nichol S.T. Sin Nombre Virus mRNA Synthesis. Virology, 1996. 224: pp. 139-149
40. Schmaljohn C.S., Nichol S.T. Bunyaviridae. Fields Virology - 5th Edition. Philadelphia: Lippincott Williams and Wilkins, 2007. pp. 1581-1602
41. Muranyi W., Bahr U., Zeier M., van der Woude F.J. Hantavirus Infection. Journal of the American Society of Nephrology, 2005. 16: pp. 3669–3679
42. Cosgriff T.M. Mechanisms of Disease in Hantavirus Infection: Pathophysiology of Hemorrhagic Fever with Renal Syndrome. Reviews of Infectious Diseases, 1991. 13: pp. 97-107
43. Linderholm M., Ahlm C., Settergren B., Waage A., Tarnvik A. Elevated Plasma Levels of

Tumor Necrosis Factor (TNF)-alpha, Soluble TNF Receptors, Interleukin (IL)-6, and IL-10 in Patients with Hemorrhagic Fever with Renal Syndrome. The Journal of Infectious Diseases, 1996. 173: pp. 38-43

44. Brett J., Gerlach H., Nawroth P., Steinberg S., Godman G., Stern D. Tumor Necrosis Factor/cachectin Increases Permeability of Endothelial Cell Monolayers by a Mechanism Involving Regulatory G Proteins. The Journal of Experimental Medicine, 1989. 169: pp. 1977-1991

45. Mackay F., Loetscher H., Stueber D., Gehr G., Lesslauer W. Tumor Necrosis Factor α (TNF-α)-induced Cell Adhesion to Human Endothelial Cell is Under Dominant Control of One TNF Receptor Type, TNF-R55. The Journal of Experimental Medicine, 1993. 177: pp. 1277-1286

46. Mantovani A., Bussolino F., Introna M. Cytokine Regulation of Endothelial Cell Function: From Molecular Level to the Bedside. Immunology Today, 1997. 18: pp. 231-240

47. Padula P., Figueroa R., Navarrete M., Pizarro E., Cadiz R., Bellomo C., Jofre C., Zaror L., Rodriguez E., Murúa. Transmission Study of Andes Hantavirus Infection in Wild Sigmodontine Rodents. Journal of Virology, 2004. 78: pp. 11972-11979

48. Lee H., van der Groen G. Hemorrhagic Fever with Renal Syndrome. Progress in Medical Virology, 1989. 36: pp. 62-102

49. Hantavirus (also known as Hantavirus Pulmonary Syndrome and Hantavirus Disease). Revised June 2008. Retrieved June 26, 2007. Web site: http://www.state. nj.us/health/cd/manual/hantavirus.pdf

50. Dournon E., Moriniere B., Matheron S., Girard P., Gonzalez J., Hirsch F., McCormick J.B. HFRS after a Wild Rodent Bite in the Haute-Savoie and risk exposure to Hantaan-like virus in a Paris Laboratory. Lancet, 1984. 1: pp. 676-677

51. Bradshaw M.H. Hantavirus. Revised February 1994. Retrieved June 27, 2007. Website: www.oznet.ksu. edu/library/hlsaf2/MF1117.PDF

52. Vitek C.R., Ksiazek T.G., Peter C.J., Breiman R.F. Evidence against Infection with Hantaviruses among Forest and Park Workers in the Southwestern United States. Clinical Infectious Disease, 1996. 2: pp. 283-285

53. Guerrant R.L., Walker D.H., Weller P.F. Tropical Infectious Diseases – Principles, Pathogens & Practice. Volume 1. Philadelphia: Churchill Livingstone Elsevier. 2006. pp. 769-772

54. Schmaljohn C., Hjelle B. Hantaviruses: A Global Disease Problem. Emerging Infectious Diseases, 1997. 2: pp. 95-104

55. Guerrant R.L., Walker D.H., Weller P.F. Tropical Infectious Diseases – Principles, Pathogens & Practice. Volume 1. Philadelphia: Churchill Livingstone Elsevier. 2006. pp. 774-775

56. Korakap P., Avsic-Zupanc T., Osterhaus A.D.M.E., Groen J. Evaluation of Two Commercially Available Immunoassays for the Detection of Hantavirus Antibodies in Serum Samples. Journal of clinical virology, 2000. 17: pp. 189-196

57. Torrez-Martinez N., Bharadwaj M., Goade D., Delury J., Moran P., Hicks B., Nix B., Davis J.L., Hjelle B. Bayou Virus-Associated Hantavirus Pulmonary Syndrome in Eastern Texas: Identification of the Rice Rat, Oryzomys palustris, as Reservoir Host. Emerging Infectious Diseases, 1998. 4: pp. 105-111

58. Ye C., Prescott J., Nofchissey R., Goade D., Hjelle B. Neutralizing Antibodies and Sin Nombre Virus RNA After Recovery From Hantavirus Cardiopulmonary Syndrome. Emerging Infectious Disease, 2004. 3: pp. 478-482

59. Ibrahim S.M., Aitichou M., Hardick J., Blow J., O'Guinn M.L., Schmaljohn C. Detection of Crimean-Congo hemorrhagic fever, Hanta, and sandfly fever viruses by real-time RT-PCR. Methods In Molecular Biology, 2011. 665: pp. 357-368

60. Huggins J.W., Hsiang C.M., Cosgriff T.M., Guang M.Y., Smith J.I., Wu Z.O., LeDuc J.W., Zheng Z.M., Meegan J.M., Wang Q.N. Prospective Double-blind, Concurrent, Placebo-controlled Clinical Trial of Intravenous ribavirin Therapy of Hemorrhagic Fever with Renal Syndrome. The Journal of Infectious Diseases, 1994. 164: pp. 1119-1127

61. Gui X.E., Ho M., Cohen M.S., Wang Q.L., Huang H.P., Xo Q.X. Hemorrhagic Fever with Renal Syndrome: Treatment with Recombinant Alpha Interferon. The Journal of Infectious Diseases, 1987; 155: pp. 1047-1051.

62. Smee D.F., Sidwell R.W., Huffman J.H., Huggins J.W., Kende M., Verbiscar A.J. Antiviral Activities of Tragacanthin Polysaccharides on Punta Toro virus Infectiuons in Mice. Chemotherapy, 1996. 42: pp. 286-293

63. Crowley M.R., Katz R.W., Kessler R., Simpson S.Q., Levy H., Hallin G.W. Successful Treatment of Adults with Severe Hantavirus Pulmonary Syndrome with Extracorporeal Membrane Oxygenation. Critical Care Medicine, 1998. 26: pp. 409-414

64. Cho H.W., Howard C.R. Antibody responses in Humans to an Inactivated Hantavirus Vaccine (Hantavax ®). Vaccine, 1999. 17: pp. 2567-2575

65. Cho H.W., Howard C.R., Lee H.W. Review of an Inactivated Vaccine against Hantaviruses. Intervirology, 2002. 45: pp. 328-333

66. Hjelle B. Vaccines Against Hantaviruses. Expert Review of Vaccines, 2002. 1: pp. 373–384

67. Sohn Y.M., Rho H.O., Park M.S., Kim J.S., Summers P.L. Primary Humoral Immune Responses to Formalin Inactivated Hemorrhagic Fever with Renal Syndrome Vaccine (Hantavax ©): Consideration of Active Immunization in South Korea. Yonsei Medical Journal, 2001. 42: pp. 278–284

68. Choi Y., Ahn C.J., Seong K.M., Jung M.Y., Ahn B.Y. Inactivated Hantaan Virus Vaccine Derived from Suspension Culture of Vero Cells. Vaccine, 2003. 21: pp. 1867–1873

69. Dargeviciute A., Brus Sjolander K., Sasnauskas K., Kruger D.H., Meisel H., Ulrich R., Lundkvist A. Yeast-Expressed Puumala Hantavirus Nucleocapsid Protein Induces Protection in a Bank Vole Model. Vaccine, 2002. 20: pp. 3523–3531

70. Klingstrom J., Maljkovic I., Zuber B., Rollman E., Kjerrstrom A., Lundkvist A. Vaccination of C57/BL6 Mice with Dobrava Hantavirus Nucleocapsid Protein in Freund's Adjuvant Induced Partial Protection against Challenge. Vaccine, 2004. 22: pp. 4029–4034

71. McClain D.J., Summers P.L., Harrison S.A., Schmaljohn A.L., Schmaljohn C.S. Clinical Evaluation of a Vaccinia-vectored Hantaan Virus Vaccine. Journal of Medical Virology, 2000. 60: pp. 77–85

Photo Bibliography

Figure 1.6-1: Transmission electron micrograph (TEM) of numerous Hantavirus virions. Photo was taken at 4000x magnification by Cynthia Goldsmith and released by the CDC in 1993. Public domain photo

Figure 1.6-4: A photomicrograph of an atypical enlarged lymphocyte found in the blood smear from a HPS patient. The photomicrograph was taken at 1000x and released by the CDC. Public domain photo

Figure 1.6.5: Genomic protein graphics produced and released by the National Institute of Health (NIH). Public domain photo

Figure 1.6-6: Chest X-ray from a patient suffering from HPS demonstrating interstitial pulmonary edema, progressing to alveolar edema with severe bilateral involvement. Photo was taken by Dr. Loren Ketai, MD in 1994 and released by the CDC. Public domain photo

Figure 1.6-7: Photomicrograph of liver tissue from a Hantavirus pulmonary syndrome (HPS) patient. Note the high concentration of immunoblasts (lymphoblasts) within the porta triads. Photo was taken at 400x magnification in 1994 and released by the CDC. Public domain photo

The Junin virus (JUNV) is a negative sense, enveloped, single stranded bisegmented RNA virus, measuring at approximately 120 nm in diameter. The bisegmented RNA genome is designated as S (small: 3.4 kb) and L (large: 7.2 kb) segments, organized in an unique ambisense coding scheme to encode 2 opposite orientated open reading frames separated by a non-coding intergenic region, which acts as a transcription termination signal for the RNA-dependent RNA polymerase, also known as the viral L protein.[1, 2, 3] JUNV also maintain Z proteins (i.e. small matrix protein with a zinc-binding domain), nucleoproteins (NP), stable signal peptides (SSP), and two types of enveloped glycoproteins: glycoprotein 1 (GP_1, peripheral membrane glycoprotein) and glycoprotein 2 (GP_2, an integral glycoprotein). Both GP_1 and GP_2 are formed from the post-translational proteolytic cleavage of the glycoprotein precursor (GPC) by cellular subtilase SKI-1/S1P.[1, 4, 5, 6]

JUNV belongs to the genus *Arenavirus*, family *Arenaviridae* and is a member of the New World group, B-lineage of the arenaviruses, which include other highly pathogenic agents, such as the Manchupo, Guanarito and Sabia viruses (Figure 1.7-1).[4, 5, 6] JUNV is known as the etiological agent responsible for Argentine Hemorrhagic Fever (AHF). Known locally as 'mal de los rastrojos', AHF was first described in 1955 and isolated in 1959 at Junin Partido, north Buenos Aires Province, Argentina (Figure 1.7-2).[7]

JUNV is a zoonotic infection and commonly found in the organs and body fluids of rodents, such as, vasper mice (*Calomys musculinus, C. venustus, C. callidus* and *C. laucha*), the yellow pygmy rice rat (*Oligoryzomys flavescens*), the Azara's grass mouse (*Akodon azarae*), the dark field mouse (*Bolomys obscurus*) and the house mouse (*Mus musculus*).[8] Experiments have shown that newborn animals infected with JUNV displayed persistent infections without mortality, while adult animals exposed to the same dosage of virus demonstrated a highly lethal, delayed hypersensitivity reaction within their central nervous system.[9, 10] Presently, there is no evidence that arthropods play any role in the transmission of AHF, although mites have been suggested by some scientists as an intermediate vector (Figure 1.7-3).[11]

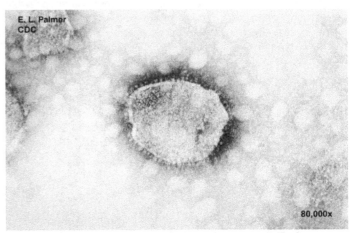

Figure 1.7-1: An electron micrograph (TEM) of a new world arenavirus

AHF is generally considered to be incapable of human to human transmission, although some scientists believe that there is the potential for such transmission to occur. For example, JUNV has been detected in oral swabs and urine samples from infected patients. Additionally, JUNV has been detected in the blood stream of patients throughout the entire febrile phase of infection. The presence of JUNV within blood and bodily fluids of patients indicates the potential for human to human transmission.[11]

Naturally occurring human infections of this disease generally occur through cuts, skin abrasions or inhalation of JUNV contaminated dust during farming or other agricultural activities.

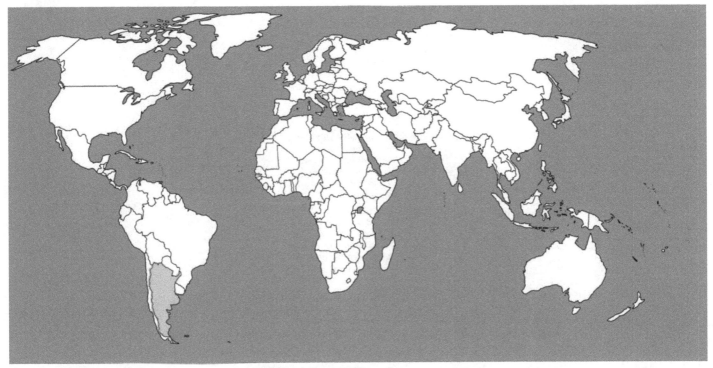

Figure 1.7-2: Distribution of Junin virus and Argentine Hemorrhagic Fever (AHF)

It is known that epithelial cells, macrophages, sinusoidal lining cells and dendritic cells are the primary targets of JUNV.[12, 13] Like all arena-viruses, JUNV is believed to gain entry into the cell by attachment of GP_1 to one or more cellular receptors, although the exact attachment proteins still remain to be elucidated. It has been reported that one of the major receptors for Old World and New World C lineages of arenaviruses are the α-dystroglycan proteins[14], however this report was contradicted by other research demonstrating that most New World arenaviruses fail to bind to this protein.[13] Recent studies indicate that other possible attachment sites for JUNV, along with other new world arenaviruses, are the transferrin receptors (TfR1), as well as, human C-type lectins DC-SIGN, L-SIGN.[1, 15, 16, 17, 18]

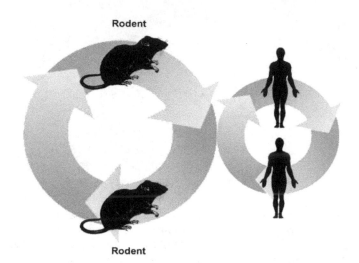

Rodent

Rodent

Figure 1.7-3: Sylvatic cycle of the Junin Virus

Subsequent to viral attachment to the membrane bounded receptor(s), clathrin-mediated endo-cytosis will bring the virion into the host cell within large, smooth-walled vesicles. Once the virus is inside the acidic environment of the endosomal vesicle, GP_2 with assistance from SSP, will mediate the fusion between the virion membrane and the endosomal membrane.

Subsequently, the nucleocapsid of the LFV virus is released into the cytoplasm of the host cell where replication of the viral genome takes place.[5, 6]

As stated previously, JUNV possesses two single stranded RNA molecules arranged in an ambisense orientation. JUNV's NP gene is encoded at the 3' end of the S RNA molecule in the complimentary sense, while the glycoprotein precursor (GPC) gene is encoded at the 5' end of the same RNA strand, in message sense. Similarly, the L protein is encoded at the 3' end of the L RNA molecule, while the zinc-finger (Z) protein is found at the 5' end of the same RNA molecule (Figures 1.7-4 and 1.7-5).[19]

The ambisense arrangement of JUNV, as well as, the genome of other arenavirus, allows for a unique mechanism to regulate gene transcription. This unique regulation allows for the transcription of genes located at the 3' of the bisegmented RNA to be expressed first, while genes lying at the 5' of the viral RNA segment (e.g. GPC and Z) cannot be expressed in the absence of viral protein synthesis. To initiate gene expression, viral capsid L protein (i.e. RNA-dependent RNA polymerase) is believed to cleave the cap and 1-7 bases from cellular messenger RNAs (mRNAs) and use these as primers to initiate the transcription of viral RNAs in a process known as "cap snatching." These non-polyadenylated viral RNAs are then translated by the host cell ribosomes to produce viral NP and L proteins (Figure 1.7-4). Transcription ends at the distal margin of the stem-loop structure found within the viral intergenomic region.[20, 21, 22]

Genes found at the 5' ends of the viral genome (e.g. GPC and Z) are not translated directly even though they are in the proper coding sense.[19, 20] Viral genomic RNAs must first go through the initial stages of replication for the expression of these genes to occur. Once the transcription of the 3' end of the viral RNA is completed, the L protein adopts a replicase mode and generates a full-length complementary antigenomic RNA (agRNA) strand from the 5' end of the viral genome. The L protein is believed to initiate RNA replication using a dinucleotide template (guanosine triphosphate cytidine monophosphate - pppGpC)

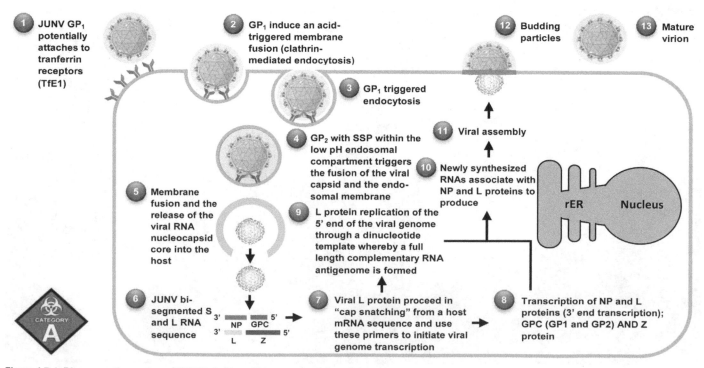

Figure 1.7-4: Diagrammatic process of JUNV infection within an eukaryotic cell

where a full length genome-complementary RNA molecule termed antigenome RNA is transcribed. The agRNA will serve as a template for the synthesis of viral mRNA in the genomic orientation. This viral mRNA will be translated to form GPC and Z protein. It has been reported that after translation, the Z protein is involved in viral particle formation where it serves as a matrix protein and interacts with the N protein, in addition to driving particle formation (Figure 1.7-4 and 1.7-5).[1, 19, 23, 24]

On the other hand, considerable post-translational processing of the GPC will take place. For example, GPC is post-translationally processed by signal peptidase to form stable signal peptide (SSP). This process is followed by the further processing of the remaining residue by the enzyme protease SKI-1/S1P to form GP_1 (45 kD) and GP_2 (38 kD). It has been reported that SSP (~5kD) is engaged in the glycoprotein expression and post-translational modification GP_1 and GP_2 by protease SKI-1/S1P, although the exact mechanism of this process requires further analysis.[5, 21] Once G_1 and G_2 is formed, these envelope glycoproteins are transported to the plasma membrane of the host cell with the

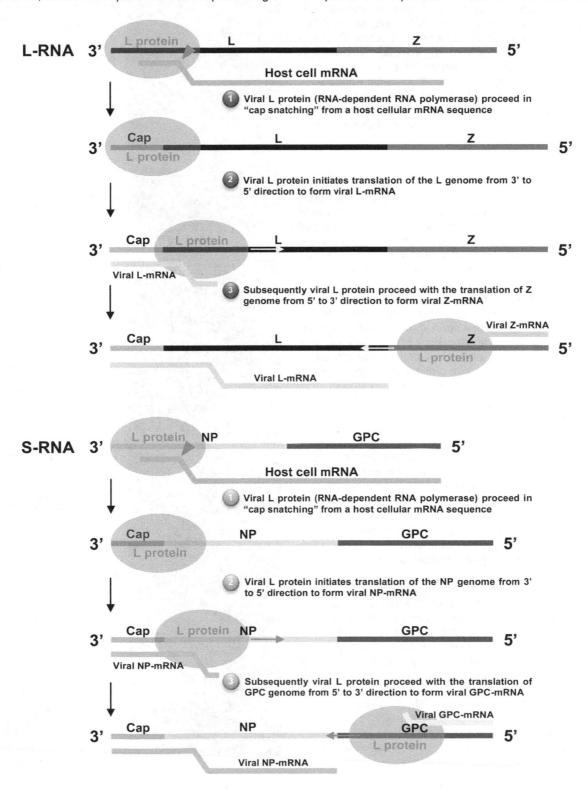

Figure 1.7-5: Diagrammatic presentation of JUNV sense and antisense viral genome transcription

73

assistance of SSP. The GP_1 tetramer will eventually form the head of the envelope spike of the LFV, while the GP_2 tetramer will form the stalk.[1, 5, 18, 19, 20, 21] It has been reported that the cytoplasmic tail of GP_2, along with SSP will interact with NP, which in turn interacts with the Z protein at the plasma membrane of the host cell. Numerous reports indicate that it is these interactions that play a critical role in the viral assembly and budding; although the exact manner of this process requires further investigation (Figure 1.8-5). [1, 5, 18, 19, 20, 25]

In 1999, Alibek wrote that Junin virus was researched and produced as a biological weapon at the Institute of Ultra-Pure Biopreparations in Leningrad, Omutninsk in Kirov, Obolensk (outside of Moscow), at the Lyubuchany Institute of Immunology in Chekhov (near Moscow), and Vector Research and Testing, located in Novosibrisk (near the small town of Koltsovo) in Siberia.[26] Based on Junin's potential of widespread person to person transmission, illness and death, the Centers for Disease Control and Prevention (CDC) in 1999 classified Junin virus as Category A biological weapon agents.[27]

SYMPTOMS

JUNV is naturally transmitted to humans from aerosolized dried excretions (saliva, feces and urine) of rodents, where the virus produces a systemic infection via the apical domain of epithelial cells in the respiratory and digestive tracts.[28] Other mechanisms, such as direct contact with contaminated materials through lesions or cuts may also expose the victim to JUNV infection.[12]

Once the virus enters the body it is believed the incubation period ranges between one to three weeks (6-14 days on average), before the onset of AHF which is indicted by fever (39°C, 102.2°F), chills, anorexia, myalgia, mild hypotension, conjunctivitis, and malaise. Gastrointestinal stress with abdominal pain, epigastric pains, nausea, vomiting, mild diarrhea and/or constipation are some of the more common symptoms.[29] In addition, during the initial stages of infection, symptoms of headache, dizziness, general weakness, irritability, lethargy, loss of appetite, photophobia, retro-orbital pains, nonproductive (dry) cough, sore throat, nasal congestion and hyporeflexia are commonly observed. Physical examination of patients may reveal flushing of the face, neck and upper chest, as well as, conjunctival congestion and periorbital edema. Oropharyngeal membranes are almost always congested, especially the blood vessels bordering the gums.[19] After the third to fifth day of the infection, patients generally begin to display symptoms of dehydration and infrequent urination. In addition, electrocardiographic examination of patients will indicate moderate bradycardia and hypotension.[11]

During the second and third weeks of infection, 70-80% of the patients begin to improve. However, the remaining patients will proceed into hemorrhagic or neurologic manifestations, shock and/or secondary bacterial infections (e.g. pneumonia and septicemia). Opportunistic fungal infections, such as thrush may also occur.[19] The hemorrhagic symptoms of disease will first appear as a petechia rash, found generally on the axilla, soft palate, and gingival margin. Progressive leucopenia (1000-2000/mm³) and thrombocytopenia (50,000-100,000/mm³) readily occur with patients suffering from AHF. Laboratory observations show that reductions of clotting factors II, VII, X and moderate decreases of clotting factors V and VII, as well as, low fibrinogen levels may lead to systemic hemorrhaging.[29]

The cause of thrombocytopenia during a JUNV infection is a question that requires further elucidation. Nonetheless, Pozner et al. (2010) indicated that the infection with JUNV did not affect megakaryocyte generation. However, the infection did trigger the release of type I interferon (IFN α/β) which caused in paracrine influences that led to abnormal platelet formation. This abnormal platelet formation is therefore theorized to be the cause of thrombocytopenia, resulting in hemorrhagic complications.[30]

Table 1: An overview of the clinical symptoms of AHF

Symptoms	+	++	+++
Fever			▪
Chills			▪
Anorexia			▪
Myalgia			▪
Conjunctivitis			▪
Malaise			▪
Flushing of the face, neck & chest			▪
Conjunctival congestion			▪
Periorbital edema			▪
Oropharynx congestion			▪
Congestion of gums			▪
Dehydration			▪
Infrequent urination			▪
Petechia rash			▪
Leucopenia			▪
Thrombocytopenia			▪
Hemorr. of nose			▪
Hemorr. of gums			▪
Hemorr. Of lungs			▪
Bloody stool			▪
Interstitial pneumontitis			▪
Diffuse alveolar damage			▪
Necrosis spleen			▪
Necrosis lymph node			▪
Atypical urine sediment		▪	
Hemoconcentrations		▪	
Hypotensive shock		▪	
Bradycardia		▪	
Hypotension		▪	
Gastrointestinal stress		▪	
Abdominal pain		▪	
Epigastric pains		▪	
Nausea		▪	
Vomiting		▪	
Mild diarrhea		▪	
Constipation		▪	
Headache		▪	
Dizziness		▪	
General weakness		▪	
Irritability		▪	
Lethargy		▪	
Loss of appetite		▪	
Photophobia		▪	
Nonproductive cough		▪	
Sore throat		▪	
Nasal congestion		▪	
Hyporeflexia		▪	
Oliguria		▪	
Anuria		▪	
Albuminuria		▪	
Asthenia		▪	
Hair loss		▪	
Irritability		▪	
Memory changes		▪	
Hematuria	▪		

+ Rare ++ Common +++ Frequent

Hemorrhages will appear in the form of nose bleeds, bleeding gums and bloody stool, which indicates hemorrhage in the stomach and intestines. Hemorrhages may affect various organs while the resulting necrosis could vary from modest and focal to substantial and multifocal. For example, the lungs will display varying extent of hemorrhages, along with interstitial pneumontitis and diffuse alveolar damage. Additionally, lymphoid tissue and the liver are almost always involved. Clinical reports indicate that widespread necrosis is generally observed in the splenic white pulp and the paracortical and cortical regions of the lymph nodes.[1, 31]

Abnormal urinary sediment and hemo-concentrations are also common. Severe cases of hemorrhage can lead to hypotensive shock. In addition, signs of oliguria (>500ml/24hr), which in terminal cases will lead to anuria, as well as, albuminuria (presence of albumin in the urine) and less frequently, hematuria (indicate an impairment of renal function) are also observed. It is known that a combination of the above described hemorrhagic symptoms, including renal impairment, results in death within 48 to 72 hours.[29] Severe neurological manifestations generally begin with mental confusion, marked ataxia, increased irritability and bodily tremors. These initial symptoms are generally followed by delirium, generalized convulsions, coma and death.[19]

Generally, 70 to 80% of patients recover after a convalescence of one to three months. During recovery, patients display transient symptoms of asthenia, hair loss, irritability, and memory changes. However, the remaining 20 to 30% of patients, within 8 to 12 days after the first onset of symptoms will suffer from severe hemorrhagic or neurological manifestations, shock, and/or secondary bacterial infections. JUNV is capable of transplacental transmission and generally results in death for both mother and fetus in the third trimester. The fatality rate for AHF is generally 15 to 30% if the symptoms are left untreated (Table 1).[32]

DETECTION

The specific symptoms of AHF are similar to those presented in patients with other infections, which may pose a problem for clinical diagnosis. Therefore, it is necessary to couple laboratory examinations with clinical diagnosis in order to accurately identify AHF. There are several methods in which JUNV may be detected in laboratories. For example, Barrera Oro et al. (1990), developed a complement-enhanced, plaque-reduction neutralization test to measure the neutralizing antibodies against JUNV in blood samples.[33] This method is effective but time consuming. Additional methods such as enzyme linked immunoassay (ELISA) are currently the most practical method for rapidly detecting JUNV specific IgG and IgM in infected individuals. This assay yielded ~1% false positives and 0.05% false negatives during clinical trials (a similar result when compared with plaque-reduction neutralization test).[34] Furthermore, indirect immunofluorescence antibody (IIF) tests for IgM and IgG specific antibodies for JUNV are commonly used by laboratories. This test is generally used about 10 days after the onset of the initial symptoms of AHF.[35]

RT-PCR assay is used for early detection of JUNV infections. RT-PCR is extremely sensitive when compared to the laboratory tests described previously and can detect low viremia within the first 8 days after the onset of initial AHF symptoms. This is important because the introduction of convalescent plasma for AHF patients has to be initiated within the first 8 days of infection in order to be effective.[1, 36]

Recently, novel monoclonal antibodies to the NPs of both LFV and JUNV were developed and used in sandwich antigen-capture ELISA. The results from this newly developed method showed promise, as it has been reported to be sensitive and specific.[37]

TREATMENT

As with all hemorrhagic fevers, supportive therapy is the mainstay of treatment. Sedatives should be used for pain relief, careful maintenance of fluids and electrolytes are essential. Intramuscular injections should be avoided due to the possibility of uncontrollable bleeding at the venous puncture sites. In addition, administering acetylsalicylic acid (e.g. Aspirin) and non-steroid anti-inflammatory drugs should always be avoided. Clinicians may prescribe acetaminophen to combat fever and inflammatory symptoms. If consumptive coagulopathy occurs, infusions of heparin, clotting factors, as well as, platelet may be lifesaving measures. In an effort to prevent secondary infections, broad spectrum antibiotics may also be administered.[19]

Introduction of convalescent plasma for AHF patients has shown a reduction in the mortality of patients from 15 to 30% to 1 to 2% if initiated within the first 8 days of infection.[38] Generally, two to three units (depending on the titer of neutralizing antibodies) of convalescent plasma are needed per patient of which a dosage of approximately 3000 therapeutic units of neutralizing antibodies per kilogram of body weight are needed.[39] Nonetheless, this form of treatment is associated with late neurological complications of undeter-mined origin in ~10% of survivors.[40, 41] Although convalescent plasma treatment is a good treatment for treating AHF, the difficulties in maintaining adequate plasma reserves for potential AHF outbreaks are problematic.

Administering ribavirin has been shown to be effective in treating AHF. Laboratory experiments have shown that ribavirin, in low doses inhibited the cytopathic effect of JUNV in Vero cell lines five days post infection. At higher concentrations, ribavirin reduced the viral load to undetectable levels.[42] In separate studies, AHF infected guinea pigs and rhesus macaques were treated with ribavirin. The antiviral agent showed some positive result, as viral replication within the host was delayed, however, deaths were still seen.[43, 44] Presently, evaluations with ribavirin in AHF afflicted humans have yielded positive results. If AHF is suspected, it is suggested that ribavirin should be given while waiting for the confirmation of the diagnosis. The suggested initial dose is 30 mg/kg intravenously (maximum dosage of 2g/kg). This initial dose is followed by 16 mg/kg intravenously (maximum 1g/kg per dose) every 6 hours for 4 days and finally, 8 mg/kg intravenously (maximum of 500 mg/kg per dose) every 8 hours for the remaining 6 days. In the event of mass casualties, oral ribavirin could be given. For patients weighing more than 75 kg, the initial dosage should be 2000 mg/kg (loading) followed by 600 mg/kg twice daily for 10 days. For patients weighing less than 75 kg (including children), initial dosage is 30 mg/kg (loading) followed by 15 mg/kg (divided into two doses) every day for 10 days.[45]

Presently, the only vaccine that has been tested and approved for use in Argentina is Candid #1. Candid #1 vaccine strain was developed from XJ strain of JUNV by United States Medical Institute of Infectious Diseases (USAMRIID) and the Argentine Ministry of Health and Social Action between 1992 to 1999. The initial field test of this live-attenuated vaccine involved 6500 male agricultural workers in endemic regions of Argentina. The effectiveness of this new vaccine during clinical trials is estimated at 98.1%. At present, this vaccine is widely used in Argentina for the prevention of AHF.[1, 46, 47]

DIFFERENTIAL DIAGNOSIS

During the first week of AHF infection, the clinical symptoms are nonspecific and may be easily confused with several

Table 2: An overview of the differential diagnosis of AHF. Hint: Dengue Fever (DF), Dengue hemorrhagic fever (DHF), Hantavirus pulmonary syndrome (HPS), Leptospirosis (Lepto), Rocky Mountain spotted fever (RMSF)

Symptoms	AHF	DF	DHF	HPS	Lepto	RMSF
Fever	■	■				■
Chills	■				■	
Anorexia	■	■		■		■
Myalgia	■	■		■		■
Conjunctivitis	■	■				
Malaise	■	■	■			■
Flushing of the face & neck	■					
Flushing of the upper chest	■					
Conjunctival congestion	■	■			■	■
Periorbital edema	■					
Congestion of oropharynx	■					
Congestion of the gums	■					
Dehydration	■					
Infrequent urination	■		■			
Petechia rash	■	■			■	■
Leucopenia	■	■				
Thrombocytopenia	■	■				■
Hemorrhage of nose & gums	■	■				
Bloody stool	■	■				
Abnormal urinary sediment	■				■	
Hemoconcentrations	■		■			
Hypotensive shock	■	■				■
Bradycardia	■	■				
Hypotension	■		■		■	■
Gastrointestinal stress	■					
Abdominal pain	■	■				■
Nausea	■	■			■	■
Vomiting	■	■		■	■	■
Mild diarrhea	■	■		■		
Constipation	■					
Headache	■	■	■		■	■
Dizziness	■					
General weakness	■	■				■
Irritability	■					
Lethargy	■					
Loss of appetite	■	■				
Photophobia	■	■				■
Nonproductive cough	■			■	■	■
Sore throat	■					
Nasal congestion	■					
Hyporeflexia	■					
Oliguria	■		■			
Anuria	■					
Albuminuria	■				■	
Asthenia	■					
Hair loss	■					
Irritability	■					
Memory changes	■					
Hematuria	■	■	■		■	

acute febrile conditions such as dengue, dengue hemorrhagic fever, hantavirus pulmonary syndrome, hepatitis, influenza, malaria (only considered in endemic areas), mononucleosis, leptospirosis, rickett-sioses, toxoplasmosis, and typhoid fever. AHF may also be confused with other diseases with hemorrhagic and neurological manifestations such as rheumatic diseases and blood dyscrasias.[19]

Most often clinical diagnosis alone cannot differentiate JUNV infection from other infections with similar symptoms. Therefore, laboratory diagnosis is essential in the confirmation of JUNV diagnosis (Table 2).

References

1. Meyer B.J., Southern P.J. Sequence heterogeneity in the termini of lymphocytic choriomeningitis virus genomic and antigenomic RNAs. Journal of Virology, 1994. 68: 7659-7664

2. Tortorici M.A., Albarino C.G., Posik D.M., Ghiringhelli P.D., Lozano M.E., Rivera Pomar R., Romanowski V., Arenavirus nucleocapsid protein displays a transcriptional antitermination activity in vivo. Virus Research, 2001, 73: pp. 41-55

3. Grant A., Seregin A., Huang C., Kolokoltsova O., Brasier A., Peters C., Paessler S. Junín Virus Pathogenesis and Virus Replication. Viruses, 2012. 4: pp. 2317-2339

4. Clegg J.C. Molecular Phylogeny of the Arenaviruses. Current Topic in Microbiology and Immunology, 2002. 262: pp. 1-24

5. Saunders A.A., Ting J.P.C., Meisner J., Neuman B.W., Perez M., de la Torre J.C., Buchmeier M.J. Mapping the Landscape of the Lymphocytic Choriomeningitis Virus Stable Signal Peptide Reveals Novel Functional Domains. Journal of Virology, 2007. 81: pp. 5649-5657

6. Buchmeier M.J., de la Torre J-C., Peters C.J. Arenavirisae: The Viruses and their Replication. Field's Virology. Fourth Edition. Philadelphia: Lippincott, Willams and Wilkins. 2007. pp. 1635-1668

7. Parodi A.S., Greenway D.J., Rugiero H.R., Frigerio M., De La Barrera J.M., Mettler N., Garzon F., Boxaca M., Guerrero L., Nota N. Concerning the Epidemic Outbreak in Junin. El Dia Medico, 1958. 30: pp. 2300-23001

8. Chiappero M.B., Gardenal C.N., Panzetta-Dutari M. Isolation and Characterization of Microsatillite Markers in Calomys musculinus (Muridae, Sigmodontinae, Phyllotini), the natural Reservoir of Junin Virus. Molecular Ecology Notes, 2005. 5: pp. 593-595

9. Vitullo A.D., Hodara V.L., Merani M.S. Effect of Persistent Infection with Junin Virus on Growth and Reproduction of its Natural Reservoir, Calomys musculinus. American Journal

of Tropical Medicine and hygiene, 1987. 37: pp. 663 - 669

10. Campetella O.E., Galassi N.V., Barrios H.A. Junin Virus-induced Non-specific Suppressor Cells Interact with Unrelated Antigen-specific Suppressor cells. Immunology, 1991. 74: pp. 14-19

11. Maiztegui J.T. Clinical and Epidemiological Patterns of Argentine Haemorrhagic Fever. Bulletin of the World Health Organization, 1975. 52: pp. 567-575

12. Weissenbacher M.C., Laguens R.P., Coto C.E. Argentine Hemorrhagic Fever. Current Topic in Microbiology and Immunololgy, 1987. 134: pp. 79–116

13. Cordo S.M., y Acuña M.C., Candurra N.A. Polarized Entry and Release of Junín Virus, a New World Arenavirus. Journal of General Virology, 2005. 86: pp. 1475-1479

14. Cao W., Henry M.D., Borrow P., Yamada H., Elder J.H., Ravkov E.V., Nichol S.T., Compans R.W., Campbell K.P., Oldstone M.B. Identification of α-dystroglycan as a Receptor for Choriomeningitis Virus and Lassa Fever Virus. Science, 1998. 282: pp. 2079-2081

15. Flanagan M. L., Oldenburg J., Reignier T., Holt N., Hamilton G.A., Martin V.K., Cannon P.M. 2008. New World Clade B Arenaviruses can use Transferrin Receptor 1 (TfR1)-dependent and -independent Entry Pathways, and Glycoproteins from Human Pathogenic Strains are associated with the use of TfR1. The Journal of Virology, 2008. 82: pp. 938-948

16. Radoshitzky S. R., Abraham J., Spiropoulou C.F., Kuhn J.H., Nguyen D., Li W., Nagel J., Schmidt P.J., Nunberg J.H., Andrews N.C., Farzan M., Choe H. 2007. Transferrin Receptor 1 is a Cellular Receptor for New World Haemorrhagic Fever Arenaviruses. Nature, 2007. 446: pp. 92-96

17. Radoshitzky S. R., Kuhn J.H., Spiropoulou C.F., Albarino C.G., Nguyen D.P., Salazar-Bravo J., Dorfman T., Lee A.S., Wang E., Ross S.R., Choe H., Farzan M.. 2008. Receptor Determinants of Zoonotic Transmission of New World Hemorrhagic Fever Arenaviruses. Proceedings of the National Academy of Sciences of the United States of America, 2008. 105: pp. 2664-2669

18. Martinez M.G., Bialecki M.A., Belouzard S., Cordo S.M., Candurra N.A., Whittaker G.R. Utilization of human DC-SIGN and L-SIGN for entry and infection of host cells by the New World arenavirus, Junín virus. Biochemical and Biophysical Research Communications, 2013. 441: pp. 612–617

19. Guerrant R.L., Walker D.H., Weller P.F. Tropical Infectious Diseases – Principles, Pathogens & Practice. Volume 1. Philadelphia: Churchill Livingstone Elsevier. 2006. pp. 734-755

20. Bishop D. Arenaviridae and their Replication. Virology. Second Edition. New York: Raven Press. 1990. pp. 1231-1243

21. Garcin D., Kolakofsky D. Tacaribe Arenavirus RNA Synthesis In Vitro is Primer Dependent and Suggests an Unusual Model for the Initiation of Genome Replication. The Journal of Virology, 1992. 66: pp. 1370-1376

22. Meyer B.J., Southern P.J. Concurrent Sequence Analysis of 5' and 3' RNA termini by Intramolecular Circularization Reveals 5' Nontemplated Bases and 3' Terminal Heterogeneity for Lymphocytic Choriomeningitis Virus mRNAs. The Journal of Virology, 1993. 67: pp. 2621-2627

23. Garcin D., Kolakofsky D. A Novel Mechanism for the Initiation of Tacaribe Arenavirus Genome Replication. The Journal of Virology, 1990. 64: pp. 6196-6203

24. Eichler R., Strecher T., Kolesnikova L., Characterization of the Lassa Virus Matrix Protein Z: Electron Microscopic Study of Virus-like Particles and Interaction with the Nucleoprotein (NP). Virus Research, 2004. 100: pp. 249-255

25. Yun N.E., Walker D.H. Pathogenesis of Lassa Fever. Viruses, 2012. 4: pp. 2031-2048

26. Alibek K. Biohazard. New York: Dell Publishing. 1999. pp. 42

27. Hemorrhagic Fever Viruses (VHF). Updated January 10, 2008. Retrieved July 24, 2008. Web Site: http://www. upmc-biosecurity.org/website/focus/agentsdiseases/fact _sheets/vhf.html

28. Cordo S., Acuna M.C., Candurra N.A. Polarized Entry and Release of Junin Virus, a New World Arenavirus. Journal of General Virology, 2005. 86: pp. 1475-1479

29. Oldstone M.B. Arenaviruses I – The Epidemiology, Molecular and Cell Biology of Arenaviruses. Current Topics In Microbiology and Immunology. New York: Springer-Verlag, 2002. pp. 67

30. Pozner R.G., Ure A.E., de Giusti C.J., D'Atri L.P., Italiano J.E., Torres O., Romanowski V., Schattner M., Ricardo M. Gómez R.M. Junín Virus Infection of Human Hematopoietic Progenitors Impairs In Vitro Proplatelet Formation and Platelet Release via a Bystander Effect Involving Type I IFN Signaling Public Library of Science, Pathology, 2010. 6: pp. e1000847

31. Reiss C.S. Neurotropic Viral Infections. Cambridge: Cambridge University Press. 2008. pp. 81

32. Harrison L.H., Halsey N.A., McKee K.T., Peters C.J., Oro J.G.B., Briggiler A.M., Feuillade M.R., Maiztegui J.I. Clinical Case Definition for Argentine Hemorrhagic Fever. Clinical Infectious Diseases, 1998. 28: pp. 1091-1094

33. Barrera Oro J.G., McKee K.T., Spisso J., Mahlandt B.G., Maiztegui J.I. A Refined Complement-enhanced Neutralization Test for Detecting Antibodies to Junin Virus. Journal of Viological Methods, 1990. 29: pp. 71 - 80

34. Riera L.M., Feuillade M.R., Saavedra M.C., Ambrosio A.M. Evaluation of an Enzyme Immunosorbent Assay for the Diagnosis of Argentine Haemorrhagic Fever. Acta Virologica, 1997. 41: pp. 305 - 310

35. Jahrling P.B. Arenaviruses and filoviruses. Diagnostic Procedures for Viral, Rickettsial, and Chlamydial Infections. 6th Edition. Washington DC: American Public Health Association Inc., 1989. pp. 857 – 891

36. Lozano M.E, Enria D., Maiztegui J.I., Grau O., Romanowski V. Rapid Diagnosis of Argentine Hemorrhagic Fever by Reverse Transcriptase PCR-based Assay. Journal of Clinical Microbiology, 1995; 33: pp. 1327 - 1332

37. Fukushi S., Tani H., Yoshikawa T., Saijo M., Morikawa S. Serological Assays Based on Recombinant Viral Proteins for the Diagnosis of Arenavirus Hemorrhagic Fevers. Viruses, 2012. 4: pp. 2097-2114

38. Oldstone M.B. Arenaviruses II – The Epidemiology, Molecular and Cell Biology of Arenaviruses. Current Topics in Microbiology and Immunology. New York: Springer-Verlag, 2002. pp. 240

39. Enria D.A., Briggiler A.M., Fernandez N.J., Levis SC, Maiztegui JI. Importance of Dose of Neutralising Antibodies in Treatment of Argentine Haemorrhagic Fever with Immune Plasma. Lancet, 1984. 2: pp. 255 - 256

40. Maiztegui J.I., Fernandez N.J., de Damilano A.J. Efficacy of Immune Plasma Treatment of Argentine Hemorrhagic Fever and Association between Treatment and a Late Neurologic Syndrome. Lancet, 1979. 2: pp. 1216–1217

41. Enria D., Franco S.G., Ambrosio A., Vallejos D., Levis D., Maiztegui J. Current Status of the Treatment of Argentine Hemorrhagic Fever. Medical Microbiology and immunology, 1986. 175: pp. 173-176

42. Rodríguez M., McCormick J.B., Weissenbacher M.C. Antiviral Effect of Ribavirin on Junin Virus Replication in Vitro. Revista Argentina de Microbiologia, 1986. 18: pp. 69-74

43. Kenyon R.H., Canonico P.G., Green D.E., Peters C.J. Effects of Ribavirin and Tributylribavirin on Argentine Hemorrhagic Fever (Junin Virus) Guinea Pigs. Antimicrobial Agents and Chemotherapy, 1986. 29: pp. 521-523

44. McKee K.T., Huggins J.W., Trahan C.J., Mahland B.G. Ribavirin Prohylaxis and Therapy for Experimental Argentine Hemorrhagic Fever. Antimicrobial Agents and Chemotherapy, 1988. 32: pp. 1304-1309

45. Ciottone G.R. Disaster Medicine. Philadelphia:Mosby Elsevier. 2006. pp. 666

46. Franz D.R., Jahrling P.B., Friedlander A.M., McClain D.J., Hoover D.L., Bryne W.R., Pavlin J.A., Christopher G.W., Eitzen E.M. Clinical Recognition and Management of Patients Exposed to Biological Warfare Agents. The Journal of American Medical Association, 1997. 278: pp. 399-411

47. Maiztegui J.I., McKee K.T. Jr., Barrera Oro J.G., Harrison L.H., Gibbs P.H., Feuillade M.R., Enria D.A., Briggiler A.M., Levis S.C., Ambrosio A.M. Halsey N.A., Peters C.J. Protective efficacy of a live attenuated vaccine against argentine hemorrhagic fever. AHF study group. The Journal of Infectious Diseases, 1998. 177: pp. 277-283.

Photo Bibliography

Figure 1.7-1: An electronmicrograph of a New World arenavirus. This photomicrograph was taken by E. L. Palmer at 80,00x magnification and released by the CDC. Public domain photo
Figure 1.7-4: Virus graphics designed by Los Alamos National Security of the United States Department of Energy. Public domain photo

Lassa fever virus (LFV) is an enveloped, single-stranded, bisegmented, ambisense RNA virus that belongs to the genus *Arenavirus*, family *Arenaviridae*. LFV is a member of the Old World group of arenavirus, which includes Lymphocytic Choriomeningitis virus, Mopeia virus, Mobala virus, Merino Walk virus and the Ippy virus (Figure 1.8-1).[1, 2]

LFV is a zoonotic infection that is transmitted by rodents to humans and is responsible for the highly pathogenic Lassa fever (LF), an acute viral hemorrhagic fever. The most common carrier of LFV is the multimammate rat (*Mastomys natalensis*), which is indigenous to equatorial Africa.[3] These LFV infected rodents become lifelong asymptomatic carriers, and excrete the virus particles through urine, feces, saliva, respiratory secretions and blood (Figure 1.8-2).[4]

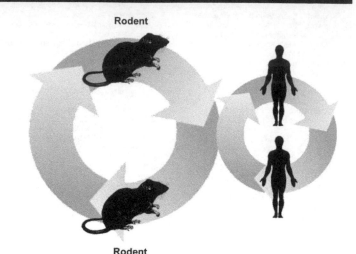

Rodent

Rodent

Figure 1.8-2: Sylvatic cycle of Lassa Fever Virus (LFV)

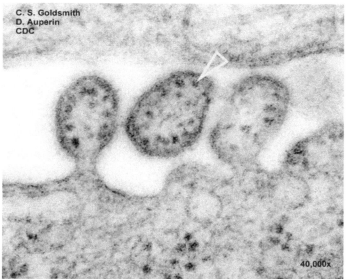

C. S. Goldsmith
D. Auperin
CDC

40,000x

Figure 1.8-1: An electron micrograph (TEM) of a number of Lassa fever virus virions (indicated by the arrow) adjacent to some cell debris

LF was first described in Sierra Leone during the 1950s, but the LFV was not isolated until 1969 when two missionary nurses died from the infection in the town of Lassa, located in the Yedseram River Valley (Jos Plateau), Northern Nigeria.[5] Subsequently, isolated cases of LF and/or outbreaks have been documented in Liberia, Sierra Leone, Guinea, Nigeria and Mali, while serological evidence of LFV has been found in neighboring countries such as the Central African Republic and the Democratic Republic of Congo.[6, 7, 8, 9, 10] Due to the prevalence of international air travel, importation of LFV into regions of the world has also been documented (Figure 1.8-3).[11, 12, 13]

Presently, it is estimated that LFV is responsible for an estimated one to four hundred thousand infections annually, of which, five thousand cases result in fatalities.[14]

There are numerous LFV strains of known. These strains

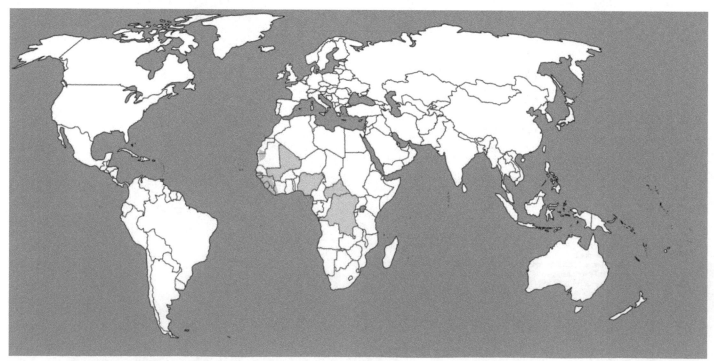

Figure 1.8-3: Distribution of Lassa Fever Virus (LFV)

have been isolated from different geographical locations and demonstrate significant variations in genetic, serologic and pathogenic characteristics. All of the LFV strains are subdivided into four phylogenetic lineages (I-IV). Lineage I-III are found in Nigeria, while IV is located in Guinea, Liberia, and Sierra Leone.[11, 15, 16, 17]

It is known that mononuclear phagocytes, such as Kupffer cells, alveolar macrophages, monocytes and dendritic cells, in addition to endothelial cells, hepatocytes, mesothelial cells and endocrine cells of the adrenal gland, ovary, uterus, placenta and

breasts are targets for LFV.[18, 19]

LFV has two single-stranded RNA genomic segments, the large (L) and small (S).[20] In the viral particle, the molar ratio of the S to L RNA segments is approximately 2:1 and the 5' terminus of both segments contains a tri- or diphosphate group but lacking a cap structure.[21]

The S RNA segment is approximately 3.4kb and contains 2 genes that encode the nucleoprotein (NP) located at the 3' end and the glycoprotein precursor (GPC) located at the 5' end in

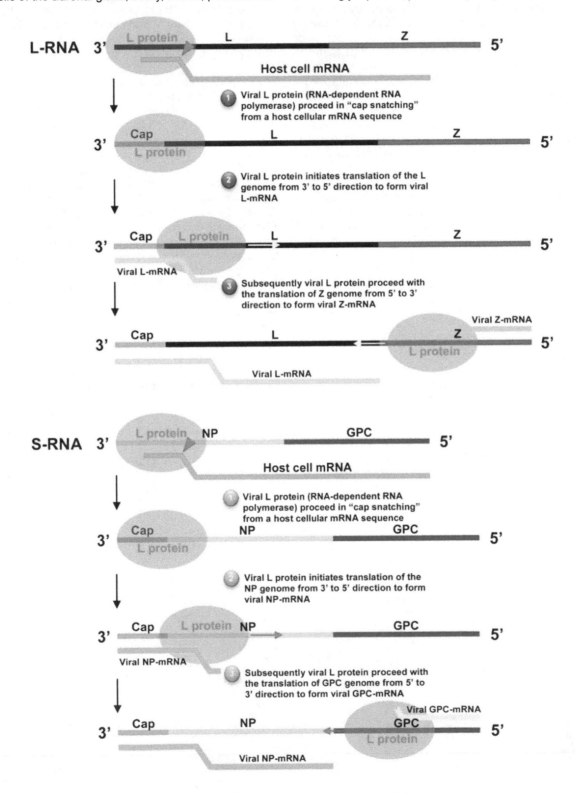

Figure 1.8-4: Diagrammatic examination of LFV sense and antisense (ambisense) viral genome transcription

ambisense arrangement.[22, 23, 24, 25, 26]

The L RNA segment is approximately 7.2 kb and encodes the viral RNA dependent RNA polymerase (L protein) located at the 3' end. Additionally, the L segment also codes the zinc-binding (Z) protein (a small protein with a zinc-binding domain) located at the 5' end. Both of these proteins are involved in the regulation of transcription and replication of LFV (Figure 1.8-4).[27, 28, 29]

Like all arenaviruses, LFV gains entry into cells via GP_1 attachment to various membrane bounded receptor of the host cell. These receptors include O-mannosylated dystroglycan, Axl, Tyro3, dendritic cell-specific intercellular adhesion molecule 3-grabbing nonintegrin (DC-SIGN) and liver and lymph node sinusoidal endothelial calcium-dependent lectin (LSECtin).[30, 31] Once the GP_1 and the host cellular receptor complex is formed, the virus is brought into the cell via clathrin-mediated endocytosis. Once the virus is within the acidic environment of the endosomal vesicle, the GP_2 with assistance from SSP will mediate the fusion between the virion membrane and the endosomal membrane. Subsequently, the nucleocapsid of the LFV virus is released into the cytoplasm of the host cell where replication of the viral genome takes place.[27, 32]

The ambisense arrangement of the LFV genome, as well as, the genome of other arenaviruses, allows for a unique mechanism to regulate gene transcription. This unique regulation allows for the transcription of genes located at the 3' of the bisegmented RNA are expressed first, while genes lying at the 5' of the viral RNA segment (e.g. GPC and Z) cannot be expressed in the absence of viral protein synthesis.[33] Gene expression is initiated when the viral L protein cleave the cap and one to seven bases from the host cellular messenger RNAs (mRNAs) and uses these primers to initiate transcription of subgenomic mRNAs in a process known as "cap snatching."[34, 35] These non-polyadenylated viral RNAs are then translated by the host cell ribosomes to produce viral NP and L proteins (Figure 1.8-4). Transcription ends at the distal margin of the stem-loop structure found within the viral intergenomic region.[36, 37]

Genes found at the 5' ends of the viral genome (e.g. GPC and Z) are not translated directly even though they are in the proper coding sense. Once the transcription of the 3' end of the viral RNA is completed, the L protein adopts a replicase mode and generates a full-length complementary antigenomic RNA (agRNA) from the 5' end of the viral genome. The L protein is believed to initiate RNA replication using a dinucleotide template (guanosine triphosphate cytidine monophosphate - pppGpC) where a full length genome-complementary RNA molecule, termed antigenome RNA (agRNA), is transcribed. agRNA will serve as a template for the synthesis of viral mRNA in the genomic orientation. This viral mRNA will be translated to form GPC and Z protein. It has been reported that after translation, the Z protein, is involved in viral particle formation where it serves as a matrix protein and interacts with the N protein, in addition to driving particle formation.[19, 37, 38]

On the other hand, considerable posttranslational processing of the GPC will take place. For example, the GPC is post-translationally processed by signal peptidase to form stable signal peptide (SSP). This process is followed by the posttranslational cleavage of the remaining residue by the enzyme protease SKI-1/S1P to form GP_1 (45 kD) and GP_2 (38 kD). It has been reported that SSP (~5kD) is engaged in the glycoprotein expression and post-translational modification GP_1 and GP_2 by protease SKI-1/S1P although the exact mechanism of this process requires further analysis.[27] Once G_1 and G_2 is formed, these envelope glycoproteins are transported to the plasma membrane of the host cell with the assistance of SSP. The GP_1 tetramer will eventually form the head of the envelope spike of the LFV, while the GP_2 tetramer will form the stalk.[24, 25, 26, 27]. It has been reported that the cytoplasmic tail of GP_2, along with SSP, will interact with NP, which in turn interacts with the Z protein at the plasma membrane of the host cell. Numerous reports indicated that it is these interactions that play a critical role in the viral assembly and budding; although the exact manner of this process requires further investigation (Figure 1.8-5).[27, 38]

LFV is a potential biological warfare agent due to its lethality, high infectivity by the aerosol dispersal as shown in animal models, and possibility for efficient replication in tissue culture.[39] In Alibek's book, *Biohazard*, he wrote that Lassa fever virus was researched

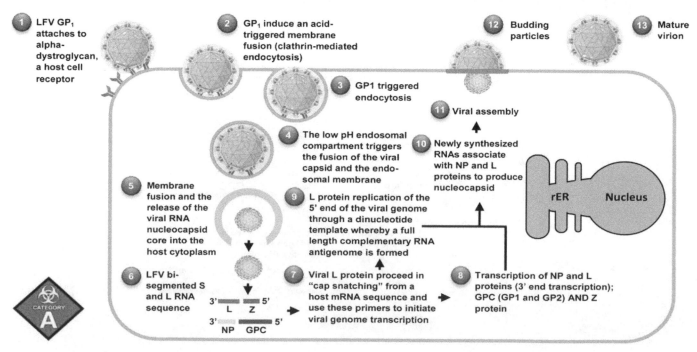

Figure 1.8-5: Diagrammatic process of LFV infection within an eukaryotic cell

and produced at the institute of Ultra-Pure Biopreparations in Leningrad, Omutninsk in Kirov, Obolensk outside of Moscow, the Lyubuchany Institute of Immunology in Chekhov near Moscow, and Vector Research and Testing, located in Novosibrisk (near small town of Koltsovo) in Siberia.[40] Based upon LFV's potential to cause widespread, person to person transmission, illness and death, the Centers for Disease Control and Prevention (CDC) in 1999 classified LFV as Category A biological weapon agents.[41]

SYMPTOMS

Due to the ubiquitous presence of multimammate rats in households in equatorial Africa, exposure to LFV is pervasive. Infection by LFV generally occurs through the inhalation of dried and aerosolized urine and/or excrement particles from infected rodent carriers. Additionally, infection may also occur through the ingestion of LFV particles in contaminated food or by consuming the multimammate rat as a delicacy.[42] Less commonly, LFV may also be spread through cuts or open wounds that may come into contact with exposure to rodent contaminated materials.[43] Like other types of viral hemorrhagic fever, once an individual is infected with LFV they possess the potential to infect others with whom they come into contact. For example, LFV can be isolated from blood, feces, urine, saliva, vomit and semen samples of infected individuals for 30 days or more after initial infection. Infections can also occur through direct contact with contaminated blood and bodily fluids. Health care workers are especially at risk when proper sanitation, safety and sanitary procedures are not properly followed.[44]

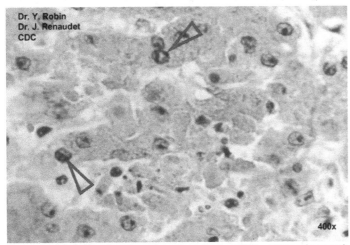

Figure 1.8-6: Hematoxylin-and-eosin-stained (H&E) photo-micrograph showing the cytoarchitectural changes in liver tissue from a Lassa fever patient. Note the zone of acidophilic necrosis, and numbers of pycnotic nuclei (indicated by the arrow)

LFV is indiscriminant in its infection. LFV infections are seen in both sexes and in all age groups. Approximately 80% of LFV infections are mild or asymptomatic. Only the remaining 20% of patients develop a severe, multisystem disease that requires hospitalization and 15% (overall case fatality rate is at 1%) of these patients succumb to the infection.[45]

Once infected, LFV proceeds through an asymptomatic incubation period that lasts 3 to 21 days.[1] The onset of the disease is indicated by high fever (40°C or 104°F), headaches, arthralgia, myalgia (back and abdominal pains), asthenia, anorexia and malaise. Within a few days after the initial onset of symptoms, patients may also experience sore throat (with or without visible pharyngitis), dysphagia, dry cough, bilateral conjunctival injection, retrosternal chest pains, diarrhea, nausea, vomiting and abdominal pains.[19, 37, 46, 47] Occasionally, some

patients may also show signs of facial and cervical edema (caused by inflamed lymph nodes), proteinuria, subconjunctival hemorrhage, periorbital edema, pulmonary edema, ascites, pleural and pericardial effusions and epistaxis.[1, 37, 47]

Table 1: An overview of the clinical symptoms of LF

Symptoms	+	++	+++
Fever			■
Headaches			■
Arthralgia			■
Myalgia			■
Asthenia			■
Malaise			■
Sore throat			■
Dysphagia			■
Cough			■
Conjunctivitis			■
Retrosternal chest pains			■
Diarrhea			■
Nausea			■
Vomiting			■
Abdominal pains			■
Facial edema		■	
Cervical edema		■	
Proteinuria		■	
Subconjunctival bleeding		■	
Periorbital edema		■	
Pleural effusions		■	
Pericardial effusions		■	
Pulmonary edema		■	
Ascites		■	
Epistaxis		■	
Blooding from the mouth		■	
Mucosal bleeding		■	
Hematemesis		■	
Bloody diarrhea		■	
Enlarged kidneys		■	
Inflamed kidneys		■	
Enlarged liver		■	
Inflamed liver		■	
Elevate respiration rates		■	
Hypotension		■	
Hypertension		■	
Thrombocytopenia		■	
Leucopenia		■	
Hyperuraemia		■	
Tachycardia		■	
Pericardial effusions		■	
Aseptic meningitis		■	
Encephalitis		■	
Global encephalopathy		■	
Seizures		■	
Deafness		■	
Shock		■	
Tremor		■	
Disorientation		■	
Delirium		■	
Respiratory stress		■	
Coma		■	
Hair loss		■	
Gait disturbances		■	
Petechial rash	■		
Maculopapular rash	■		
Swollen baby syndrome	■		

+ Rare ++ Common +++ Frequent

Signs of blood emission from the mouth and various other mucosal surfaces, hematemesis and bloody diarrhea are also observed in some severely affected individuals. These emissions are generally caused by capillary lesions in the stomach and small intestines. In some patients, liver and kidneys are often enlarged, inflamed and painful when palpated. In patients with an enlarged and inflamed liver, some cyroarchitectural changes may be found in tissue samples with acidophilic necrosis and pycnotic nuclei (Figure 1.8-6). Other microscopic findings include splenic necrosis, mild interstitial pneumontitis, alveolar edema, lymph node histiocytosis with mitosis, gastrointestinal mucosal petechiae, injury to the renal tubules and interstitial nephritis.[8, 37, 19] Infrequently, petechial and maculopapular rashes are observed on light-skinned patients but not on dark-skinned patients.[1, 42, 45, 47]

During the later stages of LF (six to ten days after the initial signs of the infection) some severely infected patients may exhibit elevated respiration rates, hypotension, hypertension, thrombo-cytopenia, leucopenia, hyperuraemia, tachy-cardia and pericardial effusions. Neurological manifestations of the disease such as aseptic meningitis, encephalitis, and global encephalo-pathy accompanied by seizures may also appear. In 29% of cases, deafness (sensor-ineural hearing deficit) appears during the later stages of disease or in early stages of convalescence.[19, 37, 46, 48, 49] It has been documented that approximately 50% of these patients recover some hearing functions after one to three months of convalescence. Presently, it is not known if the neurological manifestations are caused directly by the LFV or is a result of secondary immune-response. Shock, tremor, disorientation, delirium, seizure, respiratory stress, multi-organ failure and coma may also occur in the late stages of the infection and generally result in death.[37, 50, 51]

During pregnancy, LF causes a relatively high rate of maternal death (~29%). Mortality is more likely when LF occurs during the third trimester of pregnancy. Fetal and neonatal loss have been reported at 87%, while the fatality rate nearing 100% for fetuses in the third trimester.[46, 48, 52] LF infections in children are known to cause a clinical feature known as "swollen baby syndrome". This condition is characterized by systemic edema, abdominal distension and widespread bleeding. It has been estimated that children suffering from this condition has a fatality rate of ~80%.[45, 47]

LF is an acute illness that generally subsides after one to four weeks, but recovery may take months. Common symptoms reported during conval-escence are transient hair loss and gait disturbances.[51] Examine Table 1 for an overview of clinical symptoms of LF.

DETECTION

Due to the nature of the LF, the specific symptoms are similar to several other diseases such as malaria, yellow fever, typhoid, as well as, hemorrhagic fevers, such as Ebola and Marburg, and may pose a problem for clinical diagnosis.[43] The usual approach for clinicians is to exclude other common febrile diseases (e.g. malaria, typhoid fever etc.) through their respective treatments. However, by the time LF is finally diagnosed, the opportunity to treat the disease may be fatally delayed.[53] Therefore, it is necessary to couple laboratory tests with clinical diagnosis in order to accurately identify a LFV infection in a timely manner.

The classic method for detecting LFV is by inoculating Vero cells with serum, in addition to cerebral spinal fluid, throat swabs, pleural fluid, urine or blood samples from infected patients. LFV generally induces a conspicuous cytopathic effect on a confluent monolayer of cells within 96 hours.[43] Subsequent tests to specifically identify LFV is done by immunofluorescence using

LFV specific antibodies or through direct identification by using an electron microscopy. This manner of LFV detection is still favored by some, as it is not sensitive to the variations of the viral genome, a problem shared by RT-PCR tests. Nonetheless, the major disadvantage of these methodologies are that they requires longer periods of time and the availability of a Level 4 laboratory.[11]

LFV can also be identified through a combination of ELISA for LFV specific antibodies.[54] Bausch et al. (2000), have reported that ELISA for LFV antigen and IgM are 88% sensitive and 90% specific for an acute infection, respectively. Patients that have been admitted to the hospital generally have already developed antibodies to LFV. For example, it is estimated that 53% of patients will possess LFV specific IgG, while 67% will develop LFV specific IgM. The ELISA is easy to perform, offers quick turnaround time and has the advantage of providing a diagnosis via a single serum sample without the need for sophisticated laboratories.[55]

RT-PCR tests would be the method of choice for rapid early detection of LFV [51], however, the problem of LFV strain variation, extended processing time and cross contamination exists due to the need for additional manipulations.[57] LFV antigens generally exist in the blood stream during the early stages (approximately by day 3-9) of the infection and gradually disappear after the appearance of IgM antibodies. Only in terminally ill patients will LFV antigens persist throughout the course of the infection.[58]

A procedure of using PCR products and intercalating dyes in real time was reported by Gunther et al. (2004). This method reportedly allows for the rapid measurement of LFV RNA concentrations in serum and various other bodily fluids, allowing the clinician to utilize it as a prognostic tool.[1] Recently, novel monoclonal antibodies to the NPs of both LFV and JUNV were developed and used in a sandwich antigen-capture ELISA. The results from this newly develop method showed promise as it has been reported to be sensitive and specific.[59]

TREATMENT

All persons suspected of LFV should be admitted to isolation facilities and their body fluids and excreta properly disposed. As with any hemorrhagic fever, general supportive therapy is the mainstay of treatment for patients suffering from LF. Sedatives (e.g. opiates) should be administered to patients for pain relief and careful maintenance of fluids and electrolytes are essential. It is necessary for the clinician to carefully monitor the patient's blood pressure and control the possibility of seizures. Moreover, due to the permeability of blood vessels, clinicians must carefully monitor fluid infusions and potential pulmonary edema.[58] Intramuscular injections should be avoided due to the possibility of uncontrollable bleeding (e.g. hematomas). In addition, administering acetylsalicylic acid (Aspirin) and non-steroid anti-inflammatory drugs for fever should always be avoided. Clinicians may prescribe acetaminophen to combat fever and inflammatory symptoms. In an effort to prevent secondary infections, broad spectrum antibiotics may also be administered. In the case of both renal and respiratory distress, clinicians are advised to provide patients with renal dialysis and mechanical ventilation, respectively.[60]

Treating patients with Lassa fever-convalescent plasma did not significantly reduce mortality in any of the high-risk groups studied; however, early intravenous administration of antiviral agent ribavirin have reduced the mortality rate.[58] In clinical studies, ribavirin treatment of patients with a high risk of a fatal outcome demonstrated that the antiviral agent reduced the fatality rate from 55% to 5%.[1] In the treatment of pregnant patients (late in the third trimester), it is imperative to note that the fetus has a negligible chance of survival and all efforts should be concentrated on saving the life of the mother. Therefore, abortion of the fetus may be necessary, if spontaneous abortion does not occur. Subsequent to the abortion, the mother should receive the same aggressive ribavirin treatment as other LF patients.[61]

In 2005, a team of US and Canadian scientists developed an experimental vaccine that reportedly provided full protection to nonhuman primates after challenges with a lethal dose of LFV.[62] Nonetheless at present, there is no vaccine against LFV approved or available for use in humans.[1]

DIFFERENTIAL DIAGNOSIS

The specific symptoms of LF are similar to malaria, yellow fever, typhoid, leptospirosis, and hemorrhagic fevers, such as Ebola and Marburg. These similarities may pose a problem for clinical diagnosis.[43] The usual approach for clinicians is to exclude other common febrile diseases (e.g. malaria, typhoid fever etc.)

Table 2: Differential diagnosis of Lassa fever and other related bacterial and viral infections. Note: Yellow fever (YF), Leptospirosis (Lepto), Typhoid fever (TF), Ebola hemorrhagic fever (EHF), Marburg hemorrhagic fever (MHF)

Symptoms	LF	Malaria	YF	Lepto	TF	EHF	MHF
Fever	■	■	■	■	■	■	■
Headaches	■	■	■	■	■	■	■
Arthralgia	■					■	■
Myalgia	■	■	■	■	■	■	■
Asthenia	■	■			■	■	■
Malaise	■	■	■	■	■	■	■
Sore throat	■					■	■
Dysphagia	■						
Cough	■	■		■		■	
Conjunctivitis	■		■	■		■	
Diarrhea	■	■		■	■	■	■
Nausea	■	■	■	■	■	■	■
Vomiting	■	■	■	■	■	■	■
Abdominal pains	■	■	■	■		■	■
Facial edema	■						
Cervical edema	■						
Proteinuria	■						■
Subconjunctival hemorrhage	■						
Retrosternal chest pains	■			■		■	
Periorbital edema	■						
Pleural effusions	■						
Pericardial effusions	■						
Epistaxis	■				■	■	■
Blood emission - mouth	■						
Blood from mucosal surfaces	■		■	■			
Hematemesis	■		■				
Bloody diarrhea	■						
Enlarged and inflamed kidneys	■					■	
Enlarged and inflamed liver	■	■				■	
Elevated respiration rates	■						
Hypotension	■					■	■
Hypertension	■						
Thrombocytopenia	■					■	■
Leucopenia	■				■	■	■
Hyperuraemia	■						
Tachycardia	■					■	
Pericardial effusions	■						
Aseptic meningitis	■			■			
Encephalitis	■		■		■		
Global encephalopathy	■		■				
Seizures	■	■					
Deafness	■						
Shock	■	■				■	■
Tremor	■						
Disorientation	■						
Delirium	■	■	■		■		■
Respiratory stress	■						
Coma	■	■				■	■
Hair loss	■						
Gait disturbances	■						
Petechial rash	■		■			■	■
Maculopapular rash	■					■	
Swollen baby syndrome	■						

through their respective treatments. However, by the time LF is finally diagnosed, the opportunity to treat the disease has been fatally delayed.[53] Therefore, it is necessary to couple laboratory tests with clinical diagnosis in order to accurately identify a LFV infection in a timely manner (Table 2).

References

1. Gunther S., Lenz O. Lassa Virus. Critical Reviews in Clinical Laboratory Science, 2004. 4: pp. 339-390
2. Bowen M.D., Peters C.J., Nichol S.T. Phylogenic Analysis of the Arenaviridae: Patterns of Virus Evolution and Evidence for Cospeciation between arenaviruses and their Rodent Host. Molecular Phyogenetics and Evolution, 1997. 8: pp. 301-316
3. Keenlyside R.A., McCormick J.B., Webb P.A., Smith E., Elliott L., Johnson K.M. Case-control Study of Mastomys natalensis and Humans in Lassa Virus-infected Households in Sierra Leone. American Journal of Tropical Medicine and Hygiene, 1983. 32: pp. 829-837
4. McCormick J.B. Epidemiology and Control of Lassa Fever. Current Topics in Microbiology and Immunology, 1987. 134: pp. 69-78
5. Frame J.D., Baldwin J.M., Gocke D.J., Troup J.M. Lassa Fever, a New Virus Disease of Man from West Africa. Clinical Description and Pathological Findings. American Journal of Tropical Medicine and Hygiene, 1970. 19: pp. 670-676
6. Monath T.P., Mertens P.E., Patton R., Moser C.R., Baum J.J., Pinneo L., Gary G.W., Kissling R.E. A hospital Epidemic of Lassa Fever in Zorzor, Liberia, March-April 1972. American Journal of Tropical Medicine and Hygiene, 1973. 22: pp. 773-779
7. Monath T.P., Maher M., Casals J., Kissling R.E., Cacciapuoti A. Lassa Fever in the Eastern Province of Sierra Leone, 1970-1972. Clinical Observations and Virological Studies on Selected Hospital Cases. American Journal of Tropical Medicine and Hygiene, 1974. 23: pp. 1140-1149
8. Bausch D.G., Demby A.H., Coulibaly M., Kanu J., Goba A., Bah A., Condé N., Wurtzel H.L., Cavallaro K.F., Lloyd E., Baldet F.B., Cissé S.D., Fofona D., Savané I.K., Tolno R.T., Mahy B., Wagoner K.D., Ksiazek T.G., Peters C.J., Rollin P.E. Lassa Fever in Guinea: Epidemiology of Human Disease and Clinical Observations. Vector Borne and Zoonotic Diseases, 2007. 1: pp. 269-281
9. Richmond J.K., Baglole D.J. Lassa fever: epidemiology, clinical features, and social consequences. British Medical Journal, 2003. 327: pp. 1271-1275
10. Peterson A.T., Moses L.M., Bausch D.G. Mapping Transmission Risk of Lassa Fever in West Africa: The Importance of Quality Control, Sampling Bias, and Error Weighting. Public Library of Science One, 2014. 9: pp. e100711
11. Gunther S., Emmerich P., Laue T., Kuhle O., Asper M., Jung A., Grewing T., Meulen J., Schmitz H. Imported Lassa Fever in Germany: Molecular Characterization of a New Lassa Virus Strain. Emerging Infectious Diseases, 2000. 5: pp. 466-476
12. Macher A.M., Wolfe M.S. Historical Lassa fever reports and 30-year clinical update. Emerging Infectious Disease, 2006. 12: pp. 835–837
13. Center for Disease Control and Prevention. Lassa Fever Reported in U.S. Traveler Returning from West Africa. Contact investigation under way; risk to other travelers considered extremely low. Released April 4, 2014. Retrieved November 4, 2014. Website: http://www.cdc.gov/media/releases/2014/p0404-lassa-fever.html
14. Bossi P., Tegnell A., Baka A., Van Loock F., Hendriks J., Werner A., Maidhof H., Gouvras G. Bichat guidelines for the Clinical Management of Haemorrhagic Fever Viruses and Bioterrorism-related Haemorrhagic Fever Viruses. EuroSurveilance, 2004. 9: pp. E11 - E12
15. Clegg J.C., Wilson S.M., Oram J.D. Nucleoside Sequence of the S RNA of Lassa Virus (Nigerian Strain) and Comparative Analysis of Arenavirus Gene Products. Virus Research, 1991. 18: pp. 151-164
16. Bowen M.D., Rollin P.E., Ksiazek T.G., Hustad H.L., Bausch D.G., Demby A.H., Bajani M.D., Peters C.J., Nichol S.T. Genetic Diversity among Lassa Virus Strains. Journal of Virology, 2000. 74: pp. 6992-7004
17. Lashley F.R., Durham J.D. Emerging Infectious Diseases: Trends and Issues. New York: Springer Publishing Company. 2002. pp. 121-123
18. Lukashevich I. S., Maryankova R., Vladyko A.S., Nashkevic N., Koleda S., Djavani M., Horejsh D., Voitenok N.N., Salvato M.S. Lassa and Mopeia Virus Replication in Human Monocytes/Macrophages and in Endothelial Cells: Different Effects on IL-8 and TNF- α gene Expression. Journal of Medical Virology, 1999. 59: pp. 552-560
19. Baize S., Kaplon J., Faure C., Pannetier D., Georges-Courbot M-C., Deubel V. Lassa Virus Infection of Human Dendritic Cells and Macrophages is Productive but Fails to Activate Cells. The Journal of Immunology, 2004. 172: pp. 2861-2869
20. Lukashevich I. S., Stelmakh T. A., Golubev V. P., Stchesljenok E. P., Lemeshko, N. N. Ribonucleic acids of Machupo and Lassa Viruses. Archives of Virology, 1984. 79: pp. 189-203
21. Adewuyi G.M., Fowotade A., Adewuyi B.T. Lassa Fever: Another Infectious Menace. African Journal of Clinical and Experimental Microbiology, 2009. 10: pp. 144-155
22. Clegg J. C. S., Oram J. D. Molecular Cloning of Lassa Virus RNA: Nucleotide Sequence and Expression of the Nucleocapsid Protein Gene. Virology, 1985. 114: pp. 363-372
23. Auperin, D. D., Sasso, D. R. & McCormick, J. B. Nucleotide sequence of the glycoprotein gene and intergenic region of the Lassa virus S genome RNA. Virology, 1986. 154: pp. 155-167
24. Buchmeier M.J., Southern P.J., Parekh B.S., Wooddell M.K., Oldstone M.B. Site-specific Antibodies Define a Cleavage Site Conserved Among Arenavirus GP-C Glycoproteins. The Journal of Virology, 1987. 61: pp. 8982-8985
25. Hufert F.T., Lüdke W., Schmitz H. Epitope Mapping of the Lassa Virus Nucleoprotein using Monoclonal Anti-Nucleocapsid Antibodies. Archives of Virology, 1989. 106: pp. 201-212
26. Burns J., Buchmeier M. Glycoprotein of the Arenaviruses. The Arenaviridae. 1993. New York: Plenum Press. pp. 17-35
27. Saunders A.A., Ting J.P.C., Meisner J., Neuman B.W., Perez M., de la Torre J.C., Buchmeier M.J. Mapping the Landscape of the Lymphocytic Choriomeningitis Virus Stable Signal Peptide Reveals Novel Functional Domains. Journal of Virology, 2007. 81: pp. 5649-5657
28. Salvato, M. S. Molecular Biology of the Prototype Arenavirus, Lymphocytic Choriomeningitis Virus. The Arenaviridae. 1993. New York: Plenum Press. pp. 133-156
29. Lukashevich I.S., Djavani M., Shapiro K., Sanchez A., Ravkov E., Nichol S.T., Salvato M.S. The Lassa Fever Virus L gene: Nucleotide Sequence, Comparison, and Precipitation of a Predicted 250 kDa Protein with Monospecific Antiserum. Journal of General Virology, 1997. 78: pp. 547–551
30. Cao W., Henry M.D., Borrow P., Identification of Alpha-dystroglycan as a Receptor for Lymphocytic Choriomeningitis Virus and Lassa Fever Virus. Science, 1998. 282: pp. 2079-2081
31. Shimojima M., Ströher U., Ebihara H., Feldmann H., Kawaoka Y. Identification of Cell Surface Molecules Involved in Dystroglycan-Independent Lassa Virus Cell Entry. Journal of Virology, 2012. 86: pp. 2067-2078
32. Buchmeier M.J., Bowen M.D.P.C.J. Arenaviridae: The Virus and Their Replication. Field's Virology. 4th Edition. 2001. Philadelphia: Lippincott, Williams and Wilkins. Pp. 1635-1668
33. Bishop D. Arenaviridae and their Replication. Virology. Second Edition. New York: Raven Press. 1990. pp. 1231-1243
34. Garcin D., Kolakofsky D. Tacaribe Arenavirus RNA Synthesis In Vitro is Primer Dependent and Suggests an Unusual Model for the Initiation of Genome Replication. The Journal of Virology, 1992. 66: pp. 1370-1376
35. Meyer B.J., Southern P.J. Concurrent Sequence Analysis of 5' and 3' RNA termini by Intramolecular Circularization Reveals 5' Nontemplated Bases and 3' Terminal Heterogeneity for Lymphocytic Choriomeningitis Virus mRNAs. The Journal of Virology, 1993. 67: pp. 2621-2627
36. Meyer B.J., Southern P.J. Concurrent sequence analysis of 5' and 3' RNA termini by intramolecular circularization reveals 5' nontemplated bases and 3' terminal heterogeneity for lymphocytic choriomeningitis virus mRNAs. Journal of Virology, 1993, 67: pp. 2621-2627
37. Yun N.E., Walker D.H. Pathogenesis of Lassa Fever. Viruses, 2012. 4: pp. 2031-2048
38. Guerrant R.L., Walker D.H., Weller P.F. Tropical Infectious Diseases – Principles, Pathogens & Practice. Volume 1. Philadelphia: Churchill Livingstone Elsevier. 2006. pp. 737
39. Franz D.R., Jahrling P.B., Friedlander A.M., McClain D.J., Hoover D.L., Byrne W.R., Pavlin J.A., Christopher G.W., Eitzen E.M. Clinical Recognition and Management of Patients Exposed to Biological Warfare Agents. The Journal of American Medical Association, 1997. 278: pp. 399-411
40. Alibek K. Biohazard. New York: Dell Publishing. 1999. pp. 118
41. Hemorrhagic Fever Viruses (VHF). Updated January 10, 2008. Retrieved July 24, 2008. Web Site: http://www. upmcbiosecurity.org/website/focus/agents_diseases/fact_sheets/hf.html
42. Guerrant R.L., Walker D.H., Weller P.F. Tropical Infectious Diseases – Principles, Pathogens & Practice. Volume 1. Philadelphia: Churchill Livingstone Elsevier. 2006. pp. 742
43. Ogbu O., Ajuluchukwu E., Uneke C.J. Lassa Fever in West African Sub-region: an Overview. Journal of Vector Borne Disease, 2007. 44: pp. 1-11
44. Fisher-Hoch S.P., Tomori O., Nasidi A., Perez-Oronoz G.I., Fakile I., Hutwagner L., McCormick J.B. Review of Cases of Nosocomial Lassa Fever in Nigeria: the High Price of Poor Medical Practice. British Medical Journal, 1995. 311: pp. 857-859
45. Aufiero P., Karabulut N., Rumowitz D., Shah S., Nsubuga J., Piepszak B., Salter R.D., Bresnitz E., Lacy C.R., Robertson C., Tan C., Tan E.T. Imported Lassa Fever. New Jersey: Center for Disease Control and Prevention (CDC). Morbidity and Mortality Weekly Report, 2004. 53: pp. 894-897
46. Viral Hemorrhagic Fevers Caused by Arenaviruses. Institute for International Cooperation in Animal Biologics. Iowa State University. Updated February 23, 2010. Retrieved March 24, 2010. Web site: http://www.cfsph.iastate.edu/Factsheets/pdfs/viral_hem_orrhagic_fever_arenavirus.pdf
47. Guerrant R.L., Walker D.H., Weller P.F. Tropical Infectious Diseases – Principles, Pathogens & Practice. Volume 1. Philadelphia: Churchill Livingstone Elsevier. 2006. pp. 744
48. Update on Lassa Fever in West Africa. Weekly Epidemiological Record, 2005; 10: pp. 86-88
49. Cummins D., McCormick J.B., Bennett D., Samba J.A., Farrar B., Machin S.J., Fisher-Hoch S.P. Acute Sensorineural Deafness in Lassa Fever. Journal of the American Medical Association, 1990 264: pp. 2093-2096
50. Lassa Fever. World Health Organization. Fact Sheet N°179. Revised April 2005. Web Site: http://www.who.int/mediacentre /factsheets/fs179/en/
51. Liao B.S., Byl F.M., Adour K.K. Audiometric Comparison of Lassa Fever Hearing Loss and Idiopathic Sudden Hearing Loss: Evidence for Viral Cause. Archives of Otolaryngology Head & Neck Surgery, 1992. 106: pp. 226-229
52. Richmond J.K., Baglole D.J. Lassa Fever: Epidemiology, Clinical Features, and Social Consequences. British Medical Journal, 2003. 327: pp. 1271-1275
53. Demby A.H., Chamberlain J., Brown D.W.G., Clegg C.S. Early Diagnosis of Lassa Fever by Reverse Transcription-PCR. Journal of Clinical Microbiology, 1994. 32: pp. 2898-2903
54. Schmitz H., Wolf H.R. Use of Monoclonal Antibody for the Detection of Lassa Virus Antibody and Antigen in Patients with Lassa Fever. Medical Microbiology and Immunology, 1986. 175: pp. 181-182
55. Bausch D.G. , Rollin P.E., Demby A.H., Coulibaly M., Kanu J., Conteh AS., Wagoner K.D., McMullan L.K., Bowen M.D., Peters C.J., Ksiazek T.G. Diagnosis and Clinical Virology of Lassa Fever as Evaluated by Enzyme-Linked Immunosorbent Assay, Indirect Fluorescent-Antibody Test, and Virus Isolation. Journal of Clinical Microbiology, 2000. 38: pp. 2670-2677
56. Johnson K.M., McCormick J.B., Webb P.A., Smith E.S., Elliott L.H., King I.J. Clinical Virology of Lassa Fever in Hospitalized Patients. Journal of Infectious Diseases, 1987. 155: pp. 456-464
57. Trapper S.G., Conaty A.L., Farrar B.B., Auperin D.D., McCormick J.B., Fisher-Hoch S.P. Evaluation of the Polymerase Chain Reaction for Diagnosis of Lassa Virus Infection. American Journal of Tropical Medicine and Hygiene, 1993. 49: pp. 214-221
58. Guerrant R.L., Walker D.H., Weller P.F. Tropical Infectious Diseases – Principles, Pathogens & Practice. Volume 1. Philadelphia: Churchill Livingstone Elsevier. 2006. pp 748
59. Fukushi S., Tani H., Yoshikawa T., Saijo M., Morikawa S. Serological Assays Based on Recombinant Viral Proteins for the Diagnosis of Arenavirus Hemorrhagic Fevers. Viruses, 2012. 4: pp. 2097-2114
60. Management of Patients with Suspected Viral Hemorrhagic Fever: Center for Disease Control and Prevention (CDC). Morbidity and Mortality Weekly Report, 1988. 37: pp. 1-16
61. McCormick J.B., King I.J., Webb P.A., Scribner C.L., Craven R.B., Johnson K.M., Elliott L.H., Belmont-Williams R. Lassa Fever. Effective Therapy with Ribavirin. New England Journal of Medicine, 1986. 314: pp. 20-26
62. Sibbald B. Lassa Fever Vaccine. Canadian Medical Association Journal, 2005. 173: pp. 243

Photo Bibliography

Figure 1.8-1: An electron micrograph (TEM) of a number of Lassa Fever virus virions adjacent to some cell debris. Photo was taken by C. S. Goldsmith, D. Auperin and was released by the CDC. Public domain photo

Figure 1.8-5: Virus graphics designed by Los Alamos National Security of the United States Department of Energy. Public domain photo

Figure 1.8-7: Hematoxylin-Eosin-stained (H&E) photo-micrograph depicting the cytoarchitectural changes found in a liver tissue specimen extracted from a Lassa fever patient. Photo was taken by Dr. Yves Robin and Dr. Jean Renaudet, Arbovirus Laboratory at the Pasteur Institute in Dakar, Senegal; World Health Organization and released by the CDC. Public domain photo

The Machupo virus (MACV) is an enveloped ambisense RNA virus, composed of a bisegmented genome, belonging to the genus *Arenavirus* in the family *Arenaviridae*. It is a member of the New World group, and B-lineage of the arenaviruses which include other highly pathogenic agents such as the Junin, Guanarito and Sabia viruses (Figure 1.9-1).[1]

MACV is a zoonosis, naturally transmitted to humans by *Calomoys callosus,* the Vesper mouse and is responsible for causing Bolivian hemorrhagic fever (BHF), also referred to as Black Typhus.[2] In laboratory studies, female *Calomys spp.* infected with MACV at birth displayed chronic infection and are sterile at maturity.[3, 4] Adult animals infected with Machupo virus demonstrated a split response: 50% showed chronic viremia and viruria, while 50% developed neutralizing antibodies and cleared of infection (Figure 1.9-2).[4, 5]

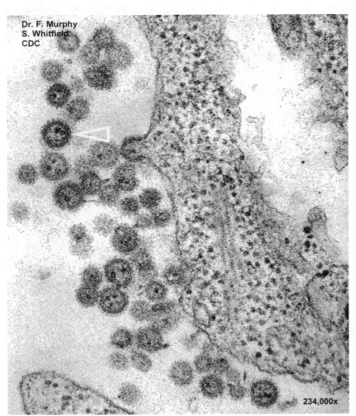

Figure 1.9-1: Electron micrograph (TEM) of Machupo virus (MACV) in human splenic tissue. Please note the arrow which indicates one MACV

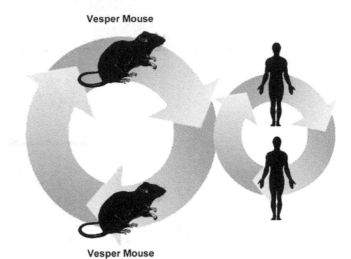

Figure 1.9-2: Sylvatic cycle of Machupo Virus (MACV) the caustic agent of Bolivian hemorrhagic fever (BHF)

BHF was first identified in 1959, in rural regions of Beni, Bolivia. By 1963, the virus itself was isolated by Johnson *et al.* from patients suffering from an acute hemorrhagic fever in San Joaquin, Bolivia.[6, 7] From 1958 to 1962, there were 470 reported cases of BHF, with 142 fatalities (30% fatality rate) (Figure 1.9-3).[8] It is believed that the pathogenesis of all arenavirus

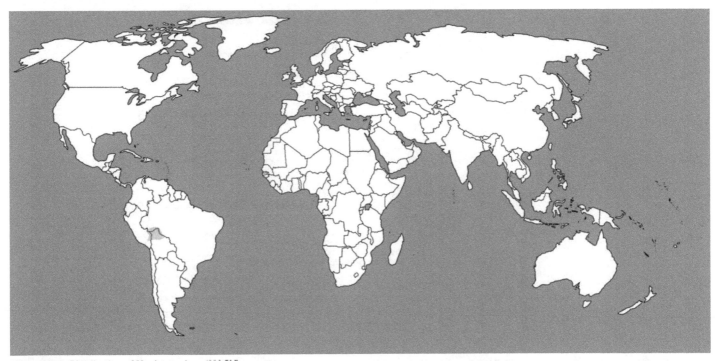

Figure 1.9-3: Distribution of Machupo virus (MACV)

infections, including MACV, involves an initial session of replication at the site of infection. The hilar lymph nodes, lungs and parenchymal organs are considered important sites for viral growth. Although pneumonic foci are not usually present, interstitial infiltration and edema may occur during the course of infection. Macrophages are generally the first and most prominent cells targeted by MACV, although as the infection spreads, additional cell types will also become involved. Cells such as monocytes, dendritic cells, endothelial cells, hepatocytes, and adrenal cortical cells will also support the replication of these viruses. It has been reported that many epithelial structures readily contain viral antigen and nucleic acids.[9, 10] The bisegmented RNAs of the MACV genome are designated as L (approximately 7.2 kb) and S (approximately 3.4 kb). The L (large) segment encodes an RNA-dependent polymerase (L protein) and a zinc finger matrix protein (Z protein). Both of these proteins are involved in the regulation of transcription and replication of MACV (Figure 1.9-4). The S (small) segment encodes the nucleoprotein (NP) and the viral glycoprotein precursor GPC.[11, 12] Like all arenaviruses, the MACV L protein is encoded at the 3' end of the L RNA segments, while the zinc-finger (Z) protein is found at the 5' end of the same RNA segment. The NP gene of MACV is encoded at the 3' end of the S RNA segment in the antisense, while the glycoprotein precursor (GPC) gene is encoded at the 5' end of the same RNA strand in message sense.[4, 10, 11, 12]

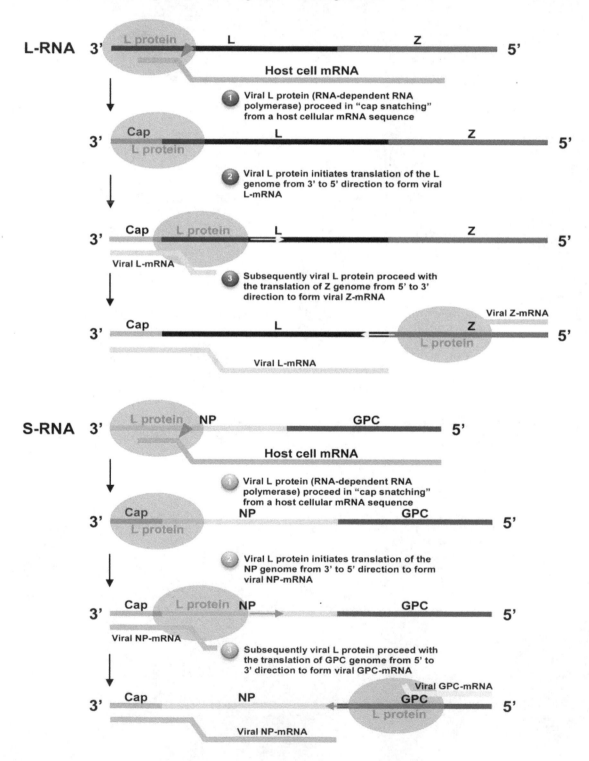

Figure 1.9-4: Diagrammatic examination of MACV sense and antisense (ambisense) viral genome transcription

The ambisense arrangement of the MACV genome, similar to other arenavirus genomes, provides a unique mechanism for regulating gene transcription. It has been reported that genes lying at the 3' end of the bisegmented RNAs are expressed first, while genes located at the 5' end cannot be expressed in the absence of protein synthesis.[4, 13] Gene expression is initiated as the viral L protein cleaves the 3' cap and one to seven bases from cellular messenger RNAs (mRNAs) and uses these primers to initiate transcription of subgenomic viral mRNAs in a process also known as "cap snatching."[4, 14, 15] Subsequently, these non-polyadenylated viral mRNAs are translated by host cell ribosomes to produce viral NP and L proteins. Transcription ends at the distal margin of the stem-loop structure found within the viral intergenomic region.[16]

Genes found at the 5' ends of the viral genome (e.g. GPC and Z) are not translated directly even though they are in the proper coding sense. Once the transcription of the 3' end of the viral RNA is completed, the L protein adopts a replicase mode and generates a full-length complementary antigenomic RNA (agRNA) from the 5' end of the viral genome. The L protein initiates RNA replication at the 5' end of the viral genome through a dinucleotide template (guanosine triphosphate cytidine monophosphate - pppGpC) where a full length genome-complementary RNA species, the antigenome, is transcribed. These newly synthesized RNAs are believed to associate with the NP and L proteins in the cytoplasm to produce the nucleocapsids.[4, 17] Subsequent to translation, the Z protein is involved in viral particle formation where it serves as a matrix protein and interacts with the N protein, as well as, driving virion formation.[4, 16]

On the other hand, considerable posttranslational processing of the GPC will take place. For example, the GPC is post-translationally processed by signal peptidase to form stable signal peptide (SSP). This process is followed by the posttranslational cleave of the remaining residue by the enzyme protease SKI-1/S1P to form GP_1 (45 kD) and GP_2 (38 kD). It has been reported that SSP (~5kD) is engaged in the glycoprotein expression and post-translational modification GP_1 and GP_2 by protease SKI-1/S1P although the exact mechanism of this process requires further analysis.[12, 16, 18] Once G_1 and G_2 is formed, these envelope glycoproteins are transported to the plasma membrane of the host cell with the assistance of SSP. The GP_1 tetramer will eventually form the head of the envelope spike of the LFV, while the GP_2 tetramer will form the stalk.[12, 16, 18] It has been reported that the cytoplasmic tail of GP_2, along with SSP, will interact with NP, which in turn interacts with the Z protein at the plasma membrane of the host cell. Numerous reports indicate that it is these interactions that play a critical role in the viral assembly and budding; although the exact manner of this process requires further investigation (Figure 1.9-5).[4, 12, 16, 18, 19, 20]

Recent studies have demonstrated that MACV GP_1 attaches to the transferrin receptor (TfR1) of the host cell.[12, 19, 20, 21, 22] Once viral attachment occurs, the virus utilizes clathrin-mediated endocytosis to gain entry into the host cell. Within the large smooth-walled endocytotic vesicles, the acidic environment and the viral membrane glycoprotein GP_2 mediate fusion between the virion envelope and the endosomal membrane. Once the fusion of the membranes has taken place, the viral nucleocapsid is released into the cytoplasm where replication takes place (Figure 1.9-5).[11, 12]

MACV is an effective biological warfare agent due to its lethality, high infectivity by the aerosol route as demonstrated in animal models, and its ease of propagation in tissue culture.[24] As described by Alibek (1999), Machupo virus was designated as N4 and was researched and produced at the Institute of Ultra-Pure Biopreparations in Leningrad, Omutninsk in Kirov, Obolensk outside of Moscow, the Lyubuchany Institute of Immunology in Chekhov (near Moscow), and Vector Research and Testing in Novosibrisk (near the small town of Koltsovo) in Siberia.[10, 25] Based upon MACV's potential for widespread person to person transmission, illness and death, the Centers for Disease Control and Prevention (CDC) in 1999 classified MACV as Category A biological weapon agents.[26]

SYMPTOMS

MACV is transmitted to humans via the aerosolized dried excretions, such as saliva, feces and urine from infected rodents. Other manners of transmission, such as direct contact

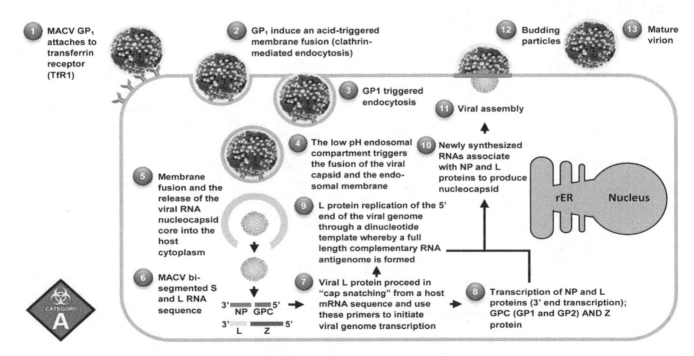

Figure 1.9-5: Diagrammatic process of MACV infection within an eukaryotic cell

with contaminated materials via lesions or cuts, or through ingestion of contaminated foods could also result in infection.[27, 28] In 1994, a broken test tube containing MACV contaminated blood was accidentally aerosolized in a centrifuge and a laboratory technician was exposed to the virus. Within 11 days, the technician developed BHF. Only after aggressive ribavirin treatment did the technician recover from the disease.[8]

Table 1: An overview of the clinical symptoms of BHF

Symptoms	+	++	+++
Fever			■
Fatigue			■
Severe frontal headaches			■
Oral ulcerations			■
Painful sore throat			■
Cough			■
Dizziness			■
Nausea			■
Vomiting			■
Bruises			■
Myalgias			■
Arthralgia			■
Lymphadenopathy			■
Malaise			■
Petechiae rash			■
Conjunctival injection			■
Retro-orbital pains			■
Photophobia			■
Asthenia			■
Prostration			■
Abdominal pains			■
Anorexia			■
Proteinuria			■
Anuria			■
Dehydration			■
Hemo. instabilities			■
Oral mucosal bleeding		■	
Nasal mucosal bleeding		■	
Bleeding from the eyes		■	
Hematemesis		■	
Hematochezia		■	
Melena		■	
Hematuria		■	
Bronchi bleeding		■	
Pulmonary bleeding		■	
Pleural effusion		■	
Ascites		■	
Thrombocytopenia		■	
Leukopenia		■	
Confusion		■	
Cerebellar tremors		■	
Gait abnormalities		■	
Hyporeflexia		■	
Tongue tremors		■	
Deafness		■	
Seizures	■		
Shock	■		
Coma	■		
Respiratory alkalosis	■		
Metabolic acidosis	■		
Jaundice	■		

+ Rare ++ Common +++ Frequent

Cases of person to person transmission through contaminated body fluids were reported in 1971 at Cochabamba hospital, located in central Bolivia. Again, in 1994, a Magdalena farmer transmitted MACV to his family members which led to six fatalities.[4, 29, 30] It has also been reported that transmission via sexual contact during convalescence is an additional possible manner of virus transmission.[31]

The replication of the MACV occurs mainly in lymphoid tissues. The evidence of this is seen in the large amounts of viral antigens present and by the presence of lymphocytopenia and lymphocyte depletion in the spleen and the lymph nodes.[4] The incubation period of BHF is approximately one to two weeks and the initial symptoms mirror flu-like conditions similar to that of other South American Hemorrhagic fevers (e.g. Argentine hemorrhagic fever). Patients initially exhibit high fever (approximately 39°C or 102.2°F), fatigue, severe frontal headaches, oral ulcerations, painful sore throat, cough, dizziness, nausea, and vomiting. Patients also develop symptoms such as bruises, myalgias (lower back pains), arthralgia, general lymphadenopathy and malaise. Other symptoms may include the development of petechiae rash (dysesthesia of the skin), conjunctival injection, retro-orbital pains, photophobia, asthenia, prostration, abdominal pains, anorexia, proteinuria, anuria, dehydration and hemodynamic instabilities.[26, 32, 33]

Within seven days after the onset of symptoms, hemorrhagic manifestations will appear, where mucosal bleeding from oral mucous membranes (e.g. gingivorrhagia) and the nasal passages are commonly seen. Other hemorrhagic symptoms such as bleeding from the eyes, intestines (e.g. hematemesis, hematochezia and melena), genitourinary (e.g. hematuria) and broncho-pulmonary tracts may also appear.[4, 29, 32, 33] Occasionally, patients may develop pleural effusion, ascites, seizures, shock and coma. Neurological manifestations are common including confusion, cerebellar tremors, gait abnormalities, hyporeflexia, tongue tremors and deafness. If the patient experiences seizures and comas, the prognosis is poor.[32, 33] During the latter stages of infection, patients may develop respiratory alkalosis, and metabolic acidosis, which eventually results in death. Clinical laboratory tests may show thrombocytopenia (<130,000 cells/mm^3), leukopenia (<3,900 cells/mm^3), and hematuria.[34] It has been reported that in cases of nosocomial outbreak located at a high altitude, patients also developed jaundice and had high mortality (Table 1).[4, 28]

DETECTION

Like other arenaviruses, the pathogenesis of BHF can easily be misdiagnosed as Argentine hemorrhagic fever (AHF) or other viral hemorrhagic fevers.[35] Other differential diagnosis may include typhoid fever, hepatitis, infectious mononucleosis, leptospirosis, hanta pulmonary syndrome (HPS), dengue fever (DF), malaria, and rickettsioses especially during the first week after the initial onset of symptoms.[32, 36]

The classic approach to BHF identification is virus isolation, which uses suckling hamsters for intracerebral inoculation or cell cultures (such as Vero cells) and indirect fluorescent assay (IFA) with confirmatory serological neutralization tests.[28, 32, 37] Nonetheless, these methods for detecting MACV require a biosafety level 4 laboratory. BHF viral antigens, as well as, virus specific IgM and IgG have been detected through enzyme linked immunoassay (ELISA) in blood or tissue samples.[8, 38] A four-fold rise in expected antibody titers should be observed or MACV specific IgM should be detected if the patient is infected with MACV. Nonetheless, cross-reaction between MACV and other arenaviruses may occur. Virus neutralization tests are very specific and can also be used. However, the antibodies detected with the neutralization tests may appear in the sera or blood too late to be useful as immediate diagnostic method. Presently, ELISA is the most effective and practical method for rapidly detecting MACV infection.[4, 28, 32] Diagnostic RT-PCR tests are not commercially available, although procedures have been published. Nonetheless, the use of these assays in a clinical environment is extremely limited.[28, 33, 39]

TREATMENT

As with any hemorrhagic fever, supportive therapy is the mainstay of treatment.[32] Sedatives should be administered to patients for pain relief and careful maintenance of fluids and electrolyte are essential. Intramuscular injections should be avoided due to the possibility of uncontrollable bleeding. In addition, the use of acetylsalicylic acid (e.g. Aspirin) and non-steroid anti-inflammatory drugs for fevers should always be avoided. Clinicians may prescribe acetaminophen to combat fever and inflammatory symptoms. If consumptive coagulopathy occurs, infusions of heparin, clotting factors, as well as, platelets may be lifesaving. In an effort to prevent secondary infections, broad spectrum antibiotics may also be administered.

Introduction of convalescent plasma in uncontrolled trials for BHF patients have been performed. This treatment should initiate prior to the ninth day of illness and it has been reported to decrease the case-to-fatality ratio from ~20% to 1% in treating patients with AHF; however, the effectiveness for treating BHF still remains to be elucidated.[32, 33, 40] Administering ribavirin has

Table 2: Differential diagnosis of the early stages of BHF in comparison to examples of other bacterial and viral infections. Note: Typhoid fever (TF), hepatitis A (Hep A), hepatitis B (Hep B), infectious mononucleosis (Mono), Leptospirosis (Lepto), Hanta pulmonary syndrome (HPS), Dengue fever (DF)

Symptoms	BHF	TF	HAV	HBV	Mono	Lepto	DF	HPS
Fever	■	■	■	■	■	■	■	■
Fatigue	■	■			■		■	■
Severe frontal headaches	■	■	■	■		■	■	
Oral ulcerations	■							
Painful sore throat	■				■			
Cough	■		■				■	■
Dizziness	■							
Nausea	■	■	■	■	■	■	■	■
Vomiting	■	■	■	■	■	■	■	■
Bruises	■							
Myalgias	■				■	■	■	■
Arthralgia	■		■	■			■	
Abdominal pains	■	■						
Anorexia	■	■	■	■	■	■	■	■
General lymphadenopathy	■			■	■			
Malaise	■	■	■	■	■	■	■	
Petechiae rash	■	■	■	■	■	■	■	
Conjunctival injection	■					■	■	
Retro-orbital pains	■						■	
Photophobia	■							
Asthenia	■	■	■					
Prostration	■							
Proteinuria	■							
Anuria	■							
Dehydration	■							
Hemodynamic instabilities	■							
Oral mucosal bleeding	■					■	■	
Nasal mucosal bleeding	■				■			
Bleeding from the eyes	■							
Hematemesis	■	■				■	■	
Hematochezia	■	■				■		
Melena	■							
Hematuria	■							■
Bronchopulmonary bleeding	■					■		■
Pleural effusion	■							
Ascites	■							
Thrombocytopenia	■						■	
Leukopenia	■							
Confusion	■	■						
Cerebellar tremors	■							
Gait abnormalities	■							
Hyporeflexia	■							
Tongue tremors	■							
Deafness	■							
Seizures	■							
Shock	■							
Coma	■							
Respiratory alkalosis	■							
Metabolic acidosis	■							
Jaundice	■							

Table 3: Differential diagnosis of the later stages of BHF in comparison to other bacterial and viral infections. Note: Argentine hemorrhagic fever (AHF), Dengue hemorrhagic fever (DHF), Ebola hemorrhagic fever (EHF), Marburg hemorrhagic fever (MHF), Lassa fever (LF), Rift Valley fever (RVF), Yellow fever (YF)

Symptoms	BHF	AHF	DF/DHF	EHF	MHF	LF	RVF	YF
Fever	■	■	■	■	■	■		
Fatigue	■	■		■	■			
Severe frontal headaches	■	■	■	■	■	■		■
Oral ulcerations	■							
Painful sore throat	■	■		■	■	■		
Cough	■					■		
Dizziness	■						■	■
Nausea	■	■	■	■	■		■	■
Vomiting	■	■	■	■	■		■	■
Bruises	■		■	■	■		■	■
Myalgias	■	■	■	■	■		■	■
Arthralgia	■							
General lymphadenopathy	■							
Malaise	■	■		■	■	■		
Petechiae rash	■		■		■			
Conjunctival injection	■		■					■
Retro-orbital pains	■		■					
Photophobia	■				■		■	
Asthenia	■	■			■	■		
Prostration	■			■	■			
Abdominal pains	■		■	■	■	■		■
Anorexia	■	■	■		■		■	
Proteinuria	■	■			■			
Anuria	■	■					■	
Dehydration	■	■						
Hemodynamic instabilities	■	■		■				
Oral mucosal bleeding	■	■		■	■	■		
Nasal mucosal bleeding	■	■		■	■	■	■	■
Bleeding from the eyes	■			■			■	■
Hematemesis	■	■		■	■	■	■	■
Hematochezia	■	■	■	■	■	■	■	■
Melena	■			■				■
Hematuria	■	■		■				■
Bronchopulmonary bleeding	■		■					
Pleural effusion	■					■		
Ascites	■							
Thrombocytopenia	■		■	■			■	
Leukopenia	■	■			■			
Confusion	■					■		
Cerebellar tremors	■							
Gait abnormalities	■					■		
Hyporeflexia	■							
Tongue tremors	■							
Deafness	■							
Seizures	■			■				
Shock	■		■	■	■		■	
Coma	■			■				
Respiratory alkalosis	■							
Metabolic acidosis	■			■				
Jaundice	■							

been reported as an effective treatment for BHF and other hemorrhagic fevers. The treatment should begin before day 7 of the illness with 30 mg/kg loading dose, followed by 15 mg/kg every 6 hours for 4 days and finally 7.5 mg/kg every 8 hours for an additional 6 days.[32, 33] Nonetheless, the effectiveness of antiviral medication in the treatment of BHF requires further examination.[8]

Currently, a vaccine known as Candid 1 earned investigational new drug status and has performed well in clinical trials, with over 2000 volunteers. This vaccine has shown its effectiveness against Junin virus infections during clinical trials (estimated at 98.1% effectiveness)[41] in addition to demonstrating cross protection for Machupo virus.[29]

DIFFERENTIAL DIAGNOSIS

During the first week after the initial onset of symptoms, BHF may be difficult to differentiate from Typhoid fever, hepatitis, infectious mononucleosis, Leptospirosis, Hanta pulmonary syndrome (HPS), Dengue fever (DF), malaria, and rickettsioses.[32, 36] At the later stages, the pathogenesis of BHF can be easily misdiagnosed as Argentine hemorrhagic fever (AHF) or other viral hemorrhagic fevers such as Dengue hemorrhagic fever, Ebola hemorrhagic fever, Marburg hemorrhagic fever, Lassa, Rift Valley and Yellow fever.[35] Therefore, it is necessary to use specific laboratory tests to differentiate BHF from other known infections. Please examine Tables 2 and 3 for more information.

References

1. Clegg J.C. Molecular Phylogeny of the Arenaviruses. Current Topic in Microbiology and Immunology, 2002. 262: pp. 1-24

2. Salazar-Bravo J., Dragoo J.W., Bowen M.D., Peters C.J., Ksiazek T.G.,Yates T.L. Natural Nidality in Bolivian Hemorrhagic Fever and the Systematics of the Reservoir Species. Infection Genetics and Evolution, 2002. 1: pp. 191–199

3. Johnson K. Arenaviruses. Virology. New York: Raven Press. 1985. pp. 1033-1053

4. Guerrant R.L., Walker D.H., Weller P.F. Tropical Infectious Diseases – Principles, Pathogens & Practice. Volume 1. Philadelphia: Churchill Livingstone Elsevier. 2006. pp 734-755

5. Bowen M.D., Peters C.J., Nichol S.T. Phylogenic Analysis of the Arenaviridae: Patterns of Virus Evolution and Evidence for Cospeciation between Arenavirus and their Rodent Host. Molecular Phyogenetics and Evolution, 1997. 8: pp. 301-316

6. MacKenzie R.B., Beye H.K., Valverde L., Garron H. Epidemic Hemorrhagic Fever in Bolivia: a Preliminary Report of the Epidemiologic and Clinical Findings in a NewEpidemic Area in South America. Journal of Tropical Medicine and Hygiene, 1964. 13: pp. 620-625

7. Johnson K.M. The Discovery of Hantaan Virus: Comparative Biology and Serendipity in a World at War. The Journal of Infectious Diseases, 2004. 190: pp. 1708-1721

8. International Notes Bolivian Hemorrhagic Fever – El Beni Department, Bolivia, 1994. Morbidity and Mortality Weekly Report, 1994. 43: pp. 943-946

9. Peters C.J., Buchmeier M., Rollin P.E., Ksiazek T.G. Arenaviruses. Field's Virology. Third Edition. Volume 1. Philadelphia: Lippincott-Raven. 1996. pp. 1521-1551

10. Jahrling P.B., Marty A.M., Geisbert T.W. Viral Hemorrhagic Fevers. Medical Aspects of Chemical and Biological Warfare. Falls Church: Office of the Surgeon General, Department of the Army, United States of America. 2007. pp. 271-310

11. Buchmeier M. J., de la Torre J.C., Peters C.J. Arenaviridae: the Viruses and their Replication. Fourth edition. Philadelphia: Lippincott-Raven. 2007. pp. 1635-1668

12. Radoshitzky S.R., Longobardi L.E., Kuhn J.H., Retterer C., Dong L., Clester J.C., Kota K., Carra J., Bavari S. Machupo Virus Glycoprotein Determinants for Human Transferrin Receptor 1 Binding and Cell Entry. Public Library of Science (PLoS) ONE, 2011. 6: pp. e21398

13. Bishop D. Arenaviridae and their Replication. Virology. Second Edition. New York: Raven Press. 1990. pp. 1231-1243

14. Garcin D., Kolakofsky D. Tacaribe Arenavirus RNA Synthesis In Vitro is Primer Dependent and Suggests an Unusual Model for the Initiation of Genome Replication. The Journal of Virology, 1992. 66: pp. 1370-1376

15. Meyer B.J., Southern P.J. Concurrent Sequence Analysis of 5' and 3' RNA Termini by Intramolecular Circularization Reveals 5' Nontemplated Bases and 3' Terminal Heterogeneity for Lymphocytic Choriomeningitis Virus mRNAs. The Journal of Virology, 1993. 67: pp. 2621-2627

16. Yun N.E., Walker D.H. Pathogenesis of Lassa Fever. Viruses, 2012. 4: pp. 2031-2048

17. Garcin D., Kolakofsky D. A Novel Mechanism for the Initiation of Tacaribe Arenavirus Genome Replication. The Journal of Virology, 1990. 64: pp. 6196-6203

18. Saunders A.A., Ting J.P.C., Meisner J., Neuman B.W., Perez M., de la Torre J.C., Buchmeier M.J. Mapping the Landscape of the Lymphocytic Choriomeningitis Virus Stable Signal Peptide Reveals Novel Functional Domains. Journal of Virology, 2007. 81: pp. 5649-5657

19. Rojek J. M., Lee A.M., Nguyen N., Spiropoulou C.F., Kunz S. Site 1 Protease is Required for Proteolytic Processing of the Glycoproteins of the South American Hemorrhagic Fever Viruses Junin, Machupo, and Guanarito. The Journal of Virology, 2008. 82: pp. 6045-6051

20. Bowden T.A., Crispin M., Graham S.C., Harvey D.J., Grimes J.M., Jones E.Y., Stuart D.I. Unusual Molecular Architecture of the Machupo Virus Attachment Glycoprotein. The Journal of Virology, 2009. 83: pp. 8259–8265

21. Flanagan M. L., Oldenburg J., Reignier T., Holt N., Hamilton G.A., Martin V.K., Cannon P.M. 2008. New World Clade B Arenaviruses can use Transferrin Receptor 1 (TfR1)-dependent and -independent Entry Pathways, and Glycoproteins from Human Pathogenic Strains are associated with the use of TfR1. The Journal of Virology, 2008. 82: pp. 938-948

22. Radoshitzky S. R., Abraham J., Spiropoulou C.F., Kuhn J.H., Nguyen D., Li W., Nagel J., Schmidt P.J., Nunberg J.H., Andrews N.C., Farzan M., Choe H. 2007. Transferrin Receptor 1 is a Cellular Receptor for New World Haemorrhagic Fever Arenaviruses. Nature, 2007. 446: pp. 92-96

23. Radoshitzky S. R., Kuhn J.H., Spiropoulou C.F., Albarino C.G., Nguyen D.P., Salazar-Bravo J., Dorfman T., Lee A.S., Wang E., Ross S.R., Choe H., Farzan M.. 2008. Receptor Determinants of Zoonotic Transmission of New World Hemorrhagic Fever Arenaviruses. Proceedings of the National Academy of Sciences of the United States of America, 2008. 105: pp. 2664-2669

24. Franz D.R., Jahrling P.B., Friedlander A.M., McClain D.J., Hoover D.L., Byrne W.R., Pavlin J.A., Christopher G.W., Eitzen E.M. Clinical Recognition and Management of Patients Exposed to Biological Warfare Agents. The Journal of American Medical Association, 1997. 278: pp. 399-411

25. Alibek K. Biohazard. New York: Dell Publishing. 1999. pp. 20, 42

26. Hemorrhagic Fever Viruses (VHF). Updated January 10, 2008. Retrieved July 24, 2008. Web Site: http://www. upmcbiosecurity.org/website/focus/agents_diseases/fac sheets/vhf.html

27. Guerrant R.L., Walker D.H., Weller P.F. Tropical Infectious Diseases – Principles, Pathogens & Practice. Volume 1. Philadelphia: Churchill Livingstone Elsevier. 2006. pp 741.

28. Viral Hemorrhagic Fevers Caused by Arenaviruses. Institute for International Cooperation in Animal Biologics. Iowa State University. Updated February 23, 2010. Retrieved March 24, 2010. Web site: http://www.cfsph.iastate.edu/Factsheets/pdfs/viral_hemorrhagic_fever_arenavirus.pdf

29. Peters C.J., Kuehne R.W., Mercado R.R., Le Bow R.H., Spertzel R.O., Webb P.A. Hemorrhagic Fever in Cochabamba, Bolivia, 1971. American Journal of Epidemiology, 1974. 99: pp. 425-433

30. Kilgore P.E., Peters C.J., Mills J.N., Rollin P.E., Armstrong L., Khan A.S., Ksiazek T.G. Prospects for the Control of Bolivian Hemorrhagic Fever. Emerging Infectious Diseases, 1995. 1: pp. 97-100

31. Douglas R., Weibenga N., Couch R. Bolivian Hemorrhagic Fever Probably Transmitted by Personal Contact. American Journal of Epidemiology, 1965. 82: pp. 85-91

32. Weinstein R.S., Alibek K. Biological and Chemical Terrorism. A Guide for Healthcare Providers and First Responders. New York: Thieme Medical Publishers. 2003. pp. 70-71

33. Khardori N. Bioterrorism Preparedness. Medicine – Pubic Health – Policy. Weinheim: Wiley-VCH Verlag Gmbh & Co. KGaA. 2006. pp. 205-208

34. Aguilar P.V., Camargo W., Vargas J., Guevara C., Roca Y., Felices V., Laguna-Torres V.A., Tesh R., Ksiazek T.G., Kochel T.J. Reemergence of Bolivian Hemorrhagic Fever, 2007–2008. Emerging Infectious Diseases, 2009. 15: pp. 1526-1528

35. Peters C.J. Arenaviruses. Textbook of Human Virology. Littleton: PSG Publishing Company, 1984. pp. 513-545

36. Child P.L., MacKenzie R.B., Valverde L.R., Johnson K.M. Bolivian Hemorrhagic Fever: a Pathologic Description. Archive of Pathological and Laboratory Medicine, 1967. 83: pp. 434-445

37. Peter C.J., Webb P.A., Johnson K.M. Measurement of Antibodies to Machupo Virus by the Indirect Fluorescent Technique. Proceedings of the Society for Experimental Biology and Medicine, 1973. 142: pp. 526-531

38. Re-emergence of Bolivian Hemorrhagic Fever. Epidemiological Bulletin. Panamerican Health Organization, 1994. 15: pp. 4-5

39. Peters C. Lymphocytic Choriomeningits Virus, Lassa Virus, and the South American Hemorrhagic Fevers. Principles and Practices of Infectious Diseases. Sixth Edition. Philadelphia: Elsevier Churchill Livingstone. 2005 pp. 2090-2098

40. Harrison L.H., Halsey N.A., McKee Jr K.T., Peters C.J., Barrera Oro J.G., Briggiler A.M., Feuillade M.R., Maiztegui J.I. Clinical Case Definitions for Argentine Hemorrhagic fever. Clinical Infectious Diseases, 1999. 28: pp. 1091-1094

41. Franz D.R., Jahrling P.B., Friedlander A.M., McClain D.J., Hoover D.L., Bryne W.R., Pavlin J.A., Christopher G.W., Eitzen E.M. Clinical Recognition and Management of Patients Exposed to Biological Warfare Agents. The Journal of American Medical Association, 1997. 278: pp. 399-411

Photo Bibliography

Figure 1.9-1: Electron photomicrograph of Machupo Virus. Photograph was taken by Dr. Fred Murphy, Sylvia Whitfield at 234,000x and released by the CDC. Public domain photo
Figure 1.9.5: Viral graphics designed by the CDC. Public domain photo

The Marburg virus belongs to the genus *Marburgvirus* and is comprised of a single species, *Marburg marburgvirus* (MARV), formally known as *Lake Victoria marburgvirus*. MARV, with approximately 55% dissimilarity at the nucleotide level with Ebola virus (EBOV), is classified as one of the two members of the *Filoviridae* family.[1] The phylogenetic analysis base on the data acquired from genomic sequencing indicates that there are at least five distinct MARV lineages. Four of the five lineages are closely related with approximately 7% difference in their nucleotide sequences, while the fifth is divergent with approximately 21% difference in its nucleotide sequences. Presently, the four closely related marburgvirus lineages are classified as Musoke isolates, while the single divergent is classified as the Ravn isolate.[2, 3]

The MARV virus particle is enveloped and filamentous in shape measuring approximately 800 nm in length and 80 nm in diameter. This virus contains a linear, non-segmented, single-stranded negative sense RNA genome (~19 kb). MARV is known to be the caustic agent for Marburg Hemorrhagic Fever (MHF), a severe and fatal disease (Figure 1.10-1).

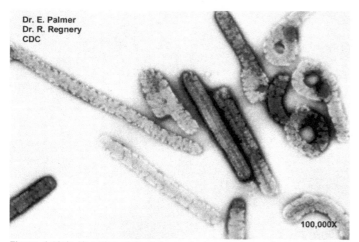

Dr. E. Palmer
Dr. R. Regnery
CDC

100,000X

Figure 1.10-1: Negative stained transmission electron micrograph (TEM), shows number of Marburg virus virions

Like EBOV, MARV is one of the most virulent pathogens on Earth. MARV (Musoke isolate) was first documented in 1967 after three coincidental outbreaks in Marburg and Frankfurt, Germany, as well as, Belgrade, former Yugoslavia. The initial MHF outbreak (primary infections) occurred in 25 laboratory employees working on polio vaccine and were exposed to the blood of African green monkeys (*Ceropithecus aethiops*) imported from Uganda. These 25 primary infections subsequently transmitted the disease to coworkers and family members, resulting in six secondary infections. The overall consequences of the outbreak were 31 infections resulting in seven fatalities.[4, 5] In 1975, an Australian traveler was infected with MARV (Musoke isolate) in Zimbabwe and subsequently transmitted the infection to his traveling companion and a health care worker in Johannesburg, South Africa. This isolated group of infections resulted in a single fatality.[6] In 1980, a French visitor to Kitum Cave, in Kenya's Mount Elgon National Park, contracted MARV (Musoke isolate) and the doctor who attempted to resuscitate the patient developed the same infection within 9 days. This isolated case resulted in a single fatality (the doctor later recovered).[7] In 1987, a 15 year old Danish boy also contracted MARV (reported Ravn isolate), during a visit to Kitum Cave and developed MHF. Unfortunately, the child died despite aggressive supportive therapy.[8] In 1990, a

single case of MARV (presumably the Musoke isolate) infection occurred in Koltsovo, Russia. Fortunately, the laboratory worker who was accidentally infected later recovered.[9] Between 1998-2000, a severe outbreak of MHF (Ravn isolate) occurred among gold mine workers and in the neighboring village of Watsa, Durba, Democratic Republic of Congo. During this outbreak, 154 people contracted the disease and 128 people died as a result (83% fatality rate).[10, 11, 12, 13] The largest MARV (Musoke isolate) outbreak occurred in 2004-2005, in Uige Province, Angola. During this outbreak, a total of 252 cases were reported, of which approximately 90% (~227) died.[14] On July 27, 2007, in the town of Ibanda, Kamwenge district of Uganda, four cases of MARV (Ravn isolate) was reported at a gold mine. The mine was promptly shutdown while the infected were isolated and treated. As a result, three miners recovered, while a single miner died of the infection.[15] Two most recent cases of MARV (Ravn isolate) occurred in 2008 when an American and Dutch tourist visited the Python Cave in Uganda. The Dutch traveler succumbed to the infection after her return to the Netherlands, while the American tourist developed only mild symptoms and survived (Figure 1.10-2).[16]

MARV is suspected to be a zoonosis, but presently the natural reservoir of this virus is not known. It is suspected that bats, belonging to the families of *Pteropodidae*, *Emballonuridae*, *Mega-dermatidae*, *Rhinolophidae* and *Vepertilionidae* fulfill this role.[13, 17] However, it is still possible that the viral reservoir may be an arthropod or plant.[18] It is believed that primary transmission of the virus from the natural reservoir(s) occurs in sub-Saharan Africa (western Kenya, Uganda and Zimbabwe).[10] Unlike its close cousin, EBOV, sites in which MARV infections occur are quite discontinuous. While EBOV tends to occur in the humid rain forests of Central and Western Africa, MARV tends to exist in the drier and more open areas of central and eastern sub Saharan Africa (Figure 1.10-3).[19]

The MARV genome is composed of a highly conserved transcriptional start and stop signal along with a 3' to 5' untranslated region and an open reading frame.[20] The Genome encodes seven structural proteins. Starting from the 3' end, the negative sense RNA encodes nucleoprotein (NP), virion protein (VP) 35, VP40, glycoprotein (GP), VP30, VP24 and finally, the polymerase (L protein) located at the 5' end.[21, 22, 23] The NP, VP30, VP35 and L protein are associated with the genomic RNA in a ribonucleoprotien complex, while the remaining proteins GP, VP24 and VP40 are associated with the viral membrane (Figure 1.10-4).[21, 24, 25, 26, 27, 28]

NP encapsulates the viral genome and antigenomic RNAs, while it serves as a viral "hub" protein and forms interactions with most other viral proteins. For example, NP's interactions between VP35 and VP30 redirect these proteins into NP-derived inclusion. NP also forms a weak interaction with VP24, which also leads to the partial relocalization of this protein into NP-derived inclusions. It is interesting to note that when NP is expressed in absence of other viral proteins, it will create the characteristic inclusion bodies that possess organized tubular structures similar to the nucleocapsids of viral infected cells.[29] NP's interactions with VP40 assist in the transport of newly synthesized nucleocapsids to the host cellular membrane. NP has been reported to enhance VP-40 induced viral budding process by recruiting Tsg 101, part of ESCRT I complex, via its C-terminal late domain motif (PSAP). Research has shown that replication and transcription activities

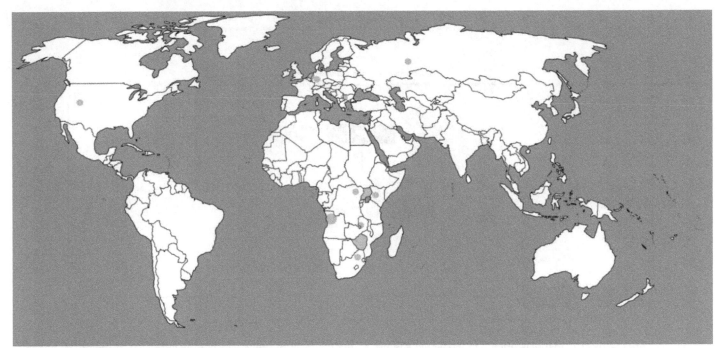

Figure 1.10-2: Distribution of Marburg virus (MARV)

in the MARV are highly dependent upon NP. NP, together with the L protein and VP35, which represent the polymerase cofactors, are sufficient for replication and transcription in an artificial MARV mini-genome system.[20, 24, 30, 31, 32, 33]

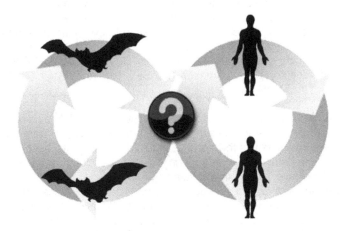

Figure 1.10-3: Possible transmission cycle of Marburg virus. This virus is efficiently transmitted among the human population through physical contact or exchange of bodily fluids without the need for an enzootic amplification. At present the sylvatic cycle of Marburg virus transmission to human is unknown

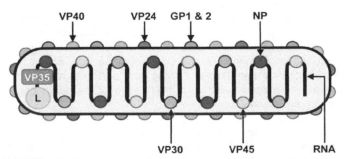

Figure 1.10-4: Internal diagram of an MARV showing structural and nucleoproteins

Unlike EBOV, the exact functionality of MARV VP30 (28

kDa) is presently unknown. Nonetheless, Fowler *et al.* (2005) demonstrated that RNAi-based down-regulation of VP30 during MARV infection produced a marked reduction in both viral protein and virion production. This discovery indicates that MARV VP30 plays a role in viral transcription and/or replication.[34]

VP40 (38 kDa) is a peripheral protein that lines the interior aspects of the virus membrane. VP40 is a matrix protein and plays an important role in the formation of the filamentous particles through the relocation of nucleocapsid from the perinuclear region to the plasma membrane of the host cell. VP40 is also involved in the recruitment of GP to the budding site and mediate virus particle release.[20, 31] Additionally, VP40 is believed to be capable of antagonizing alpha/beta interferon (IFN-α/β) and IFN-γ signaling through the inhibition of the cellular tyrosine kinase Jak1. However, the exact mechanism of this inhibition requires further investigation.[20, 35]

GP is a type I transmembrane protein that forms the viral homotrimeric spikes, which in turn, mediates host-cell receptor binding and membrane fusion.[21, 25, 26, 27, 28] The MARV GP gene encodes a single product in a continuous open reading frame. This is unlike EBOV, where the GP is encoded and subsequently processed to form a small secreted glycoprotein (sGP) and is secreted in large quantities in infected individuals. MARV GP is a precursor molecule synthesized in the rough endoplasmic reticulum of the host cell. During its transport towards the plasma membrane, it undergoes numerous post-translational modifications which include glycosylation, acetylation, and phosphorylation. At the trans-Golgi network, GP is cleaved by furin or furin-like endoproteases into two disulfide-linked subunits: the large extra membrane proteins GP_1 (160 kD) and the membrane-anchored protein GP_2 (38 kD).[20, 21, 22, 25, 26, 27, 28]

It is believed that GP plays a role in evading the host immune system. GP has been reported to counteract the antiviral activities of the IFN-inducible antiviral protein tetherin, play a role in the suppression of cytokine response, as well as, capable of inducing apoptosis of lymphocytes. However, the manner by which these actions take place requires additional research.[20, 36, 37]

93

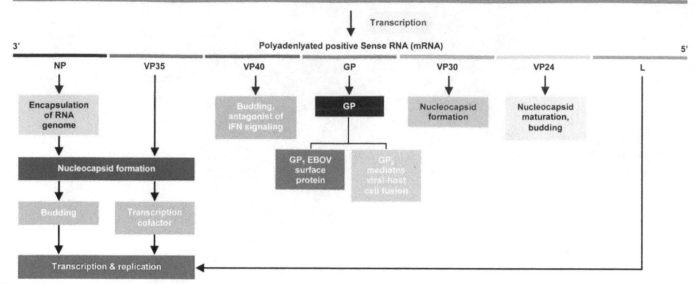

Figure 1.10-5: A diagrammatic display of the structural and nonstructural proteins encoded by MARV genome

VP24 is a minor matrix protein that is unique to the filovirus family, but its exact function remains to be elucidated. Bamberg *et al.* (2005) reported that VP24 proteins are recruited into filamentous virus-like particles generated by VP40, but this incorporation of VP24 did not alter the morphology or the budding efficiency of virus-like particles. However, when VP24 was down-regulated in MARV-infected cells, the release of viral particles was significantly reduced, although the viral transcription and replication were unaffected. Based on the data obtained, the authors deduced VP24 may act to facilitate the maturation of transport-competent nucleocapsid, in addition to assisting in the interactions between the plasma membrane of the host cell and the nucleocapsid during the budding process (Figure 1.10-4 and 1.10-5).[20, 21, 31]

As indicated previously, VP35 is a polymerase cofactor and is essential for virus transcription and replication. In conjunction with the L protein, they form the RNA-dependent RNA polymerase complex. VP35 is closely linked to NP and serves as a bridging protein between the L protein and the nucleocapsid complex. It has been reported that in VP35 down-regulated MARV-infected cells, the L protein will not associate with the nucleocapsid, which functions as the template for viral transcription and replication. [20, 24, 30] Additionally, VP35 serves as an interferon antagonist. As reported by Basler and Amarasinghe (2009), VP35 is an active competitor for the cellular kinases IKK-epsilon and TBK-1. Since both these enzymes are responsible for the phosphorylation and activation of interferon regulatory factor 3 and interferon regulatory factor 7, VP35 actively represses the transcription of the IFN gene. Furthermore, VP35 also promotes SUMOylation or post-translational modification of interferon regulatory factor 7, which also results in the repression of the transcription of the IFN gene.[38, 39]

The L protein is a major component of MARV. Together with VP35, they form the RNA-dependent RNA polymerase complex, which is essential for virus transcription and replication. Additionally, it is believed that the L proteins are responsible for capping and polyadenylation of viral mRNAs, however, the exact manner by which these actions transpire remains to be elucidated.[20, 24]

It has been reported that the asialoglycoprotein receptor (ASGP-R) located on hepatocytes, serves as the binding site for MARV. ASGP-R is a C-type lectin that binds and facilitates endocytosis of galactose containing glycol-proteins. In addition, folate receptor α, dendritic cell (DC) specific intercellular adhesion molecule (ICAM)-3-grabbing nonintegrin (DC-SIGN) expressed in immature DCs and macrophages, as well as, DC-SIGN related factors, have been reported as binding proteins for MARV. Liver/lymph node-specific intercellular adhesion molecule-3-grabbing integrin (L-SIGN), expressed on endothelial cells of the liver and the lymph nodes, has also been shown to serve as a binding protein for MARV. Other receptors that may serve as binding sites for MARV include human macrophage galactose- and *N*-acetylgalactoseamine-specific C-type lectin (hMGL), liver and lymph node sinusoidal endothelial cell C-type lectin (LSECtin), TAM receptor protein kinases Axl, DtK, Mer and Tim-1 (Table 1).[20, 40, 41, 42, 43, 44]

After MARV binds to the host cell receptor, it is widely accepted that the virus enters the cell via endocytotic pathways. There are many suspected pathways that allow MARV into the host cell. Possible pathways include macro-pinocytosis, clathrin-mediated endocytosis, caveolin-mediated endocytosis, as well as, clathrin- and caveolin-independent endocytosis.[45] Once MARV enters the endosome, exposure to the acidic pH is responsible for a conformational change in the GP, leading to the solvent accessibility of the viral fusion peptide. The fusion peptide, which is believed to exist at the N-terminus of GP_2, is then inserted into the cell membrane where it mediates virus and cell membrane fusion and the subsequent release of the viral genome into the cytoplasm, where the propagation of the virus will take place.[44, 46] It has been reported that the endosomal proteolysis of GP is also an important event in the viral-endosome fusion process. The cystine proteases (CatL and CatB) were shown to digest GP_1 in an acidic environment, which is presumed to trigger a conformational change in the GP_2 fusion peptide, linking it to the endosomal membrane drawing viral and host membranes together to induce fusion and the release of the nucleocapsid into the cytoplasm.[47]

Once the nucleocapsid is in the cytoplasm, transcription of the negative sense RNA genome is the first and most essential viral process that takes place. The initial transcription yields polyadenylated, momocistronic mRNAs in the 3' to 5' direction, from the encapsidated genomic RNA template. Viral transcription involves a process of starts (conserved start sequences) and

Table 1: List of factors that enable MARV and MARV pseudotype entry into host cell[34]

Cellular Receptors	Ligand Specificity	Cell Type
ASGP-R	Terminal Galactose	Hepatocytes
DC-SIGN	High-manose Glycans	Dendritic cell, Macrophage, Endothelial cells in liver and lymph nodes
L-SIGN	High-manose Glycans	Dendritic cell, Macrophage, Endothelial cells in liver and lymph nodes
hMGL	N-acetylgalactoseamine	Dendritic cell, Macrophage
FR-α	Follic Acid	Various Cell Types
Tyro3 (Axl, Dtk, Mer)	Gas6	Various Cell Types
LSECtin/CLEC4G	N-Acetylglucosamine	Dendritic cell, Macrophage, Endothelial cells in liver and lymph nodes

stops (polyadenylated stop sequences) as the RNA-dependent RNA polymerase complex moves along the genome.[47]

The initial expression of transcribed viral genes (antigenomic viral positive sense RNA) leads to a buildup of viral proteins (NP, VP35, VP40, GP, VP30, VP24 and L protein) in the host cell's cytoplasm. This buildup of the viral protein, especially NP, is believed to trigger a switch from transcription to replication. It has been reported that NP mRNA can be detected as early as seven hours, post infection, and peaks around 18 hours.[48, 49, 50] Additionally, the replicated antigenomic viral positive sense RNA strand serves as a template to synthesize genomic negative sense RNA molecules. Immediately after the formation of genomic negative sense RNA, it is rapidly encapsulated.[48, 49]

It has been reported that the depletion of viral proteins leads to a switch from replication to transcription and translation. Eventually, an equilibrium is reached between transcription, translation and replication, and the viral particles accumulate and are directed to the plasma membrane for virion assembly and budding (Figure 1.10-6).[49]

Experimental evidence indicates that MARV (as well as, its cousin EBOV) does not replicate in lymphocytes. However, large numbers of lymphocytes do undergo apoptosis, which explains the progressive lymphopenia and lymphoid depletion prior to the death of the patient. Although the mechanism of the apoptosis of the lymphocytes is not clearly understood, it is believed that this programmed cell death is triggered by the GP and proceeds through multiple pathways. It has been proposed that these pathways include tumor necrosis factor-related, apoptosis-induced ligand (TRAIL), Fas death receptor pathways, DC dysfunction induced by the infection and abnormal production of proapoptotic soluble mediators (e.g. nitric oxide).[20, 21, 51]

MARV, a member of the family of *Filoviruses*, is classified as a Category A biowarfare agent by the Centers for Disease Control due to its lethality, high infectivity as an aerosol as shown in animal models, and the possibility for ease of replication in tissue culture.[52] Most known human infections of MARV have been fatal, and presently there are no vaccines or therapies available that are 100% effective in combating this agent.[53] As described by Alibek (1999), MARV (Variant U) was designated as N3 and was researched and produced at the Institute of Ultra-Pure Biopreparations in Leningrad, Omutninsk in Kirov, Obolensk (outside of Moscow), the Lyubuchany Institute of Immunology in Chekhov near Moscow, and Vector Research and Testing in Novosibrisk (near the small town of Koltsovo) in Siberia.[54]

SYMPTOMS

Similar to the EBOV, secondary and tertiary transmission of MARV occurs through direct contact with contaminated blood, bodily fluids, semen, infected cell cultures or tissues, contaminated syringes, or other medical equipment.[10, 55] Evidence has shown that even direct contact with patients' clothing during the infection can spread the disease. In a report by Borchert *et al.* (2006), involving a cluster of MHF cases, including an infant, the researchers traced the generation of cases from person-to-person contact. Their research appears to indicate the person-

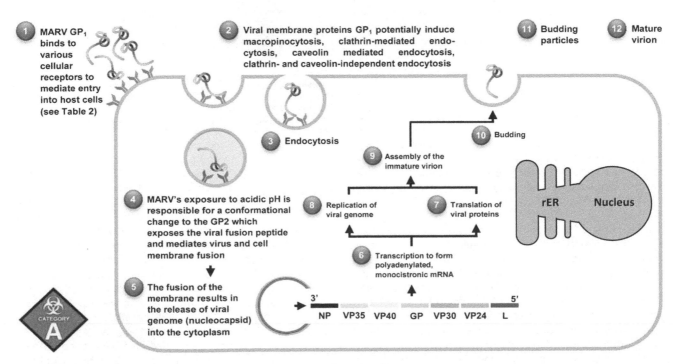

Figure 1.10-6: Diagrammatic process of Marburg virus infection within an eukaryotic cell

to-person transmission of MHF may be more common than first thought.[56] In a subsequent report by the same authors, the secondary and tertiary risks of transmission were calculated to be as high as 21% and 19%, respectively.[57]

Like the EBOV, MARV is known to infect dendritic (Langerhans) cells commonly found in the skin, but can be found in the inner linings of the respiratory and digestive tracts as well. Once infected, dendritic cells are no long able to perform their antiviral activities.[58] MARV is also known to infect monocytes and macrophages (e.g. alveolar, pleural and peritoneal macrophages), Kupffer cells, microglial cells, hepatocytes (Figure 1.10-7) and endothelial cells. In addition to the exponential growth of MARV within these cell types, the virus also initiates the secretion of significant concentrations of various chemokines and proinflamatory cytokines, which includes RANTES, monocyte chemotactic protein-1, microphage inflammatory protein-1α, tumor necrosis factor–α, interferon–γ, interleukin–6, interleukin–8 and growth related oncogenic–α.[58, 59, 60]

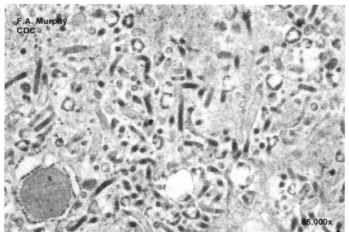

Figure 1.10-7: Transmission electron micrograph (TEM) shows numerous MARV virions in a liver tissue

Reports have indicated that the interactions between viral particles, neutrophils, other polymorphonuclear leokocytes, along with triggering receptors expressed on myeloid cells (TREMs) and Toll-like receptors (TLRs), provide another source for the release of the copious amounts of inflammatory mediators. It has been proposed that the release of pro-inflammatory cytokines can disrupt the architecture of the vascular endothelium and other tissues (Figure 1.10-8).[59, 61]

For instance, histological examinations of liver biopsies from severe cases of MHF show cyto-architectural changes in the tissue, where many of the hepatocytes are at different stages of acidophilic necrosis demonstrated by numerous Councilman's bodies. Councilman's bodies are eosinophilic globules representing hepatocytes undergoing apoptosis during a viral liver infection (Figure 1.10-9).

The incubation period of MARV is between 5 to 10 days (ranging between 2 to 19 days) before the onset of symptoms. Initial symptoms include high fever, chills, severe frontal headaches, cephalalhia and myalgia. On approximately the fifth day after the onset of symptoms, purple-red maculopapular and/or petechiae rash may appear on the patient's chest, back and stomach, followed by sore throat, pharyngitis, extreme fatigue, malaise, prostration, anorexia, nausea, vomiting, profuse diarrhea, photophobia, chest and abdominal pains.[60] Additionally, symptoms such as hiccups (developed in 5 to 18% of patients) and hypotension may also appear during this period.

[60, 61] On approximately the seventh day of infection, in addition to developing severe nausea and vomiting, hemorrhagic symptoms begin to appear. These symptoms include epistaxis, bleeding of the gums, nose, vagina; hema-temesis; melena and bleeding from sites of needle punctures.[62, 63, 64] In fatal cases of MHF, symptoms become more severe, and may include jaundice, pancreatic inflammation, sever weight loss, shock, liver failure, massive hemorrhaging and multi-organ failure.[49]

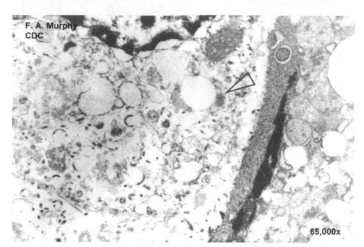

Figure 1.10-8: Transmission electron micrograph (TEM) of lung tissue from a Marburg patient in Johannesburg, South Africa, 1975. The micrograph reveals the presence of an alveolar hemorrhage in the lung tissue biopsy (arrow)

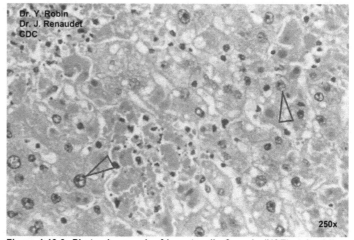

Figure 1.10-9: Photomicrograph of hematoxylin & eosin (H&E) stained liver specimen extracted from a severely MARV infected patient in South Africa. The photomicrograph shows cytoarchitectural changes where many of the hepatocytes are in different stages of acidophilic necrosis. In addition, some cells are evolving into Councilman's bodies while many basophilic bodies and early fatty changes are also found (arrows)

Leukopenia and thrombocytopenia are common laboratory abnormalities during the course of MHF, while leukocytosis may appear during the later stages of the infection. In addition, liver enzyme elevations, along with proteinuria are present during the course of MHF. In patients with advanced infections, neurological symptoms such as blindness, sudden hearing loss, paresthesia (pins and needle sensation of the skin), somnolence and delirium are also commonly observed. Eventually the patient will proceed into shock and coma. Death generally occurs six to nine days from the onset of clinical disease. Autopsy results have indicated hemorrhages of the skin, mucous membranes, visceral organs and gastrointestinal tract. In addition, histological examinations have shown necrosis in the liver, kidneys, lymphatic organs and testes. Interstitial pneumonitis has also been seen in the lungs postmortem.[62, 65] It is interesting to note that the majority of fatal cases of MHF develop clinical signs early in the infection and death generally takes place between six to nine days. Although abnormal coagulation of blood and fibrinolysis are characteristic features of MHF, it is important to note that a massive amount of blood loss is atypical. In rare cases, when substantial blood loss does occur, it is generally limited to the gastrointestinal tract. However, the total volume of blood loss has been reported to be insufficient to account for the fatality (Table 2).[63]

Table 2: An overview of the clinical symptoms of MHF

Symptoms	+	++	+++
Fever			■
Chills			■
Myalgia			■
Arthralgia			■
Malaise			■
Cephalalgia			■
Maculopapular rash			■
Petechiae rash			■
Sore throat			■
Pharyngitis			■
Extreme fatigue			■
Prostration			■
Anorexia			■
Nausea			■
Vomiting			■
Profuse diarrhea			■
Photophobia			■
Chest pains			■
Abdominal pains			■
Epistaxis			■
Bleeding of gums & nose			■
Vaginal bleeding			■
Hematemesis			■
Melena			■
Venipuncture bleeding			■
Hiccups		■	
Hypotension		■	
Jaundice		■	
Pancreatic inflammation		■	
Severe weight loss		■	
Liver failure		■	
Massive hemorrhaging		■	
Multi-organ failures		■	
Leukopenia		■	
Thrombocytopenia		■	
Liver enzyme elevations		■	
Proteinuria	■		
Leukocytosis	■		
Blindness		■	
Sudden hearing loss		■	
Paresthesia		■	
Somnolence		■	
Delirium		■	
Shock		■	
Coma		■	

+ Rare ++ Common +++ Frequent

DETECTION

The symptoms of MHF are similar to malaria, typhoid fever, rickettsial infection, leptospirosis, fulminant hepatitis, shigellosis, meningo-coccemia, arboviral fevers, dengue fever, yellow fever and other hemorrhagic fevers (e.g. EBOV), therefore, laboratory diagnostic methods are required to specifically diagnose the infection by MARV.[57, 65] For example, laboratory findings show early, profound lymphopenia and thrombo-cytopenia with a later rapid shift to neutrophilia. Elevated alanine transaminase (ALT)

and even higher elevated aspartate transaminase (AST) levels are also detected in MHF patients.[51] Nonetheless, these findings are not definitive proof of MARV infection.

Etiologic diagnosis should be sought during the acute phase of the illness when MARV is allowed to propagate in Vero cells (*Cercopithecus aethiops*, African green monkey kidney cells), particularly the E6 clone, MA-104, SW13 (human adrenal carcinoma cell line) or other primary cell cultures such as monocytes, macrophage and endothelial cells. MARV can be detected directly through electron microscopy of the tissue culture supernatants, examining the cytopathic effect or direct immunofluorescent staining of the infected cells.[2, 59, 60]

Other commonly used laboratory test for identification of MARV infections are enzyme-linked immunosorbent assay (ELISA) for identification of Marburg virus antigens and anti-Marburg IgM and IgG. Reverse transcriptase polymerase chain reaction (RT-PCR) has also been successfully utilized to detect the filovirus-specific segment of the polymerase (L protein) gene and nested primers targeting VP35 gene of the MARV have also been used.[66, 67, 68]

TREATMENT

Presently there are no direct antiviral treatments for MARV and the only available therapy is intensive supportive care of specific symptoms that develop as a result of MHF.[69] The clinician needs to closely monitor the patient's pulmonary, renal and cardiac function throughout the course of infection. Most often, in severe cases of MHF, the patient is dehydrated and in need of intravenous fluids. In addition, electrolytes and nutrition will also have to be intravenously introduced to the patient, since symptoms of nausea and vomiting will complicate ingestion.[5] Similar to the supportive therapy given to patients suffering from EHF, it is essential that the clinician closely monitor/maintain oxygen status, as well as, the blood pressure of the patient. In an effort to prevent secondary infections, broad spectrum antibiotics may also be administered. In addition, the clinicians may provide patients with replacement plasma heparin before the onset of clinical shock and may consider the use of corticosteroids for controlling inflammation.[70]

As with any type of hemorrhagic fever, intra-muscular injections should be avoided due to the possibility of uncontrollable bleeding. In addition, administering acetylsalicylic acid and non-steroid anti-inflammatory drugs for fever should always be avoided. Clinicians may prescribe acetaminophen to combat fever and inflammatory symptoms. Convalescent antiserum procedures are at times used in treating patients suffering from MHF, however, the success rate of this treatment has not yet been evaluated.[64] Ribavirin, an antiviral drug believed to interfere with the capping of viral mRNA, thereby inhibiting the replication of many RNA viruses, demonstrated no effect on MARV. Similarly, interferon demonstrated no discernable effect against MARV infections in non-human primate models.[5, 70, 71]

For years, efforts have been made to develop a vaccine against MARV. Viral nucleoproteins, glycoproteins and structural proteins, such as VP24, VP 30, VP 35 and VP 40, have been tested as vaccine candidates. Although these potential vaccines showed promise in rodent models, they failed in non-human primate models.[5] In 2006, Daddario-DiCaprio *et al.*, demonstrated that using live attenuated recombinant vesicular stomatitis virus (rVSV), expressing the transmembrane protein of MARV, showed promise as a preventive vaccine and/or as a possible postexposure treatment[51], because it completely

Table 3: A diagrammatic display of MHF in comparison with other infections with similar symptoms such as Ebola hemorrhagic fever (EHF), Dengue hemorrhagic fever (DHF), Crimean-Congo hemorrhagic fever (CCHF), Argentine Hemorrhagic Fever (AHF) and Bolivian hemorrhagic fever (BHF)

Symptoms	MHF	LF	Malaria	TF	EHF	DF/DHF	CCHF	AHF	BHF
Fever	■	■	■	■	■	■	■	■	■
Chills	■		■	■	■	■	■	■	
Malaise	■	■	■	■	■	■	■		■
Myalgia	■	■	■	■	■	■	■		
Arthralgia	■	■			■	■	■		■
Cephalalgia	■	■		■	■	■	■		■
Maculopapular rash	■				■	■			
Petechiae rash	■				■		■	■	■
Sore throat	■				■		■		■
Pharyngitis	■				■		■		
Extreme fatigue	■			■					
Prostration	■								■
Anorexia	■							■	
Nausea	■	■	■		■	■	■	■	■
Vomiting	■	■	■	■	■	■	■	■	
Profuse diarrhea	■		■		■		■	■	
Photophobia	■					■			■
Chest pains	■	■			■				
Abdominal pains	■		■	■		■		■	■
Epistaxis	■			■			■		
Bleeding of gums & nose	■	■			■		■	■	■
Vaginal bleeding	■				■		■		
Hematemesis	■				■		■		■
Melena	■	■		■	■		■		
Venipuncture bleeding	■				■				
Hiccups	■				■				
Hypotension	■	■			■	■	■	■	
Jaundice	■		■				■		■
Pancreatic inflammation	■								
Severe weight loss	■				■				
Liver failure	■				■				
Massive hemorrhaging	■	■			■	■	■		
Multi-organ failures	■				■		■		
Leukopenia	■	■		■	■	■	■	■	■
Thrombocytopenia	■	■	■	■	■	■	■	■	■
Liver enzyme elevations	■		■	■					
Proteinuria	■	■							■
Leukocytosis	■								
Blindness	■								
Sudden hearing loss	■	■							
Paresthesia	■								
Somnolence	■								
Delirium	■			■					
Shock	■	■			■		■		■
Coma	■	■	■					■	■

protected non-human primates from MARV infection.[69, 72] In 2012, Grant-Klein *et. al.* evaluated the immunogenicity, as well as, the protective efficacy of DNA vaccines. This DNA vaccine is designed to express the codon-optimized envelope glycoprotein genes of both Musoke and Ravn isolates of MARV. Using TriGrid™ electroporation device, experimental mice were intramuscular or intradermal inoculated. The results showed that the mice developed robust glycoprotein-specific antibody titers (determined by ELISA) whereby allowing the experimental animals to survive lethal MARV challenges. Further experiments will be needed to test the efficacy of this vaccine in non-human primates, as well as, in human test subjects.[20, 73]

DIFFERENTIAL DIAGNOSIS

Due to the limited data in regards to MARV infections, it is presently assumed that the differential diagnosis of MHF is very similar to EBOV infections. Similar to Ebola hemorrhagic fever

(EHF), it is assumed that in the early stages of the disease, MARV infection could be hard to differentiate from Lassa fever, malaria and typhoid fever. At the later stages, MARV infection may be difficult to differentiate from other viral hemorrhagic fevers (VHF). The VHF includes Ebola hemorrhagic fever (EHF), dengue hemorrhagic fever (DHF), Crimean-Congo hemorrhagic fever (CCHF), Argentine Hemorrhagic Fever (AHF) caused by Junin virus and Bolivian hemorrhagic fever (BHF) caused by Machupo virus. The only certain diagnosis of the particular VHF that patient or patients are infected with are through laboratory testing and confirmation (Table 3).[2, 74]

References

1. Suzuki Y. The origin and Evolution of Ebola and Marburg Viruses. Molecular Biology and Evolution, 1997. 14: pp. 800-806
2. Guerrant R.L., Walker D.H., Weller P.F. Tropical Infectious Diseases – Principles, Pathogens & Practice. Volume 1. Philadelphia: Churchill Livingstone Elsevier. 2006. pp 784-796
3. Towner J.S., Amman B.R., Sealy T.K., Reeder Carroll S,A., Comer J.A., Kemp A., Swanepoel R., Paddock C.D., Balinandi S., Khristova M.L., Formenty P.B.H., Albarino

C.G., Miller D.M., Reed Z.D., Kayiwa J.T., Mills J.N., Cannon D.L., Greer P.W., Byaruhanga E., Farnon E.C., Atimnedi P., Okware S., Katongole-Mbidde E., Downing R., Tappero J.W., Zaki S.R., Ksiazek T.G., Nichol S.T., Rollin P.E. Isolation of Genetically Diverse Marburg Viruses from Egyptian Fruit Bats. Public Library of Science (PLoS), 2009. 5: pp. e1000536

4. Martini G.A. Marburg Virus Disease. Post Graduate Medical Journal, 1973. 49: pp. 542-546
5. Hensley L.E., Jones S.M., Feldmann H., Jahrling P.B., Geisbert T.W. Ebola and Marburg Virus: Pathogenesis and Development of Countermeasures. Current Molecular Medicine, 2005. 5: pp. 761-772
6. Marburg Virus Disease – South Africa. World Health Organization. Weekly Epidemiological Record, 1975. 50: pp. 124-125.
7. Smith D.H., Johnson B.K., Isaacson M., Swanapoel R., Johnson K.M., Killey M., Bagshawe A., Siongok T., Keruga W.K. Marburg-Virus Disease in Kenya. Lancet, 1982. 1: pp. 816-820
8. Johnson E.D., Johnson B.K., Silverstein D., Tukei P., Geisbert T.W., Sanchez A.N., Jahrling P.B. Characterization of a New Marburg Virus Isolated from a 1987 Fatal Case in Kenya. Archives of Virology, 1996. 11: pp. 101-114
9. Guerrant R.L., Walker D.H., Weller P.F. Tropical Infectious Diseases – Principles, Pathogens & Practice. Volume 1. Philadelphia: Churchill Livingstone Elsevier. 2006. pp. 788
10. Bausch D.G., Borchert M., Grein T., Roth C., Swanepoel R., Libande M.L., Talarmin A., Bertherat E., Muyembe-Tamfum J-J., Tugume B., Colebunders R., Kondé K.M., Pirard P., Olinda L.L., Rodier G.R., Campbell P., Tomori O., Ksiazek T.G., Rollin P.E. Risk Factor for Marburg Hemorrhagic Fever, Democratic Republic of the Congo. Emerging Infectious Disease, 2003. 9: pp. 1531-1537
11. Bausch D.G., Nichol S.T., Muyembe-Tamfum J.J., Borchert M., Rollin P.E., Sleurs H., Campbell P., Tshioko F.K., Roth C., Colebunders R., Pirard P., Mardel S., Olinda L.A., Zeller H., Tshomba A., Kulidri A., Libande M.L., Mulangu S., Formenty P., Grein T., Leirs H., Braack L., Ksiazek T., Zaki S., Bowen M.D., Smit S.B., Leman P.A., Burt F.J., Kemp A., Swanepoel R. Marburg Hemorrhagic Fever Associated with Multiple Genetic Lineages of virus. New England Journal of Medicine, 2006. 355: pp. 909-919
12. Marburg Hemorrhagic Fever. Known Cases and Outbreaks of Marburg Hemorrhagic Fever, in Chronological Order. The Center for Disease Control and Prevention. Updated August 23, 2007. Retrieved March 30, 2010. Web site: http://www.cdc.gov/ncidod/dvrd/spb/mnpages/dispages/marburg/marburgtable.htm
13. Balter M. On the Trail of Ebola and Marburg Viruses. Science, 2000. 290: pp. 923
14. Towner J.S., Khristova M.L., Sealy T.K., Vincent M.J., Erickson B.R., Bawiec D.A., Hartman A.L., Comer J.A., Zaki S.R., Ströhe U., Gomes da Silva F., del Castillo F., Rollin P.E., Ksiazek T.G., Nichol S.T. Marburgvirus Genomics and Association with Large Hemorrhagic Fever Outbreak in Angola. Journal of Virology, 2006. 80: pp. 6497-6516
15. Outbreak Postings. Special Pathogen Branch, Center for Disease Control and Prevention. Updated October 29, 2009. Retrieved March 30, 2010. Web site: http://www. cdc.gov/ncidod/dvrd/spb/outbreaks/index.htm
16. Desjardin J., Austin C., Sabbe M., Quoilin S., Reynders D., Walsh A., Chow Y., Morgan D., Balinandi S., Downing R., Lutwama J. Imported case of Marburg hemorrhagic fever - Colorado, 2008. Morbidity and Mortality Weekly Report, 2009. 58: pp. 1377–1381
17. Peterson A.T., Carroll D.S., Mills J.N., Johnson K.M. Potential Mammalian Filovirus Reservoirs. Emerging Infectious Diseases, 2004; 10, 12: pp. 2073-2081.
18. Monath T.P. Ecology of Marburg and Ebola Viruses: Speculations and Directions for Future Research. The Journal of Infectious Diseases, 2001. 179: pp. S127-S138
19. Peterson A.T., Bauer J.T., Mills J.N. Ecological and Geographic Distribution of Filovirus Disease. Emerging Infectious Diseases, 2004. 10: pp. 40-47
20. Brauburger K., Hume A.J., Mühlberger E., Olejnik J. Forty-Five Years of Marburg Virus Research. Viruses, 2012. 4: pp. 1878-1927
21. Jahrling P.B., Marty A.M., Geisbert T.W. Viral Hemorrhagic Fevers. Medical Aspects of Chemical and Biological Warfare. Falls Church: Office of the Surgeon General, Department of the Army, United States of America. 2007. pp. 271-310
22. Sanchez A., Kiley M.P., Holloway B.P., Auperin D.D. Sequence Analysis of the Ebola virus Genome: Organization, Genetic Elements, and Comparison with the Genome of Marburg virus. Virus Research, 1993. 29: pp. 215–240
23. Sanchez A., Khan A.S., Zaki S.R., Nabel G.J., Ksiazek T.G., Peters C.J.. Filoviridae: Marburg and Ebola Viruses. Fields Virology. Fourth Edition. Philadelphia: Lippincott Williams & Wilkins. pp. 2001.
24. Mühlberger E., Lotfering B., Klenk H.D., Becker S. Three of the Four Nucleocapsid Proteins of Marburg Virus, NP, VP35 and L, are Sufficient to Mediate Replication and Transcription of Marburg Virus-Specific Monocistronic Minigenomes. The Journal of Virology, 1998. 72: pp. 8756-8764
25. Takada A., Robison C., Goto H., Anthony Sanchez A., Murti K.G., Whitt M.A., Kawaoka Y. A System for Functional Analysis of Ebola Virus Glycoprotein. Proceedings of the National Academy of Sciences of the United States of America, 1997. 94: pp. 14764–14769
26. Ito H., Watanabe S., Sanchez A., Whitt M.A., Kawaoka Y. Mutational Analysis of the Putative Fusion Domain of Ebola Virus Glycoprotein. The Journal of Virology, 1999. 73: pp. 8907–8912
27. Sanchez A., Yang Z.Y., Xu L., Nabel G.J., Crews T., Peters C.J. Biochemical Analysis of the Secreted and Virion Glycoproteins of Ebola Virus. The Journal of Virology, 1998. 72: pp. 6442–6447
28. Volchkov V.E., Feldmann H., Volchkova V.A., Klenk H-D. Processing of the Ebola Virus Glycoprotein by the Proprotein Convertase Furin. Proceedings of the National Academy of Sciences of the United States of America, 1998. 95: pp. 5762–5767
29. Kolesnikova L., Mühlberger E., Ryabchikova E., Becker S. Ultrastructural organization of recombinant Marburg virus nucleoprotein: comparison with Marburg virus inclusions. Journal of Virology, 2000. 74: pp. 3899-3904.
30. DiCarlo A. Möller P. Lander A. Kolesnikova L. Becker S. Nucleocapsid formation and RNA synthesis of Marburg virus is dependent on two coiled coil motifs in the nucleoprotein. Virology Journal, 2007 4: pp. 105.
31. Bamberg S. Kolesnikova L. Möller P. Klenk H.D. Becker S. VP24 of Marburg virus influences formation of infectious particles.Journal of Virology, 2005. 79: pp. 13421–13433
32. Dolnik O., Kolesnikova L., Stevermann L., Becker S. Tsg101 is recruited by a late domain of the nucleocapsid protein to support budding of Marburg virus-like particles. Journal of Virology, 2010. 84: pp. 7847–7856
33. Modrof J., Mortiz C., Kolesnikova L., Hartlieb B., Randolf A., Muhlberger E., Becker S. Posphorolation of Marburg Virus VP30 at Serines 40 and 42 is critical for its Interaction with NP Inclusions. Virology, 2001. 287: pp. 171-182
34. Fowler T., Bamberg S., Möller P., Klenk H.D., Meyer T.F., Becker S., Rudel T. Inhibition of Marburg virus protein expression and viral release by RNA interference. Journal of General Virology, 2005. 86: pp. 1181–1188
35. Valmas C., Basler C.F. Marburg Virus VP40 Antagonizes Interferon Signaling in a Species-Specific Manner. Journal of Virology, 2011. 85: pp. 4309–4317
36. Jouvenet N., Neil S.J., Zhadina M., Zang T., Kratovac Z., Lee Y., McNatt M., Hatziioannou T., Bieniasz P.D. Broad-spectrum inhibition of retroviral and filoviral particle release by tetherin.Journal of Virology, 2009. 83: pp. 1837–1844
37. Yaddanapudi K., Palacios G., Towner J.S., Chen I., Sariol C.A., Nichol S.T., Lipkin W.I. Implication of a retrovirus-like glycoprotein peptide in the immunopathogenesis of Ebola and Marburg viruses. The Journal of the Federation of American Societies for Experimental Biology Journal (FASEB), 2006. 20: pp. 2519–2530
38. Bosio C.M., Aman M.J., Grogan C., Hogan R., Ruthel G., Negley D., Mohamadzadeh M., Bavari S., Schmaljohn A. Ebola and Marburg Viruses Replicate in Monocyte-derived Dendritic Cells Without Inducing the Production of Cytokines and Full Maturation. The Journal of Infectious Diseases, 2003. 188: pp. 1630–1638
39. Basler C.F., Amarasinghe G.K. Evasion of interferon responses by Ebola and Marburg viruses. Journal of Interferon & Cytokine Research, 2009. 29: pp. 511-520
40. Becker S., Spiess M., Klenk H.D. The Asialoglycoprotein Receptor is a Potential Liver-Specific Receptor for Marburg Virus. Journal of General Virology, 1995. 76: pp. 393–399
41. Chan S.Y., Empig C.J., Welte F.J., Speck R.F., Schmaljohn A., Kreisberg J.F., Goldsmith M.A. Folate Receptor-Alpha is a Cofactor for Cellular Entry by Marburg and Ebola Viruses. Cell, 2001. 106: pp. 117–126
42. Takada A., Fujioka K., Tsuiji M., Morikawa A., Higashi N., Ebihara H., Kobasa D., Feldmann H., Irimura T., Kawaoka Y. Human Macrophage C-type Lectin Specific for Galactose and N-Acetylgalactosamine Promotes Filovirus Entry. The Journal of Virology, 2004. 78: pp. 2943–2947
43. Marzi A., Gramberg T., Simmons G., Moller P., Rennekamp A.J., Krumbiegel M., Geier M., Eisemann J., Turza N., Saunier B., Steinkasserer A., Becker S., Bates P., Hofmann H., Pohlmann S. DC-SIGN and DC-SIGNR Interact with the Glycoprotein of Marburg Virus and S protein of Severe Acute Respiratory Syndrome Coronavirus. The Journal of Virology, 2004. 78: pp. 12090-12095
44. Dolnik O., Kolesnikova L., Becker S. Filoviruses: Interactions with the Host Cell. Cellular and Molecular Life Sciences, 2008. 65: pp. 756-776
45. Conner S.D., Schmid S.L. Regulated Portals of Entry into the Cell. Nature, 2003. pp. 37-44
46. Earp L.J., Delos S.E., Park H.E., White J.M. The Many Mechanism of Viral Membrane Fusion Proteins. Current Topics in Microbiology and Immunology, 2005. 285: pp. 25-66
47. Chandran K., Sullivan N.J., Felbor LI, Whelan S.P., Cunningham I.M. Endosomal Proteolysis of the Ebola Virus Glycoprotein is Necessary for Infection. Science, 2005. 308: pp. 1643-1645
48. Baize S., Leroy E.M., Mavoungou E., Fisher-Hoch S.P. Apoptosis in Fatal Ebola infection. Does the Virus Toll the Bell for Immune System? Apoptosis, 2000. 5: pp. 5-7
49. Sanchez A. Kiley M.P. Identification and Analysis of Ebola Virus Messenger RNA. Virology, 1987. 157: pp.414-420
50. Knipe D.M., Howley P.M. Fields Virology. Volume 1. Philadelphia: Lippincott William & Wilkins. 2007. pp. 1410-1448
51. Bosio C.M., Aman M.J., Grogan C., Hogan R., Ruthel G., Negley D., Mohamadzadeh M., Bavari S., Schmaljohn A. Ebola and Marburg Viruses Replicate in Monocyte-derived Dendritic Cells Without Inducing the Production of Cytokines and Full Maturation. The Journal of Infectious Diseases, 2003. 188: pp. 1630–1638
52. Hemorrhagic Fever Viruses (VHF). Updated January 10, 2008. Retrieved July 24, 2008. Web Site: http://www .upmcbiosecurity.org/website/focus/agents_diseases/fact_sheets/vhf.html
53. Bray M. Defense Against Filoviruses Used as Biological Weapons. Antiviral Research, 2003. 57: pp. 53-60
54. Alibek K. Biohazard. New York: Dell Publishing. 1999. pp. 20, 42
55. Questions and Answer of Marburg Hemorrhagic Fever. Center for Disease Control. Updated August 23, 2007. Retrieved July 24, 2008. Website:http://www.cdc.gov/ncidod/dvrd/spb/mnpages/dispa ges/marburg/qa.htm
56. Borchert M., Muyembe-Tamfum J.J., Colebunders R., Mulangu S., Van der Stuyft P. A Cluster of Marburg Virus Disease Involving and Infant, Short Communication. Tropical Medicine and International Health, 2002. 7: pp. 902-906
57. Borchert M., Mulangu S., Swanepoel R., Libande M.L., Tshomba A., Kulidri A., Muyembe-Tamfum J.J., Van der Stuyft P. Serosurvey on Household Contacts of Marburg Hemorrhagic Fever Patients. Emerging Infectious Diseases, 2006. 12: pp. 433-439
58. Bosio C.M., Aman M.J., Grogan C., Hogan R., Ruthel G., Negley D., Mohamadzadeh M., Bavari S., Schmaljohn A. Ebola and Marburg Viruses Replicate in Monocyte-Derived Dendritic Cells Without Inducing the Production of Cytokins and Full Maturation. Journal of Infectious Diseases, 2003. 188: pp. 1630-1638
59. Feldmann H., Bugany H., Mahner F., Klenk H.D., Drenckhahn D., Schnittler H.J. Filovirus-induced Endothelial Leakage Triggered by Infected Monocytes/Macrophages. The Journal of Virology, 1996. 70: pp. 2208-2214
60. Stroher U., West E., Bugany H., Klenk H.D., Schnittler H.J., Feldmann H. Infection and Activation of Monocyte by Marburg and Ebola Viruses. The Journal of Virology, 2001. 75: pp. 11025-33
61. Mohamadzadeh M., Chen L., Schmaljohn A.L. How Ebola and Marburg Viruses Battle the Immune System. Nature Reviews, 2007. 7: pp. 556-567
62. Khardori N. Bioterrorism Prepardness. Medicine – Pubic Health – Policy. Weinheim: Wiley-VCH Verlag Gmbh & Co. KGaA. 2006. pp. 199-205
63. Hensley L.E., Jones S.M., Feldmann H., Jahrling P.B., Geisbert T.W. Ebola and Marburg Viruses: Pathogenesis and Development of Countermeasures. Current Molecular Medicine, 2005. 5L 761-772
64. Marburg Haemorrhagic Fever – Fact Sheet. World Health Organization. Updated March 31, 2005. Retrieved July 24, 2008. Website: http://www.who.int/csr/disease/marburg/factsheet/en/inde x.html
65. Roberts A., Kemp C. Ebola and Marburg Hemorrhagic Fevers. Journal of the American Academy of Nurse Practitioners, 2001. 13: pp. 291-292
66. Weinstein R.S., Alibek K. Biological and Chemical Terrorism. A Guide for Healthcare Providers and First Responders. New York: Thieme Medical Publishers. 2003. pp. 70-71
67. Drosten C., Gottig S., Schilling S., Asper M., Panning M., Schmitz H., Gunther S. Rapid Detection and Quantification of RNA of Ebola and Marburg Viruses, Lassa Virus, Crimean-Congo Hemorrhagic Fever Virus, Rift Valley Fever Virus, Dengue Virus, and Yellow Fever Virus by Real-Time Reverse Transcription-PCR. Journal of Clinical Microbiology, 2002. 40: pp. 2323-2330
68. Bausch D.G., Nichol S.T., Muyembe-Tamfum J.J., Borchert M., Rollin P.E., Sleurs H., Campbell P., Tshioko F.K., Roth C., Colebunders R., Pirard P., Mardel S., Olinda L.A., Zeller H., Tshomba A., Kulidri A., Libande M.L., Mulangu S., Formenty P., Grein T., Leirs H., Braack L., Ksiazek T., Zaki S., Bowen M.D., Smit S.B., Leman P.A., Burt D.J., Kemp A., Swanepoel R. Marburg Hemorrhagic Fever Associated with Multiple Genetic Lineages of Virus. The New England Journal of Medicine, 2006. 355: pp. 909-919
69. Daddario-DiCaprio K., Geisbert T., Ströher U., Geisbert J., Grolla A., Fritz E., Fernando L., Kagan E., Jahrling P., Hensley L. Postexposure Protection against Marburg Haemorrhagic Fever with Recombinant Vesicular Stomatitis Virus Vectors in Non-human Primates: an Efficacy Assessment. The Lancet , 2006. 367: pp. 1399 - 1404
70. McConnell E.A. Combating Infection. Ebola: Preparing for the worst. Nursing, 2001.31: pp. 30
71. Huggins J.W. Prospects for treatment of viral hemorrhagic fevers with ribavirin, a broad-

spectrum antiviral drug. Review of Infectious Diseases, 1989. 11: pp. S750-761

72.   Sippa N. Defending Against a Deadly Foe. Science News, 2006. 169: pp. 277-278
73.   Grant-Klein R.J., Van Deusen N.M., Badger, C.V., Hannaman D., Dupuy L.C., Schmaljohn C.S. A multiagent filovirus DNA vaccine delivered by intramuscular electroporation completely protects mice from ebola and Marburg virus challenge. Human Vaccines and Immunotherapeutics, 2012. 8: pp. 1703-1706
74.   Tomori O. Ebola: Clinical Features and Public Health Issues. The Philippine Journal of Microbiology and Infectious Diseases, 1996. 25: pp. S8-S15

Photo Bibliography

Figure 1.10-1: Negative stained transmission electron micrograph (TEM) shows a number of Marburg virus virions, which had been grown in an environment of tissue culture cells. The electron photo micrograph was taken by Dr. Erskine Palmer and Dr. Russell Regnery in 1981 and released by the CDC. Public domain photo

Figure 1.10-7: Transmission electron micrograph (TEM) demonstrates numerous Marburg virus virions in a liver tissue sample. Photo was taken in 1975 at 65,000x by Dr. Fred Murphy and released by the CDC. Public domain photo

Figure 1.10-8: Transmission electron micrograph (TEM) of lung tissue from a Marburg patient in Johannesburg, South Africa, 1975. The micrograph reveals the presence of an alveolar hemorrhage in the lung tissue biopsy.Photo was taken at 65,000x by F. A. Murphy and released by the CDC. Public domain photo

Figure 1.10-9: Photomicrograph of hematoxylin & eosin stained liver specimen extracted from a severely MARV infected patient in South Africa. The photomicrograph shows cytoarchitectural changes where many of the hepatocytes are at different stages of acidophilic necrosis. In addition, some cells are evolving into Councilman bodies while many basophilic bodies and early fatty changes are also seen. Photo was taken at 250x by Dr. Yves Robin and Dr. Jean Renaudet of the World Health Organization, Arbovirus Laboratory at the Pasteur Institute in Dakar, Senegal and released by the CDC. Public domain photo

Monkeypox viruses (MPXV) are large brick-shaped (~250 nm by 200 nm), lipid-bilayer enveloped virions, with distinctive surface tubules and a dumbbell-shaped core. MPXV exists in two distinct shapes: "C" capsular or "M" mulberry forms (Figure 1.11-1). MPXV are classified into Central African (also known as Congo Basin) and West African strains, with the former being more virulent in non-human primates. The genome of MPXV is composed of a single linear double-stranded DNA genome (dsDNA; ~191 kb) that possesses highly conserved central region coding for replication and assembly machinery, inverted terminal repeats, and covalently closed hair-pin loops at each end. The large genome of MPXV is estimated to be able to encode nearly 200 proteins.[1, 2, 3]

and in the family *Poxviridae*. Other members of the genus *Orthopoxvirus* are the causative agents of human smallpox (variola), camelpox, and cowpox.[1, 2]

The virus received its name in 1958, when it was first identified in laboratory Cynomolgus monkeys (*Macaca fascicularis*) at a research facility located in Copenhagen, Denmark.[4, 5] In nature, monkeypox is a zoonotic infection, endemic in nonhuman primates, rabbits, and wild rodents, occurring primarily in Central and West Africa. The natural reservoirs of the virus has not been conclusively identified, however, the Gambian rat (*Cricetomys emini*), elephant shrew (*Petrodromus tetradactylus*), Thomas's tree squirrel (*Funisciurus anerythrus*), Kuhl's tree squirrel (*Funisciurus congicus*), the sun squirrel (*Heliosciurus rufobrachium*) and the domestic pig (*Sus scrofa*) (1.11-2) are among the candidates.[6]

C.S. Goldsmith *et al.*
CDC

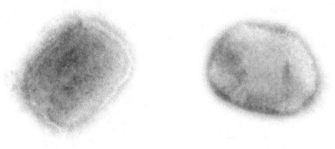

Capsular (C) Form	Mulberry (M) Form

27.500x

Figure 1.11-1: Negative stain electron micrograph showing the two forms of the monkeypox virus. On the left is the capsular (C) form which is sharply defined as a dense core surrounded by several laminated zones of differing density. On the right is the mulberry (M) form which is covered with short, whorled filaments

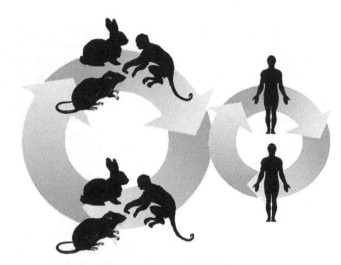

Figure 1.11-2: Sylvatic cycle of Monkeypox (MPXV)

The structure of the MPXV membrane envelope consists of well-defined surface tubules giving it a ribbed appearance. MPXV belongs to the genus *Orthopoxvirus*, subfamily *Chordopoxvirinae*

The first reported case of monkeypox infection in humans

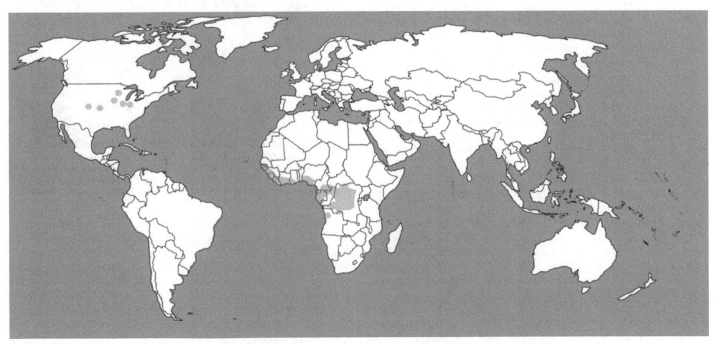

Figure 1.11-3: Distribution of Monkeypox virus (MPXV)

appeared in 1970 in the Democratic Republic of Congo (DRC, formerly Zaire) when a nine month old boy developed smallpox like symptoms, which was later identified as monkeypox.[7] Between 1970 and 1979, a total of 47 MPXV infections occurred, 38 of these cases appearing in the DRC, while the remaining infections emerged in Cameroon, Central African Republic, Cote d'Ivoire, Gabon, Liberia, Nigeria and Sierra Leone. Presently, over 450 cases of human MPXV infections have been documented in DRC.[8, 9] In June 7, 2003, 72 suspected cases of human monkeypox were identified during an outbreak in the United States (Illinois, Indiana, Kansas, Missouri, Ohio, and Wisconsin), of which, 37 cases were laboratory confirmed (Figure 1.11-3).[1,][10] These infections were traced back to infected prairie dogs (Cynomys spp.) that were exposed to infected animals imported from Africa, which were intended to be sold as exotic pets (e.g. Gambian rats, rope squirrels, dormice, etc.).[11, 12] Interestingly, humans were not directly infected by any of the rodents imported from west Africa, but were infected by the prairie dogs that were exposed to the infected African rodents. Presently, it is believed that the prairie dogs acted as amplifying hosts that facilitated the cross species infection.[13]

Initial transmission of MPXV generally occurred as a result of close contact with infected animals. The most common forms of transmission are through bites, sores, blood and contact with feces, and bodily fluids of infected animals.[1, 14] Additionally, there is evidence that indicated respiratory transmission from an infected animal to human was possible.[15] Human to human transmission is considered to be less frequent when compared to smallpox, although it is suspected to occur though exposure to oropharyngeal exudates (e.g. respiratory droplets) after prolonged face-to-face contact or through contact with virus-contaminated objects, such as bedding and/or clothing.[16, 17] Once infected, the incubation period of monkeypox is on average 12 days (ranging between 4 to 20 days).[11]

The incidences of monkeypox infections are equal in both sexes and all ages, however, data have indicated that more than 80% of human monkeypox infections occur in children less than 10 years of age (average age of children affected is 4.4 years).[18, 19]

Person to person transmission is believed to occur two to three days prior to the prodromal phase of the disease or during the appearance of the signature rash.[20] Initially, the virus accumulates at the site of inoculation and is accompanied by local inflammation. During the first week of infection, the virus spreads from the site of first infection where it enters the regional lymph nodes and subsequently spreads throughout the lymphoid organs (e.g. spleen, tonsils and bone marrow), as lymphadenopathy, followed by viremia after days 3 to 14 post infiltration. During this time, the patient will develop the signature rash, which first appears on the mucosa of the mouth and the pharynx, then spreading to the face and the forearms. Eventually, the rash proliferates to the trunk and the legs. [21, 22]

During the second week of the infection (days 8 to 23), the patients' skin erupts with lesions, evolving successively from macules, papules, vesicles, pustules, crusts to scarring (Figure 1.11-4). During this time, foci of inflammation and cellular necrosis have been observed in tonsils, lymph nodes, digestive tract, ovaries, testes, liver, kidneys and lungs. In addition, epithelial degeneration, necrosis and intracytoplasmic bodies have been detected in the mucous membrane and the skin.[22]

It is typical of the Orthopoxvirus genus for the mature virions consist of three types based upon their membrane content and location within or release from the host cell. For example,

the infectious intracellular mature virions (IMV) consist of one or two closely apposed lipoprotein bilayers, which are formed via an undetermined mechanism during an early step in virus particle assembly. [23, 24, 25] It has been shown that a large number of IMVs remain within the cytoplasm of the intact cell and are only released after host cell lysis. Nonetheless, some IMVs have been found to be released through budding.[26, 27] Other IMVs proceeds in obtaining a double membrane envelope via trans-Golgi or endosomal cisternae budding. These "wrapped" IMVs are referred to as intracellular enveloped virions (IEV). They are transported on microtubules to the periphery of the cell, where the outer IEV and plasma membranes fuse and the virion is released from the host cell.[28, 29, 30, 31, 32, 33] These externalized virions (externalized IEVs) contain one additional membrane and are commonly seen adhering to the host cellular surface at the tips of actin-containing microvilli.[34, 35] Some of these IEVs dissociate from the cell and form the last type of Orthopoxvirus virion, known as extracellular enveloped virions (EEV).[36]

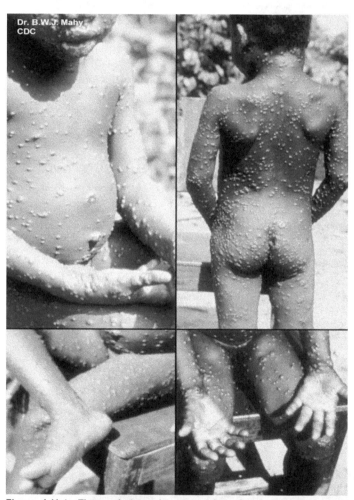

Figure 1.11-4: These photographs were taken during an outbreak of monkeypox, which took place in the Democratic Republic of the Congo (DRC), 1996 to 1997. The pictures demonstrate the characteristic maculopapular monkeypox cutaneous rash on the face, back, feet and hands of a young boy

IMV, IEV and EEV are all infectious, but due to the difference in the membrane coats and surface receptors, they are believed to bind to different cell surface receptors.[37] Research has shown that the initial attachment to the host cell surface is accomplished through interactions between viral ligands, such as A28L proteins, which are anchored to the surface of infectious IMVs and consequently lies beneath the additional membranes of IEV and EEV particles [38] and host cell surface receptors such as chondroitin sulfate or heparan sulfate.[39, 40, 41, 42] Subsequently, the virus is brought into the host cell, however, the manner by which

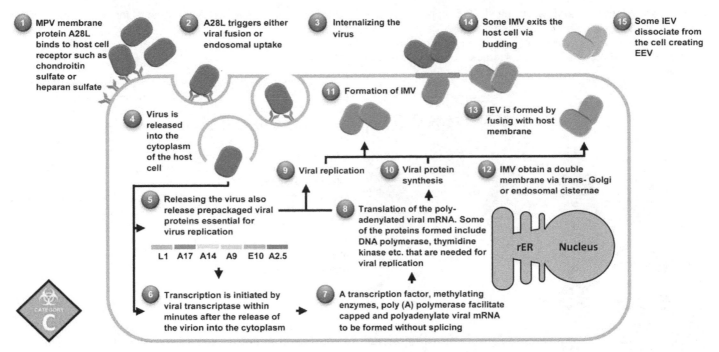

Figure 1.11-5: Diagrammatic process of Monkeypox viral infection within an eukaryotic cell

the virus transverses the host cell membrane is still unclear. Some research suggested that viral entry is mediated by a viral fusion under neutral pH conditions. Other research proposed that the entry is mediated by endosomal uptake through a macropinocytosis-like mechanism that involves actin and low pH-dependent steps.[43, 44]

Once the virus reaches the cytoplasm of the host cell, the prepackaged viral proteins and enzymatic factors that disable cell defenses are released and stimulate expression of the early viral genes.[45, 46, 47] For example, it has been reported that about a dozen viral proteins localized on the IMV membrane are essential for virus replication. These proteins include L1, A17, A14, A9, E10 and A2.5. Experiments have shown that the repression of the synthesis of any of the above proteins prevents or interrupts virion morphogenesis.[48, 49, 50, 51, 52, 53, 54]

Synthesis of early proteins promotes further uncoating, DNA replication, and the production of intermediate transcription factors.[55] Within minutes after infection, after the viral core is released into the cytoplasm, transcription is initiated by the viral transcriptase. A transcription factor, capping and methylating enzymes and poly (A) polymerase, facilitate functional capped and polyadenylated messenger RNA (mRNA) to be formed without splicing. The mRNA allows for the transcription of approximately 100 viral genes. Some of the proteins formed include: DNA polymerase, thymidine kinase and various other enzymes required for genome replication.[55, 56]

Virion assembly occurs in the cytoplasm of the host cell and the IMV moves either to the vicinity of the trans-Golgi network or to early endosomes on microtubules and obtains a double membrane. Subsequently, the double enveloped virus particle moves on microtubules to the cell surface, where the outermost membrane of the virus fuses with the plasma membrane and is released from the host cell via exocytosis. Other non-enveloped viral particles are also formed within the cytoplasm of the host cell, but they are released through the disruption of the host cell membrane rather than through exocytosis. It is known that IMV, IEV and EEV are all infectious, but it is the enveloped virions that are readily taken up by host cells and are considered to be more

important in the spread of the virus throughout the human body (Figure 1.11-5).[56]

Due to the close relationship between monkeypox and smallpox viruses, the potential remains for MPXV to be used as a biological weapon. Monkeypox causes an relatively mild illness in humans and has a low overall case fatality rate. Mathematical models were used to assess the potential for monkeypox as a bio- weapon, human-to-human transmission could not sustain this virus in the population without repeated reintroductions.[57] For this reason, the CDC does not consider monkeypox as a potential biological weapon and it is not listed as a potential biological weapon threat. Nonetheless, as indicated by Alibek (1999), the Soviet Union had weaponized this virus or engineered variant of this virus to be used as a weapon.[58] Therefore, within this text we have listed Monkeypox as a Category C biological weapon, although this virus's actual ranking requires additional investigation.

SYMPTOMS

The development of disease is preceded by a 7 to 17 days (mean 12 days) incubation period. The prodromal phase of the infection consists of rapid onset of flu-like symptoms such as high fever (39-40 °C or 102.2-104 °F), fatigue, severe headache, myalgia, malaise, anorexia, prostration, runny nose, nasal congestion, sore throat (pharyngitis), mouth sores, swollen eyelids and conjunctivitis. Additional symptoms of chills, drenching sweats, general muscular and back pains are commonly observed. Within 2-3 days after the onset of initial symptoms, lymphadenopathy is observed which is especially pronounced in the postauricular, submandibular, cervical or inguinal regions. Pronounced lymphadenopathy, which is not seen in patients suffering from smallpox, is the major symptomatic difference between these infections. Patients generally suffer from a nonproductive cough, bronchopneumonia and experience breathing difficulties. Other symptoms may include nausea, vomiting, diarrhea and dehydration. It has been reported that during the prodromal phase, patients are not considered to be contagious [22, 59, 60, 61]

The prodromal phase is followed by an exanthema (eruptive)

stage (manifestation period), which most often appears initially on the face. The exanthema stage is marked by 1 to 10 days of macular rash, which evolves into papules, blisters, pustules, umbilication, scabbing (after 2 to 4 weeks of infection) and desquamation.[22, 60, 61, 62]

Table 1: An overview of the clinical symptoms of Monkeypox

Symptoms	+	++	+++
Fever			■
Fatigue			■
Severe headache			■
Myalgia			■
Malaise			■
Anorexia			■
Prostration			■
Runny nose			■
Nasal congestion			■
Pharyngitis			■
Mouth sores			■
Swollen eyelids			■
Conjunctivitis			■
ymphadenopathy			■
Cervical lymphadeno.			■
Inguinal lymphadeno.			■
Macular rash			■
Papules			■
Blisters			■
Pustules			■
Umbilication			■
Scabbing			■
Desquamation			■
Chills		■	
Drenching sweats		■	
General muscular pain		■	
Back pain		■	
Nonproductive cough		■	
Bronchopneumonia		■	
Difficulties in breathing		■	
Nausea		■	
Vomiting		■	
Diarrhea		■	
Dehydration		■	
Encephalitis		■	

+ Rare ++ Common +++ Frequent

During development, the pustules may vary in size and can be misdiagnosed as chickenpox. In some reported cases, lesions became ulcerated, generally on the extremities (legs and arms) of the body, although they may also be present on the head (scalp), palms, sole of the feet and the trunk (Figure 1.11-6). Additionally, enanthema, resulting in nonspecific lesions and inflammation of the pharyngeal, conjunctival and genital mucosae has been reported. Lesions have also been reported in the mouth, on the tongue and on the genitalia.[61, 63] Epithelial degeneration, necrosis and intracytoplasmic bodies have been observed in the epidermis and the mucous membrane.[22]

The typical course of infection may last between 2 to 4 weeks and the fatality ranges from 10% to 15%, and generally occur during the second week of infection.[64] Fatalities tend to result from secondary infections, such as extracutaneous manifestations (secondary skin or soft-tissue infections), pneumonitis and ocular complications. Rare cases of encephalitis as a complication from MPXV infection have also been documented.[65, 66] Complete recovery is expected in most patients infected with MPXV, although hypopigmentation and later hyper-pigmentation of lesions, as well as, pitted scars from the destruction of sebaceous glands remain in over 50% of patients for two or more years (Table 1).[22]

DETECTION

Due to the nature of MPXV, the symptoms are similar to various other infections and may pose a problem for accurate clinical diagnosis. For example, MPXV infections are very similar to infections by other orthopox viruses such as chickenpox, herpes simplex virus, cowpox and smallpox (see Tables 3 and 4 for more information). Therefore, it is necessary to couple laboratory tests with clinical diagnosis in order to accurately identify MPXV infection. Electron microscopic examinations of lesions showing keratinocytes containing large numbers of mature and immature virons within the cytoplasm of the cell will signify an Orthopoxvirus infection, but cannot identify the particular species. For example, all Orthopoxvirus virions have the same brick-shaped virion morphology, so further laboratory testing is needed to differentiate one species of Orthopoxvirus from another.[56, 67]

MPXV can be isolated from skin lesions (including scabs), blood serum and/or cerebral spinal fluid. One of the most common methods of identifying MPXV particles is through immunohistochemistry using commercially available anti-monkeypox virus antibodies.[12] Serologic testing is also used to detect anti-monkeypox IgM and IgG through enzyme linked immunoassay (ELISA) via blood serum and cerebral spinal fluid (CSF) samples from patients.[56]

Specific species of Orthopoxvirus possess distinctive DNA maps. Therefore, the most accurate tests for MPXV infection are real-time and standard polymerase chain reaction (PCR) assays. PCR is capable of specific amplification of various viral genome DNA segments, followed by restriction endonuclease assays of the amplicons.[55] Another PCR method utilizes primers to target the gene sequence encoding the hemagglutinin glycoprotein which is unique to each species of Orthopoxvirus.[68, 69, 70] Additional PCR protocol targets the genes for the A-type inclusion body protein, as well as, DNA oligonucleotide microarray utilizing crmB, a cytokine response modifier (a TNF receptor homologue produced by Orthopoxvirus) gene, as the primary target has shown promise as a method of identifying the specific pox virus responsible for the infection.[71, 72]

TREATMENT

MPXV infections are generally self-limiting and medical treatment involves supportive therapies (maintenance of fluid and electrolyte balance), and the prevention and treatment of secondary infections. Although there are no FDA approved treatments for MPXV infections, there are a few potential options that may prove to be beneficial to patients suffering from the disease.[56]

Ribavirin, an antiviral compound designed to inhibit inosine monophosphate dehydrogenase, has been suggested as one possible treatment.[56] A second antiviral compound, cidofovir, used in the treatment for adverse effects of smallpox vaccinations, as well as, treating patients with HIV, suffering from cytomegalovirus retinitis, has been suggested as another treatment protocol.[73] Cidofovir (also known as Vitide or hydroxypropyl methylcellose phthalate- HPMPC), is a nucleotide analog, designed to selectively inhibit the production of viral DNA in various orthopoxvirus.[61] Cidofovir must be administered intravenously accompanied by probenecid and intravenous fluid hydration to avoid renal toxicity.[19] In an experiment performed by Stittelaar et al. (2006), using macaque monkeys challenged

Table 2: Clinical feature comparison between orthopoxvirus infections[65]

Disease Characteristics	Monkeypox	Smallpox	Chickenpox
Recent contact with exotic animals	Yes	No	No
Recent exposure to patients with vascular rash	Possible	Yes	Yes
Previous vaccination against smallpox	10-15%	Rare	Yes
Incubation periods (days)	10-14	10-14	14-16
Prodromal phase (days)	1-3	2-4	0-2

Table 3: Clinical feature comparison between orthopoxvirus infections[65]

Physical Examination	Monkeypox	Smallpox	Chickenpox
Prodromal fever and malaise	Yes	Yes	Yes (mild)
Lymphadenopathy	Yes	No	No
Centrifugal distribution of skin lesions	80%	100%	0%
Centripedal distribution of skin lesions	5%	0%	100%
Depth of skin lesions	Superficial	Deep	Superficial
Monomorphic evolution of skin lesions	80%	100%	0%
Pleiomorphic evolution of skin lesions	20%	0%	100%
Desquamation (days after onset)	22-24	14-21	6-14
Lesions on the palms and soles	Common	Common	Rare

with lethal doses of MPXV, cidofovir along with an experimental antiviral medication called HPMPO-DAPy, reduced the mortality rate in the infected experimental animals.[74] Presently, an oral form of Cidofovir is under development and has demonstrated some promise in laboratory tests in orthopoxvirus infected mice.[75]

The smallpox vaccine has been reported to afford protection against MPXV infections or drastically reduce the severity of infection.[60, 76] It is reported by Jezek et al. (1987), that patients requiring intensive care were more common in nonvaccinated (73.9%) than in vaccinated (39.5%) patients.[70] There are many different smallpox vaccines available, under many different names. One common vaccine, Dryvax (NYCBOH vaccine - calf-lymph vaccine), is administered intraepidermally by bifurcated needle (15 perpendicular insertions within a 5mm area) and has been suggested to be helpful in preventing MPXV infections.[62] Mukinda et al. (1996), reported that vaccination for smallpox 3-19 days prior to MPXV exposure is approximately 85% effective in preventing the infection.[77, 78]

DIFFERENTIAL DIAGNOSIS

As mentioned previously, the clinical presentation of MPXV infection is very similar to that of chickenpox and that of smallpox,

Table 4: Differential diagnosis of Monkeypox and other related diseases. Differential diagnosis includes: chickenpox (CP), smallpox (SP), Cowpox (COP), Genital herpes (GP), shingles and measles

Symptoms	MPXV	CP	SP	COP	GP	Shingles	Measles
Fever	■	■	■	■	■	■	■
Chills	■	■	■	■		■	
Fatigue	■	■	■	■	■	■	■
Severe headache	■	■	■	■	■	■	
Myalgia	■	■	■	■	■		■
Malaise	■	■	■	■	■		■
Anorexia	■	■	■	■	■		
Nausea	■	■	■				■
Vomiting	■	■	■				
Diarrhea			■				
Prostration			■				
Runny nose	■	■					■
Nasal congestion	■						■
Sore throat (pharyngitis)	■				■		■
Mouth sores	■		■				
Swollen eyelids	■		■				
Conjunctivitis	■		■				■
Lymphadenopathy	■						
Macular rash	■	■	■	■	■	■	■
Papules	■	■	■	■	■	■	
Blisters	■	■	■	■	■	■	
Pustules	■	■	■	■	■	■	
Umbilication	■		■	■			
Scabbing	■	■	■	■	■	■	
Desquamation	■	■	■	■		■	
Drenching sweats	■		■				
General muscular pain	■	■	■	■	■		■
Nonproductive cough	■						■
Bronchopneumonia	■						■
Difficulties in breathing	■				■		■
Encephalitis	■		■				■

cowpox, and herpes simplex viruses I and II. In addition, diseases such as orf and bovine stomatitis (caused by parapoxviruses) can produce localized skin lesions that are similar in appearance to that of MPXV infected patients and may initially confuse diagnosis. Therefore, definitive diagnosis of MPXV requires laboratory confirmation such as electron microscopy, PCR, IgM and IgG ELISA, immunofluorescent antibody assay, and histopathologic analysis. Please examine Tables 2, 3 and 4 for more information.

References

1. Monkeypox Backgrounder. American Veterinary Medical Association. January 18, 2007. Retrieved March 30, 2010. Website:http://www.avma.org/reference/backgrounders/monkeypox_backgrounder.pdf
2. Shetty N., Tang J.W., Andrews J. Infectious Sisease: Pathogenesis, Prevention and Case Studies. Hoboken: Wiley-Blackwell Publishing. 2009. pp. 568-571
3. Kugelman J.R., Johnston S.C., Mulembakani P.M., Kisalu N., Lee M.S., Koroleva G., McCarthy S.E., Gestole M.C., Wolfe N.D., Fair J.N., Schneider B.S., Wright L.L., Huggins J., Whitehouse C.A., Wemakoy E.O., Muyembe-Tamfum J.J., Hensley L.E., Palacios G.F., Rimoin A.W. Genomic Variability of Monkeypox Virus among Humans, Democratic Republic of the Congo. Emerging Infectious Diseases, 2014. 20: 232-239
4. Von Magnus P., Anderson E.K., Peterson K.B., Birch-Anderson A. A Pox-Like Disease in Cynomolgus Monkeys. Acta Pathologica et Microbiologica Scandinavica, 1959. 46: pp. 156-176
5. Gillette B. Monkeypox Outbreak Lessons: More Awareness, Funding Needed. Dermatology Times, 2006. 27: pp. 46-47
6. Hutin Y., Williams R., Malfait P., Pebody R., Loparev V.N., Ropp S.L. Outbreak of Human Monkeypox, Democratic Republic of Congo, 1996 to 1997. Emerging Infectious Diseases, 2001. 7: pp. 434-438
7. Ladnyj I.D., Ziegler P., Kima E. A Human Infection Caused by Monkeypox Virus in Basankusu Territory, Democratic Republic of Congo.. Bulletin of the World Health Organization, 1972. 46: pp. 593-597
8. Breman J., Kalisa-Ruti M., Steniowski V., Zanotto E., Gromyko A., Arita I. Human Monkeypox, 1970-1979. Bulletin of the World Health Organization, 1980. 46: pp. 165-182
9. Hutin Y.J.F., Williams R.J., Malfait P., Pebody R.L., Vladamir N., Ropp S.L., Rodriguez, M, Knight J.C., Tshioko, F.K., Khan A.S., Szczeniowski M.V., Esposito J.J. Outbreak of Human Monkeypox, Democratic Republic of Congo, 1996-1997 (Statistical Data Included). Emerging Infectious Diseases, 2001. 7: pp. 434-438
10. Snow M. On Alert for Monkeypox. Nursing, 2005. 35: pp. 1
11. Melski J., Reed K., Stratman E., Graham M.B., Fairley J., Edmiston C., Kehl K.S., Foldy S.L., Swain G.R., Biedrzycki P., Gieryn D., Ernst K., Schier D., Tomasello C., Ove J., Rausch D., Healy-Haney N., Kreuser N., Wegner M.V., Kazmierczak J.J., Williams C., Bostrom H.H., Davis J.P., Ehlenfeldt R., Kirk C., Dworkin M., Conover C., Teclaw R., Messersmith H., Sotir M.J., Huhn G., Fleischauer A.T. Multistate Outbreak of Monkeypox – Illinois, Indiana, and Wisconsin, 2003. Center for Disease Control and Prevention (CDC). Morbidity and Mortality Weekly Report, 2003. 52: pp. 537-540
12. Guarner J., Johnson B., Paddock C., Shieh W-J., Goldsmith C.S., Reynolds M.G., Damon I.K., Regnery R.L., Zaki S.R. Monkeypox Transmission and Pathogenesis in Prairie Dogs. Emerging Infectious Diseases, 2004. 10: pp. 426-431
13. Parker S., Buller R.M. A review of experimental and natural infections of animals with monkeypox virus between 1958 and 2012. Future virology, 2013. 8: pp. 129–157
14. Reynolds M.G., Davidson W.B., Curns A.T., Conover C.S., Huhn G., Davis J., Wegner M., Croft D.R., Newman A., Obiesie N.N., Hansen G.R., Hays P.L., Pontones P., Beard B., Teclaw R., Howell J.F., Braden Z., Holman R.C., Karem K.L., Damon I.K. Spectrum of Infection and Risk Factor for Human Monkeypox, United States, 2003. Emerging Infectious Diseases, 2007. 13: pp. 1332-1339
15. Hammarlund E., Lewis M.W., Carter S.V., Amanna I., Hansen S.G., Strelow L.I., Wong S.W., Yoshihara P., Hanifin J.M., Slifka M.K. Multiple diagnostic techniques identify previously vaccinated individuals with protective immunity against monkeypox. Nature Medicine, 2005. 11: pp. 1005–1011.
16. Rimoin A.W., Kisalu N., Kebela-Ilunga B., Mukaba T., Wright L.L., Formenty P., Wolfe N.D., Shongo R.L., Tshioko F., Okitolonda E., Muyembe J.J., Ryder R.W., Meyers H. Endemic Human Monkeypox, Democratic Republic of Congo, 2001-2004. Emerging Infectious Diseases, 2007. 13: pp. 934-937
17. Fleischauer A.T., Kile J.C., Davidson M., Fischer M., Karem K.L., Teclaw R., Messersmith H., Pontones P., Beard B.A., Braden Z.H., Cono J., Sejvar J.J., Khan A.S., Damon I., Kuehnert M.J. Evaluation of Human-to-Human Transmission of Monkeypox from Infected Patients to Health Care Workers. Clinical Infectious Diseases, 2005. 40: pp. 689-694
18. Jezek Z., Szczeniowski M., Paluku K.M., Mutombo M. Human Monkeypox: Clinical Features of 282 Patients. The Journal of Infectious Diseases, 1987. 156: pp. 293-298
19. Nalca A., Rimoin A.W., Bavari S., Whitehouse C.A. Reemergence of Monkeypox: Prevalence, Diagnostics and Countermeasures. Clinical Infectious Diseases, 2005. 41: pp. 1765-1771
20. Fenner F. Fields Virology – Poxviruses Third edition. Philadelphia: Lippincott-Raven Press. 1996. pp. 2693-2702
21. Shchelkunov S.N., Marennikova S.S., Moyer R.W. Orthopoxviruses Pathogenic for Humans. New York: Springer Science and Business Media. 2005. pp. 166-168
22. Breman J.G. Monkeypox: An Emerging Infection for Humans? Emerging Infections 4. Chapter 5. Washington D.C.: American Society for Microbiology (ASM) Press. 2000. pp. 45-67
23. Hollinshead M., Vanderplasschen A., Smith G.L., Vaux D.J. Vaccinia Virus Intracellular Mature Virions Contain only One Lipid Membrane. Journal of Viology, 1999. 73: pp. 1503-1517
24. Risco C., Rodriguez J.R., Lopez-Iglesias C., Carrascosa J.L., Esteban M., Rodriguez D. Endoplasmic Reticulum-Golgi Intermediate Compartment Membranes and Vimentin Filaments Participate in Vaccinia Virus Assembly. Journal of Viology, 2002. 76: pp. 1839-1855
25. Sodeik B., Doms R.W., Ericsson M., Hiller G., Machamer C.E., van't Hof W., van Meer G., Moss B., Griffiths G. Assembly of Vaccinia Virus: Role of the Intermediate Compartment Between the Endoplasmic Reticulum and the Golgi Stacks. The Journal of Cell Biology, 1993. 121: pp. 521-541
26. Meiser A., Sancho C., Krijnse Locker J. Plasma Membrane Budding as an Alternative Release Mechanism of the Extracellular Enveloped Form of Vaccinia Virus from HeLa Cells. Journal of Viology, 2003. 77: pp. 9931-9942
27. Tsutsui K. Release of Vaccinia Virus from FL Cells Infected with the IHD-W Strain. Journal of Electron Microscopy, 1983. 32: pp. 125-140
28. Hiller G., Weber K. Golgi-Derived Membranes that Contain an Acylated Viral Polypeptide are Used for Envelopment. Journal of Viology, 1985. 55: pp. 651-659
29. Schmelz M., Sodeik B., Ericsson M., Wolffe E.J., Shida H., Hiller G., Griffiths G. Assembly of Vaccinia Virus: the Second Wrapping Cisterna is Derived from the Trans-Golgi Network. Journal of viology, 1994. 68: pp. 130-147
30. Tooze J., Hollinshead M., Reis B., Radsak K., Kern H. Progeny Vaccinia and Human Cytomegalovirus Particles Utilize Early Endosomal Cisternae for Their Envelopes. European Journal of Cell Biology, 1993. 60: pp. 163-178
31. Geada M. M., Galindo I., Lorenzo M.M., Perdiguero B., Blasco R. Movements of Vaccinia Virus Intracellular Enveloped Virions with GFP Tagged to the F13L Envelope Protein. Journal of General Viology, 2001. 82: pp. 2747-2760
32. Hollinshead M., Rodger G., Van Eijl H., Law M., Hollinshead R., Vaux D.J., Smith G.L. Vaccinia Virus Utilizes Microtubules for Movement to the Cell Surface. The Journal of Cell Biology, 2001. 154: pp. 389-402
33. Rietdorf J., Ploubidou A., Reckmann I., Holmström A., Frischknecht F., Zettl M., Zimmerman T., Way M. Kinesin-Dependent Movement on Microtubules Precedes Actin Based Motility of Vaccinia Virus. Nature Cell Biology, 2001. 3: pp. 992-1000
34. Blasco R., Moss B. Role of Cell-Associated Enveloped Vaccinia Virus in Cell-to-Cell Spread. Journal of Viology, 1992. 66: pp. 4170-4179
35. Stokes G. V. High-Voltage Electron Microscope Study of the Release of Vaccinia Virus from Whole Cells. Journal of Viology, 1976. 18: pp. 636-643
36. Boulter E. A., Appleyard G. Differences Between Extracellular and Intracellular Forms of Poxvirus and Their Implications. Progress in Medical Virology, 1973. 16: pp. 86-108
37. Vanderplasschen A., Smith G.L. A Novel Virus Binding Assay Using Confocal Microscopy: Demonstration that Intracellular and Extracellular Vaccinia Virions Bind to Different Cellular Receptors. Journal of Viology, 1997. 71: pp. 4032-4041
38. Senkevich T.G., Ward B.M., Moss B. Vaccinia Virus Entry into Cells Is Dependent on a Virion Surface Protein Encoded by the A28L Gene. Journal of Virology, 2004. 78: pp. 2357-2366
39. Carter G.C., Law M., Hollinshead M., Smith G.L. Entry of the Vaccinia Virus Intracellular Mature Virion and its Interactions with Glycosaminoglycans. Journal of General Viology, 2005. 86: pp.1279-1290
40. Hsiao J.C., Chung C.S., Chang W. Vaccinia Virus Envelope D8L Protein Binds to Cell Surface Chondroitin Sulfate and Mediates the Absorption of Intracellular Mature Virions to Cells. Journal of Viology, 1999. 73: pp. 8750-8761
41. Chung C.S., Hsiao J.C., Chang Y.S., Chang W. A27L Protein Mediates Vaccinia Virus Interaction with Cell Surface Heparan Sulfate. Journal of Viology, 1998. 72: pp. 1577-1585
42. Lin C.L., Chung C.S., Heine H.G., Chang W. Vaccinia Virus Envelope H3L Protein Binds to Cell Surface Heparan Sulfate and is Important for Intracellular Mature Virion Morphogenesis and Virus Infection In Vitro and In Vivo. Journal of Viology, 2000. 74: pp. 3353-3365
43. Abdulnaser A., Hammamieh R., Hardick J., Ait Ichou M., Jett M., Ibrahim S. Gene Expression Profiling of Monkeypox Virus-Infected Cells Reveals Novel Interfaces for Host-Virus Interactions. Virology Journal, 2010. 7: pp. 173-191
44. Vanderplasschen A., Hollinshead M., Smith G.L. Intracellular and Extracellular Vaccinia Virions Enter Cells by Different Mechanisms. J Gen Virol 1998, 79(Pt 4):877-887
45. Munyon W., Paoletti E., Grace J.T. Jr: RNA Polymerase Activity in Purified Infectious Vaccinia Virus. Proceedings of the National Academy of Sciences United States of America, 1967. 58: pp. 2280-2287
46. Kates J.R., McAuslan B.R. Poxvirus DNA-Dependent RNA Polymerase. Proceedings of the National Academy of Sciences United States of America, 1967, 58: pp. 134-141
47. Da Fonseca F., Moss B. Poxvirus DNA Topoisomerase Knockout Mutant Exhibits Decreased Infectivity Associated with Reduced Early Transcription. Proceedings of the National Academy of Sciences United States of America, 2003. 100: pp. 11291-11296
48. Ravanello M. P., Hruby D.E. Conditional Lethal Expression of the Vaccinia Virus L1R Myristylated Protein Reveals a Role in Virus Assembly. Journal of Viology, 1994. 68: pp. 6401-6410
49. Rodríguez D., Esteban M., Rodríguez J.R. Vaccinia Virus A17L Gene Product is Essential for an Early Step in Virion Morphogenesis. Journal of Viology, 1995. 69: pp. 4640-4648
50. Yuwen H., Cox J.H., Yewdell J.W., Bennink J.R., Moss B. Nuclear Localization of a Double-Stranded RNA-Binding Protein Encoded by the Vaccinia Virus E3l Gene. Virology, 1993. 195: pp. 732-744
51. Rodriguez J. R., Risco C., Carrascosa J.L., Esteban M., Rodriguez D. Vaccinia Virus 15-Kilodalton (A14L) Protein is Essential for Assembly and Attachment of Viral Crescents to Virosomes. Journal of Viology, 1998. 72: pp. 1287-1296
52. Yeh W.W., Moss B., Wolffe E.J. The Vaccinia Virus A9 Gene Encodes a Membrane Protein Required for an Early Step in Virion Morphogenesis. Journal of Viology, 2000. 74: pp. 9701-9711
53. Senkevich T. G., Weisberg A., Moss B. Vaccinia Virus E10R Protein is Associated with the Membranes of Intracellular Mature Virions and has a Role in Morphogenesis. Virology, 2000. 278: pp. 244-252
54. Senkevich T., White C., Weisberg A., Granek J., Wolffe E., Koonin E., Moss B. Expression of the Vaccinia Virus A2.5L Redox Protein is Required for Virion Morphogenesis. Virology, 2002. 300: pp. 296-303
55. White D.O., Fenner F.J. Medical Virology. San Diego: Academic Press. 1994. pp. 31-52
56. Guerrant R.L., Walker D.H., Weller P.F. Tropical Infectious Diseases – Principles, Pathogens & Practice. Volume 1. Philadelphia: Churchill Livingstone Elsevier. 2006. pp. 621-636
57. Monkeypox backgrounder. American Vetenary Medical Association. January 18, 2007. Retrieved July 25, 2008. Web site: http://www.avma.org/reference/backgrounders/monkeypox_backgrounder.pdf
58. Alibek K. Biohazard. New York: Dell Publishing. 1999. pp.133
59. Reynolds M.G., Yorita K.L., Kuehnert M.J., Davidson W.B., Huhn G.D., Holman R.C., Damon I.K. Clinical Manifestations of Human Monkeypox Influenced by Route of Infection. The Journal of Infectious Diseases, 2006. 194: pp. 773-780
60. Basic Information about Monkeypox. Center for Disease Control and Prevention. Revised September 8, 2008. Retrieved April 1, 2010. Web Site: http://www.cdc.gov/ncidod/monkeypox/factsheet .htm
61. Bioterrorism and Emerging Infections Education. University of Alabama at Birmingham. Retrieved April 1, 2010. Website: http://www.bioterrorismuab.ahrq.gov/EI/monkeypox/Monkeypox.pdf
62. Sejvar J.J., Chowdary Y., Schomogyi M., Stevens J., Patel J., Karem K., Fischer M., Kuehnert M.J., Zaki S.R., Paddock C.D., Guarner J., Shieh W-J., Patton J.L., Bernard N., Li Y., Olson V.A., Kline R.L., Loparev V.N., Schmid D.S., Beard B., Regnery R.R., Damon I.K.. Human Monkeypox Infection: A Family Cluster in the Midwestern United States. The Journal of Infectious Diseases, 2004. 190: pp. 1833-1840
63. Peterson M.W., Graham M.B., Fairley J., Gunkel J. Monkeypox. eMedicine. Revised April 11, 2006. Retrieved September 1, 2008. Website: http://www.emedicine.com /derm/

topic937.htm

64. Guerrant R.L., Walker D.H., Weller P.F. Tropical Infectious Diseases – Principles, Pathogens & Practice. Volume 1. Philadelphia: Churchill Livingstone Elsevier. 2006. pp. 621

65. Di Giulio D.B., Eckburg P.B. Human Monkeypox: an Emerging Zoonosis. The Lancet Infectious Diseases, 2004. 4: pp. 15-25

66. Jezek Z., Szczeniowski M., Plauku M., Putombo M., Grab B. Human Monkeypox: Clinical Features of 282 Patients. The Journal of Infectious Diseases, 1987. 156: pp. 293–298

67. Bayer-Garner I.B. Monkeypox Virus: Histologic, Immunohistochemical and Electron-microscopic Findings. Journal of Cutaneous Pathology, 2005. 32: pp. 28-34

68. Ropp S.L., Jin Q., Knight J.C., Massung R.F., Esposito J.J. PCR Strategy for Identification and Differentiation of Small Pox and Other Orthopoxviruses. Journal of Clinical Microbiology, 1995. 33: pp. 2069-2076

69. Shchelkunov S., Totmenin A., Safronov P., Shchelkunov S.N., Totmenin A.V., Safronov P.F., Mikheev M.V., Gutorov V.V., Ryazankina O.I., Petrov N.A., Babkin I.V., Uvarova E.A., Sandakhchiev L.S., Sisler J.R., Esposito J.J., Damon I.K., Jahrling P.B., Moss B. Analysis of the Monkeypox Genome. Virology, 2002. 297: pp. 172-194

70. Jezek Z., Marennikova S., Mutumbo M., Nakano J., Paluku K., Szczeniowski M. Human Monkeypox: a Study of 2,510 Contacts of 214 Patients. The Journal of Infectious Diseases, 1986. 154: pp. 551–555

71. Lapa S., Mikheev M., Shchelkunov S., Mikhailovich V., Sobolev A., Blinov V., Babkin I., Guskov A., Sokunova E., Zasedatelev A., Sandakhchiev L., Mirzabekov A. Species-level Identification of Othropoxviruses with an Oligonucleotide Microchip. Journal of Clinical Microbiology, 2002. 40: pp. 753-757

72. Weaver J.R., Isaacs S.N. Monkeypox virus and insights into its immunomodulatory proteins. Immunological Reviews, 2008. 225: pp. 96–113

73. Guerrant R.L., Walker D.H., Weller P.F. Tropical Infectious Diseases – Principles, Pathogens & Practice. Volume 1. Philadelphia: Churchill Livingstone Elsevier. 2006. pp. 628.

74. De Clercq E. Cidofovir in the Treatment of Poxvirus Infections. Antiviral Research, 2002. 55: pp. 1-13

75. Stittelaar K.J., Neyts J., Naesens L., van Amerongen G., van Lavieren R.F., Holy A., De Clercq E., Neisters H.G.M., Fries E., Maas C., Mulder P.G.H., van der Zeijst B.A.M., Osterhaus A.D.M.E. Antiviral Treatment is more Effective than Smallpox Vaccination upon Lethal Monkeypox Virus Infection. Nature, 2006. 439: pp. 745-748

76. Quenelle D.C., Collins D.J., Wan W.B., Beadle J.R., Hostetler K.Y., Kern E.R. Oral Treatment of Cowpox and Vaccina Virus Infections in Mice with Ether Lipid Esters of Cidofovir. Antimicrob Agents and Chemotherapy, 2004. 48: pp. 404-412

77. Downie A., McCarthy K. The Viruses of Variola, Vaccina, Cowpox and Ectromelia: Neutralization Tests on the Chorio-allantois with Unabsorbed and Absorbed Immune Sera. The British Journal of Experimental Pathology, 1950. 31: pp. 789–796

78. Mukinda V.K., Mweme G., Kilundu M., Heymann D.L., Khan A.S., Esposito J.J. Re-emergence of Human Monkeypox in Zaire in 1996. The Lancet, 1997. 349: pp. 1449-1450

Photo Bibliography

Figure 1.11-1: Negative stained electron micrograph showing the two forms of the monkeypox virus. On the left is the capsular (C) form which is sharply defined, dense core surrounded by several laminated zones of differing density. On the right is the mulberry (M) from which is covered with short, whorled filaments. Electron micrograph photo was taken by Cynthia S. Goldsmith, Inger K. Damon, and Sherif R. Zaki in 2003 and released by the CDC. Public domain photo

Figure 1.11-4: These photographs were taken during an outbreak of monkeypox, which took place in the Democratic Republic of the Congo (DRC), 1996 to 1997. The pictures demonstrate the characteristic maculopapular cutaneous monkeypox rash on the face, back, feet and hands of a young boy. Photograph was taken by Dr. B.W.J. Mahy of the World Health Organization (WHO) and was released by the CDC. Public domain photo

Rift Valley Fever virus (RVFV) is an enveloped virion with a trisegmented, single stranded RNA genome (Figure 1.12-1). RVFV belongs to the genus *Phlebovirus* of the family *Bunyaviridae*.[1]

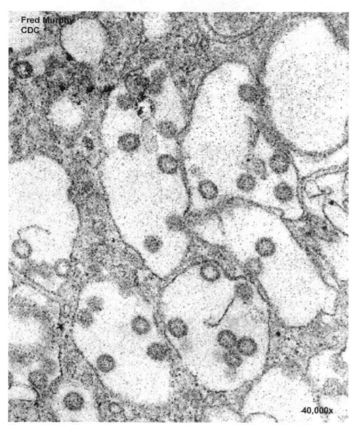

Figure 1.12-1: Transmission electron micrograph (TEM) of Rift Valley Fever Virus particle in mouse liver cell

RVFV is a zoonotic, arthropod-borne infection that causes Rift Valley Fever (RVF). RVF occurs primarily in domestic animals, mainly sheep, cattle and goats, but also affects humans (Figure 1.12-2).[2] RVF is characterized by high mortality rates in young animals and can cause spontaneous abortions in pregnant ruminants.[3] RVFV was first isolated in 1930 at Rift Valley, Kenya (Lake Naivasha), during an enzootic epidemic of fatal hepatic necrosis (hepatitis) and spontaneous abortion in sheep.[4] During 1977, RVFV caused an epidemic in 200,000 people, reportedly resulting in the deaths of 598 individuals in the Nile River Delta and Valley of Egypt.[5] In 1987 and 1988, RVFV caused an epidemic in the Islamic Republic of Mauritania, involving approximately 1200 people.[6] During 1993 and 1994, a simultaneous outbreak of RVF occurred in Egypt, Zimbabwe and Senegal involving 600-1500 individuals.[7] In 1997, an outbreak of this disease among ruminants appeared in Egypt but fortunately no human infections were reported.[8] Between 1997 and 1998, the RVFV occurred in Kenya, where an estimated 89,000 people were infected resulting in 478 fatalities.[9] In 2000, an outbreak was reported on the Red Sea Coast of Saudi Arabia and Yemen with 800 and 1000 reported cases respectively.[10] In 2003, another simultaneous outbreak of RVF occurred in Egypt and Mauritania that resulted in a total of 375 reported human cases.[7] Between November 2006 to May 2007, World Health Organization (WHO) reported a total of 1663 cases of RVF in Kenya, Tanzania, Somalia and Sudan (Figure 1.12-2, Table 1).[11, 12]

Table 1: Cases of RVF and fatality ratio of RVF between November 2006 to May 2007

Location	Cases of RVF	Fatalities	Case Fatality
Kenya	684	155	23%
Tanzania	264	109	41%
Somalia	114	51	45%
Sudan	601	211	35%

In 2010, a total of 30 laboratory-confirmed human cases were recorded in Mauritania, of which three fatalities were reported. During that same year an outbreak among ruminants appeared in South Africa, fortunately no human cases were reported.[13, 14] Finally, in 2012, another outbreak occurred in Mauritania. A total of 41 human cases were confirmed which resulted in 13 fatalities.[15]

RVFV has been isolated in 23 species of mosquitoes[16] belonging to 5 different genera: *Culex*, *Anopheles*, *Eretmapodites*, *Mansonia* and *Aedes*. Although, other biting insects such as midgets, flies and ticks (e.g. *Culicoides* spp., *Simulium* spp., *Rhipicephalus* spp. etc.) are also suspected vectors.[2, 3] The assumption that mosquitoes as the main vector for spreading the disease among livestock is supported by the fact that livestock epizootics occurs after heavy rainfall and flooding, when there is a peak in the mosquito population.[17]

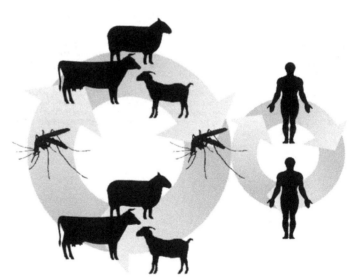

Figure 1.12-2: Sylvatic cycle of Rift Valley Fever Virus

Transmission of RVFV to humans occurs through direct exposure via arthropod bites, aerosolized virions, contaminated blood, tissue and bodily fluids.[2] Additionally, RVFV have also been detected in raw milk which could indicate that transmission of the disease through ingestion is another possibility. Furthermore, RVFV is also found in human semen, thus sexual transmission of the disease may also be possible.[18] Once infected, the incubation period in humans is approximately two to six days before the onset of symptoms.[19]

RVFV particles measure 90 to 110 nm in diameter and are surrounded by a lipid envelope containing G_N and G_C glycoproteins, which form membrane surface subunits. These subunits are 5 to 8 nm in length and regularly arranged.[20, 21] Corresponding to each of the three genomic segments (L, M and S), are viral ribonucleoproteins (RNP) in a pseudo-helical

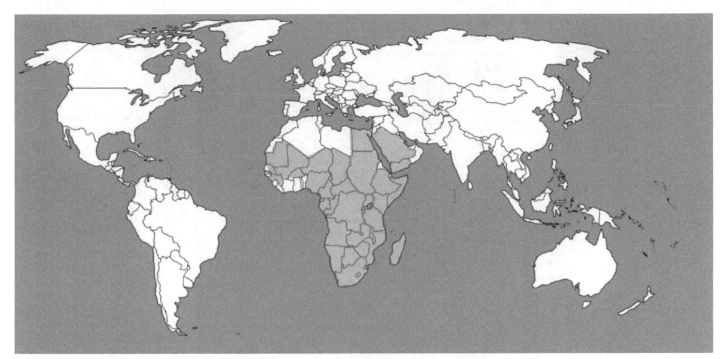

Figure 1.12-3: Distribution of Rift Valley Fever Virus (RVFV). The map shows both human & livestock outbreaks

arrangement. RNP are associated with numerous copies of the nucleoprotein (N) and the RNA dependent RNA polymerase (L) which are packaged into the virion.[20, 21]

During natural transmission cycle of RVFV, the virus is introduced into an individual through arthropod bites, and the dermal dendritic cells (DCs) are the first immunological cell to encounter the incoming virus. Located throughout the cellular surface of DCs are the DC-specific intercellular adhesion molecule 3-grabbing nonintegrin (DC-SIGN), a C-type lectin receptors that are exploited by the viral G_N and G_C glycoproteins to gain entry into the host cell. It has been reported that other cell lines possessing DC-SIGN such as macrophages, endothelial cells in liver and lymph nodes, etc. are also susceptible to early infection. DC-SIGN is a type II membrane protein that binds to a high-mannose N-glycans of the viral glycol-proteins G_N and G_C through their C-terminal carbohydrate recognition domain (CDR). Once the RVFV attaches to the host cell surface via a few DC-SIGN receptors, the virus proceeds through a process known as "receptor recruitment," where it gathers more DC-SIGNs to the virus surface, generating a receptor-rich microdomain. This microdomain is required to activate a signaling pathway that triggers the endocytotic uptake of the receptor cluster and the virus particle.[22, 23, 24]

Recent research has indicated that the DC-SIGN microdomain triggers clathrin-mediated endo-cytosis in order for the RVFV particles to gain entry into the host cell.[22, 23, 24] Within 5-10 minutes after internalization, RVFV separates from DC-SIGN receptors within the endosome via acid-induced disassembly (pH below 6.5 - 6.7). Subsequently the encapsulated genome is released into the cytoplasm. Once the encapsulated RVFV enters the cytoplasm of the host cell, virus immediately replicates and encodes for proteins. In Vero cells, RVFV has been shown to complete the reproductive cycle within 13 hours.[25, 26]

The genome of the RVFV consists of large (L), medium (M) and small (S) segments. The L and M segments are of negative sense, where the L segment codes for RNA-dependent RNA polymerase and the M segment codes for a precursor polyprotein to the glycoproteins G_N and G_C, as well as, for two nonstructural

proteins, 14K and 78K.[27] The S segment possesses two open reading frames that do not overlap. The open reading frames (ORF) of the S segment are separated by an intergenic region that is crucial for proper transcription termination. The S segment uses an ambisense strategy to code for the nucleocapsid protein (N), a non-specific single-stranded RNA binding protein (NSRNAssBS), while the nonstructural protein (NS) is translated in the positive sense orientation. These proteins are synthesized from the subgenomic viral complementary and viral positive sense mRNA, respectively. It has been reported that the viral genome S segment (vRNA) serves as a transcriptional template for the subgenomic N-encoding mRNA, while the replication intermediate (cRNA or antigenome) is utilized to generate subgenomic mRNA coding for NS.[28] In contrast with vRNA and cRNA, viral mRNAs are capped with 5' extensions acquired through a process known as "cap snatching" and use these as primers to initiate transcription; however, there is no poly (A) tail added at the 3' end (Figures 1.12-4 and 1.12-5).[2, 29]

Like all negative sense viruses, the RVFV genome transcription and replication occurs only when the N and L proteins form a complex known as ribonucleoproteins (RNPs).[30, 31] The L protein acts as both transcriptase and replicase, but requires the N protein in order to function properly. Once the viral proteins are translated, oligomerization of viral glycoproteins occur in the rough endoplasmic reticulum (rER), and these products are then transported to the Golgi apparatus.[32, 33, 34]

Unlike most other RNA viruses that use a matrix protein to package the RNPs and the subsequent release of virus, RVFV along with others in the *Bunyaviridae* family do not encode a matrix protein. Therefore, some other actions must be taken place to ensure the proper packaging of the RVFV virions. In a report published in 2011, Piper *et al.* proposed that the RVFV viral genomic RNA "is not merely a passenger within the virion, but acts like a stimulus for virion formation."[32] The authors suggested that the genomic segments located at the termini of the viral RNA are complimentary and could form a dsRNA structure which may contain the sequences needed for the proper packaging of the RVFV virions, as well as, promoter regions for initiation of transcription and replication. It is speculated that these

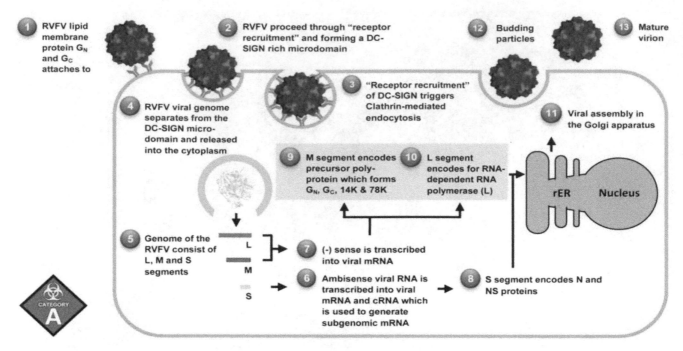

Figure 1.12-4: Diagrammatic process of Rift Valley Fever virus infection within an eukaryotic cell

sequences are recognized by multiple G_N, which acts in place a matrix protein. Once attached, G_N begins to recruit G_c, RdRp, N and genomic RNA into virions.[32]

Reports have indicated that the interactions between the encapsidated genomic segments and multiple G_N proteins cause a change in membrane curvature that leads to virus particle budding into the Golgi lumen where the maturation of the virion takes place. It is interesting to note that viral assembly and maturation will only occur when all three segments of the viral genome are present prior to budding into the Golgi apparatus.[32, 33, 34]

The manner by which the mature virions are released from the host cell remains to be elucidated. Some reports have stated that the matured virions are released via exocytosis (fusion of the plasma membrane with virion-filled Golgi elements).[35]Other reports have indicated that the release of mature particles are through the disintegration (lysis) of infected Vero cells *in vitro* (Figure 1.12-4). [36, 37, 38]

During the 1960's, the American biological warfare program at Fort Detrick researched the possibilities of weaponizing 22 microorganisms, including RVFV. RVFV is capable of being transmitted through an initial aerosol release and subsequently transmitted through mosquito vector (e.g. genus *Aedes* spp., *Anopheles* spp., *Culex* spp. etc.).

RVFV has the capability of being dormant in mosquito eggs for years and can potentially cause serious damage to humans and livestock resulting in long-term health effects and economic destruction. The weaponization of RVFV was terminated with President Nixon's executive order, signed November 25, 1969.[39, 40]

SYMPTOMS

RVFV is transported from the site of inoculation to the regional lymph nodes through lymphatic drainage. Early viral replication takes place within the lymph nodes which results in a primary viremia. Subsequently, RVFV is spread through the blood stream to various target organs.[41,]

The prodromal phase of infection usually results in an asymptomatic infection or mild to moderate flu-like symptoms. The symptoms include fever (99.5° F or 37.5° C),[7] headaches, malaise, dizziness, anorexia, myalgia, muscular and back pain and liver abnormalities.[2, 42] In some cases, patients experience stiffness of the neck, photo-phobia, nausea and vomiting. Most patients recover spontaneously within two days, or up to a week after the onset of symptoms, although convalescence may require up to three weeks (Table 2).[17, 19] However, in a small number of patients (<8%), the disease progresses into a hemorrhagic fever (<1%), meningoencephalitis (<1%) or retinitis (ocular) form (~0.5-2%).[43]

The initial symptoms of the hemorrhagic form of RVF will generally appear two to four days after the initial inoculation. These initial symptoms encompasses severe liver impairment, which includes jaundice.[2]

Although RVFV is known to infect hepatocytes, other organs are also affected. RVFV causes rapid hepatocellular changes progressing to liver necrosis. The primary foci of necrosis within the hepatocytes consist of dense aggregates of cytoplasmic and nuclear debris. Various reports have indicated that the destruction of the hepatocytes is so severe that most of the typical architecture of the liver is lost. Other tissues that are affected by RVFV include the spleen, adrenocortical cells, the glomeruli of the kidneys and the brain (Figure 1.12-6).[2]

Patients suffering from the hemorrhagic form of the disease will also develop vomiting, hematochezia and increased volumes of sputum. Additionally, patients will also develop ecchymoses, bleeding gums, nose bleeds (epistaxis), menorrhagia and uncontrollable bleeding from venipuncture sites. This illness will continue to progress and soon patients will develop disseminated intravascular coagulation, anemia, leucopenia, thrombocytopenia, kidney failure and hepatitis (e.g. abnormal liver transaminases). Many patients die as a result of gastrointestinal hemorrhage, oliguria and anuria within three to six days after the onset of the hemorrhagic symptoms.[19] The case fatality rate

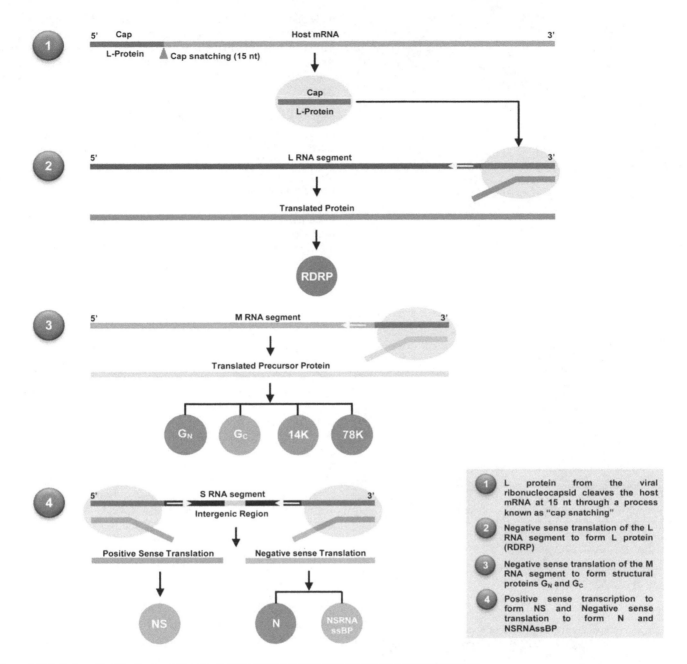

Figure 1.12-5: A diagrammatic display of the structural and nonstructural proteins encoded by RVFV genome

for patients suffering from RVFV induced hemorrhagic fever is approximately 50% and death generally occurs six days after the initial onset of hemorrhagic symptoms (Table 3).[2]

Table 2: An overview of initial clinical symptoms of RVFV infection

Symptoms	+	++	+++
Fever			■
Headaches			■
Malaise			■
Dizziness			■
Anorexia			■
Myalgia			■
Back pain			■
Liver abnormalities			■
Stiffness of the neck			■
Photophobia			■
Nausea			■
Vomiting			■

+ Rare ++ Common +++ Frequent

The initial symptoms of the meningoencephalitis form of the disease will generally appear one to four weeks after the first sign of RVF. Symptoms of this form of the disease include intense headaches, memory loss, hallucinations, confusion, disorientation, vertigo with cerebral-spinal fluid pleocytosis, convulsions and lethargy which eventually advance into a coma.[11, 19] Fatalities from this form of RVF are extremely rare, nonetheless, survivors may acquire residual brain damage (Table 4).[44, 45]

In ~10% of survivors, retinopathy occurs about 7 to 20 days after the primary fever,[14] which also involves retinal lesions. Patients suffering from this form of disease generally report blurred or decreased vision, which may resolve after 10 to 12 weeks. In some cases, macular exudate-like lesions, retinal detachment and retinitis have been reported.[44, 45, 46, 47] However, if the lesions occur on the macula densa or the retina, 50% of patients may suffer from permanent loss of vision. Nonetheless, fatalities resulting from this form of RVF are extremely rare (Table 4).[11]

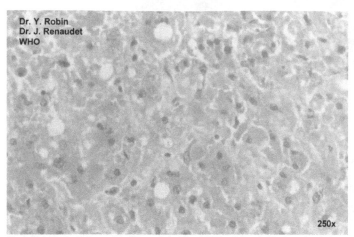

Dr. Y. Robin
Dr. J. Renaudet
WHO

250x

Figure 1.12-6: A hematoxylin and eosin (H&E) stained photo-micrograph depicts the cytoarchitectural changes found in a liver tissue sample extracted from a Rift Valley fever patient. This photomicrograph demonstrates acidophilic necrosis, which was leading to the formation of amorphous eosinophilic masses resembling Councilman's bodies

Table 3: An overview of the clinical symptoms of hemorrhagic RVFV infection

Symptoms	+	++	+++
Jaundice			■
Bloody stool			■
Bloody vomit			■
Bloody sputum			■
Ecchymoses			■
Bleeding gum			■
Bloody nose			■
Menorrhagia			■
Venipuncture bleeding			■
Intravascular coagulation			■
Anemia			■
Leucopenia			■
Thrombocytopenia			■
Kidney failure			■
Hepatitis			■
Gastrointestinal bleeding			■
Oliguria			■
Anuria			■

+ Rare ++ Common +++ Frequent

Table 4: An overview of the clinical symptoms of meningoencephalitis RVFV

Symptoms	+	++	+++
Intense headaches			■
Memory loss			■
Hallucinations			■
Confusion			■
Disorientation			■
Vertigo			■
CSF pleocytosis			■
Convulsions			■
Lethargy			■
Comatose			■
Retinal lesions			■
Blurred vision			■
Macular densa lesions			■
Retinal detachment			■
Retinitis			■

+ Rare ++ Common +++ Frequent

DETECTION

In addition to recognizing clinical and biological features of RVFV, this virus can be isolated from samples of blood, liver, and postmortem samples of nervous tissues from the brain of infected individuals.[48] RVFV can be easily isolated via intracerebral inoculation of blood samples or organ biopsies in baby mice, Vero cell (green monkey kidney) cultures or mosquito cells (e.g. *Aedes pseudoscutellaris*).[49, 50] At present, virus isolation is still considered to be the method of choice for demonstrating RVFV activity.[2]

RVFV antigens and RNA can be detected by immuno-histochemistry and/or reverse trans-cription polymerase chain reaction (RT-PCR) assays.[51, 52, 53] The RT-PCR assay is designed to target the NSs coding region of the smallest segment (S) of the tripartite, negative-sense, single stranded RNA genome of RVFV from human and animal sera.[13, 15, 54]

In convalescing patients, enzyme-linked immunoassay (ELISA) may also be used to confirm the presence of IgM antibodies to the virus, as well as, used to detect a rise in IgG levels.[13, 15, 44, 55]

TREATMENT

Presently, there is no established treatment for Rift Valley Fever. RVFV infections are generally self-limiting and medical treatment generally involves supportive therapies (maintenance of fluid and electrolyte balance) and the prevention and treatment of secondary infections. Nonetheless, in experimental animal models, treatment with ribavirin with a loading dose of 50 mg/kg followed by 10 mg/kg at 8 hour intervals for 9 days suppressed viremia in RVF-infected rhesus monkeys and reduced virus titres in infected cell cultures. In addition, the passive antibody and interferon inducer polyriboinosinicpolyribocytidylic acid complexed with poly-L-lysine and carboxy-methylcellulose have demonstrated protective effects in experimental animal models.[56] Morrill *et al.* (1989), reported that recombinant or lymphoblastoid human IFN- doses of 5×10^3 units/kg of body weight daily for 5 days have been demonstrated to suppress RVFV viremia and disease in rhesus monkeys.[57]

Presently, there is no vaccine approved by the U.S. Food and Drug Administration. Nonetheless, Spik *et al.* (2006), have shown that DNA vaccines offer tremendous promise in animal models. The authors have shown that RVFV−NSm constructs (RVFV nonstructural M segment, the fourth in-frame translation initiation codon), which express viral M genome region and encodes the envelope glycoproteins Gn and Gc, were highly immunogenic in mice and elicited protective immunity.[58] In 2013, Warimwe *et al.* successfully used a replication deficient chimpanzee adenovirus vector, ChAdOx1, that encodes RVFV envelope glycoproteins G_N and G_C to induce protective immunity in mice. Nonetheless, the efficacy of this potential vaccine in humans requires additional evaluation.[59] In 1985, Caplen *et al.* generated a RVFV strain MP-12 through serial plaque passages of parental strain ZH548 in MRC-5 cells (12 times) with the addition of 5-fluorouracil, a chemical mutagen.[60] What resulted was an RVFV strain with unique genetic characteristics. MP-12 is attenuated at the M and L segments while the S segment retains its virulent phenotype. Since that time, MP-12 has been manufactured as an Investigational New Drug vaccine.[61, 62]

DIFFERENTIAL DIAGNOSIS

The differential diagnosis of RVFV includes malaria, leptospirosis (lepto), yellow fever (YF), and various other hemorrhagic fevers such as Crimean-Congo hemorrhagic fever (CCHF), Dengue fever (DF), Ebola, Lassa fever (LF), etc. Due to its similarities among hemorrhagic fevers, laboratory diagnosis is essential to determine RVFV infection.[48, 58] Please examine Table 5 for the

Table 5: Differential diagnosis of RVF and other symptomatically related diseases. Differential diagnosis includes: leptospirosis (Lepto), yellow fever (YF), Crimean–Congo hemorrhagic fever (CCHF), Dengue fever (DF), Ebola and Lassa fever (LF)

Symptoms	RVF	Malaria	Lepto	YF	CCHF	DF	Ebola	LF
Fever	■	■	■	■	■	■	■	■
Headaches	■	■	■	■	■	■	■	■
Malaise	■	■	■	■	■	■	■	■
Dizziness	■				■			
Anorexia	■						■	
Myalgia	■	■	■	■	■	■	■	
Back pain	■	■	■	■	■	■		
Liver abnormalities	■	■	■					■
Stiffness of the neck			■					
Photophobia	■		■					
Nausea	■	■	■	■	■	■	■	■
Vomiting	■	■	■	■	■	■	■	■
Jaundice	■	■	■					
Bloody stool	■				■		■	■
Bloody vomit	■			■			■	
Bloody sputum	■		■				■	
Ecchymoses	■				■		■	
Bleeding gum	■		■		■		■	■
Bloody nose	■		■				■	
Menorrhagia	■							
Venipuncture bleeding	■							
Intravascular coagulation	■	■	■					
Anemia	■	■			■		■	■
Leucopenia	■	■			■	■		■
Thrombocytopenia	■	■			■	■	■	
Kidney failure	■	■	■	■	■		■	■
Hepatitis	■	■	■		■			
Gastrointestinal bleeding	■							
Oliguria	■		■	■				
Anuria	■							
Memory loss	■							
Hallucinations				■			■	■
Confusion				■			■	■
Disorientation				■				■
Vertigo	■	■			■			■
CSF pleocytosis	■							
Convulsions	■	■						
Lethargy	■							
Comatose	■	■		■	■			■
Retinal lesions	■							
Blurred/decrease vision	■							
Macular densa lesions	■							
Retinal detachment	■							
Retinitis			■					

symptomatic comparison of various diseases.[2, 63, 64]

References

1. Vialat P., Billecocq A., Kohl A., Bouloy M. The S Segment of Rift Valley Fever Phlebovirus (Bunyaviridae) Carries Determinants for Attenuation and Virulence in Mice. Journal of Virology, 2000. 74: pp. 1538–1543

2. Guerrant R.L., Walker D.H., Weller P.F. Tropical Infectious Diseases – Principles, Pathogens & Practice. Volume 1. Philadelphia: Churchill Livingstone Elsevier. 2006. pp. 756-761

3. The Center for Food Security and Public Health, College of Veterinary Medicine Iowa State University. Rift Valley Fever – Infectious Enzootic Hepatitis of Sheep and Cattle. Revised May 31, 2007. Retrieved January 21, 2008. Website: http://www.cfsph.ia state. edu/Factsheets/pdfs/rift_valley_fever.pdf

4. Daubney R., Hudson J.R., Garnham P.C. Enzootic Hepatitis of Rift Valley Fever: an Undescribed Virus Disease of Sheep, Cattle and Man from East Africa. East African Journal of Pathology and Bacteriology, 1931; 34: pp. 545-579

5. Meegan J.M., Shope R.E. Emerging Concept on Rift Valley Fever. Perspective in Virology, 1981; 11: pp. 267-387.

6. Digoutte J.P., Peters C.J. General Aspects of the 1987 Rift Valley Fever Epidemic in Mauritania. Research in Virology, 1989; 140: pp. 27-30

7. Drake J.M., Hassan A.N., Beier J.C. A statistical model of Rift Valley fever activity in Egypt. Journal of Vector Ecology, 2013. 38: pp. 251-259

8. Authur R.R., El-Sharkawy M.S., Cope S.E., Botros B.A., Oun S, Morrill J.C., Shope R.E., Hibbs R.G., Darwish M.A., Imam I.Z. Recurrence of Rift Valley Fever in Egypt. Lancet, 1993. 342: pp. 1149-1150

9. Nguku P., Sharif S., Omar A., Nzioka C., Muthoka P., Njau J., Dahiye A., Galgalo T., Mwihia J., Njoroge J., Limo H., Mutiso J., Kalani R., Sheikh A., Nyikal J., Mutonga D., Omollo J.,

Guracha A., Muindi J., Amwayi S., Langat D., Owiti D., Mohammed A., Musaa J., Sang R., Breiman R., Njenga K., Feikin D., Katz M., Burke H., Nyaga P., Ackers M., Gikundi S., Omballa L., Nderitu N., Wamola R., Wanjala S., Omulo J., Richardson D., Schnabel S., Martin V., Hoel D., Hanafi H., Weiner M., Onsongo J., Kojo T., Duale M., Hassan A., Dabaar M., Njuguna C., Yao M., Grein T., Formenty P., Telfer B., Lepec R., Feldmann H., Grolla A., Wainwright S., Lederman E., Farnon E., Rao C., Kapella B.K., Gould H. Rift Valley Fever Outbreak – Kenya, November 2006 - January 2007. Morbidity and Mortality Weekly Report, 2007. 56: pp. 73-76

10. Fagbo S.F. The evolving Transmission Patterns of Rift Valley Fever in the Arabian Peninsula. Annals of New York academy of science, 2002. 969: pp. 201-204

11. World Health Organization. Rift Valley Fever in Kenya Somalia and the United Republic of Tanzania. Revised May 9, 2007. Retrieved January 21, 2008. Website: http://www.who.int/csr/don/ 2007_05_09/en/index.html

12. World Health Organization. Rift Valley Fever - Update 4. Revised December 21, 2007. Retrieved January 21, 2008. Website: http://www.who.int/csr/don/2007_12_21 /en/index.html

13. Faye O., Ba H., Ba Y., Freire C.C.M., Faye O., Ndiaye O., Elgady I.O., Zanotto P.M.A., Diallo M., Sall A.A. Reemergence of Rift Valley Fever, Mauritania, 2010. Emerging Infectious Diseases, 2014. 20: pp. 300-303

14. Métras R., Baguelin M., Edmunds W.J., Thompson P.N., Kemp A., Pfeiffer D.U., Collins L.M., White R.G. Transmission Potential of Rift Valley Fever Virus over the Course of the 2010 Epidemic in South Africa. Emerging Infectious Diseases, 2013. 9: pp. 916-924

15. Sow A., Faye O., Ba Y., Ba H., Diallo D., Faye O., Loucoubar C., Boushab M., Barry Y., Diallo M., Sall A.A. Rift Valley Fever Outbreak, Southern Mauritania, 2012. Emerging Infectious Diseases, 2014. 20: pp. 296-299

16. Elwan M.S., Sharaf M.H., Gameel K., El-Hadi E., Arthur R. Rift Valley Fever Retinopathy: Observations in a New Outbreak. Annals of Saudi Medicine, 1997. 17: pp. 377-380

17. Rift Valley Fever – East Africa, 1997-1998. Morbidity and Mortality Weekly Report, 1998. 47: pp. 261-264

18. State of New Jersey Department of Agriculture. Rift Valley Fever. 2006. Revised 2003. Retrieved January 21, 2008. Website: www.state.nj.us/agriculture/divisions/ah/diseases/riftvalley.html

19. Guerrant R.L., Walker D.H., Weller P.F. Tropical Infectious Diseases – Principles, Pathogens & Practice. Volume 1. Churchill Livingstone Elsevier. Philadelphia, 2006. pp. 758

20. Ellis D.S., Simpson D.I.H., Stamford S., Wahab K.S.E.A., Rift Valley Fever Virus: Some Ultrastructural Observations on Material from the Outbreak in Egypt 1977. Journal of General Virology, 1979. 42: pp. 329–337

21. Pepin M., Bouloy M., Bird B.H., Kemp A. Paweska J. Rift Valley Fever Virus (Bunyaviridae: Phlebovirus): an Update on Pathogenesis, Molecular Epidemiology, Vectors, Diagnostics and Prevention. Veterinary Research, 2010. 41: pp. 61-101

22. Svajger U., Anderluh, M., Jeras, M., Obermajer, N. (2010). C-type lectin DC-SIGN: an Adhesion, Signalling and Antigen-Uptake Molecule that Guides Dendritic Cells in Immunity. Cellular Signalling, 2010. 22: pp. 1397–1405

23. Lozach P-Y., Kühbacher A., Meier R., Mancini R., Bitto D., le Bouloy M., Helenius A. DC-SIGN as a Receptor for Phleboviruses. Cell Host and Microbe, 2011. 10: pp. 75–88

24. Neumann A.K., Thompson N.L., Jacobson K. Distribution and Lateral Mobility of DC-SIGN on Immature Dendritic Cells – Implications for Pathogen Uptake. Journal of Cell science, 2008. 121: pp. 634–643

25. Guo Y., Feinberg H., Conroy E., Mitchell D.A., Alvarez R., Blixt O., Taylor M.E., Weis W.I., Drickamer K. Structural Basis for Distinct Ligandbinding and Targeting Properties of the Receptors DC-SIGN and DC-SIGNR. Nature Structural & Molecular Biology, 2004. 11: pp. 591–598

26. Tabarani G., Thépaut M., Stroebel D., Ebel C., Vivès C., Vachette P., Durand D., Fieschi F. DC-SIGN Neck Domain is a pH-sensor Controlling Oligomerization: SAXS and Hydrodynamic Studies of Extracellular Domain. The Journal of Viological Chemistry, 2009. 284: pp. 21229–21240

27. Bouloy M., Janzen C., Vialat P., Khun H., Pavlovic J., Huerre M., Haller O. Genetic Evidence for an Interferon-Antagonistic Function of Rift Valley Fever Virus Nonstructural Protein NSs. Journal of Virology, 2001. 75: pp. 1371–1377

28. Garcia S., Crance J.M., Billecocq A., Peinnequin A., Jouan A., Bouloy M., Garin D. Quantitative Real-Time PCR Detection of Rift Valley Fever Virus and Its Application to Evaluation of Antiviral Compounds. Journal of Clinical Microbiology, 2001. 39: pp. 4456–4461

29. Flick R., Bouloy M. Rift Valley Fever Virus. Current Molecular Medicine, 2005. 5: pp. 827-834

30. Jin H., Elliott R.M. Characterization of Bunyamwera Virus S RNA that is Transcribed and Replicated by the L Protein Expressed from Recombinant Vaccinia Virus. Journal of Virology, 1993. 67: pp. 1396–1404

31. Lopez N., Muller R., Prehaud C., Bouloy M. The L Protein of Rift Valley Fever Virus Can Rescue Viral Ribonucleoproteins and Transcribe Synthetic Genome-Like RNA Molecules. Journal of Virology, 1995. 69: pp. 3972–3979

32. Piper M.E., Sorenson D.R., Gerrard S.R. Efficient Cellular Release of Rift Valley Fever Virus Requires Genomic RNA. Public Library of Science One, 2011. 6: pp. e18070

33. Liu L., Celma C.C.P, Roy P. Rift Valley Fever Virus Structural Proteins: Expression, Characterization and Assembly of Recombinant Proteins. Virology Journal, 2008. 5: pp. 81-93

34. Gerrard S.R., Nichol S.T. Characterization of the Golgi Retention Motif of Rift Valley Fever Virus G_N Glycoprotein. Journal of Virology, 2002. 76: pp. 12200-12210

35. Pettersson R. F., Melin L. 1996. Synthesis, Assembly and Intracellular Transport of Bunyaviridae Membrane Proteins. The Bunyaviridae. Berlin: Springer-Verlag. 1996. p. 159-188

36. Gerrard S.R., Rollin P.E., Nichol S.T. Bidirectional Infection and Release of Rift Valley Fever Virus in Polarized Epithelial Cells. Virology, 2002. 301: pp. 226-35

37. Ellis D.S., Shirodaria P.V., Fleming E., Simpson D.I.H. Morphology and Development of Rift Valley Fever Virus in Vero Cell Cultures. Journal of Medical Virology, 2005. 24: pp. 161-174

38. Gerrard S.R., Nichol S.T. Characterization of the Golgi Retention Motif of Rift Valley Fever Virus G_N Glycoprotein. Journal of Virology, 2002. 76: pp. 12200-12210

39. Alibek K. Biohazard. New York: Dell Publishing. 1999. pp. 234

40. Swanepoel R., Coetzer J.A.W. 1994. Rift Valley fever. Infectious Diseases of Livestock with Special Reference to Southern Africa, Volume 1. Cape Town: Oxford University Press. 1994. pp. 687-717

41. Smith D.R., Steele K.E., Shamblin J., Honko A., Johnson J., Reed C., Kennedy M., Chapman J.L., Hensley L.E. The pathogenesis of Rift Valley fever virus in the mouse model. Virology, 407: pp. 256–267

42. Rift Valley Fever Fact Sheet. Center for Disease Control and Prevention. Retrieved July 25, 2008. Web Site: http://www.cdc.gov/ncidod/dvrd/spb/mnpages/dispages/Fact_Sheets/Rift%20Valley%20Fever%20Fact%20Sheet.pdf

43. World Health Organization. Rift Valley Fever. Revised September 2007. Retrieved July 25, 2008. Web Site: http://www.who.int/mediacentre/factsheets/fs207/en/

44. Peters C.J. Emergence of Rift Valley Fever. Factors in the Emergence of Arbovirus Diseases. Paris: Elsevier. 1997. pp. 253

45. Freed I. Rift Valley Fever in Man Complicated by Retinal Changes and Loss of Vision. South African Medical Journal, 1951. 25: pp. 930-932

46. Schrire L. Macular Changes in Rift Valley Fever. South African Medical Journal, 1951. 25: pp. 926-30

47. Joubert J.D.S., Ferguson A.L., Gear J. Rift Valley Fever in South Africa: the Occurrence of Human Cases in the Orange Free State, the North-Western Cape Province, the Western and Southern Transvaal: Epidemiological and Clinical Findings. South African Medical Journal, 1951. 25: pp. 890-891

48. Guerrant R.L., Walker D.H., Weller P.F. Tropical Infectious Diseases – Principles, Pathogens & Practice. Volume 1. Churchill Livingstone Elsevier. Philadelphia, 2006. pp. 759

49. Digoutte J.P., Jouan A., Le Guenno B., Riou O., Philippe B., Meegagn J., Ksiasek T.G., Peters C.J. Isolation of the Rift Valley Fever Virus by Inoculation into Aedes pseudoscutellaris Cells: Comparison with other Diagnostic Methods. Research in Virology, 1989. 140: pp. 31-41

50. Crabtree M.B., Crockett R.J.K, Bird B.H., Nichol S.T., Erickson B.R., Biggerstaff B.J., Horiuchi K., Miller B.R., Infection and Transmission of Rift Valley Fever Viruses Lacking the NSs and/or NSm Genes in Mosquitoes: Potential Role for NSm in Mosquito Infection. Public Library of Science (PloS) Neglected Tropical Diseases, 2012. 6: pp. e1639

51. Drosten C., Gottig S., Schilling S., Asper M., Panning M., Schmitz H., Gunther S. Rapid Detection and Quantification of RNA of Ebola and Marburg Viruses, Lassa Virus, Crimean-Congo Hemorrhagic Fever Virus, Rift Valley Fever Virus, Dengue Virus, and Yellow Fever Virus by Real-Time Reverse Transcription-PCR. Journal of Clinical Microbiology, 2002. 40: pp. 2323-2330

52. Garcia S., Crance J.M., Billecocq A., Peinnequin A., Jouan A., Bouloy M., Garin D. Quantitative Real-Time PCR Detection of Rift Valley Fever Virus and its Application to Evaluation of Antiviral Compounds. Journal of Clinical Microbiology, 2001. 39: pp. 4456-4461

53. Ibrahim M.S., Turell M.J., Knauert F.K., Lofts R.S. Detection of Rift Valley Fever Virus in Mosquitoes by RT-PCR. Molecular and Cellular Probes, 1997. 11: pp. 49-53

54. Sall A. A., Thonnon J., Sène O.K., Fall A., Ndiaye M., Baudez B., Mathiot C., Bouloy M. Single-Tube RT-PCR for Detection of Rift Valley Fever Virus in Human and Animal Sera. Journal of Virological Methods, 2001. 91: pp. 85–92.

55. Paweska J.T., Burt F.J., Anthony F., Smith S.J., Grobbelaar A.A., Croft J.E., Ksiazek T.G., Swanepoel R. IgG-sandwich and IgM-capture Enzyme-Linked Immunosorbent Assay for the Detection of Antibody to Rift Valley Fever Virus in Domestic Ruminants. Journal of Virological Methods, 2003. 113: pp. 103-112

56. Peters C.J., Reynolds J.A., Slone T.W. Jones D.E., Stephen E.L. Prophylaxis of Rift Valley Fever with Antiviral Drugs, Immune Serum, an Interferon Inducer, and a Macrophage Activator. Antiviral research, 1986. 6: pp. 285-297

57. Morrill J.C., Jennings G.B., Cosgriff T.M., Gibbs P.H., Peters C.J. Prevention of Rift Valley Fever in Rhesus Monkeys with Interferon-Alpha. Reviews of infectious diseases, 1989. 11: pp. S815-S825

58. Spik K., Shurtleff A., McElroy A.K., Guttieri M.C., Hooper J.W., Schmaljohn C. Immunogenicity of Combination DNA Vaccines for Rift Valley Fever Virus, Tick-Borne Encephalitis Virus, Hantaan Virus, and Crimean Congo Hemorrhagic Fever Virus. Vaccine, 2006. 24: pp. 4657–4666

59. Warimwe G.M., Lorenzo G., Lopez-Gil E., Reyes-Sandoval A., Cottingham M.G., Spencer A.J., Collins K.A., Dicks M.D.J., Milicic A., Lall A., Furze J., Turner A.V., Hill A.V.S., Brun A., Gilbert S.C. Immunogenicity and efficacy of a chimpanzee adenovirus-vectored Rift Valley Fever vaccine in mice. Virology Journal, 2013. 10: pp. 349

60. Caplen H, Peters CJ, Bishop DH. 1985. Mutagen-directed attenuation of Rift Valley fever virus as a method for vaccine development. J. Gen. Virol. 66:2271–2277

61. Lokugamage N., Freiberg A.N., Morrill J.C., Ikegami T. Genetic Subpopulations of Rift Valley Fever Virus Strains ZH548 and MP-12 and Recombinant MP-12 Strains. Journal of Virology, 2012. 86: pp. 13566–13575

62. Lihoradova O.A., Indran S.V., Kalveram B., Lokugamage N., Head J.A., Gong B., Tigabu B., Juelich T.L., Freiberg A.N., Ikegami T. Characterization of Rift Valley Fever Virus MP-12 Strain Encoding NSs of Punta Toro Virus or Sandfly Fever Sicilian Virus. Public Library of Science (PloS) Neglected Tropical Disease, 2013. 7: pp. e2181.

63. Updated Interim Infection Control and Exposure Management Guidance in the Health-Care and Community Setting for Patients with Possible Monkeypox Virus Infection. Center for Disease Control and Prevention. Revised September 5, 2008. Retrieved December 10, 2011. Website: http://www.cdc.gov/ncidod /monkeypox/pdf/mpoxinfectioncontrol.pdf

64. Nalca A., Rimoin A.W., Bavari S., Whitehouse C.A. Reemergence of Monkeypox: Prevalence, Diagnostics, and Countermeasures. Clinical Infectious Disease, 2005. 41: pp. 1765-1771

Photo Bibliography

Figure 1.12-1: Transmission electron micrograph (TEM) of Rift Valley Fever Virus. The electron micrograph was taken by Dr. Fred Murphy in 1975 and released by the CDC. Public domain photo

Figure 1.12-3: Virus graphics is designed and released by the National Institute of Health. Public domain photo

Figure 1.12-4: A hematoxylin and eosin (H&E) stained photo-micrograph depicts the cytoarchitectural changes found in a liver tissue sample from a RVF patient. This photomicrograph demonstrates acidophilic necrosis, which was leading to the formation of amorphous eosinophilic masses resembling Councilman bodies. This photomicrograph was taken at 250x magnification by Dr. Yves Robin and Dr. Jean Renaudet in 1980. This photomicrograph was released by the Arbovirus Laboratory at the Pasteur Institute in Dakar, Senegal; World Health Organization and the CDC. Public domain photo

Tick-Borne Encephalitis virus (TBEV), also known as Russian Spring-Summer encephalitis virus, is endemic in Europe and many parts of Asia (Figure 1.13-1). TBEV is the causative agent of Tick-Borne Encephalitis (TBE), a potentially fatal neurological infection.[1]

Between the years of 1974 to 2003, a 400% increase in TBE morbidity occurred in Europe and an increase in the geographical spread of TBEV into previously uninfected areas, involving approximately 19 different European countries.[2, 3] During the last two decades (1990 to 2009), an annual means incidence of 2,815 human TBE has been calculated for Europe, while the annual means incidence of 5,682 human TBE has been calculated for Russia.[4]

TBEV was discovered in 1937 during an expedition in Far-East Russia led by Lev Zilber searching for the etiological agent of acute encephalitis associated with tick bites. TBEV is a zoonotic arbovirus and a member of the virus genus *Flavivirus*, of the family *Flaviviridae*.[5] TBEV is an enveloped flavivirus, with an unsegmented, positive (+) sense RNA genome. [6, 7]This genomic RNA consists of an open reading frame that encodes three structural glycoproteins: C, M, and E glycoproteins, and seven nonstructural proteins: NS1, NS2A, NS2B, NS3, NS4A, NS4B and NS5.[1, 5]

Through phylogenetic analysis, TBEV has been classified into three subtypes: European subtype, (Neudoerfl strain), Far Eastern subtype (prototype Sofjin strain) and Siberian subtype (Vasilchenko strain). The European subtype is known to cause Central European encephalitis, while the Far Eastern and the Siberian subtypes are known to cause Russian Spring-Summer encephalitis (Figure 1.13-2).[8, 9, 10]

Although the pathogenesis of the three subtypes share relatively similar clinical course, it has been reported that the long-term consequence and mortality rate of the subtypes demonstrates pronounced dissimilarities. For example, the European subtype (Neudoerfl strain), is generally associated with milder form of the disease with ~30% of patients suffering from neurological

sequelae and a mortality rate estimated at ~1 to 2%. The Siberian subtype (Vasilchenko strain) associate more frequently with chronic or progressive disease and has a mortality rate estimated at ~8%. Finally, the Far Eastern subtype (Sofjin strain) is generally associated with a severe disease course with higher rates of severe neurological sequelae and a mortality rate that exceeds 20%.[8, 11, 12]

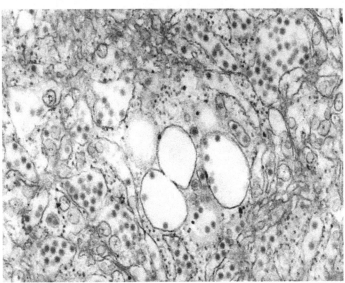

Figure 1.13-1: Negatively-stained transmission electron micrograph (TEM) revealing the presence of numerous Tick-Borne encephalitis (TBE) virions

The mature virions of TBEV are icosahedral particles that contain centrally arranged nucleocapside surrounded by supercapside lipoprotein envelope which consists of phosphor-lipids and virus specific glycoprotein.[13] The TBEV virion is approximately 50 nm (~40 to 60 nm) in diameter and possesses an electron dense core enclosed within a lipid bilayer containing E (envelope) and M (membrane) glycoproteins.[14]

The infection cycle of TBEV is initiated after the binding of E protein to the host cell receptor; the primary receptor being

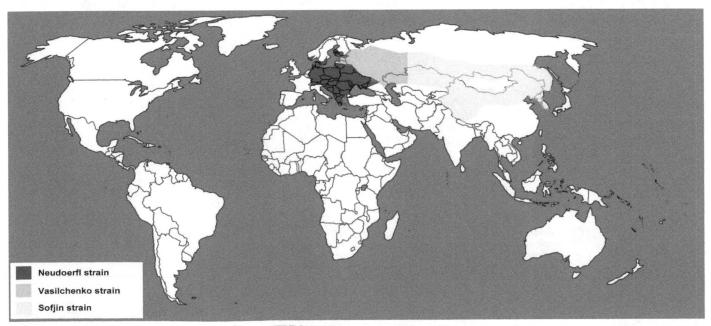

Neudoerfl strain
Vasilchenko strain
Sofjin strain

Figure 1.13-2: Distribution of Tick-Borne Encephalitis virus (TBEV)

heparan sulfate and human laminin-binding protein (LBP).[15, 16, 17, 18] Once binding has occurred, the virus is transported into the host cell via clathrin-mediated endocytosis. Within the acidic environment of the endosome, the protonation of a conserved histidine residue (His323) on the E protein found at the interface between domain I and III occurs. The protonation causes an E protein conformation change from dimer to trimmers, which results in the fusion of the endosomal membrane with the viral membrane. Once the fusion occurrs, the viral nucelocapsid is released into the cytoplasm (Figure 1.13-3).[15, 16, 17, 19, 20, 21]

Once the TBEV genome gains entry into the cytoplasm, the positive sense viral RNA genome immediately undergoes translation and replication of positive sense RNA viruses, which occurs in association with the membrane structures of the rough endoplasmic reticulum (rER). The translation of the TBEV genome is initiated when the host cellular ribosome at the rER locates the initiation codon of the viral RNA.[22]

The genome of the TBEV consists of a positive sense, single stranded RNA approximately 11 kb in length. The TBEV genome, like the genome of other positive sense viruses, is similar in structure to host cellular mRNA. The TBEV positive sense RNA genome possesses a 5' type 1, 7-methyl guanosine cap, 5' untranslated region, a single open reading frame (5' to 3' direction), and a 3' untranslated region.[23] Like most flaviviruses, Vasilchenko and Sofjin strains do not possess a poly-adenylated (poly-A) tail. It is presumed that with the absence of a poly-A tail, TBEV follows a different mechanism for translation when compared to the cellular mRNAs. However at present, the exact mechanisms remain to be elucidated.[23] However, with the Neudoerfl strain, an internal poly A tail has been found within the 3' untranslated region. The occurrence of two different types of 3' untranslated region among the strains of a single virus type is remarkable although the significance of which is presently unknown.[22, 24, 25]

The open reading frame of the TBEV encodes a viral polyprotein (~3400 amino acids). Once formed, this polyprotein transverses the rER membrane at several locations dictated by hydrophobic signal sequences. On the cytoplasmic side, the polyprotein will be processed by NS3/NS2B complex, NS2A and NS5, while within the lumen of the rER, the polyprotein will be cleaved by host's signal peptidases and furin. This post-translation processing will produce three structural proteins: capsid (protein C) protein, prM (precursor molecule of membrane protein M) and envelope (E) protein, as well as, seven nonstructural proteins: NS1 (glycosylated protein), NS2A, NS2B (protease), NS3 (helicase, protease and nucleoside triphosphatase), NS4A, NS4B and NS5 (RNA-dependent RNA polymerase) (Figure 1.13-2). These structural and nonstructural proteins are essential components in the formation of the viral replication complex (Figure 1.13-3 and Figure 1.13-4).[22, 23, 26, 27, 28]

Subsequent to the formation of the replication complex, the positive-sense viral RNA will be used to produce more viral polyproteins or used in the formation of a negative-sense viral RNA. This negative-sense RNA will serve as a template to develop new positive-sense viral genomic RNAs that could be used to produce more viral proteins or become incorporated into new viral particles (Figure 1.13-3).[22, 23]

After the formation of the new positive sense TBEV RNA, the addition of the RNA cap is a critical process for the TBEV genome. This RNA cap allows the viral RNA to be efficiently translated by the cellular translational machinery, along with providing protection from the exonucleases of host cells during forthcoming infections. TBEV genomic RNA is modified at the 5' end to generate a type 1 cap structure (me[7]-GpppA-me[2]) through the enzymatic actions of RNA triphosphatase (RTPase) which is found within the helicase domain of NS3 and guanylyltransferase (Gtase), 2'-O methyl-transferase (2'-OMTase) and N7-methyl-transferase (Guanine-N7-Mtase) which are found on the N-terminal capping enzyme domain of NS5. Please note that the C-terminal domain of the NS5 functions as the TBEV RNA dependent RNA polymerase.[29]

Once the RNA cap is added to the positive-sense viral genomic particles, the C-protein is packaged with the viral RNAS genome to form nucleocapsids. These newly formed nucelocapsids are then translocated into the lumen of the rER. Subsequently, the various proteins, nucleocapsid, prM and E protein are assembled

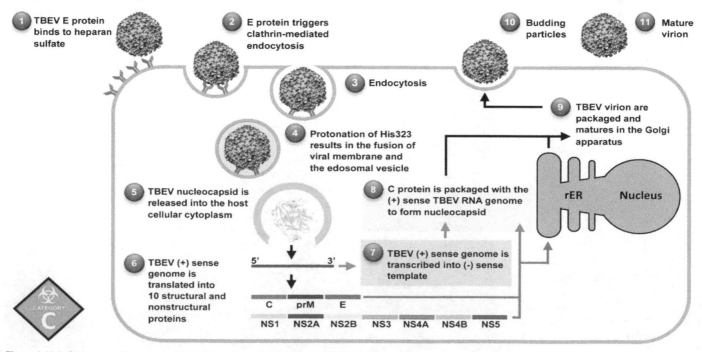

Figure 1.13-3: Diagrammatic process of Tick-Borne Encephalitis virus (TBEV) infection within an eukaryotic cell

within the lumen and forms immature virions. Subsequently, these immature virions are then transported to the Golgi apparatus via host secretory pathway in acidic vesicles. Within the low pH vesicle, prM is cleaved by host cell enzyme furin to produce M protein. Within the Golgi, the M protein and E protein is reorganized into fusion-competent homodimers. This final reorganization marks the last maturation of the virus. Finally, the matured virus is released from the cell through fusion of the transport vesicles with the host cell plasma membrane (Figure 1.13-2). [20, 30, 31, 32, 33]

The proteins formed from the cleavage of the polyprotein translated plays a part in the formation of the replication complex and are essential for the proper function of the virus. As mentioned previously, the open reading frame encodes three structural glycoproteins: C, M, and E glycoproteins, and seven nonstructural proteins: NS1, NS2A, NS2B, NS3, NS4A, NS4B and NS5 (Figure 1.13-4). [1, 5]

Protein C (11kDa) along with the viral genome, form the TBEV nucleocapsid. During viral production and assembly, protein C plays a major role in the assembly of virion particles within the host cell. For example, it has been reported that the carboxy-terminal of protein C, which is anchored to the rough endoplasmic reticulum (rER), acts as a signal sequence that instigates the translocation of precursor protein prM into the lumen of the rER. During the latter stages of viral assembly, viral proteases NS2B (which cleave the carboxy-terminal of protein C) and the action of host cell signalase allows the subsequent release of amino terminus of prM from the rER. [34, 35]

Viral structural Protein M (8 kDa) is synthesized via furin-dependent cleavage from a larger precursor molecule prM. Prior to cleavage, prM and E form heterodimers. These heterodimers are then incorporated into immature virions and assembled in the rER. The presence of prM in these immature virions prevents them from undergoing low-pH-induced rearrangements during intracellular transport through the acidic compartments. However, the precise function of TBEV protein M remains to be elucidated. [36]

Instead of forming spikes, viral structural E protein (54 kDa) exists as a flat dimer extending in a head-to-tail homodimer (parallel) direction to the viral membrane. In recent years, E protein has been the focus of various researches mainly due to its exposed residue that is important for antibody binding and systemic immune response. It has been reported that E protein is essential for virion binding to host cell receptors and that it is the mild acidic conditions during membrane fusion that induce a rearrangement of the envelope structure where the E protein dimers are converted to trimers. [37, 38, 39, 40] Researchers have proposed that the two oligomeric states of the TBEV E protein reveal the dual functional nature of this protein where the dimeric form is required for receptor recognition, while the trimeric form is necessary for membrane fusion and the eventual release of the nucleocapsid into the cytoplasm of the host cell. In addition, E protein has also been reported to be involved in virion formation where it has the ability to form envelope recombinant sub-viral particles (RSPs) with prM within the rER. [36, 37, 38, 39, 40, 41]

NS1 is an extensively glycosylated protein that has a molecular weight of ~47 kDa. NS1 exists in both an intracellular and extracellular form. It has been shown that NS1 evokes an intense host immune response and may have important implications for the development of vaccines for TBEV. [38, 39] It is believed that NS1 is involved with antibody-dependent enhancement of infection (ADE) where the generated host immune response can enhance

viral replication in fragment/crystallizable (Fc) receptor-bearing cells, such as natural killer cells, macrophages, neutrophils and mast cells. [43]

Studies have indicated that proper synthesis of the NS1 requires NS2A. NS2A is understood to function as a cis-acting proteinase to cleave NS1-NS2A polyprotein junction. [44, 45] It is believed that NS2B functions as a protease, residing on the cytoplasmic side of the membrane of rER and separates mature protein C from its carboxy-terminal anchor. This cleavage exposes a recognition sequence for the host protease signalase and subsequently liberates the amino terminus of protein prM by cleaving off the signal sequence. The result of the enzymatic process produces an anchorless, mature C protein and frees the prM which is essential for proper processing and export of E protein. [46] Additionally, it is believed that NS2B is a cofactor for the NS3 enzymatic activities. For example, it has been reported that the N-terminal region of NS3 contains the catalytic residue of the serine protease which requires NS2B as a cofactor in order for the proper functioning of the enzyme. [47, 48]

NS3 protein possesses numerous functions depending on the region of the protein. For example, at the helicase domain, NS3 possesses RNA triphosphatase (RTPase) while at the N-terminal region, NS3 functions as a serine protease that is responsible for translational cleavage of viral polyprotein. As mentioned previously, the serine protease activities of NS3 requires NS2B as a cofactor to function properly. [15, 29, 49, 50]

Lindenbach *et al.* (2001, 2007) reported that the NS4A protein plays a role in the rearrangement of the rER membrane for viral replication. Additionally, NS4A participates in the replication of viral RNA via assembling replicase component at the rER membrane. [34, 37]

Although NS4B is part of the replication complex, its exact role has been a source of debate. It has been reported that NS4B is located at RNA replication sites and plays various roles in regulating virus replication. Additionally, it has also been implicated in the inhibition of interferons in other Flaviviruses such as Dengue Fever Virus. [22]

Like NS3, NS5 is also a multifunctional protein. At the C-terminus, NS5 is a RNA-dependent RNA polymerase, while at the N-terminus a guanylyltransferase (Gtase) and a characteristic motif of *S*-adenosyl-L-methionine-dependent methyltransferases (methyltrans-ferase core) exists. The methyltransferase core exhibits a (nucleoside-2'-O-)-methyltransferase activity and is responsible for methylating the 5' cap of the viral RNA genome. On immunological aspect, NS5 has recently been identified as an interferon antagonist where it possesses the ability to inhibit STAT1 phosphorylation in response to interferon and its association with interferon receptor complexes. [29, 51, 52]

It is known that rodents such as yellow-necked field mice (*Apodemus flavicollis*) and bank voles (*Clethrionomys glareolus*) are reservoirs for this virus, while the tick species, *Ixodes ricinus*, is the vector for European subtype and *Ixodes persulcatus* is the vector for the Far Eastern and Siberian subtypes. [53, 54]

TBEV is transferred between ticks via co-feeding, whereby the infected tick transmits the virus to a non-infected tick when they are feeding in very close proximity on the rodent. Humans become infected with TBEV via infected tick bites or through the consumption of infected unpasteurized milk. It has been reported that TBEV can be isolated from the milk of goats for 5 to 25 days following infection, while the infectivity survives in various milk

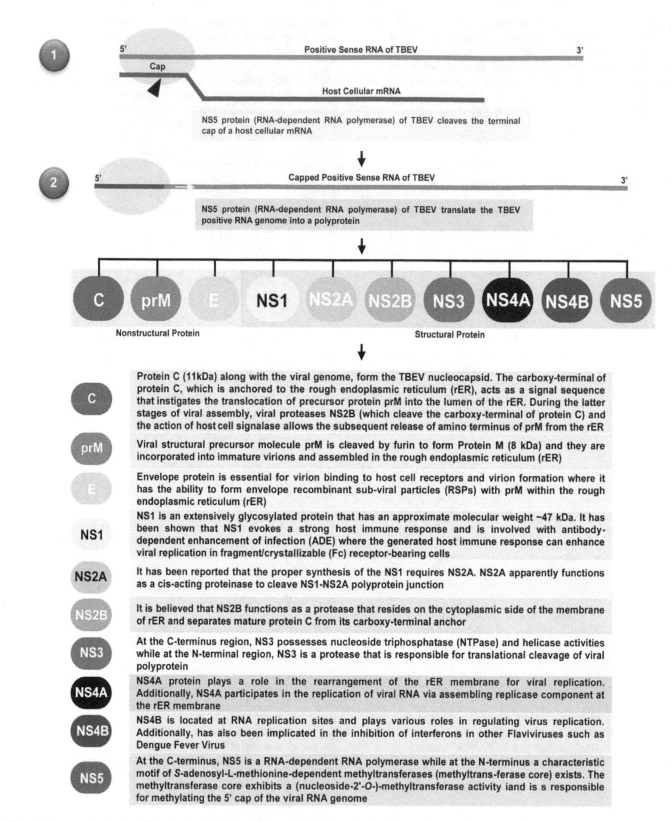

1.13-4: A diagrammatic display of the structural and nonstructural proteins encoded by TBEV genome

products such as yogurt, cheese and butter (Figure 1.13-5).[55, 56, 57, 58]

After invading the circulatory and lymphatic systems, the virus begins to replicate in the epithelium of the vessels, as well as leukocytes. The migration of the leukocytes brings the virus into various organs such as liver, kidneys and spleen etc. The invasion of the CNS occurs via hematogenic or neuronal matter, involving the direct centripetal spread among the nerves and transmigration through the olfactory tract.[59] Generally, the TBEV affects the motor neurons of the anterior horn, located in the cervical part of the spinal cord and the soft membranes of the brain. From this point, the virus invades the cerebral spinal fluid and spreads throughout the CNS. It is known that the virus influences the intensity of neuronal death and degree of pathological changes of the neuroglial cells.[45]

As described by Alibek, (1999), TBEV was researched by the

Biopreparat located at institute of Ultra-Pure Biopreparations in Leningrad, Omutninsk in Kirov, Obolensk outside of Moscow, the Lyubuchany Institute of Immunology in Chekhov near Moscow, and Vector research. The testing of this virus was completed at Novosibrisk (small town of Koltsovo) located in Siberia.[60] Unfortunately, little is known about the potential of TBEV as a biological weapon, therefore, the CDC has listed this virus as a potential biological weapon (Category C).

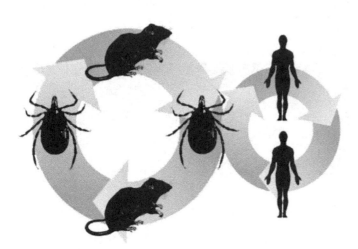

Figure 1.13-5: Sylvatic cycle of Tick-Borne Encephalitis virus (TBEV)

SYMPTOMS

On average the incubation period of Tick Borne Encephalitis (TBE) lasts between 7 to14 days and is asymptomatic. After the incubation period, a biphasic febrile illness quickly follows. The initial phase lasts approximately 2 to 4 days and is followed by the viremic phase.[61] Early symptoms of the initial phase include fatigue, malaise, anorexia, headache, pain in the neck, shoulders, and the lower back that lasts 1 to 2 days. Classical symptoms of TBE appear suddenly but patients generally can recall the exact hour of onset. The classic symptoms include a sudden elevation of temperature (38 to 39 C°; 100.4 to 102.2 F°), nausea and vomiting.[4] After approximately 8 days of remission, the second viremic phase of the disease occurs in 20 to 30% of patients and involves the central nervous system.[61]

During the viremic phase, muscular pains become severe and are localized in the neck, shoulder, lower spine and limbs. At times, fasciculation and a sense of numbness may appear in one of the patient's limbs. For some individuals, meningeal symptoms, such as neck stiffness, also develop during this early period of the TBE and may include symptoms such as shortness of breath, flushing of the face, neck and upper part of the body.[61] As reported by Gritsun et al. (2003), TBEV infections could produce a variety of symptoms that can be differentiated into various forms of TBE (Table 1).[1, 62]

The first form, also known as the Febrile TBE, will demonstrate no neurological symptoms and signs of damage to the CNS. The Febrile form occurs in about one third of all recognized TBEV infections and patients can develop a fever that reaches 39 °C (102.2 °F). Additionally, some patients may experience severe muscle pains, numbness and fasciculations. The febrile form lasts anywhere from a few hours to ~5 days and generally results in the complete recovery of the patient.[1, 62]

The second and the most common form of TBE is the Meningeal TBE. Meningeal TBE demonstrates a similar clinical course as the Febrile but exhibits more severe symptoms. Patients generally complain of very strong headaches, stiffness of the neck, nausea and frequent vomiting. Additionally, patients may also become photophobic coupled with eye pains. Fever developed during this period may reach 39 °C (102.2 °F) that lasts between 7 to14 days with gradual recovery.[1, 62]

Table 1: An overview of the clinical symptoms of classical TBE

Symptoms	+	++	+++
Fatigue			■
Malaise			■
Anorexia			■
Headache			■
Neck pain			■
Shoulder pain			■
Lower back pain			■
Fever			■
Nausea			■
Vomiting			■
Severe muscular pains		■	
Numbness		■	
Stiffness of the neck		■	
shortness of breath		■	
Flushing of the face		■	
Flushing of the neck		■	
Upper thoracic flushing		■	

+ Rare ++ Common +++ Frequent

The third form, also known as the Meningoencephalitic type, and occurs less frequently but displays severe symptoms coupled with damage to the CNS. Patients suffering from the Meningoencephalitic form are generally very weak and drowsy, while hallucinations leading to unconsciousness develop frequently. Symptoms that occur during this period include fibrillar contractions, bradycardia, bradykinesia, stomach bleeding, hyperkinesia, hemiparesis, hemiplegia, and at times, patients may experience epileptic fits. It is reported that fatalities are associated with approximately 30% of patients suffering from the Meningoencephalitic form. Hemiplegia is irreversible in survivors of this form of TBE, especially in older patients. Convalescence is very slow for patients recovering from Meningoencephalitic form of TBE. During recovery, patients demonstrate signs of nervous exhaustion, malaise and frequent mood changes (Table 2).[1, 62]

Table 2: An overview of the clinical symptoms of Meningoencephalitic TBE

Symptoms	+	++	+++
General weakness			■
Drowsy			■
Hallucination			■
Unconsciousness			■
Fibrillar contractions			■
Bradycardia			■
Bradykinesia			■
Stomach bleeding			■
Hyperkinesia			■
Hemiparesis			■
Hemiplegia			■
Epileptic fits		■	

+ Rare ++ Common +++ Frequent

The fourth form, known as Poliomyelitic TBE, is characterized by a prodromal period in which patients experience fatigue, periodic muscle contractions and weakness/numbness in one limb which later develops into a paralytic disorder. During the 1 to 4 days of the febrile period, patients may experience paresis of the neck, shoulder and upper limbs which may last 2 weeks to several months. After 2 to 3 weeks the muscles of patients may begin to atrophy, and at times, patients may also develop paralysis of the lower limbs. Convalescence is very slow for patients and only half show partial recovery from the neurological injuries. More commonly, the slow and progressive deterioration of the patient will be observed by clinicians (Table 3).[1, 62]

Table 3: An overview of the clinical symptoms of the Poliomyelitic TBE

Symptoms	+	++	+++
Fatigue			■
Muscle spasms			■
Weakness in one limb			■
Numbness in one limb			■
Paralytic disorder		■	
Paresis of the neck		■	
Shoulder & upper limb paresis		■	
Atrophy	■		
Lower limb paralysis	■		

+ Rare ++ Common +++ Frequent

The fifth form, also known as the Polyradiculoneuritic type, is characterized by painful damage to the peripheral nerves of infected individuals. The Polyradiculoneuritic form of TBE is biphasic with the first phase demonstrating symptoms within 3 to 7 days. The symptoms associated with the initial phase include fever, headache, elevated temperature (38 to 39 °C; 100.4 to 102.2 °F), insomnia, vomiting and muscular pains in the limbs. The initial phase is followed by a period in which the temperature of the patient returns to normal (7–14 days following the onset of initial symptoms). The second phase begins with fever, symptoms of damage to the CNS, meningeal and focal neurological symptoms. Patients suffering from Polyradiculoneuritic type of TBE generally experience a complete recovery (Table 4).[1]

Table 4: An overview of the clinical symptoms of the Polyradiculoneuritic TBE

Symptoms	+	++	+++
Fever			■
Headache			■
Insomnia			■
Vomiting			■
Muscular pains (limbs)			■

+ Rare ++ Common +++ Frequent

The sixth form, known as the Chronic type, is generally associated with patients suffering from infection with the Siberian and Far Eastern subtypes of the virus. The chronic type of the disease has symptoms that develop during the main course of the disease, where the patient experiences gradual deterioration for months or even years. Symptoms include Kozshevnikov's epilepsy, progressive neuritis of the shoulder plexus, lateral sclerosis, dispersed sclerosis, a Parkinson-like disease and progressive muscle atrophy. This condition is commonly associated with mental deterioration that may lead to severe dementia and/or death. Hyperkinesia (abnormal increase in muscle activity) is frequently encountered especially among individuals less than 16 years of age (Table 5).[1, 62]

Table 5: An overview of the clinical symptoms of Chronic TBE

Symptoms	+	++	+++
Kozshevnikov's epilepsy			■
Progressive neuritis			■
Dispersed sclerosis			■
Parkinson-like disease			■
Muscle atrophy			■
Mental deterioration			■
Severe dementia			■

+ Rare ++ Common +++ Frequent

DETECTION

Accurate diagnosis of TBEV infection must be accomplished through laboratory confirmation due to its non-specific clinical features. Generally the method of choice utilized is through the demonstration of specific IgM and IgG serum antibodies by enzyme-linked immuno-sorbent assay (ELISA). Cerebrospinal fluid specific anti-bodies can be found 50% of the time during the early onset of the disease. Nonetheless, by the tenth day of the illness and in almost all cases at the time of hospitalization, TBEV antibodies are invariably detectable. IgM antibodies are known to be detectable up to 10 months or longer in some rare cases, while IgG antibodies persist for the entire life of the patient.[63] It is possible to isolate TBEV or specific nucleic acid directly from the patient's blood or cerebrospinal fluid during the first viremic phase of the disease via reverse-transcriptase polymerase chain reaction (RT-PCR). Post mortem examination may yield TBEV directly from the patient's brain and other organs.[64] Recently, a TBEV-specific (subtype-specific) reverse transcriptase-loop-mediated isothermal amplification (RT-LAMP) has been developed to target the consensus sequences of NS1 and the E genes of each subtype. Experimental results indicate

Table 6: Differential diagnosis of classic TBE and other symptomatically related diseases such as Subacute Sclerosing Panencephalitis (SSPE), Rasmussen's encephalitis (RE), Venezuelan Equine Encephalitis (VEE), Eastern Equine Encephalitis (EEE), Viral Meningoencephalitis (VM) and Cruetzfeld-Jacob disease (CJD)

Symptoms	Classical TBE						
	TBE	SSPE	RE	VEE	EEE	VM	CJD
Fatigue	■					■	
Malaise	■			■	■	■	
Anorexia	■					■	
Headache	■			■	■	■	
Neck pain	■			■	■	■	
Shoulder pain	■			■	■	■	
Lower back pain	■			■	■	■	
Fever	■			■	■	■	
Nausea	■			■	■	■	
Vomiting	■			■	■	■	
Severe muscular pains	■	■		■	■	■	
Numbness	■						
Stiffness of the neck	■	■			■	■	■
Shortness of breath	■						
Flushing of the face	■						
Flushing of the neck	■						
Upper thoracic flushing	■						

that RT-LAMP provides a rapid, highly sensitive, methodology for the detection of TBEV and its subtypes.[65]

TREATMENT

Presently, there are no antiviral treatments or effective post-exposure immunizations for TBE available. The only manner to prevent this viral infection is though immunization. There are two vaccines available in Europe, but unfortunately they are not approved by the FDA and are unavailable in the United States.

The two vaccines are FSME-Immun New (Baxter Vaccine AG, former Immuno AG, Vienna, Austria) and Encepur (Chiron Behring GmbH & Co. KG, Marburg, Germany).[66] Both vaccines consist of complete inactivated virions and regardless of the subtype of the TBEV the individual encounters, there is cross-protection of the vaccine produced to protect individuals from being infected.[67, 68] The two available vaccines have demonstrated to be safe and highly effective in inducing seroconversion and neutralizing antibodies.[69, 70] Mass vaccination programs have occurred in Austria and between the years of 1979 and 2002, the cases of

Table 7: Differential diagnosis of polyradiculoneuritic TBE and other symptomatically related diseases such as Subacute Sclerosing Panencephalitis (SSPE), Rasmussen's encephalitis (RE), Venezuelan Equine Encephalitis (VEE), Eastern Equine Encephalitis (EEE), Viral Meningoencephalitis (VM) and Cruetzfeld-Jacob disease (CJD)

Polyradiculoneuritic TBE							
Symptoms	TBE	SSPE	RE	VEE	EEE	VM	CJD
Fever	■	■		■	■	■	
Headache	■			■		■	
Insomnia	■						
Vomiting	■			■	■	■	
Muscular pains in the limbs	■	■			■	■	

Table 8: Differential diagnosis of meningoencephalitic TBE and other symptomatically related diseases such as Subacute Sclerosing Panencephalitis (SSPE), Rasmussen's encephalitis (RE), Venezuelan Equine Encephalitis (VEE), Eastern Equine Encephalitis (EEE), Viral Meningoencephalitis (VM) and Cruetzfeld-Jacob disease (CJD)

Meningoencephalitic TBE							
Symptoms	TBE	SSPE	RE	VEE	EEE	VM	CJD
General weakness	■			■			
Drowsy	■						
Hallucination	■						■
Unconsciousness	■			■	■	■	
Fibrillar contractions	■						
Bradycardia	■						
Bradykinesia	■						
Stomach bleeding	■						
Hyperkinesia	■	■					
Hemiparesis	■		■			■	
Hemiplegia	■		■			■	
Epileptic fits	■						

Table 9: Differential diagnosis of poliomyelitic TBE and other symptomatically related diseases such as Subacute Sclerosing Panencephalitis (SSPE), Rasmussen's encephalitis (RE), Venezuelan Equine Encephalitis (VEE), Eastern Equine Encephalitis (EEE), Viral Meningoencephalitis (VM) and Cruetzfeld-Jacob disease (CJD)

Poliomyelitic TBE							
Symptoms	TBE	SSPE	RE	VEE	EEE	VM	CJD
Fatigue	■						
Muscle spasms	■	■					■
Weakness in one limb	■				■		■
Numbness in one limb	■				■		■
Paralytic disorder	■		■	■	■	■	■
Paresis of the neck	■		■	■	■	■	■
Paresis of the shoulder and	■				■		
Paresis of the upper limbs	■		■	■	■	■	■
Atrophy	■			■	■		
Paralysis of the lower limbs	■				■	■	■

Table 10: Differential diagnosis of chronic TBE and other symptomatically related diseases such as Subacute Sclerosing Panencephalitis (SSPE), Rasmussen's encephalitis (RE), Venezuelan Equine Encephalitis (VEE), Eastern Equine Encephalitis (EEE), Viral Meningoencephalitis (VM) and Cruetzfeld-Jacob disease (CJD)

Chronic TBE							
Symptoms	TBE	SSPE	RE	VEE	EEE	VM	CJD
Kozshevnikov's epilepsy	■		■				
Progressive neuritis	■	■					
Dispersed sclerosis	■						
Parkinson-like disease	■	■					
Muscle atrophy	■						
Mental deterioration	■	■	■		■		■
Severe dementia	■	■					■

TBE dropped from 677 to 60 (a 95.6 % protection rate).[71]

The conventional inoculation schedule for both available vaccines consists of three injections with an interval of one to three months between the first and second injections and an interval of 9 to 12 months between the second and third injections. Serological testing shows that protective antibody levels are present as early as 2 weeks following the second vaccination. In an effort to maintain long-term immunity, the first booster injection should be administered as early as 12 to 18 months and again at 36 months following the primary immunization.[66]

DIFFERENTIAL DIAGNOSIS

Differential diagnosis of TBE includes Subacute Sclerosing Panencephalitis (SSPE) and Rasmussen's encephalitis (RE). SSPE may occur subsequent to Rubella (measles) infection which is believed to be caused by an abnormal immune response to measles or maybe caused by a mutant form of the Rubeola virus (red measles). Other diseases that should be included in the differential diagnosis are Venezuelan Equine Encephalitis (VEE), Eastern Equine Encephalitis (EEE), and Viral Meningoencephalitis (VM). In addition, prion diseases such as Cruetzfeld-Jacob disease (CJD) and Gerstmann-Strussler-Scheinker syndrome should also be considered in the differential diagnosis. Please see Tables 6 to 10 for more information.

References

1. Gritsun T.S., Lashkevich V.A., Gould E.A. Tick-Borne encephalitis. (2003). Antiviral Research, 2003. 57: pp. 129-146
2. Süss J. Tick-Borne Encephalitis in Europe and beyond – the Epidemiological Situation as of 2007. Eurosurveillance, 2008. 13: pp.18916
3. Charrel R.N., Attoui H., Butenko A.M., Clegg J.C., Deubel V., Frolova T.V., Gould E.A., Gritsun T.S., Heinz F.X. Labuda M., Lashkevich V.A., Loktev V., Lundkvist A., Lvov D.V., Mandl C.W., Niedrig M., Papa A., Petrov V.S., Plyusnin A., Randolph S., Süss J., Zlobin V.I., de Lamballerie X. Tick-borne virus diseases of human interest in Europe. Clinical Microbiology and Infection, 2004. 10: pp. 1040–1055
4. Süss J. Tick-bourne encephalitis, epidemiology, risk areas, and virus strains in Europe and Asia – an overview. Ticks and Tick-borne Diseases, 2011. 2: pp. 2-15
5. Frey S., Essbauer S., Zöller G., Klempa B., Weidmann M., Dobler G., Pfeffer M. Complete Genome Sequence of Tick-Borne Encephalitis Virus Strain A104 Isolated from a Yellow-Necked Mouse (Apodemus flavicollis) in Austria. Genome A, 2013. 1: pp. e00564-13
6. Mandl C.W. Steps of the tick-borne encephalitis virus replication cycle that affect neuropathogenesis. Virus Research, 2005. 111: pp. 161-174
7. Ebert R.A. Progress in Encephalitis Research. Hauppauge: Nova Science Publishers. 2005. pp. 33
8. Suzuki Y. Multiple Transmission of Tick-Borne Encephalitis Virus between Japan and Russia. Genes and Genertic Systems, 2007. 82: pp. 187-195
9. Ecker M., Allison S.L., Meixner T., Heinz F.X. Sequence Analysis and Genetic Classification of Tick-Borne Encephalitis Virus from Europe and Asia. Journal of General Virology, 1999. 80: pp. 179-185
10. Grard G. Moureau G., Charrel R.N., Lemasson J.J., Gonzalez J.P., Gallian P., Gritsun T.S., Holmes E.C., Gould E.A., de Lamballerie X. Genetic Characterization of Tick-Borne Flaviviruses: New Insight into Evolution, Pathogenetic Determinants and Taxonomy. Virology, 2007. 361: pp. 80-92
11. Lindquist L., Vapalahti O. Tick-bourne encephalitis. Lancet, 2008. 371: pp. 1861-1871
12. Magill A.J., Strickland G.T., Maguire J.H., Ryan E.T., Solomon T. Hunter's Tropical Medicine and Emerging Infectious Disease. Amsterdam, Netherlands: Saunders Elsevier. 2013. pp. 370
13. Gresikova M., Kaluzova M. Biology of Tick-Borne Encephalitis Virus. Acta Virologica, 1997. 41: pp. 115-124
14. Schalich J., Allison S.L., Stiasny K., Mandl C.W., Kunz C., Heinz F.X. Recombinant Subviral Particles from Tick-borne Encephalitis Virus are Fusogenic and Provide a Model System for Studying Flavivirus Envelope Glycoprotein Functions. Journal of Virology, 1996 70: pp. 4549-4557
15. Mandl C.W. Heinz F.X., Stockl E., Junz C. Genome Sequence of Tick-Borne Encephalitis Virus (Western Subtype) and Comparative Analysis of Nonstructural Proteins with other Flavoviruses. Virology, 1989. 173: pp. 291-301
16. Milan L., Kozuch O., Zuffová E., Elecková E., Hails R.S., Nuttall P.A. Tick-Borne Encephalitis Virus Transmission between Ticks Cofeeding on Specific Immune Natural Rodent Hosts. Virology, 1997. 235: pp. 138-143
17. Kroschewski H., Allison S.L., Heinz F.X., Mandl C.W. Role of heparan sulfate for attachment and entry of tick-borne encephalitis virus. Virology, 2003. 308: pp. 92–100
18. Malygin A.A., Bondarenko E.I., Ivanisenko V.A., Protopopova E.V., Karpova G.G., Loktev V.B. C-terminal fragment of human laminin-binding protein contains a receptor domain for venezuelan equine encephalitis and tick-borne encephalitis viruses. Biochemistry (Moscow), 2009. 74: pp. 1328-1336
19. Chu J.J. H., Ng M.L. Infectious entry of West Nile Virus Occurs Through a Clathrin-Mediated Endocytic Pathway. Journal of Virology, 2004. 78: pp. 10543–10555
20. Fritz R., Stiasny K., Heinz F.X. Identification of Specific Histidines as pH Sensors in Flavivirus Membrane Fusion. The Journal of Cell Biology, 2008. 183: pp. 353–361
21. Allison, S. L., Schalich, J., Stiasny, K., Mandl, C. W., Kunz, C. & Heinz, F. X. Oligomeric Rearrangement of Tick-Borne Encephalitis Virus Envelope Proteins Induced by an Acidic pH. Journal of Virology, 1995. 69: pp. 695–700
22. Melik W. Molecular characterization of the Tick-borne encephalitis virus. Environments and replication. Stockholm: Universitetsservice US-AB. 2012. pp. 18-25
23. Kofler R.M., Hoenninger V.M., Thurner C., Mandl C.W. Functional Analysis of the Tick-Borne Encephalitis Virus Cyclization Elements Indicates Major Differences between Mosquito-Borne and Tick-Borne Flaviviruses. Journal of Virology, 2006. 80: pp. 4099-4113
24. Mandl C.W., Kunz C., Heinz F.X. Presence of poly(A) in a flavivirus: significant differences between the 3' noncoding regions of the genomic RNAs of tick-borne encephalitis virus strains. Journal of Virology, 1991. 65: pp. 4070-4077
25. Mandl C.W., Holzmann H., Meixner T., Rauscher S., Stadler P.F., Allison S.L., Heinz F.X. Spontaneous and Engineered Deletions in the 3' Noncoding Region of Tick-Borne Encephalitis Virus: Construction of Highly Attenuated Mutants of a Flavivirus. Journal of Virology, 1998. 72: pp. 2132-2140
26. Mansfield K.L., Johnson N., Phipps L.P., Stephenson J.R., Fooks A.R., Solomon T. Tick-Borne Encephalitis Virus – a Review of an Emerging Zoonosis. Journal of General Virology, 2009. 90: pp. 1781-1794
27. Furuichi Y., Shatkin A. J. (2000). Viral and Cellular mRNA Capping: Past and Prospects. Advances in Virus Research, 2000. 55: pp. 135–184
28. Heinz F.X., Mandl C.W. The Molecular Biology of Tick-Borne Encephalitis Virus. Review Article. Acta Pathologica, Microbiologica et Immunologica Scandinavica, 1993. 101: pp. 735-745
29. Henderson B.R., Saeedi B.J., Campagnola G., Geiss B.J. Analysis of RNA Binding by the Dengue Virus NS5 RNA Capping Enzyme. Public Library of Science (PLoS) One, 2011. 6: pp. e25795
30. Best S.M., Morris K.L., Shannon J.G., Robertson S.J., Mitzel D.N., Park G.S., Boer E., Wolfinbarger J.B., Bloom M.E. Inhibition of Interferon-Stimulated JAK–STAT Signalling by a Tick-Borne Flavivirus and Identification of NS5 as an Interferon Antagonist. Journal of Virology, 2005. 79: pp. 12828–12839
31. Murphy F. Togavirus Morphology and Morphogenesis. The Togaviruses. Biology, Structure, Replication. New York: Academic Press. 1980. pp. 241–316
32. Hernandez L.D., Hoffman L.R. Wolfsberg T.G., White J.M. Virus-Cell and Cell-Cell Fusion. Annual Review of Cell and Developmental Biology, 1996. 12: pp. 627-661
33. Chambers T.J., Hahn C.S., Galler R., Rice C.M. Flavivirus Genome Organization, Expression, and Replication. Annual Review of Microbiology, 1990. 44: pp. 649–688
34. Lindenbach B. D., Rice C. M. Flaviviridae: The Viruses and Their Replication. Fields Virology, 4th Edition. Philadelphia: Lippincott Williams & Wilkins. 2001. pp. 991-1041
35. Kofler R.M., Heinz F.X., Mandl C.W. Capsid Protein C of Tick-Borne Encephalitis Virus Tolerates Large Internal Deletions and is a Favorable Target for Attenuation of Virulence. Journal of Virology, 2002. 76: pp. 3534-3543
36. Schalich J., Allison S.L., Stiasny K., Mandl C.W., Kunz C., Heinz F.X. Recombinant Subviral Particles from Tick-Borne Encephalitis Virus are Fusogenic and Provide a Model System for Studying Flavivirus Envelope Glycoprotein Functions. Journal of Virology, 1996. 70: pp. 4549–4557
37. Lindenbach B.D., Thiel H-J., Rice C.M. Flaviviridae: the Viruses and Their Replication. Fields Virology, 5th Edition. Philadelphia, PA: Lippincott Williams & Wilkins. 2007. pp. 1101-1152
38. Rey F.A., Heinz F.X., Mandl C., Kunz C., Harrison S.C. The Envelope Glycoprotein from Tick-Borne Encephalitis Virus at 2 Å Resolution. Nature, 1995. 375: pp. 291–298
39. Orlinger K.K., Hoenninger V.M., Kofler R.M., Mandl C.W. (2006). Construction and Mutagenesis of an Artificial Bicistronic Tick-Borne Encephalitis Virus Genome Reveals an Essential Function of the Second Transmembrane Region of Protein E in Flavivirus Assembly. Journal of Virology, 2006. 80: pp. 12197–12208
40. Allison S.L., Stadler K., Mandl C.W., Kunz C., Heinz F.X. Synthesis and Secretion of Recombinant Tick-Borne Encephalitis Virus Protein E in Soluble and Particulate Form. Journal of Virology, 1995. 69: pp. 5816–5820
41. Vorovitch M. F., Timofeev A.V., Atanadze S.N., Tugizov S.M., Kushch A.A., Elbert L.B. pH-Dependent Fusion of Tick-Borne Encephalitis Virus with Artificial Membranes. Archives of Virology, 1991. 118: pp.133–138
42. Aleshin S.E., Timofeev A.V., Khoretonenko M.V., Zakharova L.G., Pashvykina G.V., Stephenson J.R., Shneider A,M., Altstein A.D. Combined prime-boost vaccination against tick-borne encephalitis (TBE) using a recombinant vaccinia virus and a bacterial plasmid both expressing TBE virus non-structural NS1 protein. BioMedical Central (BMC) Microbiology, 2005. 5: pp. 45
43. Jacobs S. C., Stephenson J. R., Wilkinson G. W. G. High-Level Expression of the Tick-Borne Encephalitis Virus NS1 Protein by Using an Adenovirus-Based Vector: Protection Elicitedin a Murine Model. Journal of Virology, 1992. 66: pp. 2086-2095
44. Falgout B., Chanock R., Lai C.J. Proper Processing of Dengue Virus Nonstructural Glycoprotein NS1 Requires the N-terminal Hydrophobic Signal Sequence and the Downstream Nonstructural Protein NS2A. Journal of Virology, 1989. 63: pp.1852-1860
45. Hiroyuki H., Lai C-J. Cleavage of Dengue Virus NS1-NS2A Requires an Octapeptide Sequence at the C Terminus of NS1. Journal of Virology, 1990. 64: pp. 4573-4577
46. Schrauf S., Schlick P., Skern T., Mandl C.W. Functional Analysis of Potential Carboxy-Terminal Cleavage Sites of Tick-Borne Encephalitis Virus Capsid Protein. Journal of Virology, 2008. 82: pp. 2218–2229
47. Gorbalenya A. E., Donchenko A.P., Koonin E.V., Blinov V.M. N-Terminal Domains of Putative Helicases of Flavi- and Pestiviruses may be Serine Proteases. Nucleic Acids Research, 1989. 17: pp. 3889–3897
48. Chambers T. J., Weir R.C., Grakoui A., McCourt D.W., Bazan J.F., Fletterick R.J., Rice C.M. 1990. Evidence that the N-Terminal Domain of Nonstructural Protein NS3 from Yellow Fever Virus is a Serine Protease Responsible for Site-Specific Cleavages in the Viral Polyprotein. Proceedings of the National Academy of Sciences United States of America, 1990. 87: pp. 8898–8902
49. Lorenz I.C., Kartenbeck J., Mezzacasa A., Allison S.L., Heinz F.X., Helenius A. Intracellular Assembly and Secretion of Recombinant Subviral Particles from Tick-Borne Encephalitis Virus. Journal of Virology, 2003. 77: pp. 4370–4382
50. Wengler G., Wengler G. The Carboxy-Terminal Part of the NS3 Protein of the West Nile Virus Flavivirus can be Isolated as a Soluble Protein after Proteolytic Cleavage and Represents an RNA-Stimulated NTPase. Virology, 1991. 184: 707–715
51. Chambers, T. J., Weir, R. C., Grakoui, A., McCourt, D. W., Bazan, J. F., Fletterick, R. J. & Rice, C. M. Evidence that the N-terminal Domain of Non-Structural Protein NS3 from Yellow Fever Virus is a Serine Protease Responsible for Site-Specific Cleavages in the Viral Polyprotein. Proceedings of the National Academy of Science United States of America, 1990. 87: pp. 8898–8902
52. Egloff M-P., Benarroch D., Selisko B., Romette J-L., Canard B. An RNA Cap (nucleoside-2'-O-) -Methyltransferase in the Flavivirus RNA Polymerase NS5: Crystal Structure and Functional Characterization. The EMBO Journal, 2002. 21: pp. 2757–2768
53. Stadler K., Allison S.L., Schalich J., Heinz F.X. (1997). Proteolytic Activation of Tick-Borne Encephalitis Virus by Furin. Journal of Virology 71, 8475–8481
54. Hayasaka D., Ivanov L., Leonova G.N., Goto A., Yoshii K., Mizutani T., Kariwa H., Takashima I. Distribution and Characterization of Tick-borne Encephalitis Viruses from Siberia and Far-Eastern Asia. Journal of General Virology, 2001. 82: pp. 1319-1328
55. Labuda M., Jones L.D., Williams T. Danielova V., Nuttall P.A. Efficient Transmission of Tick-Borne Encephalitis Virus between Cofeeding Ticks. Journal of Medical entomology,

1993. 30: pp. 295-299

56. Dumpis U., Crook D., Oksi J. Tick-Borne Encephalitis. Clinical Infectious Diseases, 1999. 28: pp. 882–890

57. Shapoval A.N. The Prophylaxis of Tick-borne Encephalitis. Moscow: Medicine, 1977. pp. 47

58. Ebert R.A. Progress in Encephalitis Research. Hauppauge: Nova Science Publishers. 2005. pp.46

59. Gaunt M. W., Sall A. A., de Lamballerie X., Falconar A. K. I., Dzhivanian T. I., Gould E. A. Phylogenetic Relationships of Flaviviruses Correlate with Their Epidemiology, Disease Association and Biogeography. Journal of General Virology, 2001. 82: pp. 1867–1876

60. Alibek K. Biohazard. New York: Dell Publishing. 1999. pp. 42-281

61. Center for Disease Control. Tick-Borne Encephalitis. Fact Sheet. Revised August 21, 2005. Retrieved November 20, 2014. Web Site: http://www.cdc.gov/ncidod/dvrd/spb/pdf/Tickborne_Encephalitis_Fact_Sheet.pdf

62. Scheld W.M., Marra C.M., Whitley R.J. Infections of the Central Nervous System. Philadelphia: Wolters Kluwer Health, 2014. pp. 227-228

63. Ebert R.A. Progress in Encephalitis Research. Hauppauge: Nova Science Publishers. 2005. pp. 11

64. Holzmann H. Diagnosis of Tick-Borne Encephalitis. Vaccine, 2003. 21: pp. S36-S40

65. Hayasaka D., Aoki K., Morita K. Development of simple and rapid assay to detect viral RNA of tick-borne encephalitis virus by reverse transcriptase-loop-mediated isothermal amplification. Virology Journal, 2013. 10: pp. 68

66. Rendi-Wagner P. Risk and Prevention of Tick-Borne Encephalitis. Journal of Travel Medicine, 2004. 11: pp. 307-312

67. Holzmann H., Vorobyova M.S., Ladyzhenskaya I.P., Ferenczi E., Kundi M., Kunz C., Heinz F.X. Molecular Epidemiology of Tick-borne Encephalitis Virus: Cross-protection Between European and Far Eastern Subtypes. Vaccine, 1992. 10: pp. 345–349

68. Klockmann U., Krivanee K., Stephenson J.R., Hilfenhaus J. Protection against European Isolates of Tick-borne Encephalitis Virus after Vaccination with a New Tick-borne Encephalitis Vaccine. Vaccine, 1991. 9: pp. 210–212

69. Barret P.N., Schober-Bendixen S., Ehrlich H.J. History of TBE Vaccines. Vaccine, 2003. 21: pp. S1/41–S1/49

70. Zent O., Beran J., Jilg W., Mach, T., Banzhoff, A. Clinical Evaluation of a Polygeline Free Tick-Borne Encephalitis Vaccine for Adolescents and Adults. Vaccine, 2003. 21: pp. 738–741

71. Kunz C. Epidemiology of Tick-borne Encephalitis and the Impact of Vaccination on the Incidence of Disease. Symposium in Immunology. Berlin: Springer-Verlag, 1996. pp. 143–149

Photo Bibliography

Figure 1.13-1: Negatively-stained transmission electron micrograph (TEM) revealed the presence of numerous tick-borne encephalitis (TBE) virions. Photo was taken by Dr. Fred Murphy; Sylvia Whitfield in 1975 and released by the CDC. Public domain photo

Variola virus, also known as the smallpox virus, is one of the greatest scourges in human history. Smallpox, the disease that variola virus causes, is theorized to be responsible for the downfall of at least three empires as it maimed, disfigured, blinded and/or killed their defenseless citizens.[1] Variola has no known animal reservoir or any other organisms as carriers of the virus, as it only infects humans (Figure 1.14-1).

During the prodromal phase, the mucous membranes in the oral cavity, as well as, the pharynx are infected, followed by the invasion of the virus of the capillary epithelium of the dermal layer in skin, leading to the development of lesions.[8, 9] Subsequently, the virus spreads to other lymphatic tissues, such as the spleen, in addition to cells of other organs such as the liver, bone marrow and lung.[8]

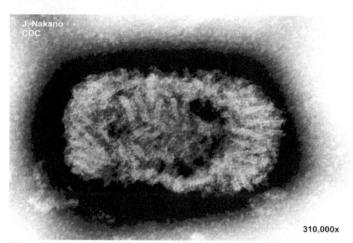

Figure 1.14-2: Highly magnified, negatively stained transmission electron micrograph (TEM), shows a single smallpox (variola) virus particle

Figure 1.14-1: Transmission of smallpox virus, which demonstrates no animal reservoir

Variola is believed to have first appeared around 10,000 BC, during the time of the first agricultural settlements in northeast Africa.[2] The earliest evidence of smallpox is found on the faces of Egyptian mummies (18th to 20th Egyptian Dynasties, 1570 to 1085 BC) and the most notable example of this are the remains of Ramses V who died of this disease as a young man in 1157 BC.[3] From Africa, smallpox spread into Asia and Europe, where it became an endemic infection.[4] In the early 16th century, smallpox began to be imported to the Americas, where it decimated the native American tribes and is presumed to be one of the main cause behind the fall of both Aztec and Incan Empires.[5]

Variola is categorized in the genus *Orthopoxvirus*, subfamily *Chordopoxvirinae*, of the family *Poxviridae* and is the largest and most complex of all known viruses.[6] Variola is a single, linear, double stranded DNA virus (~130 to 375-kb pairs), with a characteristic brick-shape structure and a diameter of approximately 250 to 300 nm. Variola possesses a double membrane that is acquired from the host Golgi apparatus with the outer membrane composed of irregularly arranged tubular lipoprotein subunits and several virus-specific polypeptides. The outer membrane of variola encloses a dumbbell shaped core which contains its viral dsDNA and associated proteins (Figure 1.14-2 and Figure 1.14-3).[7]

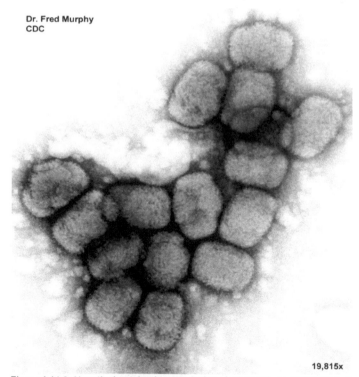

Figure 1.14-3: Negatively-stained transmission electron micrograph (TEM) of variola viruses

After aerosol exposure, the virus enters the respiratory tract, immediately seeds the mucous membranes and passes rapidly into the regional lymph nodes. Initial replication of the virus takes place within the lymph nodes, which is quickly followed by viremia. Viremia occurs for a short period before a latent interval of 4 to 14 days where the virus multiplies in the reticulo-endothelial system. This latent interval will then be followed by another period of viremia, which precedes the prodromal phase.

The variola virus enters the host cell via the fusion of the virion and the host cellular membrane. Presently, the exact manner by which the virus traverses the host cell membrane is unclear. Some research suggests that viral entry is mediated by a viral fusion under neutral pH conditions. Others have indicated that entry is mediated by endosomal uptake via a macro-pinocytosis-like mechanism, involving actin and low pH-dependent steps.[10, 11,] [12] Nonetheless, once the virus reaches the cytoplasm of the host cell, the virus releases prepackaged viral proteins and enzymatic factors that disable cell defenses and stimulate expression of early genes.[10, 13, 14, 15]

Within minutes, after the viral core is released into the cytoplasm, transcription is initiated by the viral transcriptase. A transcription factor, capping and methylating enzymes and poly (A) polymerase facilitates the formation of functional capped and polyadenylated messenger RNA (mRNA) without splicing. The mRNA allows for the transcription of approximately 100 genes. Some of the proteins formed include DNA polymerase, thymidine kinase and numerous other enzymes required for genome replication. Coupled these newly synthesized proteins with various variola membrane bounded proteins, such as L1, A17, A14, A9, E10 and A2.5, the replication of the viral dsDNA occurs. It is understood that the newly replicated dsDNA provides a template for the synthesis of intermediate and late classes of viral mRNA.[6, 16, 17, 18, 19, 20, 21, 22, 23, 24, 25]

Virion assembly occurs in the cytoplasm of the host cell and the immature intracellular virus moves either to the vicinity of the trans-Golgi network or early endosomes on microtubules and obtains a double membrane. Subsequently, the double enveloped virus moves via microtubules to the cell surface where the outermost double membrane of the virus fuses with the plasma membrane and is released from the host cell via exocytosis. Other viral particles are also formed within the cytoplasm of the host cell, but they are released through the disruption of the host cell membrane rather than through exocytosis. It is known that both enveloped and non-enveloped forms of the smallpox virus are equally infectious, but it is the enveloped virus that is readily taken up by cells and is considered to be more important in the spread of the virus throughout the human body.[6]

Typically in Orthopox viruses there are three types of mature virions depending upon their membrane content, location within and how they have been moved outside of the host cell. For example, the infectious intracellular mature virions (IMV) have one or two closely apposed lipoprotein bi-layers which are formed by an undetermined mechanism during an early step in virus assembly.[26, 27, 28] It has been demonstrated that a great number

of the IMVs remain within the cytoplasm of the intact cell and are only released after host cell lysis. Nonetheless, some IMVs have been shown to be released through budding through the host cell plasma membrane.[29, 30] Other IMVs proceed in obtaining a double membrane via trans-Golgi or endosomal cisternae. These "wrapped" IMVs, also referred to as intracellular enveloped virions (IEV), are transported on microtubules to the periphery of the cell where the outer IEV and plasma membranes fuse.[31, 32, 33, 34, 35, 36] These externalized IEVs possess an additional membrane and are commonly seen adhering to the host cell surface at the tips of actin-containing microvilli.[37, 38] Some of these IEVs dissociate from the cell and form the last *Orthopoxvirus* type, known as extracellular enveloped virions (EEV) (Figure 1.14-4).[39]

IMV, IEV and EEV are different due to their membrane coat receptors, but they are all equally virulent. It has been reported that due to their differences in membrane coats and surface receptors, they bind to different host cell surface receptors.[40]

Recent research has shown that the initial attachment to the host cell surface is accomplished through interactions between various viral ligands (e.g. A26L, A27L, A28L, D3 and H3 proteins), which are anchored to the surface of infectious IMV and consequently lie beneath membranes of IEV and EEV,[41] and with the host cell surface receptors, such as, laminin, chondroitin sulfate and/or heparan sulfate (Table 1).[11, 42, 43, 44, 45]

Table 1: Variola attachment proteins

Attachment	kDa	Properties
A26L	58	Binds to Laminin
A27L	13	Binds to heparin sulfate
A28L	81	Binds to heparin & chondroitin sulfate
D3	35	Binds to chondroitin sulfate
H3	38	Binds to heparin sulfate

There are two strains of smallpox: Variola Major and Variola Minor. Variola Major is the most common form of smallpox and is the more severe form of this disease.[46] Variola Major has an overall fatality rate of 30 to 50%, among those who are unvaccinated and 3% in vaccinated individuals.[47] The last case of Variola Major occurred in Bangladesh in 1975. Variola Minor causes a less

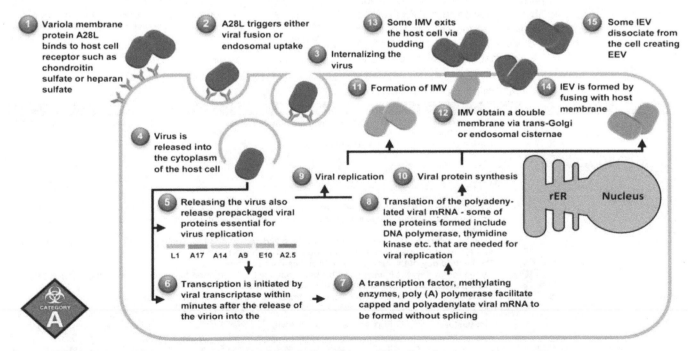

Figure 1.14-4: Diagrammatic process of smallpox virus (variola) infection within an eukaryotic cell

common type of smallpox and has less than 1% fatality rate.[48, 49] The last case of Variola Minor occurred in Somalia in 1977.[50]

There are four subtypes of Variola Major: ① Ordinary Variola Major, which occurs in 90% or more of cases; ② Modified Variola Major, is a mild type of smallpox that occurs in previously vaccinated individuals; ③ Flat Variola Major and ④ Hemorrhagic Variola Major. Both Flat Variola Major and Hemorrhagic Variola Major are rare and very severe forms of smallpox infection. It has been estimated that the Ordinary and Modified Variola Major have an approximate overall fatality rate of 30%, while individuals suffering from Flat and Hemorrhagic Variola Major have nearly 100% fatality rate.[51, 52]

Natural transmission of the variola virus results when virus-containing aerosol droplets from the oral, nasal, or pharyngeal mucosa are inhaled by individuals who are in close contact with patients that are developing the signature smallpox rash. Transmission is most frequent during the first week of exanthema.[6] It has been estimated that inhaling approximately 10 to 100 variola viruses can result in infection.[53] Smallpox can also be spread through direct contact with the scabs or pus from the skin lesions caused by Variola where high titers of the virus are found.[54]

Once infected, the Variola virus multiplies in the lymph nodes. During this initial phase, which lasts 3 to 4 days, the patient is asymptomatic. This initial phase is followed by further viral development in the spleen, bone marrow and the lymphatics which results in a second viremia that lasts 8 to 10 days. The second phase is followed by the prodromal stage where the first sign of fever and toxemia appears.[55]

Smallpox is considered to be one of the most dangerous biological weapons, due to its infectivity in an aerosol form, high human-to-human transmission rate, as well as, its high mortality rate. Because of the discontinuation of the world wide vaccination program and the declaration of its eradication by the World Health Organization, this disease is becoming more dangerous with each passing day.[56] Put simply, "a world no longer protected from smallpox was a world newly vulnerable to the disease."[55] The Soviet Union, who first proposed the smallpox eradication campaign to the World Health Organization in 1958, saw the potential of smallpox as a biological weapon subsequent to its eradication. Therefore in 1967, Soviets collected a strain of Indian smallpox (a subtype of Variola Major) that was highly virulent and

was stable enough to maintain its infectivity over a long period of time. They dubbed this strain India-1967 or India-1 and began mass producing it as a biological weapon. Subsequent to the weaponization of India-1, the Soviets redesignated the biological weapon as N1. The Soviet military's standing order was to maintain the stockpile of the agent at 20 tons and was stored at army facilities in Zagorsk.[57]

SYMPTOMS

The incubation period for Ordinary Variola Major is approximately 12 days (7 to 17 days). Patients during this time are asymptomatic and are not contagious. The incubation period, followed by an immediate onset of flu-like symptoms, also known as the prodromal phase, lasts 2 to 5 days with symptoms of high fever (33 to 40 C°; 101 to 104 F°), chills, sweats, malaise, prostration, headache, backache, body ache and myalgia. In addition, symptoms of nasal congestion, pharyngitis, mouth sores, swollen eyelids and conjunctivitis are also common symptoms. Less commonly, patients may develop anorexia, abdominal pains, diarrhea, nausea and vomiting.[47, 58] These initial symptoms are followed by the early rash stage (e.g. exanthema), where the development of maculopapular rash appears on the mucosa of the mouth, tongue, pharynx, face, and the forearms before it spreads to the trunk and legs (Figure 1.14-5).[59]

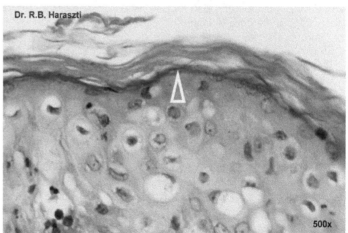

Dr. R.B. Haraszti

500x

Figure 1.14-5: A photomicrograph showing the histopathologic cytoarchitectural changes, which manifest inside the confines of a smallpox, variola maculopapular lesion. Note the reduction in the normal thickness of the stratum corneum (arrow), which at first glance from a macroscopic appearance may appear exophytic in nature, but is really pseudoexophytic

Table 2: Example of symptoms and corresponding time period of smallpox infection

Approximate Time Period	Symptoms
0 to 17 days	· Exposure to the virus is followed by an incubation period during which people do not have any symptoms and may feel fine · During this time, people are not contagious
18 to 22 days	· Prodrome phase is the start of the contagious period of the disease. The initial symptoms include fever, malaise, head and body aches, fatigue and vomiting · The fever is usually high, in the range of 101 to 104 degrees Fahrenheit · At this time, people are usually too sick to carry on their normal activities
23 to 27 days	· A rash emerges first as small red spots on the tongue and in the mouth. These spots develop into sores that break open and spread large amounts of the virus into the mouth and throat. At this time, the person is the most contagious · A rash appears on the skin, starting on the face and spreading to the arms and legs and then to the hands and feet (complete spread throughout the body within 24 hours) · By the third day of the rash, the rash becomes raised bumps · By the fourth day, the bumps fill with a thick, opaque fluid and often have a depression in the center that looks like a bellybutton. (This is a major distinguishing characteristic of smallpox) · Fever often will rise again at this time and remain high until scabs form over the bumps
28 to 32 days	· The bumps become pustules
33 to 37 days	· The pustules begin to form a crust and then scab
38 to 42 days	· The scabs begin to fall off, leaving marks that eventually becomes pitted scars
43+ days	· The person is contagious to others until all of the scabs have fallen off

With the appearance of the rash, the fever generally falls and marks a short period during which the patient feels better. However, the appearance of the rash also marks the period when the patient is most contagious.[49]

Within 1 to 2 days, the rash becomes vesicular, then round, tense and deeply embedded pustules are formed. This marks the beginning of the pustular rash phase when the fever will rise again and will remain high for approximately 5 days until the scabs form over the pustules (Figure 1.14-6). Patients during this period are still highly infectious. The pustular rash phase is followed by the resolving scab phase when the scabs begin to fall off, whereby leaving marks on the skin that may become pitted scars. This phase lasts approximately 6 days and the patient remains contagious until all of the scabs have fallen off.[58, 60] Examine Table 2 for a breakdown of the symptoms and chronology of smallpox infection.

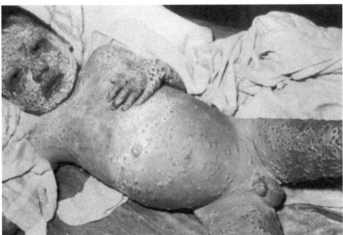

Figure 1.14-6: This photograph shows a 7 year old male displaying the characteristic maculopapular rash, which had spread over all the body regions

Both Variola Major and Variola Minor share relatively similar clinical course. As indicated previously, Variola Minor is the less common form of the disease. Comparatively, Variola Minor exhibits lower intensity in both rash and fever, as well as, other symptoms.[61]

Modified Smallpox demonstrates fewer lesions and expresses an accelerated clinical course compared with the Ordinary Variola Major. Modified Smallpox generally appears in previously vaccinated individuals. For example, in the Rao sub-form of the Modified Smallpox, 25% is found in individuals that had prior vaccination while only 2% were seen in unvaccinated patients. Patients suffering from this form of the disease will experience the same pre-eruptive symptoms, but the fever will subside by the 6th or 7th day. The lesions will be more superficial, fewer in numbers and evolve more quickly by comparison. The lesions will not develop pustules and will be encrusted by the 10th day. The Modified Form of smallpox is rarely, if ever, fatal and is easily confused with symptoms of the chicken pox.[62]

Flat-type Variola Major, also known as malignant smallpox, was so named because the lesions of the patients remain soft, flat to the skin, and velvety to the touch at the time of vesiculation.[4] Presently, it is still not known why certain patients develop this form of disease. For patients suffering from Flat-type Variola Major, a severe prodromal phase lasts approximately 3 to 4 days, accompanied by prolonged high fever and severe symptoms of toxemia.[63] Flat-type disease is generally associated with lesions that develop slowly and do not progress to the pustular

phase. By day 7 to 8 after the onset of fever, these lesions possess hemorrhages in their base and the central flattened portions appear black or dark purple, while pulmonary edema is also observed. An extensive enanthem, a rash that appears inside the body, is usually present on the tongue, hard palate and the rectal mucosa. The color of the lesions will turn ashen gray approximately 24 to 48 hours prior to death. Respiratory complications are commonly observed with patients suffering from this form of disease (Table 3 and Figure 14-7).[62]

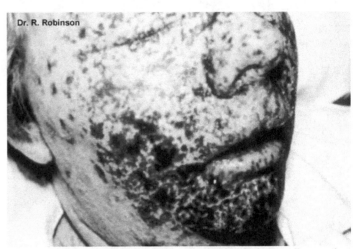

Dr. R. Robinson

Figure 1.14-7: This photograph shows a 35 year-old female smallpox patient suffering from a malignant Variola Major rash. The photograph was taken on the tenth day posteruption; this rash included hemorrhagic papules, but did not display vesicles. This patient died on the twelfth day post onset

Historically, Flat-type accounts for 5%–10% of all cases and the majority of these cases (approximately 72%) are in children, 14 years old or younger, as well as pregnant women. Cases of this form of smallpox are rare in vaccinated individuals, while the fatality rate for unvaccinated individuals is estimated to be as high as 96.5%.[62] In rare cases where the patient survives (patients suffering from Flat-type generally do not survive), the lesions disappear without forming scabs.[4, 64]

There are two types of Hemorrhagic (Purpura Variolosa) Variola Major: Early and Late Hemorrhagic Variola Major. Both types are accompanied by high mortality rates and generally appear more commonly in adults than children, and also appear more frequently in vaccinated individuals. Unlike a Ordinary Variola Major infection where the viremia subsides after the appearance of the rash, the pathogenesis of the hemorrhagic form demonstrate continuous high grade viremia throughout the course of infection.[62]

Early Hemorrhagic Type is commonly seen in both vaccinated and unvaccinated adults and is almost always fatal. It has been reported that 88% of the individuals that contract this disease are over the age of 14.[62] Pregnant women are highly susceptible to this form of smallpox. The Early Hemorrhagic Type is characterized by hemorrhaging in the skin and/or mucous membranes before the appearance of the rash. Patients suffering from this form of hemorrhagic smallpox display severe symptoms of toxemia, a sudden onset of headache and backache and are generally restless, anxious and pale in appearance. These individuals will generally remain conscious until death. Petichial rash may appear, however it is usually confined to the groin area, extending to the upper thighs while a generalized erythema usually appears on the second day after the onset of fever. Sixty percent of patients will suffer from subconjunctival hemorrhages, which may be accompanied by bleeding gums, hematemesis, hemoptysis, hematuria, melena and/or epistaxis. Approximately

70% of women suffering from the Early Hemorrhagic Type will display vaginal bleeding. Death generally occurs around the 6th day after the onset of fever. Autopsy results indicate that heart failure and pulmonary edema are the causes of death rather than hemorrhagic symptoms (Table 3).[62]

Table 3: An overview of the clinical symptoms of smallpox infections

Symptoms	+	++	+++
High fever			■
Chills			■
Sweats			■
Malaise			■
Prostration			■
Exhaustion			■
Headache			■
Backache			■
Body aches			■
Myalgia			■
Fatigue			■
Nasal congestion			■
Sore throat			■
Mouth sores			■
Swollen eyelids			■
conjunctivitis			■
Exanthema (early rash)			■
Maculopapular rash			■
Papules			■
Blisters			■
Vesicular rash			■
Umbelication			■
Desquamation			■
Pustular rash			■
Hemorrhaged lesions			■
Scabbing			■
Pitted scars			■
Toxemia			■
Hemorrhaged lesions			■
Pulmonary edema			■
Enanthem			■
Respira. complication			■
Non-scabbed lesions			■
Hemorrhage of the skin			■
Mucous mem. hemorr.			■
Petichial rash			■
Generalized erythema			■
Subconjunct. hemorr.			■
Bleeding gums			■
Hematemesis			■
Hemoptysis			■
Hematuria			■
Melena			■
Epistaxis			■
Vaginal bleeding			■
Heart failure			■
Pulmonary edema			■
Anorexia		■	
Abdomianl pains		■	
Diarrhea		■	
Nausea		■	
Vomiting		■	

+ Rare ++ Common +++ Frequent

■ General Variola symptoms
■ Symptom for Modified & Flat-type (No pustules)
■ Symptoms for Flat-type Variola
■ Symptoms for Early and Late Hemorrhagic Variola

Patients suffering from the Late Hemorrhagic Type will develop a severe and prolonged prodromal phase lasting approximately 4 to 5 days. Late Hemorrhagic smallpox is characterized by hemorrhaging in the skin and/or mucous membranes after the appearance of the rash (Figure 1.14-8).[62] The pre-eruptive stage of this disease demonstrates high fever (40 C°; 104 F°) and severe constitutional signs which continue even after the appearance of the rash. The lesions start as macules and turn into papules, which may have hemorrhages in their base, giving them a plateau-like appearance. These rashes appear to be symmetrical and a localized rash appears in the groin and along the flanks to the axillae. Fifty five percent of the patients suffer from subconjuntival hemorrhages and 60% of the females display vaginal bleeding. Late Hemorrhagic Type smallpox is fatal in 90% to 95% of cases. Death usually occurs between day 8 and 9 of the fever. Late Hemorrhagic Type smallpox also occurs more often in adults (individuals over 14 years of age), with higher frequencies noted in pregnant women (Table 3).[62]

DETECTION

In order to provide an accurate diagnosis, vaccinated healthcare providers will need to swab the patient's pharynx and/or open skin lesions (e.g. pustule contents, material from the base of the scab) to obtain samples of the virus.[54] These swabs will then be sent to a biosafety level 4 (BSL-4) laboratory to examine the acquired samples.[65]

However, in order not to cause unnecessary panic, the clinical features of smallpox should be used to classify persons presenting with suspected smallpox into one of three categories: those with high, moderate, and low risk of having smallpox. Highly specific laboratory testing should only be reserved for patients in the high-risk category, in an effort to minimize the number of false-positive test results. [65, 66, 67]

Diagnosis of poxvirus infection can be rapidly confirmed through electron microscope examination of virus particles in vesicular fluid, pustular fluid or scabs. All Orthopoxvirus virions have the same "brick shaped," appearance, therefore, electron microscopy can only provide a rapid form of initial diagnosis and cannot differentiate the various types of Orthopoxvirus.[6]

Smallpox is commonly misdiagnosed as Varicella zoster virus (VZV; herpes virus type 3 or chickenpox), therefore, a process of elimination and the utilization of VZV diagnostic tests may give a rapid resolution to the type of infection. The most useful VZV diagnostic test is direct fluorescent antibody screening where a positive for VZV, will likely be a negative for smallpox virus.[6] A second method of rapid diagnosis for smallpox infection is the Tzanck smear, which is also a method for VZV identification. A positive Tzanck smear confirms either a VZV or HSV (herpes simplex virus) infection, ruling out variola virus infection.[65, 66, 67]

For diagnostic purposes, poxvirus samples are generally grown in chorioallantoic membranes (CAM) of 10 to 12 day old domestic chicken embryos. Cultured on CAM, each of the four types of orthopox viruses develop distinctive pocks, characteristic of their species, allowing accurate diagnosis (Figure 1.14-9).[67]

It is known that each species of Orthopoxvirus possesses a distinctive DNA map that can be identified though polymerase chain reaction (PCR) amplification of various specific viral genome DNA segments followed by restrictive endonuclease assays of the PCR products.[68] Two additional PCR methods are available to identify the variola virus. The first utilizes primers that target the unique hemagglutinin glycoprotein gene.[69] The second PCR method targets the gene for the acidophilic-type inclusion body (A-type) protein. Through previous research using enzyme analysis and blot hybridizations each species of *Orthopoxvirus* has specific deletions of A-type inclusion body protein genes, therefore, these are used to allow discrimination between the viral species.[70, 71]

Data show that real-time PCR can produce definitive results within two to four hours of specimen submission and the specificity of the test is greater than 99%. In the light of this technical advancement, World Health Organization suggests that these tests be made available to as many countries as possible in order to maintain global surveillance for smallpox.[72]

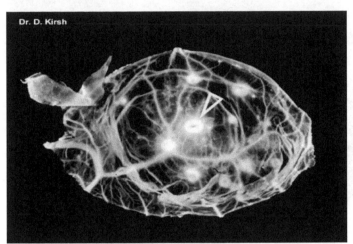

Figure 1.14-9: A photograph revealing smallpox virus pocks on the chorioallantoic membrane of a developing chicken embryo. An example of the smallpox virus pock is indicated by the arrow

TREATMENT

Dryvax©, a vaccine made by Wyeth Laboratories™, has been available for over 20 years. Dryvax© is a lyophilized live virus preparation of infectious vaccinia virus that induces a protective response to variola virus and other *Orthopoxviruses*. To date, it is still the best method of preventing smallpox infection. Due to the current climate of terroristic actions around the world, the United States has increased the number of doses of smallpox vaccine in its stockpile. However, this vaccine, which is harvested from bovine is not sterile and may be allergenic to select individuals.[73] Dryvax© is delivered via scarification, which involves dipping a bifurcated needle (a needle with two points at the end) into the vaccine and poking the tip of the needle into the skin over

the deltoid muscle, or the posterior aspect of the arm over the triceps muscle repeatedly. Successful vaccination is marked by the typical Vaccinia reaction, indicated by a visible papule by day 3 and further develops into a blister-like pustule by day 7 to 10. Redness and swelling of the vaccination site usually appear after 8 to 12 days. Patients may suffer swelling of the local lymph nodes, as well as, a low grade fever and exhaustion. Nonetheless, by approximately 21st day, the pustule will resolve with scab separation.[74]

Efforts are being made in creating a new, live cell-culture-derived smallpox vaccine. Currently, over 200 million doses of cell-culture-derived smallpox vaccine are available, and Acambis™ is under contract with the federal government to maintain this level of supply until 2020.[75, 76]

There is no specific treatment for patients suffering from smallpox. Nonetheless, cidofovir (hydroxypropyl methylcellulose phthalate), its cyclic derivative, and ribavirin have demonstrated significant inhibition patterns when administered during early stages of illness in laboratory animals, although the effectiveness of this treatment has not been proven in humans.[74] Both cidofovir and its cyclic derivative inhibit viral DNA polymerase, while ribavirin inhibits the actions of viral inosine monophosphate dehydrogenase.[68]

Corneal lesions due to smallpox may be treated topically with topical idoxuridine. Topical antiviral drops or ointments are given every 4 hours for 7 to 10 days.[77, 78] Antibodies to the vaccinia virus called Vaccinia immune globulin (an experimental medication) is designed to stimulate the immune system to react against the vaccinia virus and in turn aid to develop immunity towards smallpox. Vaccinia immune globulin may help people who have certain serious reactions to the smallpox vaccine, but does not appear to offer a survival benefit when given to patients during the incubation or active-disease stages of smallpox.[79, 80] The mainstay of treatment for patients suffering from smallpox is supportive therapy, whereby fluids, electrolytes and nutrition are maintained. Many methods ranging from physically abrading the pustules to painting the skin with gentian violet have been used in reducing the physical appearance of skin lesions. However, none has proven to be effective.[67]

DIFFERENTIAL DIAGNOSIS

Symptoms displayed by smallpox are easily confused with a

Table 4: List of conditions that may be confused with smallpox

Conditions	Clinical Clues and Features
Varicella	Most common found in children under 10 years of age and usually does not have a prodrome phase
Disseminated herpes zoster	Most commonly found in immunocompromised patients. The rash resembles that of the varicella and it usually begins in dermatomal distribution
Impetigo	Impetigo caused by *Streptococcus pyogenes* or *Staphylococcus aureus* possesses classic symptoms of honey-colored crusted plaques with bullae, although it may begin as vesicles. The rash is regionally distributed and is not disseminated. Patients are generally asymptomatic
Drug eruptions	Caused by exposure to medication and the rash is often generalized
Contact dermatitis	Itching and localized rash that suggest external contact with allergens
Erythema multiforme	This condition may include Stevens-Johnson Syndrome. Major forms involve mucous membrane and conjunctivae, which may display target lesions or vesicles
Enteroviral infection	This condition may include Hand, Foot and Mouth Disease. Patients contracting this disease develop fever and mild pharyngitis, which begins 1-2 days before appearance of rash. The lesions may first appear maculopapular, but evolve into whitish-grey, tender, flat, oval-shaped vesicles mainly found peripherally on the hands, feet, and mouth
Disseminated herpes simplex	Lesions are indistinguishable from varicella and are commonly witnessed in immunocompromised hosts
Scabies	This infection is caused by *Sarcoptes scabiei* (a mite). Major symptoms include rash and itching, but no sign of febrile symptoms. The rash generally appears in the webs of fingers, flexing surfaces of the wrists and armpits, the areolae of the breasts in females and on genitals of males, along the belt line, and on the lower buttocks
Molluscum contagiosum	This is a viral skin infection caused by *Molluscum contagiosum* virus (MCV) and generally appears in immunocompromised patients. There are 4 types of MCV, MCV-1 to -4, with MCV-1 being the most prevalent and MCV-2 seen in adults and is often sexually transmitted. Lesions caused by this virus are flesh-colored, dome-shaped, and pearly in appearance

Table 5: Differential diagnosis of small pox and other symptomatically related diseases such as varicella zoster (VZ), herpes zoster (HZ), erythema multiforme (EM), measles, allergic dermatitis (AD), meningococcemia (MEN) and acute leukemia (AL)

Symptoms	Smallpox	VZ	HZ	EM	MP	Measles	AD	Men	AL
High fever	■	■			■	■			■
Chills	■	■			■			■	
Sweats	■	■			■				■
Malaise	■	■	■	■		■		■	
Prostration	■				■				
Exhaustion	■							■	■
Headache	■				■			■	■
Backache	■	■	■					■	
Body aches	■			■		■		■	
Myalgia	■	■			■	■		■	
Fatigue	■				■			■	■
Anorexia	■	■	■		■				■
Exanthema (early rash)	■	■	■				■		
Nasal congestion	■	■			■				
Sore throat (pharyngitis)	■	■	■	■	■				
Mouth sores	■			■	■				
Swollen eyelids	■	■			■	■			
Conjunctivitis	■			■	■	■	■		
Desquamation	■				■	■	■		
Maculopapular rash	■	■		■	■				
Papules	■	■	■	■	■				
Blisters	■	■	■	■	■		■		
Vesicular rash	■	■	■	■	■	■	■		
Umbelication	■								
Pustular rash	■	■	■				■		
Hemorrhaged lesions	■					■			
Scabbing	■	■	■		■				
Pitted scars	■				■				
Toxemia	■								
Hemorrhaged lesions	■								
Pulmonary edema	■								
Enanthem	■								
Respiratory complications	■								
Non-scabbed lesions	■								
Hemorrhage of the skin	■							■	
Mucous mem. hemorrhage	■								
Petichial rash	■							■	■
Generalized erythema	■								
Subconjunct. hemorrhage	■								
Bleeding gums	■					■			■
Hematemesis	■								
Hemoptysis	■								
Hematuria	■								
Melena	■					■			
Epistaxis	■					■			■
Vaginal bleeding	■								
Heart failure	■								
Pulmonary edema	■								
Abdomianl pains	■					■			
Nausea	■	■	■		■			■	
Vomiting	■				■			■	
Diarrhea	■				■	■			

■ General Variola symptoms
■ Symptom for Modified & Flat-type (No pustules)
■ Symptoms for Flat-type Variola
■ Symptoms for Early and Late hemorrhagic Variola

variety of other diseases that are accompanied by a rash. These diseases include erythema multiforme (EM), measles, *Molluscum contagiosum* (MC) or allergic dermatitis (AD) etc. In addition, smallpox could also be confused with other forms of poxvirus infections such as varicella zoster (VZ), herpes zoster (HZ), and monkeypox (MP). It has been reported that hemorrhagic cases of smallpox are commonly misdiagnosed as meningococcemia (MEN), acute leukemia (AL) or drug toxicity (Table 4).[2, 81]

Differential diagnosis of smallpox could begin with the identification and recognition of the patterns of lesion formation. For example, the lesion formation for smallpox begins centrally and spreads to the extremities. In contrast, the lesion formation for VZ begins on the face and subsequently spreads to the trunk; HZ forms lesions around the genital region, while MC lesions are formed in non-specific locations. In addition, both smallpox and MC forms lesions at the same stage of development at a given

Table 6: Comparison of lesions between Smallpox, herpes zoster (HZ), *Molluscum contagiosum* (MC) varicella zoster (VZ)

Lesions	Smallpox	HZ	MC	VC
Begin centrally & spread to the extremities	▪			
Begin at the face & spread to the trunk				▪
Same stage of development	▪		▪	
Different stages of development		▪		▪
Unilateral distribution		▪		
Widespread distribution	▪		▪	▪

time period while HZ and VZ develops lesions at various stages at a given time period.[2, 81] Please examine Tables 4, 5, and 6 for more information.

References

1. Barquet N., Domingo P. Smallpox: The Triumph over the Most Terrible of the Ministers of Death. Annals of Internal Medicine, 1997. 127: pp. 635-642
2. Guerrant R.L., Walker D.H., Weller P.F. Tropical Infectious Diseases – Principles, Pathogens & Practice. Volume 1. Churchill Livingstone Elsevier. Philadelphia, 2006. pp. 621-622
3. Ruffer M.A., Ferguson A.R. Note on an Eruption Resembling that of Variola in the Skin of a Mummy of the Twentieth Dynasty (1200-1100 BC). Journal of Pathology and Bacteriology, 1911. 15: pp. 1-4
4. Fenner F., Henderson D.A., Arita I., Jezek Z., Ladnyi I.D. Smallpox and Its Eradication. Geneva: World Health Organization. 1988. pp. 210-217
5. McNeill W.H. Plagues and People. New York: Anchor Books. 1998. pp. 365
6. Guerrant R.L., Walker D.H., Weller P.F. Tropical Infectious Diseases – Principles, Pathogens & Practice. Volume 1. Churchill Livingstone Elsevier. Philadelphia, 2006. pp.623-625
7. Wagner E.K. and Hewlett MJ. Basic Virology. Malden. Blackwell Publishing Company, 2004. pp. 623-624
8. Breman J.G., Henderson D.A. Diagnosis and Management of Smallpox. The New England Journal of Medicine, 2002. 346: pp. 1300-1308
9. Strano A.J. Smallpox. Pathology of Tropical and Extraordinary Diseases: An Atlas. Volume 1. Washington, D.C.: Armed Forces Institute of Pathology, 1976. pp. 65-67
10. Moss B. Poxvirus Cell Entry: How Many Proteins Does it Take? Viruses, 2012. 4: pp. 688-707
11. Abdulnaser A., Hammamieh R., Hardick J., Ait Ichou M., Jett M., Ibrahim S. Gene Expression Profiling of Monkeypox Virus-Infected Cells Reveals Novel Interfaces for Host-Virus Interactions. Virology Journal, 2010. 7: pp. 173-191
12. Vanderplasschen A, Hollinshead M, Smith GL: Intracellular and Extracellular Vaccinia Virions Enter Cells by Different Mechanisms. J Gen Virol 1998, 79(Pt 4):877-887
13. White D.O., Fenner F.J. Medical Virology. San Diego: Academic Press. 1994. pp. 31-52
14. Munyon W., Paoletti E., Grace J.T. Jr: RNA Polymerase Activity in Purified Infectious Vaccinia Virus. Proceedings of the National Academy of Sciences United States of America, 1967. 58: pp. 2280-2287
15. Kates J.R., McAuslan B.R. Poxvirus DNA-Dependent RNA Polymerase. Proceedings of the National Academy of Sciences United States of America, 1967, 58: pp. 134-141
16. Da Fonseca F., Moss B. Poxvirus DNA Topoisomerase Knockout Mutant Exhibits Decreased Infectivity Associated with Reduced Early Transcription. Proceedings of the National Academy of Sciences United States of America, 2003. 100: pp. 11291-11296
17. Ravanello M. P., Hruby D.E. Conditional Lethal Expression of the Vaccinia Virus L1R Myristylated Protein Reveals a Role in Virus Assembly. Journal of Viology, 1994. 68: pp. 6401-6410
18. Rodríguez D., Esteban M., Rodriguez J.R. Vaccinia Virus A17L Gene Product is Essential for an Early Step in Virion Morphogenesis. Journal of Viology, 1995. 69: pp. 4640-4648
19. Yuwen H., Cox J.H., Yewdell J.W., Bennink J.R., Moss B. Nuclear Localization of a Double-Stranded RNA-Binding Protein Encoded by the Vaccinia Virus E3l Gene. Virology, 1993. 195: pp. 732-744
20. Rodriguez J. R., Risco C., Carrascosa J.L., Esteban M., Rodriguez D. Vaccinia Virus 15-Kilodalton (A14L) Protein is Essential for Assembly and Attachment of Viral Crescents to Virosomes. Journal of Viology, 1998. 72: pp. 1287-1296
21. Yeh W.W., Moss B., Wolffe E.J. The Vaccinia Virus A9 Gene Encodes a Membrane Protein Required for an Early Step in Virion Morphogenesis. Journal of Viology, 2000. 74: pp. 9701-9711
22. Senkevich T. G., Weisberg A., Moss B. Vaccinia Virus E10R Protein is Associated with the Membranes of Intracellular Mature Virions and has a Role in Morphogenesis. Virology, 2000. 278: pp. 244-252
23. Senkevich T., White C., Weisberg A., Granek J., Wolffe E., Koonin E., Moss B. Expression of the Vaccinia Virus A2.5L Redox Protein is Required for Virion Morphogenesis. Virology, 2002. 300: pp. 296-303
24. Moss B., de Silva F. DNA Replication and Human Disease. Poxvirus DNA Replication and Human Disease. New York: Cold Spring Harbor Laboratory Press. 2006. pp. 707–727
25. Yang Z., Reynolds S.E., Martens C.A., Bruno D.P. Porcella S.F., Moss B. Expression profiling of the intermediate and late stages of poxvirus replication. Journal of Virology, 2011. 85: pp. 9899–9908
26. Hollinshead M., Vanderplasschen A., Smith G.L., Vaux D.J. Vaccinia Virus Intracellular Mature Virions Contain Only One Lipid Membrane. Journal of Viology, 1999. 73: pp. 1503-1517
27. Risco C., Rodriguez J.R., Lopez-Iglesias C., Carrascosa J.L., Esteban M., Rodriguez D. Endoplasmic Reticulum-Golgi Intermediate Compartment Membranes and Vimentin Filaments Participate in Vaccinia Virus Assembly. Journal of Viology, 2002. 76: pp. 1839-1855
28. Sodeik B., Doms R.W., Ericsson M., Hiller G., Machamer C.E., van't Hof W., van Meer G., Moss B., Griffiths G. Assembly of Vaccinia Virus: Role of the Intermediate Compartment Between the Endoplasmic Reticulum and the Golgi Stacks. The Journal of Cell Biology, 1993. 121: pp. 521-541
29. Meiser A., Sancho C., Krijnse Locker J. Plasma Membrane Budding as an Alternative Release Mechanism of the Extracellular Enveloped Form of Vaccinia Virus from HeLa Cells. Journal of Viology, 2003. 77: pp. 9931-9942
30. Tsutsui K. Release of Vaccinia Virus from FL Cells Infected with the IHD-W Strain. Journal of Electron Microscopy, 1983. 32: pp. 125-140
31. Hiller G., Weber K. Golgi-Derived Membranes that Contain an Acylated Viral Polypeptide are Used for Envelopment. Journal of Viology, 1985. 55: pp. 651-659
32. Schmelz M., Sodeik B., Ericsson M., Wolffe E.J., Shida H., Hiller G., Griffiths G. Assembly of Vaccinia Virus: the Second Wrapping Cisterna is Derived from the Trans-Golgi Network. Journal of viology, 1994. 68: pp. 130-147
33. Tooze J., Hollinshead M., Reis B., Radsak K., Kern H. Progeny Vaccinia and Human Cytomegalovirus Particles Utilize Early Endosomal Cisternae for Their Envelopes. European Journal of Cell Biology, 1993. 60: pp. 163-178
34. Geada M. M., Galindo I., Lorenzo M.M., Perdiguero B., Blasco R. Movements of Vaccinia Virus Intracellular Enveloped Virions with GFP Tagged to the F13L Envelope Protein. Journal of General Viology, 2001. 82: pp. 2747-2760
35. Hollinshead M., Rodger G., Van Eijl H., Law M., Hollinshead R., Vaux D.J., Smith G.L. Vaccinia Virus Utilizes Microtubules for Movement to the Cell Surface. The Journal of Cell Biology, 2001. 154: pp. 389-402
36. Rietdorf J., Ploubidou A., Reckmann I., Holmström A., Frischknecht F., Zettl M., Zimmerman T., Way M. Kinesin-Dependent Movement on Microtubules Precedes Actin Based Motility of Vaccinia Virus. Nature Cell Biology, 2001. 3: pp. 992-1000
37. Blasco R., Moss B. Role of Cell-Associated Enveloped Vaccinia Virus in Cell-to-Cell Spread. Journal of Viology, 1992. 66: pp. 4170-4179
38. Stokes G. V. High-Voltage Electron Microscope Study of the Release of Vaccinia Virus from Whole Cells. Journal of Viology, 1976. 18: pp. 636-643
39. Boulter E. A., Appleyard G. Differences between Extracellular and Intracellular Forms of Poxvirus and Their Implications. Progress in Medical Virology, 1973. 16: pp. 86-108
40. Vanderplasschen A., Smith G.L. A Novel Virus Binding Assay Using Confocal Microscopy: Demonstration that Intracellular and Extracellular Vaccinia Virions Bind to Different Cellular Receptors. Journal of Viology, 1997. 71: pp. 4032-4041
41. Senkevich T.G., Ward B.M., Moss B. Vaccinia Virus Entry into Cells Is Dependent on a Virion Surface Protein Encoded by the A28L Gene. Journal of Virology, 2004. 78: pp. 2357-2366
42. Carter G.C., Law M., Hollinshead M., Smith G.L. Entry of the Vaccinia Virus Intracellular Mature Virion and Its Interactions with Glycosaminoglycans. Journal of General Viology, 2005. 86: pp.1279-1290
43. Hsiao J.C., Chung C.S., Chang W. Vaccinia Virus Envelope D8L Protein Binds to Cell Surface Chondroitin Sulfate and Mediates the Absorption of Intracellular Mature Virions to Cells. Journal of Viology, 1999. 73: pp. 8750-8761
44. Chung C.S., Hsiao J.C., Chang Y.S., Chang W. A27L Protein Mediates Vaccinia Virus Interaction with Cell Surface Heparan Sulfate. Journal of Viology, 1998. 72: pp. 1577-1585
45. Lin C.L., Chung C.S., Heine H.G., Chang W. Vaccinia Virus Envelope H3L Protein Binds to Cell Surface Heparan Sulfate and is Important for Intracellular Mature Virion Morphogenesis and Virus Infection In Vitro and In Vivo. Journal of Viology, 2000. 74: pp. 3353-3365
46. Smallpox (Variola). Utah Department of Health Bureau of Epidemiology. Revised December 2002. Retrieved July 25, 2008. Web Site: http://health.utah.gov/epi/fact_sheets/smallpox.pdf
47. Massung R.F., Liu L.I., Qi J., Knight J.C., Yuran T.E., Kerlavage A.R., Parsons J.M., Venter J.C., Esposito J.J. Analysis of the Complete Genome of Smallpox Variola Major Virus Strain Bangladesh-1975. Virology, 1994. 201: pp. 215-240
48. Loveless B.M., Mucker E.M., Hartmann C., Craw P.D., Huggins J., Kulesh D.A. Differentiation of Variola major and Variola minor Variants by MGB-Eclipse Probe Melt Curves and Genotyping Analysis. Molecular and Cellular Probes, 2009. 23: pp. 166-170
49. Smallpox Disease Overview. Center for Disease Control and prevention. Revised December 30, 2004. Retrieved July 25, 2008. Web Site: http://www.bt.cdc.gov/agent/smallpox/overview/over view.pdf
50. Potential Bioterrorism Agent: Category A. Washington State Department of Health. Revised October 2002. Retrieved August 2, 2008. Web Site: http://www.jeffersoncountypublichealth.org/pdf/ disease/smallpox.pdf
51. de Paolo C. Epidemic Disease and Human Understanding: A Historical Analysis of Scientific and Other Writings. Jefferson: McFarland & Company. 2006. pp. 215
52. Bossi P., Tegnell A., Baka A., Van Loock F., Hendriks J., Werner A., Maidhof H., Gouvras G. Bichat Guidelines for the Clinical Management of Smallpox and Bioterrorism-Related Smallpox. EuroSurveilance, 2004. 9: pp. E1- E6
53. Darling R.G., Woods, J.B. USAMRIID's Medical Management of Biological Casulties Handbook. Fifth Edition. Fort Detrick: US Army Medical Research Institute of Infectious Diseases, 2004. pp. 59-65
54. Mitra A.C., Sarkar J.K., Mukherjee M.K. Virus Content of Smallpox Scabs. Bulletin of the World Health Organization, 1974. 54: pp. 106-107
55. Riedel S. Smallpox and Biological Warfare: a Disease Revisited. Baylor University Medical Center Proceedings, 2005. 18: pp. 13–20
56. Bellamy R.J., Freedman A.R. Bioterrorism. Quarterly Journal of Medicine, 2001. 94: pp. 227-234
57. Alibek K. Biohazard. New York: Dell Publishing. 1999. pp. 20, 110-112
58. World Health Organization. Smallpox. Retrieved July 25, 2008. Web Site: http://www.who.int/mediacentre/ factsheets /smallpox/en/print.html
59. Guerrant R.L., Walker D.H., Weller P.F. Tropical Infectious Diseases – Principles, Pathogens & Practice. Volume 1. Churchill Livingstone Elsevier. Philadelphia, 2006. pp. 626-627
60. Sarkar J.K., Mitra A.C., Mukherjee M.K., De S.K. Virus Excretion in Smallpox. Bulletin of the World Health Organization, 1973. 48: pp. 523-527
61. Smallpox (Variola). The Merck Manuals. November 2005. Retrieved August 2, 2008. Web Site: http://www. merck.com/mmpe/sec14/ch193/ch193f.html
62. Khardori N. Bioterrorism Preparedness: Medicine - Public Health – Policy. Springfield: Wiley-VCH Verlag GmbH and CO. 2006. pp. 104-105
63. Atkinson W., Hamborsky J., McIntyre L., Wolfe S. Smallpox. Epidemiology and Prevention of Vaccine-Preventable Diseases. Ninth Edition. Washington DC: Public Health Foundation. 2005. pp. 281-306
64. Constantin C.M., Martinelli A.M., Foster S.O., Bonney E.A., Strickland O.L. Smallpox: a Disease of the Past? Consideration for Midwives. Journal of Midwifery and Womens

Health, 2003. 48: pp. 258-267

65.   Franz D.R., Parrott C.D., Takafuji E.T. The U.S. Biological Warfare and Biological Defense Programs. Medical Aspects of Chemical and Biological Warfare. Washington D.D.: Office of the Surgeon General Department of the Army, United States of America. 1997. pp. 425-436

66.   Seward J. F., Galil K., Damon I.,Norton S.A., Rotz L.,Schmid S.,Harpaz R.,Cono J.,Marin M.,Hutchins S., Chaves S.S.,McCauley M.M. Development and Experience with an Algorithm to Evaluate Suspected Smallpox Cases in the United States, 2002–2004. Clinical Infectious Diseases, 2004. 39: pp. 1477–83

67.   Gupta L.K., Singhi M.K. Tzanck Smear: A Useful Diagnostic Tool. Indian Journal of Dermatology, Venereology and Leprology, 2005. 71: pp. 295-299

68.   Wagner E.K. and Hewlett MJ. Basic Virology. Malden. Blackwell Publishing Company, 2004. pp. 628-629

69.   Ropp S.L., Jin Q., Knight J.C., Massung R. F., Esposito J. J. Polymerase Chain Reaction Strategy for Identification and Differentiation of Smallpox and other Orthopoxviruses. Journal of Clinical Microbiology, 1995. 33: pp. 2069-2076

70.   Meyer H., Rziha H.J. Characterization of the Gene Encoding the A-type Inclusion Protein of Camelpox Virus and Sequence Comparison with other Orthopoxviruses. Journal of General Virology, 1993. 74: pp. 1679-1684

71.   Meyer H., Pfeffer M., Rziha H.J. Sequence Alterations within and Downstream of the A-type Inclusion Protein Genes allow Differentiation of Orthopoxvirus Species by Polymerase Chain Reaction. Journal of General Virology, 1994. 75: pp. 1975-1981

72.   Smallpox Eradication: Destruction of Variola Virus Stocks. World Health Organization Executive Board EB117/33. 117th Session Provisional agenda item 4.7. January 16, 2006. Retrieved August 3, 2008. Web Site: http://www.who.int/gb/ebwha/pdf_files/EB117/B117_33-en.pdf

73.   Rosenthal S.R., Merchlinsky M., Kleppinger C., Goldenthal K.L. Developing New Smallpox Vaccines. Emerging Infectious Diseases, 2001. 7: pp. 920-926

74.   Smallpox Vaccination Method. Center for Disease Control and Prevention. Revised February 7, 2008. Retrieved August 2, 2008. Web Site: http://emergency.cdc.gov/agent/smallpox/vaccination /vaccination-method.asp

75.   Birmingham K., Kenyon G. Smallpox Vaccine Development Quickened. Nature Medicine, 2001. 7: pp. 1167

76.   Baker R.O., Bray M., Huggins J.W. Potential Antiviral Therapeutics for Smallpox, Monkeypox and Other Orthopoxvirus Infections. Antiviral Research, 2003. 57: pp. 13-23

77.   Semba R.D. The Ocular Complications of Smallpox and Smallpox Immunization. Archives of Ophthalmology, 2003. 121: pp. 715-719

78.   Pavan-Langston D. Ocular Viral Infections. Medicine Clinics of North America, 1983. 67: pp. 973-990

79.   Investigational Vaccinia Immune Globulin (VIG) Information. Center for Disease Control and Prevention. Revised January 16, 2003. Retrieved August 3, 2008. Web Site: http://www.bt.cdc.gov/agent/smallpox/ vaccination/pdf/vig.pdf

80.   Vaccinia (Smallpox) Vaccine: Recommendations of the Advisory Committee on Immunization Practices 2001. Morbidity and Mortality Weekly Report, 2001. 50: pp. 1-24

81.   J.H. McIsaac. Hospital Preparation for Bioterror. A Medical and Biomedical System Approach. Burlington: Academic Press. 2006. pp. 52

Photo Bibliography

Figure 1.14-2: Negatively-stained transmission electron micrograph (TEM) of variola viruses. Photo was taken by Dr. Fred Murphy in 1975 and released by the CDC. Public domain photo

Figure 1.14-3: Highly magnified, negatively stained transmission electron micrograph (TEM) shows a single smallpox (variola) virus particle. Photo was taken by J. Nakano in 1968 and released by the CDC. Public domain photo

Figure 1.14-5: A photomicrograph showing the histopathologic cytoarchitectural changes, which manifest inside the confines of a smallpox, variola maculopapular lesion. Note the reduction in the normal thickness of the stratum corneum (arrow), which at first glance from a macroscopic appearance may appear exophytic in nature, but is really pseudoexophytic. The photomicrograph was taken by Dr. R.B. Haraszti in 1965 and released by the CDC. Public domain photo

Figure 1.14-6: This Photograph shows a 7 year old male displaying the characteristic maculopapular rash, which had spread over all body regions. This photograph was taken by Dr. J. D. Miller in 1962 and released by the CDC. Public domain photo

Figure 1.14-7: This photograph shows a 35 year-old female smallpox patient suffering from Malignant Variola Major rash. The photograph was taken on the tenth day of post-eruption, this rash included hemorrhagic papules, but did not display vesicles. This patient died on the twelfth day post onset. The photograph was taken by Dr. R. Robinson in 1962 and released by the CDC. Public domain photo

Figure 1.14-8: This photograph depicted a bedridden smallpox patient from the Late Hemorrhagic smallpox. The skin of this patient displays what was termed a severe malignant, confluent, eruptive maculopapular rash on his face, arms and chest. This photograph was taken in 1965 by Carl Flint and released by the CDC. Public domain photo

Figure 1.14-9: A photograph revealing smallpox virus pocks on the chorioallantoic membrane of a developing chicken embryo. This photograph was taken by Dr. Kirsh and released by the CDC. Public domain photo

Venezuelan equine encephalitis virus (VEEV) belongs to the genus *Alphavirus* in the family *Togaviridae*. VEEV are small (~70 nm in diameter), enveloped, positive sense (mRNA sense), single stranded RNA viruses that cause highly virulent Venezuelan Equine Encephalitis (VEE) in equines and is readily transmitted to humans via mosquitoes.[1] Presently, there are at least 13 different VEEV subtypes and varieties known, including several different species, making up the VEE complex.[2] To date, VEEV subtype I varieties A, B, and C have caused outbreaks involving hundreds of thousands of equine and human cases. Subtype I varieties D, E, and F and II-VI are enzootic, equine avirulent strains and are not responsible for major equine outbreaks, although they have been known to cause human illness, which can be fatal (Figure 1.15-1).[3, 4]

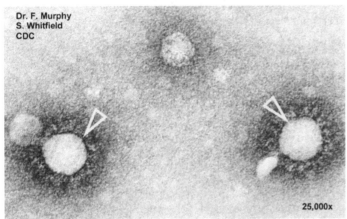

Figure 1.15-1: A negatively-stained transmission electron micrograph (TEM) of a number of Venezuelan equine encephalitis (VEE) virus virions (arrow)

The VEEV ssRNA genome (~12 kb in length) is enclosed within an icosahedral nucleocapsid surrounded by a host-cell acquired lipid bilayer. There are two integral glycoproteins that lie within the lipid bilayer: E1, which lies below the spikes adjacent to the envelope, and E2, which forms the spikes on the surface of virion. Both E1 and E2 are compiled as heterodimers into 80 trimeric spikes located on the surface of the virus.[5, 6]

There are six known antigenic subtypes of VEEV with subtypes I and III subdivided into five groups (AB, C, D, E and F) and three (A, B and C) antigenic variants, respectively.[7, 8, 9, 10, 11] VEEV exists in two distinct ecological cycles: epizootic/enzootic or endemic.

VEE was first described in Venezuela in 1936 as a disease of horses, mules, and donkeys. It has since caused numerous epizootics and epidemics in many regions of tropical Latin America.[12] Since, there are no epidemiological records of any VEE outbreaks during the nineteenth century[13], phylogenetic estimates derived from sequences of VEEV strains implicated in early outbreaks, indicate that this virus probably evolved in the early twentieth century (Figure 1.15-2).[14]

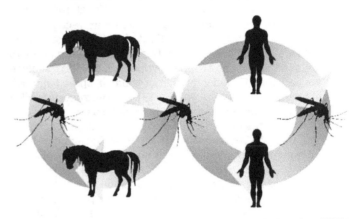

Figure 1.15-2: Sylvatic cycle of Venezuelan equine encephalitis virus (VEEV)

Although epidemiological records imply that VEE outbreaks may have begun as early as the 1920s, the first widely recognized outbreak of the disease appeared in the central river valleys of Colombia during 1935.[12] In 1936, VEE outbreaks spread into

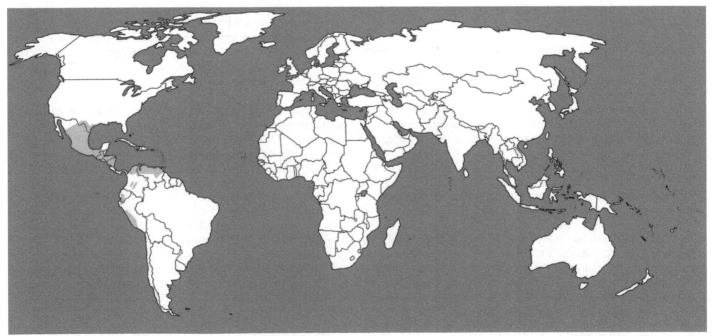

Figure 1.15-3: Distribution of Venezuelan equine encephalitis virus (VEEV)

Table 1: Examples of species and subtype of *Alphavirus* that are responsible for VEE in humans[24]

Species	Antigenic Subtype	Antigenic Variety	Clinical Syndrome	Location
Venezuelan Equine Encephalitis virus	I	AB C D E	Febrile illness, encephalitis	AB: N, C, & S. America C: S. America D: S. America E: C and S America
Mosso das Pedras virus	I	F (strain 78V3531)	None recognized	Brazil
Everglades virus	II	-	Febrile illness, encephalitis	Florida
Mucambo virus	III	A C (strain 71D1252) D (strain 407660)	A: febrile illness, myalgia C: none recognized D: febrile illness	A: S. America, Trinidad C and D – Peru
Tonate virus	III	B	Febrile illness, encephalitis	Brazil and Colorado
Pixuna virus	IV	-	Febrile illness, myalgia	Brazil
Cabassou virus	V	-	None recognized	French Guiana
Rio Negro virus	VI	-	Febrile illness, myalgia	Argentina

the Guajira Peninsula of northern Colombia and Venezuela, a desert environment populated by large numbers of mosquitoes following infrequent rainfall. From 1936 to 1938, outbreaks of this disease spread across northern Venezuela and in 1943, VEE appeared on the island of Trinidad. The connection between equine and human VEE was not established until 1954, when the human form of this infectious disease was recognized in Colombia[15] and in 1967, when VEEV was first isolated from human cases of febrile illness and fatal encephalitis in northern Venezuela.[16] In the spring of 1969, an outbreak of VEEV (subtype IAB) appeared in Ecuador and from there it spread through Central America into Mexico. In July 1971, an epizootic of VEEV (subtype IAB) occurred for the first time in Texas.[17, 18] Following almost two decades of VEE inactivity, the next outbreak occurred in Trujillo, western Venezuela (subtype IE) in December, 1992[19] and in the summer of 1993, a minor outbreak (subtype IE) was described in Chiapas State, Mexico.[20] In 1995, one of the largest VEE epizootics and epidemics (subtype IC) on record occurred, involving an estimated 75,000 to 100,000 people (resulting in ~300 deaths), began in Falcon State, Venezuela (April) and by July in Carabobo, Yaracuy, Lara, and Zulia States of Venezuela. By August a major epidemic occurred in rural areas of the Guajira Peninsula, both in Venezuela and Colombia. Sporadic human and equine VEE cases (subtype IC) continued in Trujillo, Portuguesa, Cojedes, and Guarico States, Venezuela until December 1995.[12, 21] From June to July 1996, another epizootic (subtype I-E) occurred in Oaxaca State, Mexico causing the deaths of many horses but no human fatalities were reported (Figure 1.15-3).[12]

It is known that enzootic VEEV subtypes ID-F, II-IV are generally avirulent for equines, but are pathogenic for humans and can be fatal.[22, 23] While epidemic and enzootic VEEV subtypes IAB and IC are virulent for both humans and equines, scientists have yet to discover the interepizootic maintenance cycles.[23, 24] Please examine Table 1 for more information with regards to species of *Alphaviruses* that are responsible for arborviral encephalitis.

The epidemic and epizootic transmission cycle of the VEEV involves various species of mammalian mosquitoes. *Psorophora confinnis* and *P. columbiae* are probably the most important vectors involved in outbreaks in northern South America and in the 1971 epizootic/epidemic in northern Mexico and Texas. A third vector, *Ochlerotatus sollicitans*, formerly known as *Aedes sollicitans*, also exhibited extremely high infection rates in Mexico and Texas during the 1971 outbreak.[25] In South America, the mosquito species, *Ochlerotatus taeniorhynchus*, may be the most important epizootic vector. This species is abundant in coastal areas, including the Guajira Peninsula, located on the coastal areas of Columbia where some of the largest outbreaks have occurred.[26, 27] Other suspected vectors may be *Culex*

(*Deinocerites*) spp.[28], as well as, some non-mosquito arthropods such as Black flies (suborder *Nematocera*, family *Simmuliidae*), ticks, including *Amblyomma cajennense* (*Acari: Ixodidae*) and *Hyalomma truncatum* and possibly even chicken mites (*Dermanyssus gallinae*).[29, 30, 31, 32]

VEEV gains entry into host cells either through fusion with membrane components or through receptor attachment and internalization. Due to the broad tropism of these viruses, many possible receptors may be responsible for facilitating viral entry. These possible receptors that could serve to initiate cellular entry for VEEV include the 37/67-kd laminin receptor (LAMR), dendritic cell-specific intercellular adhesion molecule-3-grabbing non-integrin (DC-SIGN), liver/lymph node-specific intercellular adhesion molecule-3-grabbing integrin (L-SIGN), and heparin sulfate.[33, 34, 35, 36, 37]

The entry of VEEV into cells is facilitated by interaction of the E2 integral glycoprotein spikes with protein receptors (e.g. LAMR) located on the surface of target cells. After VEEV binds with the host cell receptor (s), it is believed that clathrin-mediated endocytosis is the mechanism of entry. Once internalized, VEEV is delivered to early endosomes and subsequently transported to late endosomes. Within the late endosome, the E1-E2 heterodimer undergo irreversible conformational changes when exposed to the acidic environment (pH of 6 or below). This acidic environment liberates the E1 subunit from the E2 subunit, allowing the rearrangement to an E1 homotrimeric active enzyme/protein to induce fusion of the VEEV envelope with the endosome membrane. Subsequent to the fusion viral and endosomal membranes, the nucleocapsid is released and undergoes disassembly, releasing genomic RNA into the cytoplasm of the host cells (Figure 1.15-4).[38, 39]

Once inside the cytoplasm, the VEEV positive sense RNA genome is translated into two large open reading frames (ORFs). Like messenger RNA (mRNA), the VEEV genomic RNA contains a 5' methyguanylate cap structure and a 3' polyadenylate sequence. At the 5' end, two-thirds of the genome is translated directly into nonstructural (P1234) polyprotein precursor upon entry into the cytoplasm of the host cell. P1234 is later cleaved to form nsP1, nsP2, nsP3 and nsP4. At the 3' end, one-third of the remaining viral genome encodes the five viral structural polyproteins. The viral structural proteins include capsid (C), E3, E2, 6K, and E1 glycoproteins (e.g. NH_2-Capsid-E3-E2-6K-E1-COOH). During the synthesis of viral nonstructural and structural proteins, full length negative sense RNA strands are synthesized to serve as a template for the formation of viral genomic RNA (Figures 1.15-4 and 1.15-5).[6, 24, 38]

VEEV nsP1 possesses both guanine-7-methyltransferase and

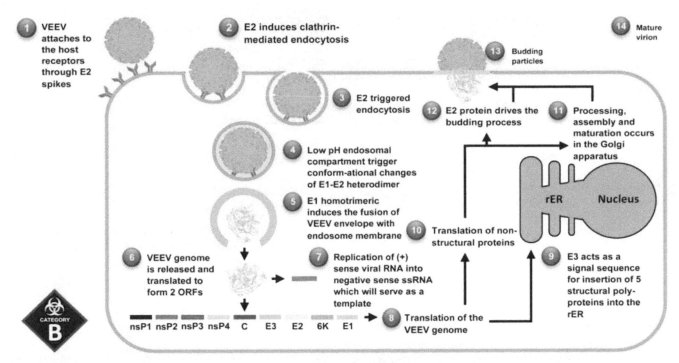

Figure 1.15-4: Diagrammatic process of Venezuelan equine encephalitis virus (VEEV) infection within an eukaryotic cell

Within the figure:

1. VEEV attaches to the host receptors through E2 spikes
2. E2 induces clathrin-mediated endocytosis
3. E2 triggered endocytosis
4. Low pH endosomal compartment trigger conform-ational changes of E1-E2 heterodimer
5. E1 homotrimeric induces the fusion of VEEV envelope with endosome membrane
6. VEEV genome is released and translated to form 2 ORFs
7. Replication of (+) sense viral RNA into negative sense ssRNA which will serve as a template
8. Translation of the VEEV genome
9. E3 acts as a signal sequence for insertion of 5 structural poly-proteins into the rER
10. Translation of non-structural proteins
11. Processing, assembly and maturation occurs in the Golgi apparatus
12. E2 protein drives the budding process
13. Budding particles
14. Mature virion

nsP1 nsP2 nsP3 nsP4 C E3 E2 6K E1

rER   Nucleus

CATEGORY B

guanylyl transferase activities, which are required for capping and methylation of viral genomic and subgenomic RNAs. [24, 40] VEEV nsP2 exhibits dual functions. At the N-terminus nsP2 it possesses helicase capabilities, while at the C-terminus it is a viral cysteine protease that regulates the processing of nonstructural polyproteins.[24, 41] The N-terminus of nsP3 shows ADP-ribose 1-phosphate phosphatase and RNA-binding activity, while the nsP4 protein serves as RNA-dependent RNA-polymerase.[38, 42]

VEEV capsid (C) protein is responsible for nucleocapsid formation. It has been reported that the C protein binds to viral genomic RNA via N- terminal arginine, lysine, and proline residues. Mutagenesis studies show a leucine zipper located within this region that is essential for the formation of nucleocapsid-like particles. It is speculated that this leucine zipper is designed to mediate dimerization during virus assembly.[38] The C-terminal of the C protein is a serine-protease domain that possesses a hydrophobic pocket for glycoprotein binding.[38, 43]

As indicated previously, the E1-E2 forms heterodimer within the lipid membrane of the virus envelope and are responsible for host cell receptor binding and subsequent acid-induced fusion of the viral and endosomal membrane.[38, 39] The E2 protein, on the other hand, is known to be a determinant of neurovirulence.[44]

The VEEV structural protein 6K is essential for viral particle assembly. 6K is believed to be involved in virion assembly at the plasma membrane before being incorporated into the virion prior to release.[38] 6K structural protein have also been reported to form cation-selective ion channels and serve as a viroporin, which alters the membrane permeability in mammalian cells.[45, 46]

The E3 structural protein of VEEV acts as a signal sequence for insertion of the five structural polyproteins into the rough endoplasmic reticulum where it is processed by host signal peptidase.[38] Once processed, the structural proteins are transported to the cell plasma membrane via the Golgi apparatus, where the virion assembly takes place. It has been reported that the interactions between the C protein and the cytoplasmic domain of the E2 protein drive the budding process whereas E1-

E2 heterodimers forms an envelope around virus particles.[43] As the virion is released from the host cell via budding, it acquires a membrane bilayer derived from the host cell plasma membrane (Figure 1.15-4).[38]

VEE is known to cause a large spectrum of disease ranging from an indistinct infection to acute encephalitis, with a viral attack rate at approximately 30%. VEEV infection in human results in a biphasic disease.[1] The infection enters the body and spreads through the lymphatic system, and causes viremia.[47] VEEV also enters the bone marrow cells via receptor-mediated endosytosis. Subsequent to the appearance of the virus in the blood stream, VEEV enters the CNS through the olfactory neuroepithelium via the brain capillary endothelial cells and the area of the olfactory system innervated by the trigeminal nerve (cranial nerve V).[48, 49] Within the CNS, VEEV begins to spread through neurons and neuroglial cells, such as astrocytes[50], where it causes cellular degeneration and cell death. It is known through the use of mouse models that the infection of astrocytes induces gene expression of two neuro-immune modulators: tumor necrosis factor-alpha (TNF-α) and inducible nitric oxide synthase (iNOS). Findings indicate that the inflammatory response, which are partly mediated by TNF- α and iNOS, may contribute to neurodegeneration following encephalitic virus infection.[50, 51] Gliosis and the intense inflammatory response are characterized by the infiltration of mononuclear cells (e.g. lymphocytes) into the CNS via blood vessels and interstitial fluids.[1] In addition, cerebral edema and apoptotic neurons associated with astrogliosis in the regions of the brain which are free of VEEV antigens could also contribute to neuro-degeneration.[50] However, the exact mechanism of infection is presently poorly understood and requires further elucidation.

Due to its infectiousness, only 10-100 pathogens are needed to infect a person. Due to VEEV's effectiveness as an incapacitating agent, the United States Biological Warfare program located at Fort Detrick researched the potential of VEEV as a biological weapon in 1964.[52] Research has shown that VEEV can be disseminated through aerosolization in dried or liquid form.[52] Investigations in regards to VEEV were also conducted at the

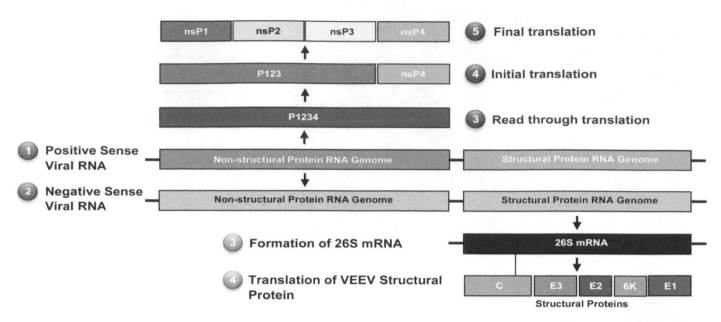

Figure 1.5-5: The protein products of VEEV positive sense viral RNA genome

Virological Center of the Ministry of Defense in the former Soviet Union.[54] According to Ken Alibek (1999), Sergei Netyosov, the Deputy Scientific Director of Vector Complex, was attempting to create a chimera by splicing VEEV genome into a Vaccinia virus. Alibek reported that in 1990, Netyosov had succeeded in combining the genome of Vaccinia and VEEV, although it was unclear if chimeric VEEV was ever mass produced for use as a bioweapon.[55]

SYMPTOMS

Patients infected with VEEV will experience symptoms ranging from infection with no symptoms, mild influenza-like symptoms, severe systematic infection, encephalitis and/or death. VEEV infections are unlike other encephalitic diseases, as they cause a systemic illness rather than a localized disease of the brain.[56]

The incubation period for VEEV is approximately 1 to 4 days. Patients with a mild infection may be asymptomatic or develop minor flu-like symptoms such as a low-grade fever, myalgias, and/or headache. Patients with moderate infections may develop fever (39 to 40 °C; 102.2 to 104 °F), intermittent chills, myalgias, back pain, headache, photophobia, vomiting, general weakness, prostration, sore throat, confusion and hypesthesia (Table 2).[57]

Table 2: An overview of the clinical symptoms of moderate VEEV infections

Symptoms	+	++	+++
Fever			■
Myalgias			■
Headache			■
Intermittent chills			■
Back pain			■
Headache			■
Photophobia			■
Vomiting			■
General weakness			■
Prostration			■
Sore throat			■
Confusion			■
Hypesthesia			■

+ Rare ++ Common +++ Frequent

Patients suffering from a severe infection of VEEV will develop

fever, lethargy, severe headaches, chills, dizziness, body aches, myalgia, chills, nausea, vomiting, retroorbital pains and prostration.[58] Other common symptoms include inflammation of the throat, cervical lymphadenitis, and tenderness of the abdominal region. These initial symptoms may subside after several days, but there is a chance that they may reappear. Severe neurological symptoms such as seizures occur in approximately 4 to 14% of cases and generally appear in children. Patients that developed encephalitis with subsequent symptoms of convulsions, paralysis and coma have a fatality rate of 10 to 25% (Table 3).[59, 60]

Table 3: An overview of the clinical symptoms of severe VEEV infections

Symptoms	Rare	Common	Frequent
Lethargy			■
Severe headaches			■
Chills			■
Dizziness			■
Body aches			■
Myalgia			■
Chills			■
Nausea			■
Vomiting			■
Retroorbital pains			■
Prostration			■
Throat inflammation		■	
Cervical lymphadenitis		■	
Abdomianl tenderness		■	
Seizures	■		
Convulsions	■		
Paralysis	■		
Coma	■		

DETECTION

Definitive diagnosis of VEEV through viral particle isolation from patient serum is most successful during the first three days of illness. The serum is tested for virus by intracerebral inoculation of newborn mouse, and by the inoculation of Vero and C6/36 cells.[61, 62] Typically, titers of 10^3 to 10^6 plaque-forming units/mL of virus are easily isolated.[21] Pharyngeal swabs can also be used to isolate samples of the viruses but with lower isolation titers.[62] Reverse transcription polymerase chain reaction (RT-PCR) has

Table 4: Differential diagnosis of VEEV and other symptomatically related diseases such as Dengue fever (DF), viral hepatitis (VH), influenza, leptospirosis (Lepto), malaria, Q fever, St. Louis encephalitis (St. LE), West Nile Encephalitis (WNE)

Symptoms	VEEV	DF	VH	Influenza	Lepto	Malaria	Q Fever	St. LE	WNE
Fever	■	■	■	■	■	■	■	■	■
Myalgias	■	■	■	■	■	■	■		■
Headache	■	■		■	■	■	■	■	■
Back pain	■	■							
Photophobia	■	■							
General weakness	■							■	■
Prostration	■								
Sore throat	■			■				■	
Confusion	■					■	■	■	■
Hypesthesia	■								
Lethargy	■	■							
Chills	■	■		■	■	■	■		
Dizziness	■								
Body aches	■	■							
Nausea	■	■	■		■	■	■	■	■
Vomiting	■	■	■		■	■	■		■
Retroorbital pains	■	■							
Prostration	■								
Inflammation of the throat	■								
Cervical lymphadenitis	■	■			■				
Abdomianl tenderness	■	■	■		■				■
Seizures	■								
Convulsions	■							■	■
Paralysis	■							■	■
Coma	■					■		■	■

been successfully used to detect VEEV in human serum and throat swabs. For example, Linssen et al. (2000) utilized the RT-PCR-seminested-PCR combination to specifically amplify 342- and 194-bp fragments of the region of the 6K gene in VEEV. They reported that the sensitivity was as high as 20 RNA molecules for subtype IAB virus and 70 RNA molecules for subtype IE virus. Furthermore, three of the enzootic VEEV such as subtypes IIIB, IIIC, and IV showed the amplicon in the seminested PCR.[63] Nonetheless, the identification of specific serotype of VEEV is best achieved through enzyme linked immunoassay (ELISA). It has been reported that IgM and IgG antibodies are present in both vaccinated (two weeks post-vaccination) and naturally infected patients (after the onset of symptoms). At two weeks postinfection, there are 12 times titers of VEEV IgM antibody compared to IgG antibody titers. As described by Rosato et al. (1988), ELISA tests are very specific and sensitive for VEEV IgM and IgG antibodies and have great potential as tools for use in rapid diagnosis of acute infections. [64, 65, 66]

TREATMENT

Presently, there is no specific antiviral treatment approved for VEEV. Treatment for VEEV is limited to symptomatic and supportive therapies.[62] For example, clinicians are limited to managing symptoms such as fever, maintaining hydration and electrolyte balance, assuring adequate respiratory function, administering anticonvulsants (phenobarbital or diazepam particularly in younger patients), giving osmotic diuretics to decrease intracranial pressure and provide physical therapy when necessary. Corticosteroids and similar compounds have immunosuppressive capacities; however, this treatment method requires further trials. Antiviral compounds such as amantadine, rimantidine, chloroquine, selanazofurin, tiazofurin etc., interfere with the replication of other viruses in laboratory animal testing. Nevertheless, none of these drugs have undergone trials in humans, and none is approved for human use.[67]

Lukaszewski and Brooks (2000) have tested the effectiveness of polymer polyethylene glycol alpha interferon (PEG IFN-α) in preventing disease in animals exposed to both subcutaneous and inhalational VEEV. These researchers have shown that the treatment with PEG IFN-α prevents the excessive inflammatory immune response to VEEV infection observed in untreated mice.[68]

In 2014, Chung et al. reported that a quinazolinone compound, CID15997213, showed promising antiviral activity in vitro and in vivo with low toxicity. CID15997213 is alphavirus-specific and targets nsP2. It is believed to hinder viral replication. Although this compound showed promise as a therapeutic drug, additional testing and analysis are required.[69]

Vaccines for VEE are presently only accessible through the United States Department of Defense Joint Vaccine Acquisition Program and have yet been approved for use in the general population. The first vaccine, also known as TC-83 (strain TC-83 or comparable compound V3526), is composed of live-attenuated VEEV (Trinidad donkey strain: TrD subtype IAB) and is sufficient to protect most humans and horses for life. Nonetheless, vaccination with TC-83 does not elicit antibodies that protect against the various subtypes of VEEV and thereby does not provide any cross-protection.[67, 70] The second vaccine, also known as C84, was developed to accommodate individuals who do not seroconvert or produce the necessary antibodies after receiving the TC-83 vaccine. C84 is an inactivated TC-83, and is well tolerated by individuals who received it. However, its protection is relatively short-lived and far less effective against aerosol challenge in animal models.[71]

DIFFERENTIAL DIAGNOSIS

In the absence of neurological symptoms, as in most cases of VEEV infection, clinical diagnosis of disease is difficult, since the signs of the disease are indistinguishable from a number of other viral and bacterial infections including arenaviruses, cytomegalovirus, Dengue fever (DF), viral hepatitis (VH), herpes simplex encephalitis, influenza, leptospirosis (Lepto), malaria, bacterial meningitis, Q fever, St. Louis encephalitis (St. LE), West Nile Encephalitis (WNE), yellow fever, Colorado tick fever, and the early prodromal phase of measles (Table 4).[61, 62]

References

1. Sharma A., Bhattacharya B., Puri R.K., Maheshwari R.K. Venezuelan Equine Encephalitis Virus Infection Causes Modulation of Inflammatory and Immune Response Genes in Mouse Brain. Biomed Central Genomics, 2008. 9: pp. 289-300
2. Aguilar P.V., Greene I.P., Coffey L.L., Medina G., Moncayo A.C., Anishchenko M., Ludwig G.V., Turell M.J., O'Guinn M.L., Lee J., Tesh R.B., Watts D.M., Russell K.L., Hice C., Yanoviak S., Morrison A.C., Klein T.A., Dohm D.J., Guzman H., Travassos da Rosa A.P.A., Guevara C., Kochel T., Olson J., Cabezas C., Weaver S.C. Endemic Venezuelan Equine Encephalitis in Northern Peru. Emerging Infectious Diseases, 2004. 10: pp. 880-888
3. Oberste M.S., Weaver S.C., Watts D.M., Smith J.F. Identification and Genetic Analysis of Panama-genotype Venezuelan Equine Encephalitis Virus Subtype ID in Peru. American Journal of Tropical Medicine and Hygiene, 1998. 58: pp. 41–46
4. Johnson K.M., Shelokov A., Peralta P.H., Dammin G.J., Young N.A. Recovery of Venezuelan Equine Encephalomyelitis Virus in Panama. A Fatal Case in Man. American Journal of Tropical Medicine and Hygiene, 1968.17: pp. 432–440
5. Hunt A.R., Frederickson S., Maruyama T., Roehrig J.T., Blair C.D. The First Human Epitope Map of the Alphaviral E1 and E2 Proteins Reveals a New E2 Epitope with Significant Virus Neutralizing Activity. Public Library of Science (PLoS) Neglected Tropical Diseases, 2010. 4: pp. e739
6. Strauss E.G., Strauss J.H. Structure and Replication of the Alphavirus Genome. In The Togaviridae and Flaviviridae. New York: Plenum Press. 1986. pp. 35-90
7. Young N.A., Johnson K.M. Antigenic Variants of Venezuelan Equine Encephalitis Virus: Their Geographic Distribution and Epidemiological Significance. American Journal of Epidemiology, 1969. 89: pp. 286-307
8. France J.K., Wyrick B.C., Trent D.W. Biochemical and Antigenic Comparisons of the Envelope Glycoproteins of Venezuelan Equine Encephalomyelitis Virus Strains. Journal of General Virology, 1979. 44: pp. 725-740
9. Kinney R.M., Trent D.W., France J.K. Comparative Immunological and Biochemical Analyses of Viruses in the Venezuelan Equine Encephalitis Virus Complex. Journal of General Virology, 1983. 64: pp.135-147
10. Calisher C.H. Kinney R.M., De Souza Lopez O., Trent D.W., Monath T.P., Francy D.B. Identification of a New Venezuelan Equine Encephalitis Virus from Brazil. American Journal of Tropical Medicine and Hygiene, 1982. 31: pp. 1260-1272
11. Calisher C.H., Monath T.P., Mitchell C.J., Sabatrini M.S., Cropp C.B., Kerschiner J., Hunt A.R., Lazuick J.S. Arbovirus Investigations in Argentina, 1977 1980. III. Identification and Characterization of Viruses Isolated, Including New Subtypes of Western and Venezuelan Equine Encephalitis Viruses and Four New Bunyaviruses (Las Malayos, Resistencia, Barranqueras, and Antequera). American Journal of Tropical Medicine and Hygiene, 1985. 34: pp. 956-965
12. Weaver S.C., Ferro C., Barrera R., Boshell J, Navarro JC. Venezuelan Equine Encephalitis. Annual Review of Entomology, 2004. 49: 141-174
13. Walton T.E., Grayson M.A. Venezuelan Equine Encephalomyelitis. The Arboviruses: Epidemiology and Ecology. Volume IV. Boca Raton: Chemical Rubber Company Press. 1988. pp. 203-231
14. Powers A.M., Oberste M.S., Brault A.C. Rico-Hesse R., Schmura S.M., Smith J.F., Kang W., Sweeney W.P., Weaver S.C. Repeated Emergence of Epidemic/Epizootic Venezuelan Equine Encephalitis from a Single Genotype of Enzootic Subtype ID Virus. Journal of Virology, 1997. 71: pp. 6697–6705
15. Sanmartin-Barberi C., Osorno-Mesa E. Human Epidemic in Colombia Caused by the Venezuelan Equine Encephalomyelitis Virus. American Journal of Tropical Medicine and Hygiene, 1954. 3: pp. 283-291
16. Briceno Rossi A.L., Rural Epidemic Encephalitis in Venezuela Caused by a Group A Arbovirus (VEE). Progress in Medical Virology, 1967. 9: pp. 176–203
17. Sudia W.D., Newhouse V.F. Epidemic Venezuelan Equine Encephalitis in North America: a Summary of Virus-Vector-Host Relationships. American Journal of Epidemiology, 1975. 101: pp. 1-13
18. Zehmer R.B., Dean P.B., Sudia W.D., Calisher C.H., Sather G.E., Parker R.L. Venezuelan Equine Encephalitis Epidemic in Texas, 1971. Health Services Reports, 1974. 89: pp. 278-282
19. Rico-Hesse R., Weaver S.C., de Siger J., Medina G., Salas R.A.. Emergence of a New Epidemic/Epizootic Venezuelan Equine Encephalitis Virus in South America. Proceedings of the National Academy of Sciences of the United States of America, 1995. 92: pp. 5278–5281
20. Oberste MS, Fraire M, Navarro R, Zepeda C, Zarate ML, Ludwig G.W., Kondig J.F., Weaver S.C., Smith J.F., Rico-Hesse R. Association of Venezuelan Equine Encephalitis Virus Subtype IE with two Equine Epizootics in Mexico. American Journal of Tropical Medicine and Hygiene, 1998. 59: pp. 100–107
21. Weaver S.C., Salas R., Rico-Hesse R., Ludwig G.V., Oberste M.S., Boshell J., Tesh R.B. Re-emergence of Epidemic Venezuelan Equine Encephalomyelitis in South America.VEE Study Group. The Lancet, 1996. 348: pp. 436–440
22. Johnson K.M., Shelokov A., Peralta P.H. Dammin G. J., Young N.A. Recovery of Venezuelan Equine Encephalomyelitis Virus in Panamá. A Fatal Case in Man. American Journal of Tropical Medicine and Hygiene, 1968. 17: pp. 432-440
23. Franck P.T., Johnson K.M. An Outbreak of Venezuelan Encephalitis in Man in the Panama Canal Zone. American Journal of Epidemiology, 1971. 94: pp. 487-495
24. Guerrant R.L., Walker D.H., Weller P.F. Tropical Infectious Diseases – Principles, Pathogens & Practice. Volume 1. Churchill Livingstone Elsevier. Philadelphia, 2006. pp. 832-834
25. Sudia W.D., Newhouse V.F., Beadle I.D., Miller D.L., Johnston J.G. Jr, Young R., Calisher C.H., Maness K. Epidemic Venezuelan Equine Encephalitis in North America in 1971: Vector Studies. American Journal of Epidemiology, 1975. 101: pp. 17–35
26. Kramer L.D., Scherer W.F. Vector Competence of Mosquitoes as a Marker to Distinguish Central American and Mexican Epizootic from Enzootic Strains of Venezuelan Equine Encephalitis Virus. American Journal of Tropical Medicine and Hygiene, 1976. 25: pp. 336–46
27. Turell M.J., Ludwig G.V., Beaman J.R. Transmission of Venezuelan Equine Encephalomyelitis Virus by Aedes sollicitans and Aedes taeniorhynchus (Diptera: Culicidae). Journal of Medical Entomology, 1992. 29: pp. 62–65
28. Grayson M.A., Galindo P. Experimental Transmission of Venezuelan Equine Encephalitis Virus by Deinocerites pseudes Dyar and Knab, 1909. Journal of Medical Entomology, 1972. 9: pp. 196–200
29. Yanoviak S.P., Aguilar P.V., Lounibos L.P., Weaver S.C. Transmission of a Venezuelan Equine Encephalitis Complex Alphavirus by Culex (Melanoconion) gnomatos (Diptera: Culicidae) in Northeastern Peru. Journal of medical entomology, 2005. 42: pp. 404-408
30. Linthicum K.J., Gordon S.W., Monath T.P. Comparative Infections of Epizootic and Enzootic Strains of Venezuelan Equine Encephalomyelitis Virus in Amblyomma cajennense (Acari: Ixodidae). Journal of Medical Entomology, 1992. 29: pp. 827–31
31. Navarro J-C, Medina G., Vasquez C., Coffey L.L., Wang E., Suárez A., Biord H., Salas M., Weaver S.C. Postepizootic Persistence of Venezuelan Equine Encephalitis Virus, Venezuela. Emerging Infectious Diseases, 2005. 11: pp. 1907-1915
32. Durden L.A., Linthicum K.J., Turell M.J. Mechanical Transmission of Venezuelan Equine Encephalomyelitis Virus by Hematophagous Mites (Acari). Journal of Medical Entomology, 1992. 29: pp. 118-21
33. Scheiman J., Tseng J-C., Zheng Y., Meruelo D. Multiple Functions of the 37/67-kd Laminin Receptor Make It a Suitable Target for Novel Cancer Gene Therapy. Molecular Therapy, 2010. 18: pp. 63–74
34. Klimstra W. B., Ryman K. D., Johnston R. E. Adaptation of Sindbis Virus to BHK Cells Selects for Use of Heparan Sulfate as an Attachment Receptor. Journal of Virology, 1998. 72: pp. 7357–736
35. Bernard K., Klimstra W. B., Johnston R. E., Mutations in the E2 Glycoprotein of Venezuelan Equine Encephalitis Virus Confer Heparan Sulfate Interaction, Low Morbidity, and Rapid Clearance from Blood of Mice. Virology, 2000. 276: pp. 93–103
36. Heil M., Albee A., Strauss J., Kuhn R. J. An Amino Acid Substitution in the Coding Region of the E2 Glycoprotein Adapts Ross River Virus to Utilize Heparan Sulfate as an Attachment Moiety. Journal of Virology, 2001. 75: pp. 6303–6309
37. Klimstra W. B., Nangle E. M., Smith M. S., Yurochko A. D., Ryman K.D. DC-SIGN and L-SIGN can act as Attachment Receptors for Alphaviruses and Distinguish between Mosquito Cell- and Mammalian Cell-Derived Viruses. Journal of Virology, 2003. 77: pp. 12022–12032
38. Leung J. Y-S., Ng M.M-L., Chu J.J.H. Replication of Alphaviruses: A Review on the Entry Process of Alphaviruses into Cells. Advances in Virology, 2011. 2011: pp. 1-9
39. Kolokoltsov A. A,. Fleming E. H, Davey R. A., Venezuelan Equine Encephalitis Virus Entry Mechanism Requires Late Endosome Formation and Resists Cell Membrane Cholesterol Depletion, Virology, 2006. 347: pp. 333–342
40. Ahola T., Kääriäinen L. Reaction in Alphavirus mRNA Capping: Formation of a Covalent Complex of Nonstructural Protein nsP1 with 7-methyl-GMP. Proceedings of the National Academy of Sciences of the United States of America, 1995. 92: pp. 507–511
41. Vasiljeva L., Merits A., Auvinen P., Kääriäinen L. Identification of a Novel Function of the Alphavirus Capping Apparatus. RNA 5'-triphosphatase Activity of Nsp2. The Journal of Biological Chemistry, 2000. 275: pp. 17281–17287
42. Malet H., Coutard B., Jamal S., Dutartre H., Papageorgiou N., Neuvonen M., Ahola T., Forrester N., Gould E.A., Lafitte D., Ferron F., Lescar J., Gorbalenya A.E., de Lamballerie X., Canard B. The Crystal Structures of Chikungunya and Venezuelan Equine Encephalitis Virus nsP3 Macro Domains Define a Conserved Adenosine Binding Pocket. Journal of Virology, 2009. 83: pp. 6534–6545
43. Owen K. E., Kuhn R.J. Alphavirus Budding is Dependent on the Interaction between the Nucleocapsid and Hydrophobic Amino Acids on the Cytoplasmic Domain of the E2 Envelope Glycoprotein. Virology, 1997. 230: pp. 187–196
44. Ubol S., Tucker P. C., Griffin D. E., Hardwick J. M. Neurovirulent Strains of Alphavirus Induce Apoptosis in bcl-2-Expressing Cells: Role of a Single Amino Acid Change in the E2 Glycoprotein. Proceedings of the National Academy of Sciences of the United States of America, 1994. 91: pp. 5202–5206
45. Melton J., Ewart G., Weir R. C., Lee E. K., Board P. G., Gage P. W. Alphavirus 6K Proteins form Ion Channels," The Journal of Biological Chemistry, 2002. 277: pp. 46923–46931
46. Sanz M. A., Madan V., Carrasco L., Nieva J.L. Interfacial Domains in Sindbis Virus 6K Protein: Detection and Functional Characterization, The Journal of Biological Chemistry, 2003. 278: pp. 2051–2057
47. Grieder F.B., Davis N.L., Aronson J.F., Charles P.C., Sellon D.C., Suzuki K., Johnston R.E. Specific Restrictions in the Progression of Venezuelan Equine Encephalitis Virus-induced Disease Resulting from Single Amino Acid Changes in the Glycoproteins. Virology, 1995. 206: pp. 994-1006
48. Charles P.C., Walters E., Margolis F., Johnston R.E. Mechanism of Neuroinvasion of Venezuelan Equine Encephalitis Virus in the Mouse. Virology, 1995. 208: pp. 662-671
49. Ryzhikov A.B., Ryabchikova E.I., Sergeev A.N., Tkacheva N.V. Spread of Venezuelan Equine Encephalitis Virus in Mice Olfactory Tract. Archieves of Virology, 1995. 140: pp. 2243-2254
50. Schoneboom B.A., Fultz M.J., Miller T.H., McKinney L.C., Grieder F.B. Astrocytes as Targets for Venezuelan Equine Encephalitis Virus Infection. Journal of Virology, 1999. 5: pp. 342-354
51. Schoneboom B.A., Catlin K.M., Marty A.M., Grieder F.B. Inflammation is a Component of Neurodegeneration in Response to Venezuelan Equine Encephalitis Virus Infection in Mice. Journal of Neuroimmunology, 2000. 109: pp. 132-146
52. Franz D.R., Parrott C.D., Takafuji E.T. The U.S. Biological Warfare and Biological Defense Programs. Medical Aspects of Chemical and Biological Warfare. Washington D.D.: Office of the Surgeon General Department of the Army, United States of America. 1997. pp. 425-436
53. Weapons of Mass Destruction (WMD). GlobalSecurity.org. Revised October 23, 2007. Retrieved August 6, 2008. Web Site: http://www.globalsecurity.org /wmd/intro/bio_vee.htm
54. Alibek K. Biohazard. New York: Dell Publishing. 1999. pp. 111
55. Alibek K. Biohazard. New York: Dell Publishing. 1999. pp. 259-260
56. Krauss H., Weber A., Appel M., Enders B., Isenberg H.D., Schiefer H.G., Slenczka W., von Graevenitz A., t Zahner H. Zoonoses: Infectious Diseases Transmissible from Animals to Humans. Washington D.C. American Society for Microbiology Press. 2003. pp. 13
57. Smith J.F., Davis K., Hart M.K., Ludwig G.V., McClain D.J., Parker M.D., Pratt W.D. Viral Encephalitides. Medical Aspects of Chemical and Biological Warfare. Falls Church: Office of the Surgeon General, Department of the Army, United States of America. 1997. pp. 561-589
58. Tsai T.F., Weaver S.C., Monath T.P. Alphavirus. Clinical Virology. Washington D.C. American Society for Microbiology Press. 2002. pp. 1177
59. Bowen G.S. Fashinell T.R., Dean P.B. Gregg M.B. Clinical Aspects of Human Venezuelan Equine Encephalitis in Texas. Bulletin of the Pan American Health Organization, 1976. 10: pp. 46-57
60. Venezuelan Equine Encephalitis Virus – Material Safety Data Sheets (MSDS). Material Safety Data Sheet – infectious Substances. Health Canada 2001. Retrieved August 9, 2008. Website: http://www.phac-aspc.gc.ca/msds-ftss/msds162e-eng.php
61. Venezuelan Equine Encephalitis Virus. Bioterrorism Agent Profiles for Health Care Workers. Arizona Department of Health Services. Revised August, 2004. Retrieved August 8, 2008. Website: http://www.azdhs.gov/phs/edc/ edrp/es/pdf/veeset.pdf
62. Guerrant RL, Walker DH, Weller PF. Tropical Infectious Diseases – Principles, Pathogens & Practice. Volume 1. Philadelphia: Churchill Livingstone Elsevier. 2006. pp. 836-837
63. Linssen B., Kinney R.M. Aguilar P., Russell K.L., Watts D.M., Kaaden O.R., Pfeffer M. Development of Reverse Transcription-PCR Assays Specific for Detection of Equine

Encephalitis Viruses. Journal of Clinical Microbiology, 2000. 38: pp. 1527-1535

64. Watts D.M., Lavera V., Callahan J., Rossi C., Oberste M.S., Roehrig J.T. Wooster M.T., Smith J.F., Cropp C.B., Fentrau E.M., Karabatsos N., Gubler D., Hayes C.G. Venezuelan Equine Encephalitis Febrile Cases Among Humans in the Peruvian Amazon River Region. The American Journal of Tropical Medicine and Hygiene, 1998. 58: pp. 35–40

65. Watts D.M., Lavera V., Callahan J., Rossi C., Oberste M.S., Roehrig J.T., Cropp C.B., Karabatsos N., Smith J.F., Gubler D.J., Wooster M.T., Nelson W.M., Hayes C.G. Venezuelan Equine Encephalitis and Oropouche Virus Infections Among Peruvian Army Troops in the Amazon Region of Peru. The American Journal of Tropical Medicine and Hygiene, 1997. 56: pp. 661-667

66. Rosato R.R., Francisco F., Macasaet T., Jahrling P.B. Enzyme-Linked Immunosorbent Assay Detection of Immunoglobulins G and M to Venezuelan Equine Encephalomyelitis Virus in Vaccinated and Naturally Infected Humans. Journal of Clinical Microbiology, 1988. 26: pp. 421-425

67. Calisher C.H. Medically Important Arboviruses of the United States and Canada. Clinical Microbiology Reviews, 1994. 7: pp. 89-116

68. Lukaszewski R.A., Brooks T.J.G. Pegylated Alpha Interferon Is an Effective Treatment for Virulent Venezuelan Equine Encephalitis Virus and Has Profound Effects on the Host Immune Response to Infection. Journal of Virology, 2000. 74: pp. 5006–5015

69. Chung D-H., Jonsson C.B., Tower N.A., Chu Y-K., Sahin E., Golden J.E., Noah J.W., Schroeder C.E., Sotsky J.B., Sosa M.I., Cramer D.E., McKellip S.N., Rasmussen L., White E.L., Schmaljohn C.S., Julander J.G., Smith J.M., Filone C.M., Connor J.H., Sakurai Y., Davey R.A. Discovery of a Novel Compound with Anti-Venezuelan Equine Encephalitis Virus Activity That Targets the Nonstructural Protein 2. Public Library of Science (PLoS) Pathogens, 2014. 10: pp. e1004213

70. Fine D.L., Roberts B.A., Terpening S.J., Mott J., Vasconcelos D., House R.V. Neurovirulence evaluation of Venezuelan Equine Encephalitis (VEE) Vaccine Candidate V3526 in Nonhuman Primates. Vaccine, 2008. 26: pp. 3497-3506

71. Paessler S., Weaver S.C. Vaccines for Venezuelan equine encephalitis. Vaccine, 2009. 27: pp. D80–85

Photo Bibliography

Figure 1.15-1: A negatively-stained transmission electron micrograph (TEM) shows a number of Venezuelan equine encephalitis (VEE) virus virions, This photo was taken by Dr. Fred Murphy and Sylvia Whitfield and was released by the CDC. Public domain photo

Figure 1.15-3: Computer-generated model of the surface of an alphavirus derived by cryoelectron microscopy. Graphic was designed and released by the CDC in 2007. Public domain photo

Figure 1.15-3: Genomic protein graphics produced and released by the National Institute of Health (NIH). Public domain photo

Bacillus anthracis is a Category A biological warfare agent as listed by the Center for Disease Control. In recent years, this agent has managed to attract a substantial amount of attention due to the intentional release of *B. anthracis* spores through the United States Postal System in the autumn of 2001. These anthrax spores infected a total of 22 individuals; out of these, 11 developed cutaneous anthrax, while the remaining 11 developed the inhalational form of this disease. Out of the 11 that suffered from inhalational anthrax, five died due to the infection, generating a mortality rate of ~45%.[1, 2, 3]

Although highly publicized, the 'Anthrax Letters' was not the most devastating release of *B. anthracis* spores in history. The most deadly incident occurred on April 7, 1979, when anthrax was accidentally released from a top secret biological weapons facility in Sverdlovsk, USSR (now Yekaterinburg, Russia), which killed an estimated 66-105 people (the actual number of casualties are not known). Subsequent to the accident, the Soviet Union claimed these deaths were due to contaminated meat, and maintained this position until Russian President Boris Yeltsin finally admitted to the true nature of the deaths on May 27, 1993.[4, 5]

Full scale experimentation with *B. anthracis* (along with tularemia, plague, botulinum, smallpox, Glanders, and typhoid) as an offensive biological weapons is believed to have been initiated by the Japanese soon after World War I.[6] It is now known that since 1937, the Japanese conducted a large scale biological warfare program, which included human testing by Unit 731 in Manchuria and they stockpiled 400 kg of anthrax spores, to be used in specially designed fragmentation bombs.[7, 8] In 1943, the United States implemented its own biological warfare program, until the unilateral renouncement of the use of biological weapons in two National Security Memoranda announced in 1969, and 1970 respectively. These National Security Memoranda formally banned the production and usage of Biological weapons after ratifying the Biological Weapons Convention in 1975. Nonetheless, recognizing the threat of biological weapons is still necessary, therefore the United States maintains an active medical defense program against all known biological warfare agents.[8] The fear of biological weapon attacks were justified when, in 1995, the United States Office of Technology Assessment and at United States Senate committee hearings released the names of 17 countries that maintained active biological weapons programs. These countries are: Iran, Iraq (eliminated from the list in 2003), Libya, Syria, North Korea, Taiwan, Israel, Egypt, Vietnam, Laos, Cuba, Bulgaria, India, South Korea, South Africa, China and Russia (formally Soviet Union). It is known that many of the named nations still have highly active biological weapons research and production programs today.[9]

B. anthracis, is the microbe responsible for the zoonotic disease known as anthrax. The lifecycle of *B. anthracis* includes both vegetative and dormant morphotypes. For example, these microbes may exist as ~1 μm endospores found naturally in soil and can cause fatal disease in both livestock and humans (Figure 2.1-1). These endospores are highly resistant to heat, desiccation, oxidation and ultraviolet radiation. It has been estimated that these endospores may remain viable for up to 200 years in favorable conditions.[10]

B. anthracis endospores possess eight *gerA* family sensors that are utilized to recognize nutrients, which, in a favorable

environment will germinate into a sizable bacterium (1x3 to 10 μm) (Figure 2.1-2). *B. anthracis* are non-motile, Gram- positive, aerobic, rod shaped bacterium and belong to the genus *Bacillus*. *B. anthracis* is an obligate pathogen that has a 5.23 Mb genome, encoding 5,508 proteins.[11, 12, 13]

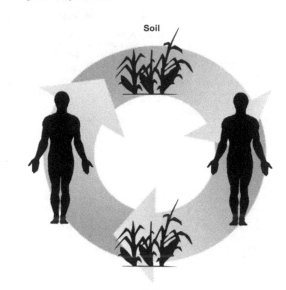

Soil

Soil

Figure 2.1-1: Transmission cycle of *B. anthracis*

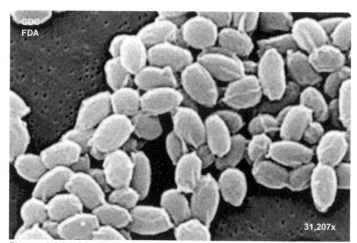

Figure 2.1-2: Scanning electron micrograph of Sterne strain anthrax endospores

The key virulence genes of this bacterium are found on its two plasmids pXO1 and pXO2, which are controlled by *atxA* and *acpA* regulatory genes.[11, 14, 15] The plasmid, pX01, is ~198 kilobase pairs (kbp) in length, the function of which is not entirely well understood. Nonetheless, a region of the pX01, also known as the pathogenic island, has been well documented. The pathogenic island of pX01 contains three genes, *pag*, *lef*, and *cya*, which encodes three distinct proteins: protective antigen (PA; 85 kDa in size), lethal factor (LF; 83 kDa in size) and the edema factor (EF; 89 kDa in size) respectively. Individually, these proteins are nontoxic, but in binary and tertiary combinations they form tripartite A-B toxin on the surfaces of mammalian cells (Figure 2.1-3).[16, 17, 18]

PA is a 735 amino acid protein composed of four domains. The first domain (domain 1), located between amino acids 1-258,

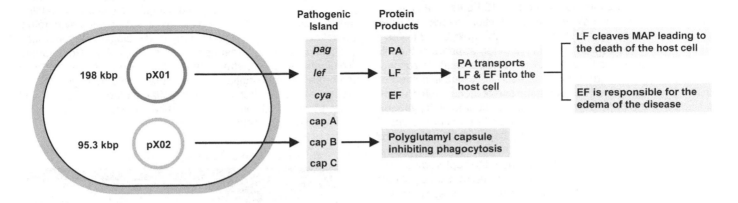

Figure 2.1-3: Virulence genes and their products of *B. anthracis*

is cleaved by the furin-like protease located on the surface of the host cell. The cleavage of domain 1 results in the release of two fragments, PA_{20} and PA_{63}. Once released, PA_{20} has no further function, while PA_{63} proceeds through heptamerization via monomer-monomer interactions and is responsible for binding to LF and EF. Domain 2, located between amino acids 259 and 487, contains a D2L2 unstructured loop which is inserted into the host membrane to form a cation-selective channel. Domain 3, located between amino acids 488-595, is involved in the heptamerization of PA_{63}. Finally, domain 4, located between amino acids 596 and 735, is responsible for binding to host cellular receptors such as tumor endothelial marker 8 (TEM8), capillary morphogenesis protein 2 (CMG2) and beta1-integrin.[19, 20, 21, 22, 23] Research indicates that TEM8 and CMG2 are found in high concentrations within the membranes of epithelial cells lining the skin, lungs and intestines; entry sites favored by *B. anthracis*.[23]

Although the mechanisms of these toxins are not fully understood, it is known that LF, a Zn^{2+}-protease, is responsible for cleaving mitogen-activated protein (MAP) kinases 1, 2 and 3, which results in the death of the host cell. EF, on the other hand, is a calcium and calmodulin-dependent adenylate cyclase that is responsible for the edema seen in diseased individuals. It is speculated that both EF and LF provide an advantage for *B. anthracis* by undermining the abilities of the host's immune system to contain *B. anthracis* infection through the destruction of phagocytes.[22, 24]

The second plasmid, pX02, is 95.3 kbp in size and encodes three genes: cap B, cap C, and cap A. These three genes encode the instructions for the synthesis of the polyglutamyl capsule, which inhibits host phagocytosis of the vegetative form of *B. anthracis* (Figure 2.1-3).[25]

There are three distinct types of infection and resultant disease that are caused by anthrax spores depending upon the location of entry of the microbes. The majority of reported cases (~95%) are cutaneous anthrax infections, occurring mostly in people who work with wool and/or animal hides. Less common is the gastrointestinal form of anthrax which transpires after the ingestion of anthrax spores through contaminated meats or other food products. Lastly, the rarest and the most serious form of infection, the inhalational form of anthrax, occurs when anthrax spores are inhaled and phagocytized by the macrophages located with the respiratory tracts.[26, 27] Although *B. anthracis* infections are extremely serious, it is important to note that there have never been a reported case of human-to-human anthrax transmission.[28]

SYMPTOMS

Cutaneous Anthrax

In cases of cutaneous anthrax, the spores are introduced through a cut, insect bite or abrasions on the epidermis (Figure 2.14). The locations of the human body that are commonly infected are generally the face, neck, hands and fingers.[12] Cutaneous anthrax mainly occurs when handling contaminated wool, as well as, other animal hair products, hides and/or leather products from infected animals.[29] Between 1944 and 2000, only 224 cases of cutaneous anthrax were identified within the United States, only nine of which occurred between 1984 to 2007.[30, 31]

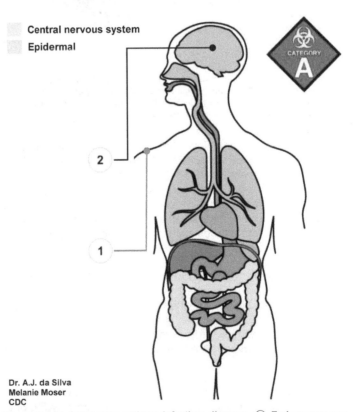

Dr. A.J. da Silva
Melanie Moser
CDC

Figure 2.1-4: Cutaneous anthrax infection diagram. ① Endospores are introduced via a cut, insect bite or abrasions upon the epidermis ② Meningitis results from an initial cutaneous anthrax infection which spread to the CNS

The incubation period of *B. anthracis* for cutaneous infection varies. There are reports that the infection may have an incubation period as short as one to seven days, although

Abdenour *et al.* (1987), reported that the incubation period of cutaneous anthrax could be as short as 12 hours or as long as 19 days.[12, 29] The initial symptoms of infection involve localized pruritus and/or painless erythema. Over the next 24-72 hours a papule lesion, a few millimeters in diameter, appears at the site of infection. During the following 24 to 48 hours, multiple painless vesicles (papules) without purulent secretions accompanied by localized red edema will appear at the site of inoculation. Pus will be present if the papules are secondarily infected with pyogenic bacteria, such as *Staphylococcus spp.* or *Streptococcus spp.*[28, 29] Within the next 24 to 72 hours, the papules will rupture and an ulcer ~0.5 to 3 cm in diameter with a black center will appear (Figure 2.1-5). Soon after its appearance, the ruptured papules will change into a black eschar ~1 to 3 cm in size. Some patients during this time are afebrile, while others display symptoms of fever, headaches, anorexia, nausea, malaise, toxemia, severe edema around the eschar and painful lymphadentitis (Table 1).[5, 12, 26, 27, 28, 32]

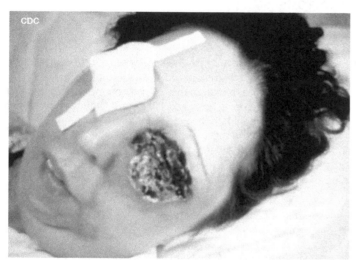

Figure 2.1-5: A female patient suffering from cutaneous *B. anthracis* infection involving her left eye. This photo was taken on the 24th day of infection. Please note the erupted papules with black center appearing on the palpebral, as well as, the surrounding epidermal tissues

Depending on the location, the edema itself could be fatal, especially if it appears around the head or neck. Severe edema is generally characterized by induration, multiple bullae and symptoms of shock. Corticosteroid therapy is generally used for patients suffering from this condition; however, in regards to patients experiencing severe edema around the head and neck region, surgical procedures such as tracheotomy may be needed to prevent asphyxiation.

It has been reported that approximately 80% of patients suffering from cutaneous anthrax will begin to recover without medical treatment within six weeks after the onset of disease; 99% of patients suffering from cutaneous anthrax will recover if antibiotic treatments are administered. Systemic complications, such as sepsis and/or meningoencephalitis are rare and may result in fatalities (Table 1).[5, 12, 26, 27, 28, 32]

Meningoencephalitis, also known as anthrax meningitis, is a rare neurological complication that occurs in approximately 5% of all known cutaneous anthrax cases, and much less commonly, from oral-oropharyngeal or gastrointestinal anthrax.[28, 32, 33, 34]

Once the microbes enter the skin, they spread to the central nervous system through the hematogenous or lymphatic routes. Patients suffering from anthrax meningitis will experience a prodromic period of approximately 1 to 6 days. Early symptoms include high fever, fatigue, headaches, myalgia, nuchal rigidity (stiff neck), chills, nausea, vomiting, confusion, irritability, seizures and delirium. Soon after the onset of initial symptoms, the patients will begin to show a rapid neurological degeneration whch almost always results in death (~6 days). Postmortem examinations demonstrate the infection is consistent with hemorrhagic meningitis, where the leptomeninges show extensive edema, hemorrhaging, inflammatory infiltrates, and Gram staining indicates the presence of Gram-positive bacilli (Figure 2.1-6 and Table 2).[28, 33, 34, 35, 36]

Table 1: An overview of the clinical symptoms of cutaneous anthrax

Symptoms	+	++	+++
Fever			▪
Headaches			▪
Anorexia			▪
Nausea			▪
Malaise			▪
Toxemia			▪
Painful lymphadentitis			▪
Severe edema at eschar			▪
Localized pruritus			▪
Painless erythema			▪
Papule lesion			▪
Black centered ulcer			▪
Black eschar			▪
Sepsis	▪		
Meningoencephalitis	▪		

+ Rare ++ Common +++ Frequent

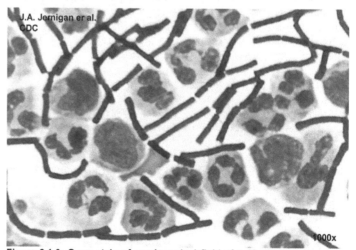

Figure 2.1-6: Gram stain of cerebrospinal fluid of a 63-year-old Caucasian photo editor from Florida demonstrating B. anthracis. Patient contracted anthrax on October 2, 2001 and died on October 5, 2001

Table 2: An overview of the clinical symptoms of anthrax meningitis. Please note that the abbreviation neuro. represents neurological

Symptoms	+	++	+++
Nuchal rigidity			▪
High fever			▪
Fatigue			▪
Headaches			▪
Myalgia			▪
Chills			▪
Nausea			▪
Vomiting			▪
Confusion			▪
Irritability			▪
Seizures			▪
Delirium			▪
Neuro. degeneration			▪

+ Rare ++ Common +++ Frequent

Oral-Oropharyngeal / Gastrointestinal Anthrax

Oral-oropharyngeal and gastrointestinal anthrax are contracted through the consumption of spore contaminated meat that is either undercooked or raw (Figure 2.1-7).[26, 37] This form of anthrax infection has been reported frequently in Africa, the Middle East and Asia, but has not been reported in the United States. Nonetheless, between 1930 and 1940, the Japanese attempted to weaponize this form of anthrax infection by distributing contaminated chocolate laced with anthrax spores to Chinese children.[38]

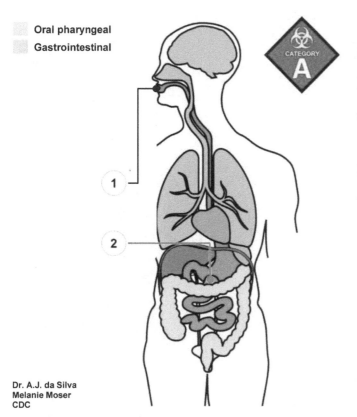

■ **Oral pharyngeal**

■ **Gastrointestinal**

Dr. A.J. da Silva
Melanie Moser
CDC

Figure 2.1-9: Oral-oropharyngeal and gastrointestinal anthrax infection diagram. ① Endospores are introduced via the consumption of tainted meats. ② Endospores are introduced via a breach within the mucosal lining

The first sign of oral-oropharyngeal anthrax appears ~48 hours after consuming contaminated meat. It is believed that the bacteria are introduced into the body through breaches in the mucosal lining. Mucosal lesions are common and generally located on the tonsils, posterior pharyngeal wall, base of the tongue, uvula, soft and hard palate, as well as, the anterior and posterior pillars of the fauces.[12, 28, 39] Once inoculated with anthrax, the lesions are initially congested and edematous. Soft tissue edema and regional lymphadenopathy are also common symptoms. By the end of the first week, the lesion will take on a whitish appearance where they undergo necrosis and ulceration. By the second week, a pseudomembrane will form over the ulcers (Figure 2.1-8).[12, 35, 39]

Patents suffering from oral-oropharyngeal anthrax generally display symptoms including cervical edema, fever, respiratory difficulties, sore throat and dysphagia.[12, 35, 39] With proper hospitalization and aggressive antibiotic treatment patients will generally recover. However, in 24 cases of oral-oropharyngeal anthrax reported in Thailand the mortality rate has been calculated to be 12.4% (3 out of 24 died), while in 1986, six cases from Turkey demonstrated a mortality rate of 50%.[39, 40] Patients that succumb to oral-oropharyngeal anthrax generally die from respiratory distress and/or septicemic toxemia (Table 3).[12]

Symptoms of gastrointestinal anthrax generally appear two to five days after ingesting spore contaminated meat. Like oral-oropharyngeal anthrax, the bacteria may be introduced through a breach of the mucosal lining.[28] Regional lymph nodes are also involved, becoming enlarged and hemorrhagic due to the infection.[41, 42, 43]

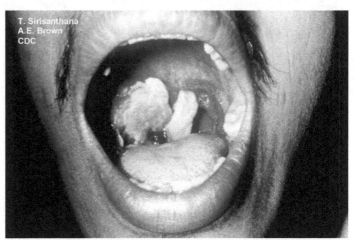

Figure 2.1-8: Patient suffering from oral-oropharyngeal Anthrax demonstrating necrosis and ulceration of the soft palate and back of the throat and over the uvula

Table 3: An overview of the clinical symptoms of oral-oropharyngeal anthrax

Symptoms	+	++	+++
Fever			■
Respiratory difficulties			■
Sore throat			■
Dysphagia			■
Mucosa lesions - tonsils			■
Pharynx (mucosa) lesion			■
Mucosa lesions - tongue			■
Mucosa lesions - fauces			■
Mucosa lesions - uvula			■
Mucosa lesions (palates)			■
Soft tissue edema			■
Lymphadenopathy			■
Necrosis of the lesions			■
Ulceration of the lesion			■
Cervical edema		■	

+ Rare ++ Common +++ Frequent

Ulcerative lesions are always seen in this form of anthrax infection. For example, multiple superficial ulcerative lesions may appear in the esophagus, stomach and/or jejunum, which may bleed, or in severe cases cause hemorrhages that may result in fatality.[39, 41, 42, 43] Ulcerative lesions found in the mid-jejunum, terminal ileum and/or cecum have a different distribution pattern in comparison with lesions found in the upper gastrointestinal tract. These lesions generally appear to be comparable to cutaneous anthrax infections, where the lesions develop in a small region or appear in few locations. These ulceration and edema will appear to be more diffuse.[39] Lesions in the lower gastrointestinal tract may lead to any or all of the following: hemorrhage, obstruction and/or perforation (Figure 2.1-9).[44, 45, 46, 47, 48] Pathologic fluid collection within the abdominal cavity, also known as ascites, may further complicate the condition. In some reported cases, the sudden shift of fluids from the vascular system to the abdominal cavity may result in shock and/or death.[39, 48, 49, 50, 51, 52]

Patients suffering from gastrointestinal anthrax display initial

143

symptoms of low-grade fever, headaches, congestion of the conjunctiva and of the face. Within 24 hours, signs of nausea, loss of appetite, fever, diffused abdominal pains with rebound tenderness, hypovolemia, vomiting of blood, constipation and/or severe diarrhea will appear.[12, 26] In some rare cases, mediastinal widening is also observed, although this symptom is typically a characteristic of inhalational anthrax (Table 4).[28]

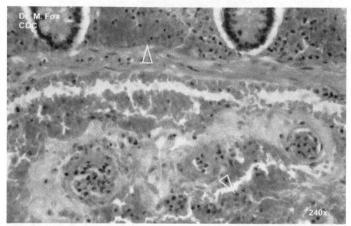

Figure 2.1-9: Photomicrograph of the small intestine in a fatal case of gastrointestinal anthrax. This micrograph reveals submucosal hemorrhage (arrows)

Table 4: An overview of the clinical symptoms of gastrointestinal anthrax. Please note that the abbreviation Gastro. represents gastrointestinal tract and hemorr. represents hemorrhages

Symptoms	+	++	+++
Fever			■
Headaches			■
Conjunctiva congestion			■
Congestion of the face			■
Nausea			■
Loss of appetite			■
Diffused abdominal pains			■
Rebound tenderness			■
Hypovolemia			■
Vomiting of blood			■
Constipation			■
Severe diarrhea			■
Lymphadenopathy			■
Lymph node hemorr.			■
Esophagus ulcer lesions			■
Stomach ulcer lesions			■
Jejunum ulcer lesions			■
Ilium ulcer lesions			■
Cecum ulcer lesions			■
Stomach hemorr. lesions			■
Jejunum hemorr. lesions			■
Ascites			■
Lower gastro. lesions			■
Gastro. obstruction			■
Gastro. perforation			■
Shock		■	
Mediastinal widening	■		
Toxemia	■		

+ Rare ++ Common +++ Frequent

Fatalities are relatively common in cases of gastrointestinal anthrax. It has been estimated that the mortality rates range from 25 to 60%. Generally, morbidity is due to blood and fluid loss and electrolyte imbalance that result in shock. Additionally, death may result from intestinal perforation and/or anthrax toxemia. Nonetheless, with proper hospitalization and aggressive antibiotic treatments, many patients will recover within 10 to 14 days after the initial onset of symptoms (Table 4).[26, 28, 53]

Inhalational Anthrax

As the name states, inhalational anthrax, also known as systemic anthrax, is contracted through the human respiratory tract and it is the most serious form of anthrax infection (Figure 2.1-10). Prior to the utilization of B. anthracis as an agent of biological terrorism, cases of inhalational anthrax was typically found in people who handled anthrax contaminated animal wool and hides.[28, 54]

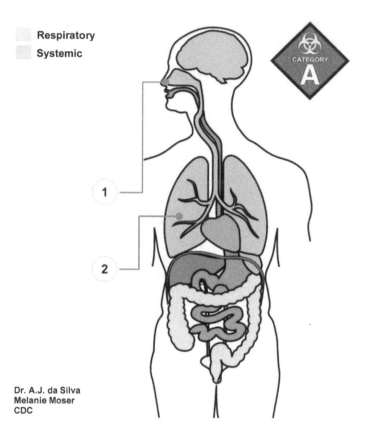

■ Respiratory
■ Systemic

Dr. A.J. da Silva
Melanie Moser
CDC

Figure 2.1-12: Inhalational anthrax infection diagram. ① The endospores enter the host via the upper respiratory tract. ② The endospores are introduced via the lower respiratory tract

Inhalation anthrax is generally fatal when contracted. B. anthracis endospores, which are approximately 1-2 µm in diameter, are deposited in the alveolar spaces of the lungs. These deposited B. anthracis endospores are then phagocitized by the alveolar macrophages and transported to the mediastinal and peribronchial lymph nodes within hours, leaving no pulmonary lesions. During transit, within the enclosed vesicles of the macrophage, the spores germinate forming vegetative bacilli, which begin to multiply and secrete toxins. Subsequently, the bacilli are transported throughout the entire body via the circulatory system. B. anthracis infection causes massive hemorrhages (e.g. hemorrhagic mediastinitis), edema and necrosis within the lymph nodes in addition to septic shock subsequent to systemic distribution (Figure 2.1-11).[12, 27, 28, 35, 55, 56]

Approximately two to five days (or ~10 days as indicated by the data from the Sverdlovsk outbreak) after exposure to anthrax endospores, the initial signs of inhalational anthrax are "flu-like" symptoms (viral upper respiratory tract infection) of mild fever, malaise, fatigue, non-productive cough and myalgia. Chest radiographs during the early stages of disease show a widened mediastinum, which is a sign of hemorrhagic mediastinitis (Figure

2.1-12). [5, 12, 28, 57]

This prodromal phase lasts approximately 48 hours, but may be as long as 6 weeks, depending on the quantity of inocula. The patient deteriorates suddenly with the development of an acute illness, which includes symptoms of acute dyspnoea, strident cough, stridor, fever, cyanosis, fever, chills, cyanosis, tachypnoea, tachycardia, fluid in the tracheobronchial tree and pleural effusion. Fifty percent of these patients will develop meningitis.

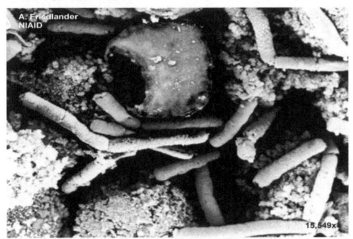

Figure 2.1-11: Color-enhanced scanning electron micrograph shows splenic tissue from a monkey with inhalational anthrax after systemic distribution. Note that the rod-shaped bacilli and an erythrocyte

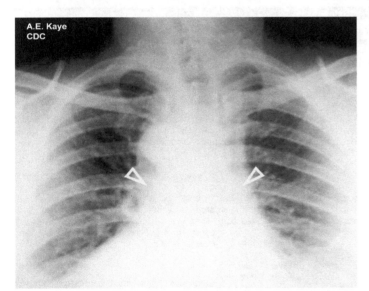

Figure 2.1-12: A posteroanterior chest x-ray was taken four months after the onset of inhalational anthrax infection in a 46 yr. old male. Note the widening of the mediastinum

Within one to two days after the initial onset of acute symptoms, the patients will become extremely disorientated, as their pulse becomes rapid and faint, while dyspnoea and cyanosis worsen. Soon after, the patient will quickly fall into shock, coma and eventually death (Table 5). [5, 12, 28, 57]

DETECTION

B. anthracis is very similar to *B. cereus*, *B. thuringiensis*, and *B. mycoides*, which are closely related group of bacilli. [28] In most laboratory tests, this group of bacteria are generally considered contaminants and are dismissed during testing, unless the physician specifically requests their analysis. *B. anthracis* is

differentiated from other bacilli by the morphological features of their colonies when cultured. *B. anthracis* can be cultured from ascites fluid, pleural effusions and cerebral spinal fluid in cases of meningo-encephalitis. Culture samples may also be isolated via fluid carefully expressed from eschar. Nonetheless, as stated by Dixon *et al.* (1999), fluids expressed from eschar are not recommended, due to the possibility that this method may cause the spread of the pathogenic bacteria. [28] Colonies of most *B. anthracis* isolates are nonhemolytic, white to gray (2–5 mm in diameter) with irregular edges, and are ground-glass in appearance (Figure 2.1-13). In addition, *B. anthracis* will develop a poly-d-glutamic acid capsule when cultured overnight on a nutrient agar, containing 0.7 % bicarbonate, at 37°C in the presence of 5 to 20% carbon dioxide. [28, 57, 58]

Table 5: An overview of the clinical symptoms of inhalational anthrax

Symptoms	+	++	+++
Fever			■
Malaise			■
Fatigue			■
Non-productive cough			■
Myalgia			■
Widened mediastinum			■
Acute dyspnoea			■
Strident cough			■
Stridor			■
Cyanosis			■
Chills			■
Cyanosis			■
Tachypnoea			■
Tachycardia			■
Fluids in trachea/ bronchi			■
Pleural effusion			■
Meningitis		■	
Shock		■	
Coma		■	

+ Rare ++ Common +++ Frequent

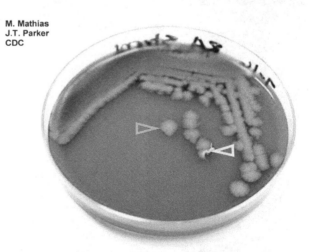

Figure 2.1-13: This photograph shows B. *anthracis* colonies grown on sheep"s blood agar (SBA) for a 24 hour period. Note the classical appearance exhibited in the colonial morphology including a ground-glass, non-pigmented texture with accompanying `comma' projections from some of the individual rough-edged colonies (arrow). Please note that a "tenacity test" had been performed using an inoculating loop, which proved positive for B. *anthracis*, causing the 'colony' to 'stand up' like beaten egg white (arrow)

By using M'Fadyean stain, blood samples from patients can be examined for *B. anthracis*, which have a pink capsule surrounding a dark blue square ended bacilli. [12, 37] Unfortunately, patients suffering from systemic disease often die prior to the completion of a positive blood culture. Bacilli may also be detected via a direct Gram stained smear of skin lesions (either vesicle or eschar), blood, or cerebrospinal fluid. Positive stains will show large Gram-positive, encapsulated, box car shaped bacilli in short chains (Figure 2.1-2).[57]

In 1985, Logan *et al.*, utilized API 50 CH and API 20E test strips (API Laboratory Products Ltd.™) to identify *B. anthracis* with high accuracy.[59] Unfortunately, serological testing can only be used retrospectively and requires both acute and convalescent sera for examination comparison. In cases of cutaneous anthrax, antibodies produced towards protective antigen and/or the bacterial capsule of *B. anthracis* develop only in 68-92% of patients.[57]

Real-time PCR testing may be used for rapid detection of *B. anthracis* spores. Detection was accomplished through hybridization of probes BaP1 (TCCAAAGCGCTATGATTTAGCAAATGT-fluorescein) and BaP2 (GGTCGCTACAAGATCAACAAGTTACAC-Phosphorylation at the 3' end) within 90 minutes.[60, 61]

Commercially available Anthrax protective antigen (PA) IgG ELISA Kits developed by GenWay™, Novus™, Calbiotech ™ and various other companies are capable of determining if an individual has been exposed to anthrax. These tests use prepared wells coated with purified PA antigen to react with anti-PA IgG specific antibodies found in the patient's serum. Once the anti-PA IgG specific antibodies are bounded to the antigen, an enzyme conjugate is added and allowed to incubate. Subsequently, the intensity of the color generated through enzymatic reactions will indicate the amount of IgG specific antibody.[62]

In 2011, Addanki *et al.* developed a rapid, highly sensitive method to detect the anthrax toxin lethal factor gene located in pXO1. Instead of capturing antibodies, the researchers utilized enzyme-linked immunosorbent assay (ELISA) to target anthrax lethal factor endopeptidase sequences located in pXO1. These endopeptidase sequences are targeted via complementary biotin conjugated oligoprobe and are subsequently visualized through streptavidin-peroxidase-based colorimetric assay. The results obtained showed promise as the method has been reported to be over 1000 times more sensitive than the standard ELISA methodology.[63]

TREATMENT

Organisms within the *Bacillus* group, with the exception of *B. anthracis*, are penicillin resistant due to their capabilities of transcribing beta-lactamases. For example, *B. cereus* possesses type I and II beta-lactamase genes that are responsible for producing enzymes that hydrolyze the beta-lactam ring, thereby inactivating the antimicrobial agent. Never-theless, Chen *et al.* (2003), found that *B. anthracis* (Sterne strain) also possess similar genes known as bla1 (a 927-nucelotide gene that is 93.8% similar to type I) and bla2 genes (a 768-nucleotide gene that is 92% similar to type II). These researchers reported that

Table 6a – Medication dosage and side effects of various treatment for cutaneous anthrax

Medication	Mechanism of Action	Side Effects	Recommended Dosage
Amoxicillin Ampicillin	Inhibits cell wall synthesis	Fever, chills, pharyngitis, headache body aches, red skin rash, severe blistering & peeling, nausea, stomach pain, diarrhea, flu-like symptoms, vomiting, anorexia, dark urine, jaundice, easy bruising or bleeding, weakness, agitation, confusion, seizure, vaginal itching or discharge	In severe cutaneous disease: ampicillin 2 g q 6h iv for 60 days. Pediatric dose: 200-400 mg/kg·24h divided q 6h. Cutaneous /postexposure prophylaxis (if strain is susceptible): amoxicillin 500 mg po q 8 h for 60 days. Pediatric dose: 20-50 mg/kg·24h divided q 8h.
Chloramphenicol	Inhibits protein synthesis	Headache, diarrhea, nausea, vomiting, fever, fatigue, pharyngitis, unusual bleeding or bruising, abdominal pain, bloating, vision changes, eye pain, rash, itching, swelling, dizziness, trouble breathing and tingling of the hands or feet	Cutaneous anthrax infections: in both adults and children: 50-100 mg/kg·d iv divided q 6h until patient stable
Ciprofloxacin (Cipro)	Inhibits the function of DNA gyrase	Headache, nausea, diarrhea, abnormal liver function, vomiting, abdominal pain/discomfort, rash, foot pain, pain in extremities, injection site reaction	In severe cutaneous disease: 600-800 mg iv q 12h for 60 days (pediatric dose: 10-15 mg/kg q 12h bid iv). In cutaneous / postexposure prophylaxis: 500 mg po bid. Pediatric dose: 10-15 mg/kg q 12h not to exceed 1 g/d for 60 days. If cutaneous disease is not related to bioterrorism, treat for 7-14 d
Clarithromycin	Inhibits protein synthesis	Headache, fever, severe dizziness, diarrhea, nausea, vomiting, stomach upset, abdominal pain, changes in taste, hearing loss, mental/mood changes, fainting, fast/irregular heartbeats, sore throat, rash, itching, swelling, trouble breathing, dark urine, yellowing of eyes or skin	Cutaneous anthrax infections: 500 mg po bid for 60 days. Pediatric dose: 15 mg/kg·24h divided q 12h for 60 days
Clindamycin	Inhibits protein synthesis	Nausea, vomiting, upset stomach, mild diarrhea, rash, itching, swelling, severe dizziness, trouble breathing, sore throat, joint pain/swelling, yellowing eyes or skin	Cutaneous anthrax infections: 450-900 mg iv q 8 h until patient is stable, then switch to 300-450 mg q 6h po for 60 d. Pediatric dose: 24-40 mg/kg·24 h iv divided q 6 h until stable, then 20-30 mg/kg·24h po divided q 6h
Doxycycline	Inhibits protein synthesis	Headaches, blurred vision, fever, nausea, diarrhea, bloody stools, severe stomach cramps, indigestion, heartburn, vomiting, photosensitivity, loss of appetite, dysphagia, rash, joint pain, feeling tired	In severe cutaneous disease: 100 mg q 12h iv for 60 days. Pediatric dose: >8 years and >45 kg, 100 mg q 12h iv; >8 years and ≤45 kg, 2.2 mg/kg q 12h iv; ≤8 years, 2.2 mg/kg q 12h iv for 60 days. Cutaneous / post-exposure prophylaxis (if strain is susceptible): 100 mg q 12h po for 60 days. Pediatric dose: >8 years and >45 kg, 100 mg q 12h po; >8 years and ≤ 45 kg, 2.2 mg/kg q 12h po; ≤8 years, 2.2 mg/kg q 12h po for 60 days. If cutaneous disease is not related to bioterrorism, treat for 7-14 d

bla1 genes encode penicillinase, while bla2 appears to be a cephalosporinase. However, *B. anthracis* poorly expresses these genes, leaving them susceptible to beta-lactam agents.[64]

The treatment of cutaneous anthrax comprises of the administration of oral potassium penicillin V. The recommended dosage of potassium penicillin V required is 30 mg/kg of body weight per day divided in four doses (one dose every six hours). In severe cases, intramuscular injection of procaine penicillin G in aqueous solution is often provided for patients. The recommended dosage of this medication is 24,000 units/kg of body weight per day divided into 2 doses, 1 dose every 12 hours. For patients who are allergic to penicillin: tetracycline, erythromycin, chloram-phenicol or ciprofloxacin can be used.[12] Please examine Tables 6a and 6b for more information regarding medication options, dosages and side effects.

The treatment of systemic anthrax infections such as

Table 6b – Medication dosage and side effects of various treatment for cutaneous anthrax

Medication	Mechanism of Action	Side Effects	Recommended Dosage
Imipenem	Inhibit cell wall synthesis	Fever, chills, headache, body aches, hallucinations, confusion, seizure, tremors, fainting, rapid heartbeats, flu-like symptoms diarrhea, sore throat, nausea, vomiting, stomach pain, heartburn	Cutaneous anthrax infections: 500 mg iv q 6h until patient is stable. Pediatric dose: 50-100 mg/kg·24h iv divided q 6h until patient is stable, then stop
Penicillin	Inhibits bacterial cell wall synthesis	Headache, diarrhea (watery or bloody), fever, chills, body aches, flu symptoms, easy bruising or bleeding, unusual weakness, severe skin rash, itching, peeling, agitation, confusion, unusual thoughts or behavior, seizure, nausea, vomiting, stomach pain, vaginal itching or discharge	In severe cutaneous: 20-30 million IU/d PCN G iv for 60 days. Cutaneous/postexposure prophylaxis (if strain is susceptible): 500 mg PCN VK q 6h po for 60 days. Pediatric dose: 50 mg/kg 24h divided q 6h. If cutaneous disease is not related to bioterrorism, treat for 7-14 days
Rifampin	Inhibits protein synthesis	Headache, fever, chills, dizziness, upset stomach, nausea, stomach pain, heartburn, drowsiness, dizziness, sore throat, dark urine, yellowing eyes or skin, rash, itching, swelling, trouble breathing	Cutaneous anthrax infections: 600 mg po or iv q d for 60 days in combination with doxycycline or ciprofloxacin. Pediatric dose: 10-20 mg/kg iv/po q 24h 60 days in combination with doxycycline or ciprofloxacin
Vancomycin	Inhibit cell wall synthesis	Ringing in the ears, hearing problems, severe dizziness, trouble breathing, easy bleeding/bruising, rash, itching/swelling, fever, persistent sore throat, diarrhea, abdominal or stomach pain/ cramping, blood/mucus in your stool	Cutaneous disease: 1 g iv q 12h until patient is stable. Pediatric dose: 15 mg/kg iv q 8h until patient is stable

Table 7a – Medication dosage, side effects of various treatment for systemic anthrax

Medication	Mechanism of Action	Side Effects	Recommended Dosage
Amoxicillin Ampicillin	Inhibits cell wall synthesis	Fever, chills, headache, body aches, sore throat, nausea, stomach pain, loss of appetite, vomiting, diarrhea that is watery or bloody, flu-like symptoms, dark urine, jaundice (yellowing of the skin or eyes), unusual weakness, agitation, confusion, seizure, vaginal itching or discharge, severe blistering, peeling, and red skin rash, easy bruising or bleeding	In inhalational, meningitis, GI anthrax infection: ampicillin 2 g q 6h iv for 60 days. Pediatric dose: 200-400 mg/kg·24h divided q 6 h. Cutaneous /postexposure prophylaxis (if strain is susceptible): amoxicillin 500 mg po q 8h for 60 days. Pediatric dose: 20-50 mg/kg·24h divided q 8h
Chloramphenicol	Inhibits protein synthesis	Headache, diarrhea, nausea, vomiting, fever, fatigue, sore throat, unusual bleeding or bruising, abdominal pain, bloating, vision changes, eye pain, rash, itching, swelling, dizziness, trouble breathing and tingling of the hands or feet	Inhalational, meningitis, GI, anthrax infections: in both adults and children: 50-100 mg/kg·d iv divided q 6h until patient stable
Ciprofloxacin (Cipro)	Inhibits the function of DNA gyrase	Headache, nausea, diarrhea, abnor-mal liver function, vomiting, abdominal pain/discomfort, rash, foot pain, pain in extremities, injection site reaction	In cases of inhalational, meningitis, GI anthrax infection: 600-800 mg iv q 12h for 60 days; pediatric dose: 10-15 mg/kg q 12h bid iv
Clarithromycin	Inhibits protein synthesis	Headache, fever, severe dizziness, diarrhea, nausea, vomiting, stomach upset, abdominal pain, changes in taste, hearing loss, mental/mood changes, fainting, fast/irregular heartbeats, sore throat, rash, itching, swelling, trouble breathing, dark urine, yellowing of eyes or skin	Inhalational, meningitis, GI anthrax infections: 500 mg po bid for 60 days. Pediatric dose: 15 mg/kg·2h divided q 12h for 60 days
Clindamycin	Inhibits protein synthesis	Nausea, vomiting, upset stomach, mild diarrhea, rash, itching, swelling, severe dizziness, trouble breathing, sore throat, joint pain/swelling, yellowing eyes or skin	Inhalational, meningitis, GI, anthrax infections: 450-900 mg iv q 8h until patient is stable, then switch to 300-450 mg q 6h po for 60 days. Pediatric dose: 24-40 mg/kg·24h iv divided q 6h until stable, then 20-30 mg/kg·24h po divided q 6h
Doxycycline	Inhibits protein synthesis	Headaches, blurred vision, fever, nausea, diarrhea, bloody stools, severe stomach cramps, indigestion, heartburn, vomiting, photosensitivity, loss of appetite, dysphagia, rash, joint pain, feeling tired	In cases of inhalational, meningitis, GI anthrax infection: 100 mg q 12h iv for 60 days. Pediatric dose: >8 years and >45 kg, 100 mg q 12h iv; >8 years and ≤ 45 kg, 2.2 mg/kg q 12h iv; ≤ 8 years, 2.2 mg/kg q 12h iv for 60 days
Imipenem	Inhibit cell wall synthesis	Fever, chills, headache, body aches, hallucinations, confusion, seizure, tremors, fainting, rapid heartbeats, flu-like symptoms diarrhea, sore throat, nausea, vomiting, stomach pain, heartburn	Inhalational, meningitis, GI, anthrax infections: 500 mg iv q 6h until patient is stable, then stop. Pediatric dose: 50-100 mg/kg·24h iv divided q 6h until patient is stable, then stop

Table 7b – Medication dosage, side effects of various treatment for systemic anthrax

Medication	Mechanism of Action	Side Effects	Recommended Dosage
Penicillin	Inhibits cell wall synthesis	Headache, diarrhea (watery or bloody), fever, chills, body aches, flu symptoms, easy bruising or bleeding, unusual weakness, severe skin rash, itching, peeling, agitation, confusion, unusual thoughts or behavior, seizure, nausea, vomiting, stomach pain, vaginal itching or discharge	Inhalational, meningitis, GI anthrax infection: 20-30 million IU/d PCN G iv for 60 days
Rifampin	Inhibits protein synthesis	Headache, fever, chills, dizziness, upset stomach, nausea, stomach pain, heartburn, drowsiness, dizziness, sore throat, dark urine, yellowing eyes or skin, rash, itching, swelling, trouble breathing	Inhalational, meningitis, GI anthrax infections: 600 mg po or iv q d for 60 days in combination with doxycycline or ciprofloxacin. Pediatric dose: 10-20 mg/kg iv/po q 24h 60 days in combination with doxycycline or ciprofloxacin
Vancomycin	Inhibit cell wall synthesis	Ringing in the ears, hearing problems, severe dizziness, trouble breathing, easy bleeding/bruising, rash, itching/swelling, fever, persistent sore throat, diarrhea, abdominal or stomach pain/ cramping, blood/mucus in your stool	Inhalational, meningitis, GI, anthrax infection: 1 g iv q 12h until patient is stable. Pediatric dose: 15 mg/kg iv q 8h until patient is stable

Table 8: Differential diagnosis of cutaneous anthrax with other diseases of similar symptoms. These diseases include brown recluse (BR) spider bite, cutaneous leishmaniasis (CL), tularemia (TU), *Staphylococcus aureus* (Staph), Scrub typhus (ST) and Rocky Mountain Spotted Fevers (RMSF)

Symptoms	Anthrax	BR	CL	TU	Staph	ST	RMSF
Fever	■	■	■	■	■	■	■
Headaches	■				■	■	■
Anorexia	■		■				■
Nausea	■	■			■		
Malaise	■						
Toxemia						■	
Painful lymphadentitis	■			■		■	
Severe edema at eschar	■	■					
Localized pruritus	■	■					
Painless erythema	■	■				■	■
Papule lesion	■	■	■				■
Black centered ulcer	■	■	■		■	■	
Black eschar	■	■				■	
Sepsis	■						

Table 9: Differential diagnosis of inhalational anthrax with other diseases of similar symptoms. These diseases include influenza, Respiratory syncytial virus (RSV), *Legionella*, bacterial pneumonia (BP), Q fever and dissecting aortic aneurysm (DAA)

Symptoms	Anthrax	Influenza	RSV	Legionella	BP	Q Fever	DAA
Fever	■	■	■	■	■	■	
Malaise	■	■	■	■	■	■	
Fatigue	■	■		■	■		■
Non-productive cough	■	■	■	■			■
Myalgia	■	■		■			■
Widened mediastinum	■						
Acute dyspnoea	■	■	■		■		■
Strident cough	■	■	■	■	■	■	
Stridor	■						
Cyanosis	■		■		■		■
Chills	■	■		■		■	
Cyanosis	■						
Tachypnoea	■						■
Tachycardia	■				■		■
Fluids in trachea/ bronchi	■						
Pleural effusion	■						■
Meningitis	■					■	
Shock	■						
Coma	■						

oropharyngeal, gastrointestinal and inhalational anthrax comprises the administration of ciprofloxacin at 400 mg or doxycycline at 100 mg intravenously every 12 hours. This same regimental treatment is also used to treat systemic anthrax sepsis.[12, 65] Please examine Tables 7a and 7b for medication options, dosages and side effects.

Work on the development of anthrax vaccines started as early as the 1880s by W.S. Greenfield and Louis Pasteur.[66] After World War II, the potential use of anthrax as a biological warfare agent prompted the United States and the United Kingdom to develop inactivated vaccines at Fort Detrick, Maryland and Porton Down, United Kingdom.[67] Various strains of *B. anthracis* were evaluated and finally the nonencapsulated, nonproteolytic mutant of Vollum strain V770-NP1-R was selected. The current available vaccine, Anthrax Vaccine Absorbed (AVA), was first licensed

Table 10: Differential diagnosis of gastrointestinal anthrax with other diseases of similar symptoms. These diseases include shigellosis, salmonellosis (Sal), Crohn's disease, *Clostridium difficile* colitis (CDC), *Campylobacter enteritis* (CE), and amebiasis

Symptoms	Anthrax	Shigellosis	Sal	Crohn's	CDC	CE	Amebiasis
Fever	■	■	■			■	
Headaches	■		■			■	
Conjunctiva congestion	■			■			
Congestion of the face	■						
Nausea	■	■	■	■	■	■	■
Loss of appetite	■	■	■	■	■		
Diffused abdominal pains	■	■	■	■	■	■	■
Abdominal tenderness	■	■	■	■	■	■	■
Hypovolemia	■						
Vomiting	■		■			■	■
Vomiting of blood	■						
Constipation	■						
Severe diarrhea	■	■	■	■	■		■
Regional lymphadenopathy	■		■	■		■	
Lymph nodes - enlargement	■		■			■	
Lymph node – hemorrhagic	■						
Ulcer-lesions - esophagus	■			■			
Ulcer-lesions - stomach	■			■		■	
Ulcer-lesions - jejunum	■						
Ulcer-lesions - ileum cecum	■	■					
Ulcerative lesions	■			■			
Hemorr. lesions - stomach	■						
Hemorr. lesions - jejunum	■						
Ascites	■			■			
Gastrointestinal obstruction	■	■	■	■	■		
Gastrointestine Perforation	■	■	■	■	■	■	
Shock	■						
Mediastinal widening	■						
Toxemia	■						

for manufacture in 1970 by the Michigan Department of Public Health and subsequently the entire production line was sold to BioPort; they are now the sole manufacturer of AVA.[66]

AVA requires the subcutaneous administration of a basic initial series of six 0.5 mL doses with subsequent doses administered at two weeks, four weeks, six months, 12 months and 18 months. Subsequent annual booster shots are required after the completion of the initial series. Between 1974 and 1989, approximately 68,000 doses were distributed. Between 1998 and 2001, more than 500,000 military personnel received approximately 2 million doses of AVA through the Anthrax Vaccine Immunization Program (AVIP), initiated by the Department of Defense[68], however, this vaccination program was not without its share of controversies. Complaints developed among a few of the vaccinated Gulf War veterans of various chronic conditions such as fever, headaches, malaise, swellings, joint pains as well as more serious conditions of hypogonadism, Stevens-Johnson syndrome and aplastic anemia, which were attributed to, but lacked identifiable relationships, AVA use. A few military personnel, at the risk of court-martial, have refused being vaccinated.[66]

DIFFERENTIAL DIAGNOSIS

Careful documentation of patient history must be made in order to properly diagnose *B. anthracis* infection. For example, patient's travels to anthrax endemic areas and/or the patient's occupation (e.g. wool, animal hide worker), which predispose them to anthrax infection, must be first considered. Other signs and symptoms that must also be carefully weighed are symptomatically similar diseases. For instance, differential diagnosis for cutaneous anthrax must include brown recluse (BR) spider bite, cutaneous leishmaniasis (CL), *Staphylococcus aureus* (Staph), tularemia

(TU), Scrub typhus (ST) and Rocky Mountain Spotted Fever (RMSF) must be considered (Table 8). For Inhalational anthrax, influenza, Respiratory syncytial virus (RSV), *Legionella*, bacterial pneumonia (BP), Q fever or dissecting aortic aneurysm (DAA - because of the widening of mediastinum, chest pains and shortness of breath) must be included in the differentially diagnosed (Table 9). For gastrointestinal anthrax, bacterial diarrhea such as shigellosis, salmonellosis (Sal), *Clostridium difficile* colitis (CDC), *Campylobacter enteritis* (CE), amebiasis and inflammatory bowel disease (IBD) such as Crohn's disease must be considered. Finally, meningeal complications resulting from anthrax, bacterial meningitis must be included with the differential diagnosis (Table 10).

References

1. Quentzel H., Spear S., Barakat L., Lustig N., Spargo K., Cartter M., Garcia J., Barden D.M., Mayo D.R., Kelley K.A., Hadler J. Update: Investigation of Bioterrorism-Related Inhalational Anthrax - Connecticut, 2001. Morbidity and Mortality Weekly Report, 2001. 50: pp. 1049–1051
2. Jernigan J.A., Stephens D.S., Ashford D.A., Omenaca C., Topiel M.S., Galbraith M., Tapper M., Fisk T.L., Zaki S., Popovic T., Meyer R.F., Quinn C.P., Harper S.A., Fridkin S.K., Sejvar J.J., Shepard C., McConnell M., Guarner J., Shieh W-J., Malecki J.M., Gerberding J.L., Hughes J.M., Perkins B.A. Bioterrorism-Related Inhalational Anthrax: the First 10 cases Reported in the United States. Emerging Infectious Diseases, 2001. 7: pp. 933–944
3. The United States Army Medical Research Institute for Infectious Diseases' Medical; Management of Biological Casualties Handbook – Sixth Edition. Fort Detrick: United States Army Medical Research Institute of Infectious Diseases. 2005. pp. 17-24
4. Alibek K. Biohazard. New York: Dell Publishing. 1999. pp. 20, 70-86
5. Anderson R.A. Outbreak: Cases in Real-World Microbiology. Washington D.C.: American Society for Microbiology Press. 2006. pp. 270-271
6. Fox L.A. Bacterial warfare: The Use of Biologic Agents in Warfare. Military Surgeon, 1933. 72: pp. 189–207
7. Williams P., Wallace D. Unit 731: Japan's Secret Biological Warfare in World War II. New York: Free Press. 1989. pp. 238
8. Franz D.R., Parrott C.D., Takafuji E.T. The U.S. Biological Warfare and Biological Defense Programs. Medical Aspects of Chemical and Biological Warfare. Chapter 19. Washington D.C.: Office of the Surgeon General Department of the Army, United States of America. 1997. pp. 425-436
9. Anthrax Fact File. Biological Weapons and Anthrax. British Broadcasting Corporation. Retrieved December 26, 2008. Website: http://news.bbc.co.uk/hi/english/static/in_depth/world/2001/anthrax/biological.stm
10. Pohanka M., Skládal P. Bacillus anthracis, Francisella tularensis and Yersinia pestis. The most important bacterial warfare agents. Folia Microbiologica, 2009. 54: pp. 263-272

11. Liu H., Bergman N. H., Thomason B., Shallom S., Hazen A., Crossno J., Rasko D. A., Ravel J., Read T. D., Peterson S. N., Yates J. III, Hanna P. C. Formation and Composition of the Bacillus anthracis Endospore. The Journal of Bacteriology, 2004. 186: pp. 164-178
12. Guerrant R.L., Walker D.H., Weller P.F. Tropical Infectious Diseases – Principles, Pathogens & Practice. Volume 1. Philadelphia: Churchill Livingstone Elsevier. 2006. pp. 488-453
13. Read T.D., Peterson S.N., Tourasse N., Baillie L.W., Paulsen I.T., Nelson K.E., Tettelin H., Fouts D.E., Eisen J.A., Gill S.R., Holtzapple E.K., Okstad O.A., Helgason E., Rilstone J., Wu M., Kolonay J.F., Beanan M.J., Dodson R.J., Brinkac L.M., Gwinn M., DeBoy R.T., Madpu R., Daugherty S.C., Durkin A.S., Haft D.H., Nelson W.C., Peterson J.D., Pop M., Khouri H.M., Radune D., Benton J.L., Mahamoud Y., Jiang L., Hance I.R., Weidman J.F., Berry K.J., Plaut R.D., Wolf A.M., Watkins K.L., Nierman W.C., Hazen A., Cline R., Redmond C., Thwaite J.E., White O., Salzberg S.L., Thomason B., Friedlande A.M., Koehler T.M., Hanna P.C., Kolstø A.B., Fraser C.M. The Genome Sequence of Bacillus anthracis Ames and Comparison to Closely Related Bacteria. Nature, 2003. 423: pp. 81-86
14. Bourgogne A., Drysdale M., Hilsenbeck S.G., Peterson S.N., Koehler T.M. Global Effects of Virulence Gene Regulators in a Bacillus anthracis Strain with both Virulence Plasmids. Infection and Immunity, 2003. 71: pp. 2736-274
15. Little S.F., Ivins B.E. Molecular Pathogenesis of Bacillus anthracis Infection. Microbes and Infection, 1999. 1: pp. 131–139
16. Park S-H., Oh H-B., Seong W-K., Kim C-W., Cho S-Y., Yoo C-K. Differential Analysis of Bacillus anthracis after pX01 Plasmid Curing and Comprehensive Data on Bacillus anthracis Infection in Macrophages and Glial Cells. Proteomic – Clinical Applications. Volume 7. Weinheim: Wiley Verlag. 2007. pp. 3743-3758
17. Leppla S.H. The Anthrax Toxin Complex. Sourcebook of Bacterial Protein Toxins. London: Academic Press. 1991. pp. 277–302
18. Rasheed M.A., Nayarisseri S.A., Yadav M., Jain A., Sharma P., Roy S., Saket S. Screening of Bacillus anthracis Plasmid Px01 Proteins to Identify Novel Antigenic Peptides-an Immunoinformatics Approach. European Journal of Biological Sciences, 2013. 5: pp. 68-76
19. Leppla S.H. Anthrax Toxin Edema Factor; a Bacterial Adenylate Cyclase that Increases Cyclic AMP Concentrations of Eukaryotic Cells. The Proceedings of the National Academy of Sciences United States of America, 1982. 79: pp. 3162–3166
20. Leppla S.H. Bacillus anthracis Calmodulin-dependent Adenylate Cyclase: Chemical and Enzymatic Properties and Interactions with Eukaryotic Cells. Advances in cyclic nucleotide research, 1984. 17: pp. 189–198
21. O'Brien J, Friedlander A., Drier T., Ezzell J., Leppla S. Effects of Anthrax Toxin Compounds on Human Neutrophils . Infection and Immunity, 1985. 47: pp. 306–310
22. Mongridge J., Mourez M., collier R.J. Involvement of Domain 3 in Oligomerization by the Protective Antigen Moiety of Anthrax Toxin. Journal of Bacteriology, 2001. 183: pp. 2111-2116
23. Ingram R. J., Harris A., Ascough S., Metan G., DoganayM., Ballie L., Williamson E.D., Dyson H., Robinson J.H., Sriskandan S., Altmann D.M. Exposure to anthrax toxin alters human leucocyte expression of anthrax toxin receptor 1. Clinical and Experimental Immunology, 2013. 173: pp. 84-91
24. Collier R.J., Young J.A. Anthrax Toxin. Annual Review of Cell and Developmental Biology, 2003. 19: pp. 45-70
25. Makins S-I., Ucluda I., Terakads N., Sasakawa C., Yoshikawa M. Molecular Characterisation and Protein Analysis of the Cap Region, which is Essential for Encapsulation in Bacillus anthracis. Journal of Bacteriology, 1989. 171: pp. 722–730
26. Anthrax. Center for Disease Control and Prevention. Retrieved August 1, 2009. Website: http://www.cdc.gov/nczved/dfbmd/ disease_listing/anthrax_gi.html
27. Salyers A., Whitt D.D. Bacterial Pathogenesis: A molecular Approach. Second Edition. Washington D.C.: American Society for Microbiology Press. 2002. pp. 333
28. Dixon T.C., Meselson M., Guillemin J., Hanna P.C. Anthrax. The New England Journal of Medicine, 1999. 341: pp. 815-826
29. Abdenour D., Larouze B., Dalichaouche M., Aouati, M. Familial Occurrence of Anthrax in Eastern Algeria. Journal of Infectious Disease, 1987. 155: pp. 1083–1084
30. Summary of Notifiable Diseases: 2007. Mortality and Morbidity Weekly Report, 2009. 56: pp. 78-85
31. Summary of Notifiable Diseases: 1994. Mortality and Morbidity Weekly Report, 1995. 43: pp. 69-80
32. Maguiña C., Flores Del Pozo J., Terashima A., Gotuzzo E., Guerra H., Vidal J.E., Legua P., Solari L. Cutaneous Anthrax in Lima, Peru: Retrospective Analysis of 71 Cases, Including Four with a Meningoencephalic Complications. Revista do Instituto de Medicina Tropical de São Paulo, 2005. 47: pp. 25-30
33. Abramova F.A., Grinberg L.M., Yampolskaya O.V., Walker D.H. Pathology of Inhalational Anthrax in 42 Cases from the Sverdlovsk Outbreak of 1979. The Proceedings of the National Academy of Sciences United States of America, 1993. 90: pp. 2291-2294
34. Tabatabaie P., Syadati A. Bacillus Anthracis as a Cause of Bacterial Meningitis. The Pediatric Infectious Disease Journal, 1993. 12: pp. 1035-1037
35. Dutz W., Kohout E. Anthrax. Pathology Annual, 1971. 6: pp. 209-248
36. Rangel R.A., Gonzalez D.A. Bacillus anthracic Meningitis. Neurology, 1975. 25: pp. 525-530
37. LaForce F.M. Anthrax. Clinical Infectious Diseases, 1994. 19: pp. 1009-1014
38. Harris S. Japanese Biological Warfare Research on Humans: a Case Study of Microbiology and Ethics. Annals of the New York Academy of Sciences, 1992. 666: pp. 21–49
39. Sirisanthana T., Brown A.E. Anthrax of the Gastrointestinal Tract. Emerging Infectious Diseases, 2002. 8: pp. 649-651
40. Doganay M., Almac A., Hanagasi R. Primary Throat Anthrax. A Report of Six Cases. Scandinavian Journal of Infectious Diseases, 1986. 18: pp. 415–419
41. Viratchai C. Anthrax Gastro-enteritis and Meningitis. Journal of the Medical Association of Thailand, 1974. 57: pp. 147–150
42. Kunanusont C., Limpakarnjanarat K., Foy J.M. Outbreak of Anthrax in Thailand. Annals Tropical Medicine Parasitology, 1990. 84: pp. 507–512
43. Perl D.P., Dooley J.R. Anthrax. Pathology of Tropical and Extraordinary Diseases. Washington: Armed Forces Institute of Pathology. 1976. p. 118–123
44. Tantajumroon T., Panas-Ampol K. Intestinal Anthrax: Report of Two Cases. Journal of the Medical Association of Thailand, 1968. 51: pp. 477–480
45. Kohout E., Sehat A., Ashraf A.M. Anthrax: a Continuous Problem in Southwest Iran. Americal Journal of the Medical Sciences, 1964. 3: pp. 565–575
46. Tantachumroon T. Pathologic Studies of Intestinal Anthrax: Report of 2 Cases. Chiang Mai Medical Bulletin, 1966. 4: pp. 135–44
47. Jena G.P. Intestinal Anthrax in Man: a Case Report. Central African Journal of Medicine, 1980. 26: pp. 253–254
48. Sirisanthana T., Jesadaporn U. Survival of a Patient with Gastrointestinal Anthrax. Chiang Mai Medical Bulletin, 1985. 24: pp. 1–5
49. Nalin DR, Sultana B, Sahunja R, Islam AK, Rahim MA, Islam M, Costa BS, Mawla N, Greenough WB 3rd. Survival of a Patient with Intestinal Anthrax. American Journal of Medicine, 1977. 62: pp. 130–132
50. Dutz W., Saidi F., Kohout E. Gastric Anthrax with Massive Ascites. Gut, 1970. 11: pp. 352–354
51. Tantajumroon T., Panas-Ampol K. Intestinal Anthrax: Report of Two Cases. Journal of the Medical Association of Thailand, 1968. 51: pp. 477–480
52. Baht P., Mohan D.N., Srinivasa H. Intestinal Anthrax with Bacteriological Investigations. The Journal of Infectious Diseases, 1985. 152: pp. 1357–1358
53. Alizad A., Ayoub E.M., Makki N. Intestinal Anthrax in a Two-Year-Old Child. The Pediatric Infectious Disease Journal, 1995. 14: pp. 394-395
54. Brachman P.S., Kaufman A.F., Dalldorf F.G. Industrial Inhalation Anthrax. Bacteriological Reviews, 1966. 30: pp. 646-659
55. Albrink W.S. Pathogenesis of Inhalation Anthrax. Bacteriological Reviews, 1961. 25: pp. 268-273
56. Guarner J, Jernigan J.A., Shieh W-J, Tatti K., Flannagan L.M., Stephens D.S., Popovic T., Ashford D.A., Perkins B.A., Zaki S.R., Inhalational Anthrax Pathology Working Group. Pathology and Pathogenesis of Bioterrorism-Related Inhalational Anthrax. American Journal of Pathology, 2003.163: pp. 701-709
57. Spenser R.C. Bacillus anthracis. Journal of Clinical Pathology, 2003. 56: pp. 182-187
58. Green B.D., Battisti L., Koehler T.M., Thorne C.B., Ivins B.E. Demonstration of a Capsule Plasmid in Bacillus anthracis. Infection and Immunity, 1985. 49: pp. 291-297
59. Logan N.A., Carman J.A., Melling J., Berkeley R.C.W. Identification of Bacillus anthracis by API Tests. Journal of Medical Microbiology, 1985. 20: pp. 75-85
60. Qi Y., Patra G., Liang X., Williams L.E., Rose S., Redkar R.J., Del Vecchio V. G. Utilization of the rpoB Gene as a Specific Chromosomal Marker for Real-time PCR Detection of Bacillus anthracis. Applied and Environmental Microbiology, 2001. 67: pp. 3720-3727
61. Drago L., Lombardi A., Vecchi E.D., Gismondo M.R. Real-time PCR Assay for Rapid Detection of Bacillus anthracis Spores in Clinical Samples. Journal of Clinical Microbiology, 2002. 40: pp. 4399
62. Addanki K.C., Sheraz M., Knight K., Williams K., Pace D.G., Bagasra O. Detection of anthrax toxin genetic sequences by the solid phase oligo-probes. Indian Journal of Medical Microbiology, 2011. 29: pp. 372-378
63. Quinn C.P., Semenova V.A., Elie C.M., Romero-Steiner S., Greene C., Li H., Stamey K., Steward-Clark E., Schmidt D.S., Mothershed E., Pruckler J., Schwartz S., Benson R.F., Helsel L.O., Holder P.F., Johnson S.E., Kellum M., Messmer T., Thacker W.L., Besser L., Plikaytis B.D., Taylor T.H. Jr, Freeman A.E., Wallace K.J., Dull P., Sejvar J., Bruce E., Moreno R., Schuchat A., Lingappa J.R., Martin S.K., Walls J., Bronsdon M., Carlone G.M., Bajani-Ari M., Ashford D.A., Stephens D.S., Perkins B.A. Specific, sensitive, and quantitative enzyme-linked immunosorbent assay for human immunoglobulin G antibodies to anthrax toxin protective antigen. Emerging Infectious Diseases, 2002. 8: pp. 1103-1110
64. Chen Y., Succi J., Tenover F.C., Koehler T.M. Beta-lactamase genes of the Penicillin-Susceptible Bacillus anthracis Sterne strain. The journal of Bacteriology, 2003. 185: pp. 823-830
65. Beatty ME, Ashford D.A., Griffin P.M., Tauxe, R. V., Sobel, J. Gastrointestinal Anthrax: Review of the Literature. Archieves of Internal Medicine, 2003. 163: pp. 2527-2531
66. Joellenbeck L.M., Zwanziger L.L., Durch J.S., Strom B.L. The Anthrax Vaccine: Is it Safe? Does it Work? Washington D.C.: The National Academies Press. 2002. pp. 48-183
67. Turnbull P.C.B. Current Status of Immunization against Anthrax: Old Vaccines May be Here to Stay for a While. Current Opinion in Infectious Diseases, 2000. 13: pp. 113-120
68. Sever J.L., Brenner A.I., Gale A.D., Lyle J.M., Moulton L.H., Ward B.J., West D.J. Safety of Anthrax Vaccine: an Expanded Review and Evaluation of Adverse Events Reported to the Vaccine Adverse Event Reporting System (VAERS). Pharmacoepidemiology and Drug Safety, 2004. 13: pp. 825-840

Photo Bibiography

Figure 2.1-2: Scanning Electron micrograph of Sterne strain anthrax endospores. This photomicrograph was taken by the CDC and released by FDA on August 29, 2007 in an article titled: Building a Stronger Defense against Bioterrorism. Public domain photo

Figure 2.1-4: Cutaneous anthrax infection diagram. The human anatomical illustration is created by Dr. Alexander J. da Silva and Melanie Moser in 2003. The illustration is released by CDC. Public domain graphics

Figure 2.1-5: A female patient suffering from *Bacillus anthracis* infection involving her left eye. This photo was taken on the 24th day of infection. Photo was taken and released by the CDC. Public domain photo

Figure 2.1-6: Gram stain of cerebrospinal fluid of a 63-year-old Caucasian photo editor from Florida demonstrating *B. anthracis*. Patient contracted anthrax on October 2, 2001 and died on October 5, 2001. The photograph was taken in October, 2001 and was published by CDC. Jernigan J.A., Stephens D.S., Ashford D.A., Omenaca C., Topiel M.S., Galbraith M., Tapper M., Fisk T.L., Zaki S., Popovic T., Meyer R.F., Quinn C.P., Harper S.A., Fridkin S.K., Sejvar J.J., Shepard C.W., McConnell M., Guarner J., Shieh W-J, Malecki J.M., Gerberding J.L., Hughes J.M., Perkins B.A., members of the Anthrax Bioterrorism Investigation Team. Bioterrorism-Related Inhalational Anthrax: The First 10 Cases Reported in the United States. Emerging Infectious Diseases, 2001. 7: pp. 933-944. Public domain photo

Figire 2.1-7: Oral-oropharyngeal and gastrointestinal anthrax infection diagram. The human anatomical illustration is created by Dr. Alexander J. da Silva and Melanie Moser in 2003. The illustration is released by the CDC. Public domain graphics

Figure 2.1-8: Patient suffering from Oral-Oropharyngeal Anthrax demonstrating necrosis and ulceration. This photograph was taken between March and April 1982 and published by CDC. Sirisanthana T., Brown A.E. Anthrax of the Gastrointestinal Tract. Emerging Infectious Diseases, 2002. 8: pp. 649-651. Public domain photo

Figure 2.1-9: Photomicrograph of the small intestine in a fatal case of gastrointestinal anthrax. Histopathology of This micrograph reveals submucosal hemorrhage. Photo was taken by Dr. Marshall Fox in 1976 and released by the CDC. Public domain photo

Figire 2.1-10: Inhalational anthrax infection diagram. The human anatomical illustration is created by Dr. Alexander J. da Silva and Melanie Moser in 2003. The illustration is released by the CDC. Public domain graphics

Figure 12.1-11: Color-enhanced scanning electron micrograph shows splenic tissue from a monkey with inhalational anthrax after system distribution. Note that the rod-shaped bacilli (yellow) and an erythrocyte (red). The scanning electron micrograph was taken by Arthur Friedlander and released by National Institutes of Health, Department of Health and Human Services. Public domain photo

Figure 12.1-12: A posteroanterior chest x-ray was taken 4 months after the onset of inhalational anthrax infection in a 46 year old male. Note the widening of the mediastinum. This photo was taken by Arthur E. Kaye in 1972 and released by the CDC. Public domain photo

Figure 2.1-13: This photograph shows B. *anthracis* colonies grown on sheep"s blood agar (SBA) for a 24 hour period. Note the classical appearance exhibited in the colonial morphology including a ground-glass, non-pigmented texture with accompanying 'comma' projections from some of the individual rough-edged colonies. Please note that a "tenacity test" had been performed using an inoculating loop, which proved positive for *B. anthracis*, causing the 'colony' to 'stand up' like beaten egg white. This photograph was taken by Megan Mathias, J. Todd Parker and released by the CDC. Public domain photo

There are a total of six species of *Brucella* that are responsible for the disease brucellosis. Brucellosis is a zoonotic disease that predominantly infects animals with humans as its accidental host. The *Brucella* species that are capable of causing disease in humans are *B. abortus* (found in sheep and goats, etc.) (Figure 2.2-1), *B. melitensis* (found in cattle), *B. suis* (found in swine) and *B. canis* (found in canines). There are two other organisms that are not pathogenic to humans, but are able to cause brucellosis in sheep (*B. ovis*) and wood rats (*B. neotomae*) (Table 1). Presently, *B. melitensis, B. abortus* and *B. suis* are categorized as Category B biological warfare weapons by the Center for Disease Control (CDC).[1, 2]

Table 1: Host specificity of *Brucella* species

Species	Animal Host	Human Pathogenicity
B. suis	Swine	Highly infectiousness
B. melotensis	Sheep, goat	Highly infectiousness
B. abortus	Cattle, bison	Moderate infectious
B. canis	Dog	Moderate infectious
B. ovis	Sheep	None
B. neotomae	Rodent	None

Brucellosis has a number of names, based on the scientists who discovered the disease, location of the disease and characteristic clinical manifestations. For example, Brucellosis is also named Bang's Disease, Undulant Fever, Malta Fever, Mediterranean Remittent Fever, Rock Fever, County Fever of Constantinople and Fever of Crete, to name a few.[1, 2, 3]

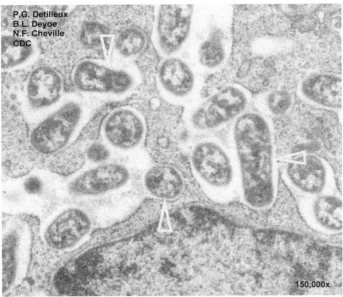

P.G. Detilleux
B.L. Deyoe
N.F. Cheville
CDC

150,000x

Figure 2.2-1: Transmission electron micrograph (TEM) of numerous *B. abortus* (arrows) coccobacilli located inside perinuclear envelope of a Vero cell

The United States began developing *B. suis* as a non-lethal (incapacitant) biological weapon in 1942 and it was field tested in 1944 and 1945 with animal targets. By the 1950s, large stockpiles of bombs (United States designation M33 munition) containing this pathogen, were a part of the United States military arsenal.[2, 4] The 1972 Convention on the Prohibition of the Development, Production and Stockpiling of Bacteriological (Biological) and Toxin Weapons and on their Destruction resulted in the elimination of the stockpile of the brucellosis biological weapons from the United States military inventory.[5]

The Soviets also experimented and produced large quantities of *Brucella* spp. as an offensive biological weapon. According to Alibek (1999), the Soviet designation of this biological weapon was L3 and the amount of Russian (former Soviet Union) stockpile of this weapon is unknown at this time.[6, 7] Nonetheless, the potential brucellosis attacks from other nations, as well as terrorist groups, remains a threat to the United States military and civilians. A 1997 model of a potential aerosol attack with *Brucella* spp. on an urban population estimated the economic impact of 477.7 million dollars per 100,000 people exposed.[8]

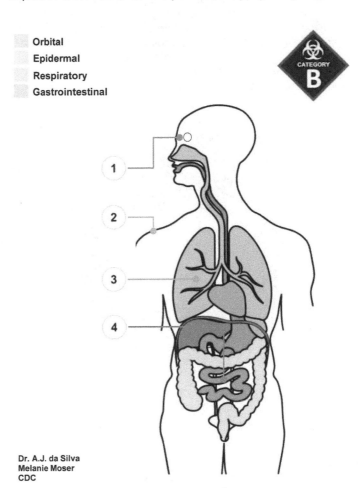

- Orbital
- Epidermal
- Respiratory
- Gastrointestinal

Dr. A.J. da Silva
Melanie Moser
CDC

Figure 2.2-2: *Brucella* **spp. infection diagram.** ① *Brucella* **spp. spores could be introduced via conjunctiva,** ② **introduced via abrasion or cuts on the epidermis.** ③ **could be introduced via the respiratory tract and/or** ④ **could be introduced via gastro-intestinal tract**

Brucella spp. are aerobic, non-motile, non-sporulating, non-toxigenic, non-fermenting, Gram negative coccobacillus, facultative intracellular parasites belonging to the α-Proteobacteria (α-2 group).[1, 2] Natural *Brucella* spp. infections in humans can be subdivided into two epidemiologically distinct profiles.

The first profile is seen in developed countries and is considered an occupational disease of meat (abattoir) workers, veterinarians and farmers (shepherds, cattleman etc.). This epidemiological form of brucellosis is generally caused by *B. abortus* and affects predominantly adult males. *B. abortus* has 7 recognized biovars (bv 1-6 and 9) with biovars 1-4 and 9 being the most commonly reported as the cause of brucellosis infections.[9] Generally, individuals contract the disease via abrasions or cuts of the skin, as well as, inoculation through the conjunctiva, respiratory and gastrointestinal tracts (Figure 2.2-2). Rarely, brucellosis may be transmitted through blood transfusions, tissue transplantation and sexual contact.[3] This first epidemiologically profile of brucellosis generally causes a mild form of disease, where no chronic form of the infection has been documented in recent years and mortality rate is less than 0.1%.[1, 10]

The second epidemiological profile involves endemic regions, such as the Mediterranean countries, Middle Eastern and Latin American countries. Brucellosis infections in these regions are generally caused by *B. melitensis*, which infects both adult males and females equally, as well as, causing ~20-25% of brucellosis infections in children. *B. melitensis* is the most virulent species of the *Brucella* genus has 3 recognized biovars (bv 1-3), with 1 and 3 being most commonly reported as the cause of brucellosis infections.[9] This infection is generally acquired via the gastrointestinal tract by the consumption of unpasteurized cheese and milk and may result in a more severe form of brucellosis; it frequently relapses into the chronic form of the disease and may result in higher mortality rate (>0.1%) (Figure 2.2-3).[1, 11, 12, 13]

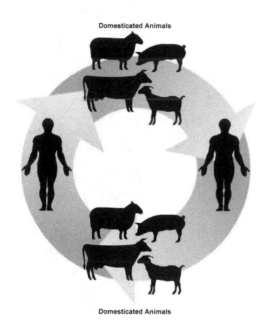

Figure 2.2-3: Sylvatic cycle of *Brucell* spp.

All species of *Brucella* are facultative intracellular parasites, which indicate that they can survive and multiply within the phagocytic cells of the host. *Brucella* infection begins after penetrating the skin and/or mucosal membrane (depending on the route of infection). For example, in the gastrointestinal tract, the organisms are engulfed by the lymphoepithelial cells of the gut-associated lymphoid tissue (GALT) and subsequently gain access to the submucosa.[1, 2, 14] Once gaining access to the host, *Brucella* spp. are rapidly phagocitized by macrophages, as well as, polymorphonuclear leukocytes and enter the lymphoid tissue draining the infection site. *Brucella* spp. utilizes these phagocytes as vehicles to proceed with bacterial fission and disseminate throughout the host especially in the lymph nodes (reticuloendothelial system), liver, spleen, mammary glands, joints, kidneys and bone marrow.[2, 3, 15, 16]

As in other Gram negative bacteria, lipopoly-saccharides (LPS) are an essential component of *Brucella* outer membrane. It is known that the LPS possess three domains: lipid A, core oligosaccharide and O polysaccharides (OPS or O-antigen). *B. melitensis*, *B. abortus* and *B. suis* exist in two variants: smooth

variant (S-LPS) which expresses O-antigen and the rough variant (R-LPS) which lacks the expression of the O-antigen. Smooth variant *Brucella* spp. inhibits the fusion of phagosomes and lysosomes within the phagocytes, depending on the level of their expression of O-antigen as a component of the LPS. The O-antigen is a homopolymer of perosamine (4, 6-dideoxy-4-formamido-D-mannopyranosyl) and is believed to prevent bactericidal activities, such as oxygen-dependent reactions and oxygen-independent reactions.[17, 18, 19, 20, 21, 22]

Once internalized, *Brucella* spp. is contained within a membrane bounded vesicle also known as *Brucella*-containing vacuoles (BCV). BCV transiently interact with early and late endosomes, and possibly lysosomes to acquire endosomal compartments markers such as early endosome antigen 1 (EEA1), guanosine triphos-phatase, Rab5, Rab7 and lysosomal-associated membrane protein 1 (LAMP-1). During these initial phases of maturation, the BCV becomes acidic thereby allowing *Brucella* spp. to express its VirB type IV secretion system (T4SS). The activation of the T4SS prompts the translocation of effector proteins to modulate membrane trafficking along the endocytic and secretory pathways.[23] In 2013, Myeni *et al.* identified 5 effector proteins: Bsp (*Brucella* secreted protein) A, BspB, BspC, BspE and BspF that are translocated through a VirB T4SS-dependent manner. Experimental result demonstrated that BspA, BspB and BspF inhibited protein secretion by the host cell, as well as, promoted its ability to replicate in macrophages and persist in the liver of infected mice. However, the exact functions of BspC and BspE require further elucidation.[24] Soon after, the BCV interacts with the subdomains (endoplasmic reticulum exit sites) of the endoplasmic reticulum (ER). At approximately 12 hours post infection, *Brucella* spp. begins to multiply within the ER-derived vesicles. At approximately 48 hours post infection, these replicative BCV are converted into LAMP-1 and Rab7 autophagic BCV which will complete the intracellular lifecycle of *Brucella* spp. and promote its cell-to-cell spreading.[22, 25]

SYMPTOMS

In aerosolized form, as few as 10-100 *Brucella* spp. bacteria, is sufficient to cause brucellosis. The incubation period for the disease is approximately 5 to 60 days while the onset of the disease may be abrupt or insidious.[1, 2, 26] Depending on the individual, the clinical presentation of brucellosis could exist in either acute (~50% of the cases), subacute or chronic form. Unfortunately, the conditions associated with the three forms of brucellosis still elicit some controversy. Due to brucellosis protean nature, a universally accepted symptomatic definition of the condition is still lacking.[1, 27] Nonetheless, it is noteworthy to indicate that *B. abortus* and *B. suis* are generally associated with the acute form of brucellosis while *B. melitensis* is generally associated with the chronic presentation.[1, 27] Please examine Table 2 for a list of symptoms and signs of 1240 patients suffering symptoms associated with *B. melitensis*.

In the acute form of the infection, patients generally complain of influenza-like and septicemic illness, as well as, non-specific symptoms such as fever (~100 °F/37.8 °C or higher), chills, profuse or patchy sweats, myalgia, malaise, fatigue, asthenia and anorexia (weight loss of 3-10 kg/6.6-22 lb within 1-2 weeks). Additional symptoms such as cough, pleuritic chest pain, dyspepsia, mild anemia and leukopenia are also frequently seen. Genitourinary involvement, such as urinary retention, orchitis, urinary tract infection, and glomerulonephritis has on rare occasions been reported. Joint pains, and back pains, peripheral arthritis and sacroileitis are also frequently seen; however, spondylitis is rarely observed (Table 3).[1, 2, 3, 28, 29]

Pityriasis alba has been reported to be a common sign among children suffering from acute brucellosis. Other cutaneous complications including rashes, erythema nodosum, nodules, papules, petechiae, purpura, cutaneous ulcers, abscesses and supportive lymphangitis are commonly seen in adults. On rare occasions and generally in association with thrombocytopenia, epitaxis, gingivorrhea, and hematuria are also observed. [1, 2, 3, 28, 29]

Table 2: Symptoms associated with *B. melitensis*[3, 29]

Symptoms	# of patients	% of cases
Fever	1040	83
Sweats	464	37
Fatigue	483	39
Joint pain	587	47
Headache	420	34
Weight loss	332	27
Abdominal pain	249	20
Orchiepididymitis	77	6
Lymphadenopathy	183	15
Splenomegaly	253	20
Hepatomegaly	172	14

Brucella endocarditis and resulting complications, such as acute myocardial infarction due to septic coronary embolisms, are extremely rare. Other unusual complications resulting from *Brucella* endocarditis, including dysrhythmias and pulmonary edemas, have also been reported. Cardiac and/or cardiac related complications are the main cause of fatalities in *Brucella* spp. infections.[30, 31, 32, 33]

Hepatic involvements, such as nonspecific hepatic inflammation, granulomatous hepatitis, and rarely cirrhosis of the liver may result (Figure 2.2-4).[26, 27] Splenomegaly and lymphadenopathy are also common occurances.[1, 2, 3, 29] Patients may also exhibit neuropsychiatric manifestations, such as dizziness, unsteady gait, depression, headaches and irritability. With proper treatment, acute brucellosis generally completes its course within two months, however, a few of the patients will relapse into subacute brucellosis.[1, 2, 3, 29]

Subacute infections generally persist between 2 to 12 months, with rare cases lasting more than a year. This form of brucellosis generally represents 25-30% of infections within endemic areas and generally indicates that the treatment for brucellosis is incomplete and/or inadequate.[1, 2, 29] Patients suffering from the subacute form of brucellosis is generally diagnosed after two months. These patients may experience undulating fever (~100 ºF/37.8 ºC or higher), as well as, some and/or all of the symptoms described for acute brucellosis. Nonetheless, there are minor dissimilarities between the two conditions. For example, arthritic involvements, peripheral arthritis, sacroileitis and spondylitis are frequently observed (Table 3). Additional symptoms of uveitis and orchi-epididymitis that rise and fall at 2 to 14 days intervals have also been reported.[1, 3]

There are two patterns of chronic brucellosis. The first is a cyclic course, similar to chronic fatigue syndrome, which is observed more frequently in women more than 40 years of age. The second

is the localized form of chronic brucellosis, which is seen equally in both sexes, but is rare in children.[1] Clinical manifestations of chronic brucellosis include intermittent fever (~100 ºF/37.8 ºC or higher), as well as, some and/or all of the symptoms described for acute brucellosis. Arthritis is the most common feature of chronic brucellosis. In young adults and children, peripheral arthritis is the most common form afflicting patients, while cases of sacroileitis and spondylitis are also frequently observed (Table 3).[1, 29, 34, 35, 36, 37, 38, 39]

Hepatic involvements are common symptoms of chronic brucellosis. The most commonly observed sign is hepatomegaly, although liver function tests are generally normal or only slightly elevated. In spite of hepatic involvements, post-necrotic cirrhosis is extremely rare. Spleno-megaly or lymphadenopathy may also be infrequently observed with chronic brucellosis (Table 4). Typical histopathological indication of recurrent brucellosis is active splenic granulomas with peripheral necrosis (Figure 2.2-5).[1, 2, 3, 29] Please examine the following section for a more in-depth discussion to the symptoms involved with brucellosis infection.

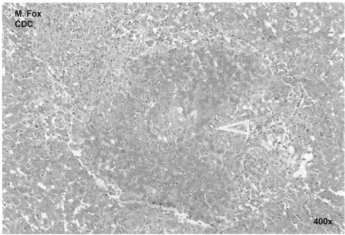

Figure 2.2-4: Histopathological photomicrograph of *Brucella suis* infection in guinea pig liver demonstrating granuloma with peripheral necrosis (arrow)

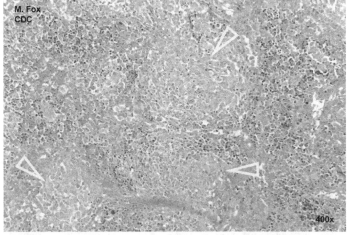

Figure 2.2-5: Histopathological photomicrograph of *Brucella suis* infection in guinea pig spleen, demonstrating 3 granulomas with peripheral necrosis (arrows)

Table 3: Types of arthritis involvements in brucellosis related to age[1]

Brucellosis	Peripheral Arthritis	Sacroileitis	Spondylitis	Age of Patients
Acute	Frequent	Frequent	Rare	Children, young adults
Subacute	Common	Frequent	Common	Children, young adults
Chronic	Rare	Rare	Frequent	Adults

Table 4: An overview of the clinical symptoms of all forms of (acute, subacute and chronic) brucellosis

Symptoms	+	++	+++
Fever and chills			▪
Undulating fever**			▪
Intermittent fever*			▪
Profuse sweats			▪
Patchy sweats			▪
Myalgia			▪
Malaise			▪
Fatigue			▪
Asthenia			▪
Anorexia			▪
Cough			▪
Pleuritic chest pain			▪
Dyspepsia			▪
Mild anemia			▪
Leukopenia			▪
Joint & back pains			▪
Peripheral arthritis***			▪
Sacroileitis***			▪
Dizziness			▪
Unsteady gait			▪
Depression			▪
Headaches			▪
Irritability			▪
Spondylitis*			▪
Hepatomegaly*			▪
Splenic granulomas*			▪
Peripheral arthritis		▪	
Sacroileitis		▪	
Pityriasis alba (children)		▪	
Rashes		▪	
Erythema nodosum		▪	
Nodules		▪	
Papules		▪	
Petechiae		▪	
Purpura		▪	
Cutaneous ulcers		▪	
Abscesses		▪	
Supportive lymphangitis		▪	
Hepatic inflammation		▪	
Granulomatous hepatitis		▪	
Splenomegaly		▪	
Lymphadenopathy		▪	
Uveitis**		▪	
Orchiepididymitis**		▪	
Urinary retention	▪		
Orchitis	▪		
Urinary tract infection	▪		
Glomerulonephritis	▪		
Spondylitis	▪		
Thrombocytopenia	▪		
Epitaxis	▪		
Gingivorrhea	▪		
Hematuria	▪		
Endocarditis	▪		
A. myocardial infarction	▪		
Septic coronary embolism	▪		
Dysrhythmias	▪		
Pulmonary edemas	▪		
Liver cirrhosis	▪		
Post-necrotic cirrhosis*	▪		
Splenomegaly*	▪		
Lymphadenopathy*	▪		

+ Rare ++ Common +++ Frequent

■ All forms   ** Subacute
* Chronic   *** Subacute & chronic

Arthritic Involvement

Peripheral arthritis may involve two forms. The first is referred to as reactive arthritis where *Brucella* spp. bacteria are not isolated from the joints. This condition is caused by high circulating immune complex levels. The second type of peripheral arthritis is known as infectious monarticular arthritis. This condition involves isolation of *Brucella* spp. bacteria from the synovial fluids of the joints.[1, 29, 34, 35, 36]

Most cases of peripheral arthritis found in young adults and children involve monarticular arthritis in the knee, hip, ankles and wrists while others may develop polyarthritis, as well as, other rheumatoid-like syndromes.[1, 29, 34, 35, 36] Other forms of arthritis, such as sacroiliitis are also observed, which is generally found in young adults of both sexes. Sacroiliitis involves inflammation of one or both sacroiliac joints. Patients suffering from this condition will experience extreme discomfort even with the slightest movements of the spine.[1, 37]

Spondylitis is generally observed in adults older than 40 years of age and is rarely observed in young adults and children suffering from the subacute form of brucellosis. This form of arthritis is caused by the inflammation of the joints between the vertebrae of the spine and often involves the sacroiliac joints. Other form of arthritis, such as osteomyelitis, bursitis and tenosynovitis has also been reported although the frequency of such syndromes is rare. [1, 34, 35, 38]

Hepatic Involvement

Hepatic involvement is also common in all forms of brucellosis, although liver function tests are generally normal or slightly elevated. Hepato-megaly is observed in 50 to 70% of all cases. Nonetheless, the cases of clinical hepatitis exist only in 3 to 6% of all cases. Mild jaundice with slightly elevated levels of bilirubin and hepatic enzymes are also occasionally observed in patients suffering from brucellosis. Depending upon the species of *Burcella* involved, histological changes may vary. For example, infections caused by *B. abortus*, may demonstrate epithelioid granulomas that are identical to sarcoidosis lesions. Brucellosis caused by *B. melitensis* may result in scattered small foci of inflammation that may resemble viral hepatitis and/or small loosely formed epithelioid granulomas with giant cells. Infections caused by *B. melitensis* result in larger aggregates of inflammatory cells that can be located within the parenchyma of the liver. These areas are generally associated with hepatic cell necrosis. In spite of hepatic involvements post-necrotic cirrhosis is extremely rare.[1, 3, 29, 40, 41, 42]

Hematologic Involvement

Anemia, leukopenia, neutropenia, lymphopenia and thrombocytopenia have been associated with brucellosis. In some reported cases, bleeding complications that were observed are associated with clotting abnormalities, such as low platelet and fibrinogen levels, as well as, extended thrombin clotting time. Severe thrombocytopenia may require steroid therapy and/or in cases lasting more than 2 months, sphenectomy may be required. If left untreated severe thrombo-cytopenia may result in fatal central nervous system hemorrhage. In rare cases, pancytopenia, cytophagocytosis, bone marrow hypoplasia, erythema nodosum has also been reported.[1, 2, 3, 43, 44, 45, 46]

Neurological Involvement

Neurobrucellosis is defined as neurological complications

connected with brucellosis infections. In general, these complications involve either acute or chronic Brucella meningitis (e.g. meningoencephalitis) or encephalitis which have been observed in 1-5% of adults, but is rarely seen in children.[1, 3, 29, 47, 48] Laboratory analysis of cerebral spinal fluid (CSF) in infected individuals rarely isolate Brucella spp. bacteria however, specific antibodies are commonly detected, as well as, elevated protein content, normal or low glucose concentration and elevated lymphocyte count. Computerized axial tomography (CAT scan) and/or magnetic resonance imaging (MRI) of individuals afflicted with meningitis generally are helpful to reveal the integrity of the epidural space as well as detecting central nervous system (CNS) lesions. Other CNS manifestations, such as cerebral vasculitis, mycotic aneurysms, brain and epidural abscesses, infarcts, hemorrhages and cerebral cerebellar ataxia are rarely observed. Peripheral nervous system complications associated with brucellosis include neuropathy, radiculopathy and Guillain-Barré syndrome, as well as, poliomyelitis-like syndrome have also been reported although they are extremely rare in occurrence .[1, 3, 29, 49, 50]

Ophthalmic Involvement

In rare cases, involving subacute and chronic brucellosis, a variety of ocular lesions have been observed. Many of the lesions are considered to be the result of the immunological response to brucellosis. Anterior or posterior uveitis is the most commonly observed manifestation of the eye and can present itself as iridocyclitis, nummular keratitis, multifocal choroiditis or optic neuritis. Other ophthalmic lesions include episcleritis and papilledema has also been observed. Panuveitis, a form of uveitis, often results in patients losing their vision. If left untreated, patients often develop secondary glaucoma, cataracts, retinal detachment, as well as, phthisis bulbi.[1, 3, 51, 52]

Cardiovascular Involvement

Endocarditis is the most commonly seen cardiovascular manifestation in patients suffering from brucellosis. This condition occurs in approximately 2% of all cases and it generally involves the aortic valve (50-70%) in most occasions, although involvement of the mitral valve has also been reported. Brucella endocarditis remains the most severe complication of brucellosis and accounts for 80% of the fatalities resulting from this infection. With proper treatment of Brucella spp. endocarditis, patients usually recover, however the infected valve will become calcified and need to be replaced. Other cardiovascular complications include aneurysms of the sinus of Valsalva, and mycotic aneurysms that generally involve the middle cerebral artery are also observed, although rarely.[1, 3, 29, 47, 48, 53, 54]

Congenital Involvement

It has been reported that brucellosis during pregnancy can lead to transplacental transmission of the bacteria leading to fetal infections and/or spontaneous abortions, although the course of the infection remains a topic of controversy.[2, 29, 55, 56] Congenitally infected infants are, at times, prematurely delivered with symptoms of fever, low birth weight, jaundice, hepatomegaly, splenomegaly, respiratory difficulties or distress. Infants suffering from brucellosis also demonstrate symptoms of hypotension, vomiting and signs of sepsis.[2, 55, 57]

DETECTION

Definitive diagnosis of Brucella spp. infection may be accomplished through culture and/or serology. Brucella spp. can be isolated from blood, bone marrow, CSF, urine, wounds, pus, or tissue cultures. Although the procedure that provides the highest yield is bone marrow culture, with a reported yield of 92%, by comparison to 72% yield with blood culture (e.g. conventional Castaneda blood cultures).[58] Unfortunately, Brucella spp. are slow growing and culture results may not be available for days, if not weeks. With patients suffering from chronic brucellosis the sensitivity of the culture can be low. Brucella spp. are identified using various standardized classification examinations such as Gram stain, modified Ziehl-Neelsen stain, growth characteristics, H_2S production, oxidase activity, and urase activity. Dye tolerance with basic fuchsin (1:50000 and 1:100000) and thionin (1:25000, 1:50000 and 1:100000) have also been utilized for identification.[29] Serum (tube) agglu-tination examination (SAT: a version of sero-agglutination) remains the standard methodology. This method reflects the presence of anti-O-antigen antibodies which is indicated by its ability to agglutinate killed Brucella spp. bacteria.[2, 59]

Enzyme-linked immunosorbent assay (ELISA) may also be used to detect the presence of anti-O-antigen antibodies. For example, the human immunoresponse towards brucellosis is characterized by the initial production of IgM isotype antibodies followed by the subsequent production of IgG isotype antibodies towards the infection. ELISA can be used to detect and measure the progression of the immunoglobulin isotopes development subsequent to the infection and treatment.[2]

Polymerase Chain Reaction (PCR) methodology utilizing ribosomal RNA (rRNA) have also been developed for clinical Brucella spp. detection. Primers for genus specific insertion sequences are in IS 711, IS650 or sections of the 16S-23S rRNA, BCPS31 and omp 2a genes. Presently, PCR identifications have not been used for direct identification of Brucella spp., nonetheless, they can provide valuable epidemiological information.[2]

TREATMENT

Effective treatment of brucellosis involves the immediate and continuous administration of antibiotics over a subscribed length of time. It is suggested that antibiotic treatment continue even if the patient demonstrates signs of spontaneous improvement. The antibiotics of choice are those that are highly active intracellularly. These antibiotics include macrolides, such as azithromycin, clarithromycin and erythromycin and have demonstrated effectiveness toward treating the infection. In addition, beta-lactam antibiotics, such as penicillin and cephalosporin, are also effective, however they are generally associated with high levels of relapse. Therefore, it is recommended that the combination of two antibiotics be used in conjunction to treat this infection.[1, 2]

Tetracycline administered at 500 mg every six hours orally for six weeks has long been the standard treatment for brucellosis. Unfortunately, this medication has a 10-20% chance of relapse with mono-therapy. In addition, the gastro-intestinal side effects of this medication may limit its use among certain patients. Doxycycline is a tetracycline analogue and is preferable, since it is only required to be given at a dose of 100 mg twice a day (orally every 12 hours for approximately six weeks) and has fewer side effects in comparison to tetracycline. However, like tetracycline, doxycycline also has a 10-20% chance of relapse.[1, 2] Please examine Table 5 for more information regarding the medication, dosage and potential side effects.

Due to the high rate of relapse with tetracycline and doxycycline, it is suggested that amino-glycosides should also be given as co-therapy for the first three weeks of treatment. For example, streptomycin administered at a dose of 1 gram per day intramuscularly has long been the treatment of choice to accompany tetracycline or doxycycline. In addition, aminoglycosides such as gentamicin have been used in place of streptomycin at a dose of 5 mg per kilogram of body weight per day intravenously or intramuscularly for 7-10 days and yielded good results with fewer side effects.[1, 2, 60, 61]

Other antibiotics such as rifampicin and trimethoprim/sulfamethoxazole (TMP/SMZ) have also been given as co-therapy in the treatment of brucellosis. For example, rifampicin

Table 5: Primary medication dosage, side effects of various treatment for brucellosis

Medication	Mechanism of Action	Side Effects	Recommended Dosage
Doxycycline	Inhibits protein synthesis	Fever, headaches, blurred vision, nausea, diarrhea, bloody stools, severe stomach cramps, indigestion, heartburn, vomiting, photosensitivity, loss of appetite, dysphagia, rash, joint pain, feeling tired	100 mg twice a day (orally every 12 hours for ~6 weeks)
Tetracycline	Inhibits protein synthesis	Fever, chills, headache, blurred vision, fever, hives, diarrhea, nausea, vomiting difficulty swallowing, difficulty breathing, hoarseness, indigestion, lingua villosa, inflammation of tongue, swellings (mouth, face, lips, or tongue), joint pain, loss of appetite, sores in the mouth, rash, sensitivity to sunlight, sore throat, stomach pain, swelling and itching of the rectum, rash, hives, itching, tightness in the chest, itching, vaginal irritation or discharge	500 mg every 6 hours orally for 6 weeks

Table 6: Co-therapy medication dosage, side effects of various treatment for brucellosis

Medication	Mechanism of Action	Side Effects	Recommended Dosage
Gentamicin	Inhibits protein synthesis	Shortness of breath, increased thirst, loss of appetite, closing of the throat, hives, swellings (lips, face, or tongue), rash, fainting, lack of urine, decreased hearing, ringing in the ears, dizziness, clumsiness, unsteadiness, numbness, skin tingling, muscle twitching, seizures, diarrhea, abdominal cramps, nausea, vomiting, rash	5 mg per kilogram of body weight per day intravenously or intra-muscularly for 7-10 days in conjunction with tetracycline and doxycycline
Rifampin	Inhibits protein synthesis	Upset stomach, heartburn, nausea, headache, drowsiness, dizziness, fever, chills, sore throat, nausea, stomach pain, dark urine, yellowing eyes or skin, rash, itching, swelling, dizziness, trouble breathing	600-900 mg/day orally
Streptomycin	Inhibits protein synthesis	Fever, swelling, rash, hives, difficulty breathing, tightness in the chest, swellings (mouth, face, lips, or tongue), decreased urination, dizziness, headache, hearing loss, hives, lightheadedness, loss of balance, muscle weakness, nausea, numbness, tingling, ringing or roaring in the ears, skin rash, vaginal irritation, vaginal discharge and vomiting	1 gram per day intramuscularly accompanying tetracycline or doxycycline
Trimethoprim / sulfamethoxazole	Inhibit successive steps in the folate synthesis pathway in bacteria	Appetite loss, nausea, vomiting, rash, hives, itching, difficulty breathing, shortness of breath, severe or persistent cough, swellings (mouth, face, lips, or tongue), skin irritation (blistering, peeling, red, or swollen skin), bloody stools, severe diarrhea, nausea, vomiting, chest pain, chills, fever, sore throat, decreased urination, depression, hallucinations, joint or muscle pain, seizures, headache, vaginal irritation or discharge	10-50 mg per kilogram of body weight per day for 3 weeks

Table 7: Therapeutic regiment for adults suffering from brucellosis

Regiment	Doxycycline	Tetracycline	Gentamicin	Rifampin	Streptomycin	TMP/SMZ	Duration
1	200 mg/d			600-900 mg/d			6 weeks
2	100 mg/12 h			600-900 mg/d			6 weeks
3	200 mg/d				1 g/d 14-21 d		6 weeks
4	100 mg/12 h		15 mg/kg/d		1 g/d 15 d		45 days
5		2 g/d			1 g/d 15-21 d		6 weeks
6		500 mg/6 h			1 g/d		6 weeks
7	100 mg/12 h				1 g/d		6 weeks
8	100 mg/12 h		5 mg/kg/d 9 d				6 weeks
9	100 mg/12 h					80 mg/400 mg	6 weeks

Table 8: Therapeutic regiment for children 8 years or younger suffering from brucellosis

Regiment	Doxycycline	Tetracycline	Gentamicin	Rifampin	Streptomycin	TMP/SMZ	Duration
1	4 mg/kg/d		5 mg/kg/d 5-7 d	10 mg/kg/d			6 weeks
2			2 mg/kg/8 h 14d			5 mg/kg/12 h	6 weeks
3			5 mg/kg/d 5 d			10-50 mg/kg/d	3 weeks
4				18 mg/kg/12 h		15 mg/kg/12 h	6 weeks
5						40 mg/kg/d	6 weeks

Table 9: Differential diagnosis of Brucellosis with other diseases of similar symptoms. These diseases are typhoid fever, malaria, Epstein-Barr virus infection (EBVI), toxo-plasmosis (Toxo), HIV infection, and tuberculosis (TB)

Symptoms	Brucellosis	Typhoid	Malaria	EBVI	Toxo	HIV	TB
Fever	■			■	■		
Undulating fever*	■	■	■				
Intermittent fever*	■						
Chills	■	■	■	■		■	■
Profuse sweats	■		■	■		■	■
Patchy sweats	■		■	■		■	■
Myalgia	■	■	■		■		
Malaise & fatigue	■	■	■	■	■		■
Asthenia	■	■	■	■	■		■
Anorexia	■	■		■			■
Cough	■	■				■	■
Pleuritic chest pain	■						■
Dyspepsia	■	■					
Mild anemia	■		■				
Leukopenia	■	■	■	■	■		■
Joint pains	■	■	■	■		■	■
Back pains	■	■	■	■		■	■
Peripheral arthritis***	■	■	■	■	■		■
Sacroileitis***	■	■		■			■
Dizziness & unsteady gait	■						
Depression	■	■					
Headaches	■	■	■	■	■	■	
Irritability	■						
Spondylitis*	■		■			■	■
Hepatomegaly*	■		■	■	■		
Splenic granulomas*	■						
Peripheral arthritis	■	■		■	■		■
Sacroileitis	■	■		■		■	■
Pityriasis alba (children)	■						
Rashes	■	■		■	■		
Erythema nodosum	■						■
Nodules	■					■	■
Papules	■	■				■	
Petechiae	■						
Purpura	■						
Cutaneous ulcers	■						
Abscesses	■						
Supportive lymphangitis	■						
Hepatic inflammation	■						
Granulomatous hepatitis	■						
Splenomegaly	■	■	■	■			
Lymphadenopathy	■	■		■	■	■	■
Uveitis**	■						
Orchiepididymitis**	■						
Urinary retention	■						
Orchitis	■						
Urinary tract infection	■						
Glomerulonephritis	■						
Spondylitis	■						
Thrombocytopenia	■				■		■
Epitaxis	■	■					
Gingivorrhea	■						
Hematuria	■						
Endocarditis	■						
A. myocardial infarction	■						
Septic coronary embolism	■						
Dysrhythmias	■						
Pulmonary edemas	■						
Liver cirrhosis	■						
Post-necrotic cirrhosis*	■						
Splenomegaly*	■	■	■	■	■	■	
Lymphadenopathy*	■	■		■	■		■

	All forms		**	Subacute
*	Chronic		***	Subacute & chronic

157

is a lipid soluable antibiotic and is highly active intracellularly. Rifampicin has been shown to be effective when it is administered at 600-900 mg/day orally in combination with doxycycline (200 mg/day orally) for 6 weeks. On the other hand, it has been shown that TMP/SMZ in a fixed ratio of 1:5 (80 mg TMP/400 mg SMZ) is highly effective against *Brucella* spp. as a co-therapy with either tetracycline or doxycycline. TMP/SMZ should be administered at 10-50 mg per kilogram of body weight per day for a 3 week period.[1, 2, 60, 61] Please see Table 6 for more information regarding the medication, dosage and potential side effects.

There are numerous antibiotic combinations for the co-treatment of brucellosis. As indicated previously, the drug combinations are instituted in an effort to prevent relapse of the disease. Please examine Tables 7 and 8 for possible therapies that have been shown to be effective against the disease for adults and children under the age of 8, respectively.

DIFFERENTIAL DIAGNOSIS

Brucellosis is at times difficult to differentially diagnose from other diseases with similar symptoms. The fever caused by brucellosis may be hard to distinguish from typhoid fever and malaria. Nonetheless, there are two distinguishing features of brucellosis fever. First, if left untreated, the fever in brucellosis shows an undulating pattern that persists for weeks before displaying an afebrile period and possible relapse. Secondly, the fever of brucellosis is commonly associated with musculoskeletal symptoms. In regards to symptomatic display of hepatosplenomegaly or lymphadenopathy caused by brucellosis, the differential diagnosis includes glandular fever–like illnesses such as Epstein-Barr virus infection (EBVI), toxo-plasmosis (Toxo), cytomegalovirus infection (CI), HIV infection, and tuberculosis (TB). In brucellosis patients displaying symptoms of osteomyelitis or septic arthritis, the differential diagnosis is TB.[1, 62] Please examine Table 9 for more information.

References

1. Guerrant R.L., Walker D.H., Weller P.F. Tropical Infectious Diseases – Principles, Pathogens & Practice. Volume 1. Philadelphia: Churchill Livingstone Elsevier. 2006. pp. 463-470
2. Purcell B.K., Hoover D.L. Friedlander A.M. Brucellosis. Medical Aspects of Biological Warfare. Chapter 9. Washington D.C.: The Surgeon General United States Army Medical Department Medical Center and School Borden Institute. 2007. pp. 185-198
3. Corbel M.J. Brucellosis in Human and Animals. Geneva: World Health Organization Press. 2006. pp. 2-12
4. Guillemin J. Biological Weapons. New York: Columbia University Press. 2005. pp.7
5. Convention on the Prohibition of the Development, Production, and Stockpiling of Bacteriological (Biological) and Toxin Weapons and their Destruction. Retrieved May 11, 2006, from United States Department of the State web site. March 26, 1975. Web site: http://www.state.gov/t/ac/trt/4718.htm
6. Alibek K. Biohazard. New York: Dell Publishing. 1999. pp. 20
7. Croddy E.A., Wirtz J.J., Larson J.A. Weapons of Mass Destruction. An Encyclopedia of Worldwide Policy, Technology, and History. Santa Barbra: ABC-CLIO Publishing. 2005. pp. 74-76
8. Kaufmann A.F., Meltzer M.I., Schmid G.P. The Economic Impact of a Bioterrorist Attack: Are Prevention and Postattack Intervention Programs Justifiable? Emerging Infectious Diseases, 1997. 3: pp. 83-94
9. Aparicio E.D. Epidemiology of brucellosis in domestic animals caused by Brucella melitensis, Brucella suis and Brucella abortus. Revue scientifique et technique / Office international des epizooties, 2013. 32: pp. 53-60
10. Spink W.W. Family Studies on Brucellosis. The American Journal of Medical Sciences, 1954. 227: pp. 128-133
11. Abo-Shehada M.N, Odeh J.S., Abu-Essud M. Abuharfeil N. Seroprevalence of Brucellosis among High Risk People in Northern Jordan. International Journal of Epidemiology, 1996. 25: pp. 450-454
12. Lunbani M.M., Dudin K.I., Sharda D.C., Ndhar D.S., Araj G.F., Hafez H.A., al-Saleh Q.A., Helin I., Salhi M.M. A Multicenter Therapeutic Study of 1100 Children with Brucellosis. The Pediatric Infectious Disease Journal, 1989. 8: pp. 75-78
13. Corbel M.J. Brucellosis: An Overview. Emerging Infectious Diseases, 1997. 3: pp. 213-221
14. Ackermann M.R., Cheville N.F., Deyoe B.L. Bovine Ileal Dome Lymphoepithelial Cells: Endocytosis and Transport of Brucella abortus Strain 19. Veterinary Pathology, 1988. 25: pp. 28-35
15. Foulongne V., Bourg G., Cazevieille C., Michaux-Charachon S., O'Callaghan D. Identification of Brucella suis Genes Affecting Intracellular Survival in an In Vitro Human Macrophage Infection Model by Signature-Tagged Transposon Mutagenesis Infection and Immunity, 2000. 68: pp. 1297-1303
16. Elsbach P. Degradation of Microorganisms by Phagocytic Cells. Reviews of Infectious Diseases, 1980. 2: pp. 106-128
17. Harmon B.G., Adams L.G., Frey M. Survival of Rough and Smooth Strains of Brucella abortus in Bovine Mammary Gland Macrophages. American Journal of Veterinary Research, 1988. 49: 1092-1097
18. Fernandez-Prada C.M., Nikolich M., Vemulapalli R., Sriranganathan N., Boyle S.M., Schurig G.G., Hadfield T.L., Hoover D.L. Deletion of wboA Enhances Activation of the Lectin Pathway of Compliment in Brucella abortus and Brucells melitensis. Infection and Immunity, 2001. 69: pp. 4407-4416
19. Del Vecchio V.G., Kapatral V., Redkar R., Patra G., Mujer C., Los T., Ivanova N., Anderson I., Bhattacharyya A., Lykidis A., Reznik G., Jablonski L., Larsen N., D'Souza M., Bernal A., Mazur M., Goltsman E., Selkov E., Elzer P.H., Hagius S., O'Callaghan D., Letesson J-J., Haselkorn R., Kyrpides N., Overbeek R. The Genome Sequence of the Facultative Intracellular Pathogen Brucella melitnesis. Proceedings of the National Academy of Sciences of the United States of America, 2002. 99: pp. 443-448
20. Riley L.K., Robertson D.C. Ingestion and Intracellular Survival of Brucella abortus in Human and Bovine Polymorphonuclear Leukocytes. Infection and Immunity, 1984. 46: pp. 224-230
21. Ugalde J.E., Czibener C., Feldman M.F., Ugalde R.A. Identification and Characterization of the Brucella abortus Phosphoglucomutase Gene: Role of Lipopolysaccharide in Virulence and Intracellular Multiplication. Infection and Immunity, 2000. 68: pp. 5716-5723
22. Hamer I., Goffin E., De Bolle X., Letesson J-J., Jadot M. Replication of Brucella abortus and Brucella melitensis in fibroblasts does not require Atg5-dependent macroautophagy. BioMed Central (BMC), 2014. 14: pp. 223
23. Starr T., Ng T.W., Wehrly T.D., Knodler L.A., Celli J. Brucella intracellular replication requires trafficking through the late endosomal/lysosomal compartment. Traffic, 2008. 9: pp. 678–694
24. Myeni S., Child R., Ng T.W., Kupko J.J. III, Wehrly T.D., Porcella S.F., Knodler L.A., Celli J. Brucella modulates secretory trafficking via multiple type IV secretion effector proteins. Public Library of Science (PLoS) Pathogens, 2013. 9: pp. e1003556
25. Starr T., Child R., Wehrly T.D., Hansen B., Hwang S., Lopez-Otin C., Virgin H.W., Celli J. Selective subversion of autophagy complexes facilitates completion of the Brucella intracellular cycle. Cell Host and Microbe, 2012, 11: pp. 33-45
26. Leach D., Ryman D.G. Biological Weapons: Preparing for the Worst. Medical Laboratory Observer Online. Revised September 2000. Retrieved September 24, 2009. Website: www.mlo-online.com/articles/sep00.pdf
27. Williams R.K., Crossley K. Acute and Chronic Hepatic Involvement of Brucellosis. Gastroenterology, 1982. 83: pp. 455-458
28. Mantur B.G., Akki A.S., Mangalgi S.S., Patil S.V., Gobbur R.H., Peerapur B.V. Childhood Brucellosis – a Microbiological, Epidemiological and Clinical Study. Journal of Tropical Pediatrics, 2004. 50: pp. 153-157
29. Mantur B.G., Amarnath S.K., Shinde R.S. Review of Clinical and Laboratory Features of Human Brucellosis. Indian Journal of Medical Microbiology, 2007. 25: pp. 188-202
30. 30. Gunes Y., Tuncer M., Guntekin U., Akdag S., Ali Gumrukcuoglu H., Karahocagil M., Ekim H. Clinical characteristics and outcome of Brucella endocarditis. Tropical Doctor, 2009. 39: pp. 85-88
31. Açar G., Ozkok A., Dönmez C., Avcı A., Alizade E., Yanartaş M. Myocardial infarction due to septic coronary artery embolism in the course of Brucella endocarditis. Herz, 2014. pp. 1-2
32. Park S.H., Choi Y.S., Choi Y.J., Cho S.H., Yoon H.J. Brucella Endocarditis with Splenic Abscess: A Report of the First Case Diagnosed in Korea. Yonsei Medical Journal, 2009. 50: pp. 142-146
33. Jubber A.S., Gunawardana D.R., Lulu A.R. Acute pulmonary edema in Brucella myocarditis and interstitial pneumonitis. Chest, 1990. 97: pp. 1008-1009
34. Gotuzzo E., Carrillo C. Infection in the Rheumatic Disease. Orlando: Grune & Stratton Incorporated. 1988. pp. 31-41
35. Gotuzzo E., Alarcón G., Bocanegra T., Carrillo C., Guerra J., Rolando I., Espinoza L. Articular Inolvement in Human Brucellosis: A Retrospective Analysis of 304 Cases. Seminars in Arthritis and Rheumatism, 1982. 12: pp. 245-55
36. Bocanegra T., Gotuzzo E., Alarcón G., Vasey F.B., Germain B.F., Espinoza L.R. Circulating Immune Complexes in Acute Typhoid Fever and Brucellosis. Clinical Research, 1981. 29: pp. 381A
37. Memish Z.A., Balkhy H.H. Brucellosis and International Travel. Journal of Travel Medicine, 2004. 11: pp. 49-55
38. Ariza J., Gudiol F., Valverde J., Pallarés R., Fernández-Viladrich P., Rufí G., Espadaler L., Fernández-Nogues F. Brucellar Spondylitis: a Detailed Analysis Based on Current Findings. Reviews of Infectious Diseases, 1985. 7: pp. 656-664
39. The Center for Food Security & Public Health. Iowa State University. Brucellosis. Revised July 19, 2009. Retrieved September 26, 2009. Website: www.cfsph.iastate. edu/Factsheets/pdfs/brucellosis.pdf
40. Sunmez S., Cagatay A., Karadeniz A., Ozsut H., Eraksoy H., Calangu S. A case of acute hepatitis due to brucellosis. Southern Medical Journal. June 1, 2006. Retrieved September 28, 2009. Website: http://www.thefreelibrary.com/A+case+of+acute+hepatitis+due+to+brucellosis-a0148139431
41. Williams R.K., Vrossley K. Acute and Chronic Hepatic Involvement of Brucellosis. Gastroenterology, 1982. 83: pp. 455-458
42. Türkdoğan M.K., Akdeniz H., Berktas M., Irmak H., Tuncer I, Algün E., Buzgan T., Seckinli M.T. Evaluation of Hepatic Involvement in Brucellosis. Eastern Journal of Medicine, 1996. 1: pp. 8-9
43. Crosby E., Llosa L., Miro Quesada M., Carrillo C., Gotuzzo E. Hematologic Changes in Brucellosis. The Journal of Infectious Disease, 1984. 150: pp. 419-424
44. Stoll D.B., Blum S., Pasquale D., Murphy S. Thrombocytopenia with Decreased Megakaryocytes. Evaluation and Prognosis. Annals of Internal Medicine, 1981. 94: pp. 170-175
45. Gurkan E., Baslamisli F., Guvenc B., Bozkurt B., Unsal C., Immune Thrombocytopenic Purpura Associated with Brucella and Toxoplasma Infections. American Journaql of Hematology, 2003. 74: pp. 52-54
46. Mazokopakis E., Christias E., Kofyeridis D., Acute Brucellosis Presenting with Erythema Nodosum. European Journal of Epidemiology, 2003. 18: pp. 913-915
47. Young E.J. Human Brucellosis. Review of Infectious Diseases, 1983. 5: pp. 821-842
48. al Deeb S.M., Yaqub B.S., Sharif H.S., Phadke J. Neurobrucellosis: Clinical Characteristics, Diagnosis and Outcome. Neurology, 35: pp. 1576-1581
49. Oliveri R.I., Matera G., FocàA., Zappia M., Aguglia U., Quattrone A. Polyradiculoneuropathy with Cerebrospinal Fluid Albuminocytological Dissociation due to Neurobrucellosis. Clinical Infectious Diseases, 1996. 23: pp. 833-834
50. Mousa A.R., Koshy T.S., Araj G.F. Marafie A.A., Muhtaseb S.A., Al-Mudallal D.S., Busharetulla M.S. Brucella Meningitis: Presentation, Diagnosis and Treatment: A Prospective Studies of Ten Cases. Quarterly Journal of Medicine, 1986. 60: pp. 873-875
51. Rolando I., Carbone A., Gotuzzo E. Carrillo C. Circulating Immune Complexes in the Pathogenesis of Human Brucellar Uveitis. Chibret International Journal of Ophthalmology, 1985. 3: pp. 30-38
52. Rolando I, Carbone A, Haro D, Gotuzzo E, Carrillo C. Retinal Detachment in Chronic Brucellosis. American Journal of Ophthalmology, 1985. 99: pp. 733-734
53. Peery T.M., Belter L.F., Brucellosis and Heart Disease. II. Fatal Brucellosis: a Review of

the Literature and Report of New Cases. The American Journal of Pathology, 1960. 36: pp. 673-697

54.   Reguera J.M., Alarcon A., Miralles F., Pachon J., Juarez C., Colmenero J.D. Brucella Endocarditis: Clinical, Diagnostic and Therapeutic Approach. European Journal of Clinical Microbiology and Infectious Diseases, 2003. 22: 647-650

55.   Lubani M.M., Dudin K.I., Sharda D.C., AbuSinna N.M., Al-Shab. T., Al-Refeai A.A., Labani S.M., Nasrallah A. Neonatal Brucellosis, 1988. 147: pp. 520-522

56.   Khan M.Y., Mah M.W., Memish Z.A. Brucellosis in Pregnate Women. Clinical infectious Diseases, 2001. 32: pp. 1172-1177

57.   Imani R., Shamsipoor E., Khadivi R. Congenital Brucellosis in an Infant. Iranian Journal of Clinical Infectious Diseases, 2007. 2: pp. 29-31

58.   Diaz R. Moriyon I. Laboratory Techniques in the Diagnosis of Human Brucellosis. Brucellosis: Vlinical and Laboratory Aspects. Boca Raton: Chemical and Rubber Company (CRC) Press. 1989. pp. 73-84

59.   Young E.J. Serologic Diagnosis of Human Brucellosis: Analysis of 214 Cases by Agglutination Tests and Review of the Literature. Reviews of Infectious Diseases, 1991. 13: pp. 359-372

60.   Isenberg D.A., Maddison P.J., Woo P., Glass D., Breedveld F.C. Oxford Textbook of Rheumatology. Third Edition. New York: Oxford University Press. 2004. pp. 649-650

61.   Kwan-Gett T.S.C., Kemp C., Kovarik C. Infectious and Tropical Diseases. St. Louis: Elsevier Mosby. 2006. pp. 114-119

62.   J.H. McIsaac. Hospital Preparation for Bioterror. A Medical and Biomedical System Approach. Burlington: Academic Press. 2006. pp. 55

Photo Bibliography

Figure 2.2-1: Transmission Electron micrograph of *B. abortus* located inside perinuclear envelope of Vero cell. The electron micrograph was taken by P.G. Detilleux, B.L. Deyoe and N.F. Cheville in Penetration and intracellular growth of Brucella abortus in nonphagocytic cells *in vitro*. Infection and Immunity, 1990. 58:pp. 2320-2328. The photo was released by National Animal Disease Center, U.S. Department of Agriculture. Public domain photo

Figure 2.2-2: *Brucella spp.* infection diagram. The human anatomical illustration is created by Dr. Alexander J. da Silva and Melanie Moser in 2003. The illustration is released by the CDC. Public domain graphics

Figure 2.2-4: Histological photomicrograph of *Brucella suis* infection in guinea pig liver demonstrating granuloma with peripheral necrosis. Photomicrograph was taken by Dr. Marshall Fox in 1976 and released by the CDC. Public domain photo

Figure 2.2-5: Histopathological photomicrograph of *Brucella suis* infection in guinea pig spleen demonstrating 3 granulomas with peripheral necrosis. Photomicrograph was taken by Dr. Marshall Fox in 1976 and released by the CDC. Public domain photo

Formally known as *Pseudomonas mallei*, *Burkholderia mallei* is the causative agent of a subcutaneous infection known as Farcy, or it can disseminate within the host to generate a serious zoonotic disease, known as Glanders. *B. mallei* is an obligate mammalian pathogen that primarily infects solipeds, such as horses, mules, donkeys, as well as, goats, camels, dogs and cats. Naturally occurring *B. mallei* infections of individuals are rare, since humans serve only as accidental hosts. Nonetheless, these infections could result in an extremely painful ailment, and at times, become life-threatening. To this date no human epidemics caused by *B. mallei* have been reported.[1, 2]

During World War I (WWI), Germany initiated the first state sponsored offensive biological warfare program with solid scientific foundation. Glanders was one of the biological weapons researched and used during the twentieth century.[3] During the war, Germany launched an ambitious biological sabotage campaign in the United States (U.S.), Mesopotamia, Norway, Russia and France. For example, in 1914, German agents inoculated horses, mules and other livestock targeted for shipment from the U.S. to the Allies in Europe. In 1916, the Germans infected many mules and horses on the Russian eastern front. Germany was successful in impairing Russian artillery movements and supply convoys through the dissemination of this pathogen. In 1917, the Germans successfully infected approximately 4500 mules used by the British forces in Mesopotamia and attempted to infect reindeer in Norway. During that same year, German agents successfully infected horses and other livestock being shipped from Argentina to India by the British forces.[3, 4, 5]

The research and development of *B. mallei* as a biological weapon did not end with the surrender of Germany on November 11, 1918, marking the end of WWI. Between the years of 1932 to 1945, Imperial Japanese forces also developed Glanders as a biological weapon at Unit 731. Under the leadership of General Shiro Ishii, the Japanese tested this biological weapon on horses, prisoners of war and civilians. During the Soviet invasion of Afganistan (1982 to 1984), alligations that Russian forces used Glanders against the Mujahedeen were publically made by the US, although these claims were never substantiated.[3, 6, 7]

The US examined Glanders as a potential biological weapon and also performed defensive research. Although *B. mallei* was never weaponized by the US, defensive research continued. For example, from 1944 to 2000, there were eight documented cases of laboratory acquired Glanders. Seven out of the eight infections were the result of mouth pipetting, while the eighth infection involved a microbiologist working with *B. mallei* without proper protective gear. All eight infections occurred at Fort Detrick, Maryland.[4, 6, 8, 9]

Presently, the United States believes that attempts are being made by nations and/or nation sponsored terrorist groups to develop an aerosolized antibiotic resistant form of *B. mallei* that could be as potent of a biological weapon as anthrax. Due to its potential use as a biological weapon, *B. mallei* has been listed as a Category B biological agent by the Center for Disease Control and Prevention.[10, 11]

B. mallei, is a Gram negative, strictly aerobic, non-motile, obligated intracellular bacillus, closely related to *B. pseudomallei*, the caustic agent of meliodosis (Figure 2.3-1). *B. mallei* is both catalase- and oxidase-positive. When stained with methylene

blue or Wright's stain, this bacillus demonstrates a safety pin appearance.[2, 9] *B. mallei* is not particular hardy in the environment and is quickly killed by drying, heat and sunlight. Nonetheless, in warm and moist environments, the organism can survive a few months. *B. mallei* is easily aerosolized and highly infectious. It has been reported that inhaling just a few *B. mallei* bacteria may cause infection in equines, humans and other susceptible species. Due to its infectiousness, laboratory experimentations on this organism requires, at minimum, a biosafety level 3 (BSL-3) environment.[2, 6, 12, 13]

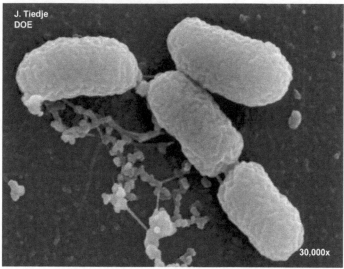

Figure 2.3-1: Scanning electronmicrograph (SEM) of *Burkholderia* spp.

Although Glanders has been eradicated from most countries, this disease is believed to be endemic in parts of Africa, the Middle East, Asia, Central and South America. It is known that equines are a reservoir and possibly an amplifying host for *B. mallei*. Glanders is transmitted by a direct bacterial invasion of the lungs through aerosolized *B. mallei*, ingestion of contaminated water, dust or through lacerated skin. *B. mallei* may also enter the human body through oral, nasal and conjunctival mucous membranes. Although a rare occurance, human to human transmission has been reported. These reported cases involve family members who were nursing the infected individuals, or through sexual transmission (Figure 2.3-2 and 2.3-3).[2, 6, 13]

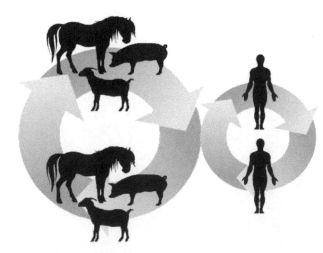

Figure 2.3-2: Sylvatic cycle of *B. mallei*

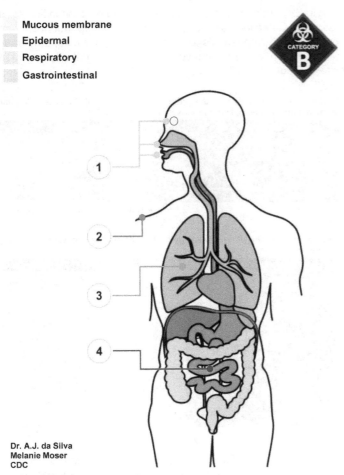

Mucous membrane
Epidermal
Respiratory
Gastrointestinal

Dr. A.J. da Silva
Melanie Moser
CDC

Figure 2.3-3: *B. mallei* infection diagram. ① Introduction of *B. mallei* spores via oral, nasal or conjunctival mucous membrane. ② Introduction of *B. mallei* spores via abrasion or cuts on the epidermis. ③ Introduction of *B. mallei* spores via respiratory tract. ④ Introduction of *B. mallei* spores via gastrointestinal tract

The *B. mallei* genome consist of 5.7Mb of DNA distributed across two chromosomes: chromosome 1 (3.5 Mb) and 2 (2.3 Mb). Whitelock *et al.* (2007) have found that most of the genes associated with virulence are on chromosome 2, while genes associated with capsule production, lipopolysaccharide bio-synthesis and metabolism are found on chromosome 1. Genomic comparisons between *B. mallei* and *B. pseudomallei* demonstrated significant homology (~99% identical between conserved genes), although the *B. mallei* genome is considerably smaller than that of *B. pseudomallei*.[14] It has been calculated that the approximately 1400 genes that are present in *B. pseudomallei* are either missing or are variant in *B. mallei* (~1.41 Mb less DNA). For example, the *B. mallei* genes that code for the flagella and chemotaxis mechanism have undergone frame shift or insertion mutations, resulting in defective proteins. It is postulated that portions of *B. mallei*'s genome have undergone active decay, possibly to further their adaptation to a lifestyle suitable within their selected mammalian hosts. Nonetheless, comparative analysis of the two bacteria have shown similar or identical genes encoding an exopolysaccharide capsule, a lipopoly-saccharide, type IV pili, type III and type VI secretion system.[14, 15, 16]

Molecular characterization of *B. mallei* has demonstrated that *wcbF* is an essential gene, responsible for the production of the exopoly-saccharide capsule. Challenges with the wild-type and mutant-type (capsule negative) *B. mallei* have shown a greater than 10^5- to 10^3-fold difference in lethal dose (LD_{50}). This work was accomplished by using animal models (Syrian Hamsters and BALB/c mice) infected by intraperitoneal and aerosol routes.

These experiments showed that this capsule protein is a key factor in virulence. In addition, the exopolysaccharide capsule has been shown to possess the ability to protect the bacterium from phagocytosis in experimentally infected guinea pigs.[6, 17, 18, 19]

The lipopolysaccharide (LPS) of *B. mallei* is composed of Lipid A, a core region and a cell wall antigen (O antigen). It is known that the Lipid A component of the LPS normally functions as a hydrophobic membrane-anchor component, responsible for stimulating a variety of pathophysiological responses in mammals.[20, 21] It has also been reported that the O antigen is effective in resisting the bactericidal effects of normal human serum (NHS), indicating that this bacterial surface structure is a key contributor to virulence.[22, 23]

Research has shown that certain strains of *B. mallei* are capable of producing an endotoxin that affects the smooth muscle cells of various internal organs. The reaction of various tissues to this endotoxin includes lymphangitis and mucous membrane erosions, as well as, the slow healing nature of some infections, a clinical symptom that corroborates this localized effect.[6]

Although Glanders is one of the oldest known infectious diseases, the molecular mechanisms by which this bacillus causes disease remains poorly defined and not well understood.[24] It is proposed that the virulence of *B. mallei* is multifactorial and there are several virulence determinants that have been identified and characterized using animals models. For example, type III secretion system (TTSS) is ancestrally related to flagella and is an essential part of the Gram-negative bacteria's protein secretion systems. BopE, a protein encoded within the *B. mallei* TTSS loci, is responsible for the necessary cytoskeleton rearrangements for epithelial and phagocytic cellular invasion.[19, 25, 26] In addition, a complex quorum-sensing network and a two-component transcriptional regulatory system (VirAG) have been shown as essential for maximal virulence in hamsters, although the genes controlled by these regulators remain to be elucidated.[14, 27] Furthermore, investigations have also focused on intracellular survival and the spread of the bacillus from the phagosomes into the cytosol, where it can use actin-based motility for intra- and intercellular spread. Research has shown that *B. mallei* use elements of the cytoskeleton to propel the bacterium through the host cytosol. These motility proteins, also known as autotransporters (BimA), are a class of bacterial proteins that mediate their own secretion and/or membrane localization.[15, 16, 26, 28, 29]

SYMPTOMS

The symptoms of *B. mallei* infection are related to the manner of their entry into the human body. For example, there are five known forms of disease: acute localized (cutaneous and mucosal), chronic localized cutaneous, acute pulmonary, chronic pulmonary and septicemia. Nonetheless, in Glanders infection of humans, one form of the disease may progress to another or a combination of the forms may occur.[1, 13]

The incubation periods are variable depending on the form of the disease and the manner that *B. mallei* enters the host. For example, the incubation period for chronic localized infections could last up to 12 weeks. On the other hand, the incubation period for acute localized infections is typically 1 to 5 days (3 to 5 days on average). Reports have indicated that left untreated, the acute localized infections could progess into septicemia within two weeks.[2, 6, 13, 30]

Similar duration as the chronic localized infections, the incubation period for for chronic pulmonary infections could also last up to

12 weeks. In contrast, an acute pulmonary infection may require anywhere from 10 to 14 days (7 to 21 days in some reports) subsequent to the introduction of the microbes. Septicemia resulting from acute pulmonary exposure may develop almost immediately after inoculation or progress within two weeks subsequent to initial contact. Nonetheless, pneumonic disease generally has a rapid onset and is almost always lethal within 10-30 days if left untreated.[2, 6, 13, 30]

Localized infections are regionally confined and generally involve the area of the body where the bacilli first entered. For example, B. mallei may enter through the oral, nasal, and ocular mucous membranes. Additionally, B. mallei may also enter through abrasions of the skin, which generally are found on the hands, forearms, face and neck.

Localized cutaneous infections are typically characterized by an inflammatory response, which includes pain and swellings at the site of the inoculation. Soon after, a 'Glanders node(s)' or blister(s) will appear at the site before gradually evolving into pus-forming nodule(s), also known as ulcerative abscess(es), that can drain for a prolonged period of time. These nodules that are formed are firm with a caseous or calcified center and may appear white or gray. At this time, the inflammation that accompanied the infection will spread into the regional lympghatics and cause lymphangitis with numerous foci of suppuration. The endotoxin produced and secreted by B. mallei will target the smooth musculature of the lymphatics, which will enhance the inflammation. Commonly, localized cutaneous infections are accompanied by a fever or a low-grade fever, chills, severe headaches, diaphoresis, malaise, generalized myalgias (particularly in the limbs, joins, neck and back), dizziness, nausea, vomiting, diarrhea, tachypnea, sore throat, chest pains, splenomegaly, abdominal pains, fatigue and altered mental states (Table 1). [2, 6, 13, 16, 30, 31, 32]

Table 1: An overview of the clinical symptoms of cutaneous Glanders

Symptoms	+	++	+++
Blister			■
Pus-forming nodules			■
Fever or low grade fever		■	
Chills		■	
Severe headaches		■	
Diaphoresis		■	
Malaise		■	
Generalized myalgias		■	
Dizziness		■	
Nausea		■	
Vomiting		■	
Diarrhea		■	
Tachypnea		■	
Sore throat		■	
Chest pains		■	
Splenomegaly		■	
Abdominal pains		■	
Fatigue		■	
Altered mental states		■	

+ Rare ++ Common +++ Frequent

With ocular involvement, excessive lacrimation, mucopurulent conjunctival discharge, blurred vision, photophobia and preauricular lymph-adenopathy are common signs. In cases involving the upper respiratory tract, the nose may become greatly inflamed and swollen, while copious amounts of mucopurulent or at times blood-tinged nasal discharge may be observed. Additionally, B. mallei may invade the nasal septum and boney tissues, causing tissue destruction and fistulae between the nasal passages. At times, the infection may spread to the lower respiratory tract and cause tracheitis and/or bronchitis. As a result, this infection can trigger cough and mucopurulent sputum production. Lymphangitis or regional lymph-adenopathy may also develop in the lymphatic pathways that drain the infected site(s) (Table 2 and Table 3). [2, 6, 13, 16, 30, 31, 32]

Table 2: An overview of the clinical symptoms of localized (ocular involvement) Glanders. Note: mucosal conjunctival (MC)

Symptoms	+	++	+++
Excessive lacrimation		■	
MC discharge		■	
Blurred vision		■	
Photophobia		■	
Lymphadenopathy		■	

+ Rare ++ Common +++ Frequent

Table 3: An overview of the clinical symptoms of localized (nasal/respiratory) Glanders

Symptoms	+	++	+++
Inflamed nose			■
Swollen nose			
Nasal discharges			■
Fistulae			■
Nasal septum damage			
Tracheitis		■	
Bronchitis		■	
Coughing		■	
Sputum production		■	
Lymphangitis		■	
Lymphadenopathy		■	

+ Rare ++ Common +++ Frequent

Mucosal and skin infections may disseminate after 1 to 4 weeks. The symptoms of disseminated infections include a papular or pustular rash that may erupt anywhere on the patient's body; while abscesses may also appear in the liver, spleen, lungs, subcutaneous tissues, as well as, muscles. Disseminated infections may also progress into pulmonary infections, chronic infections or even septicemia. It has been estimated that the mortality rate for the cutaneous and mucosal form of Glanders is as high as ~90 to 95% if left untreated. However, even with proper treatment, the mortality rate is as high as ~50%.[2, 6, 13, 16, 30, 31, 32]

The chronic form of the infection can last up to 25 years, and is generally characterized by multiple abscesses, nodules and ulcers that can be seen in various tissues. Cutaneous eruptions may appear on the body, where the extremities are often affected. This form of disease is generally milder than acute forms, with periodic reoccurrences. Various organs may be affected with the chronic form of Glanders, including the skin, subcutaneous tissues, liver, spleen, gastrointestinal tract, respiratory tract, skeletal structures, meninges, brain and skeletal muscles. Patients generally experience weight loss, lymphangitis and lymphadenopathy. The mortality rate for the chonic form of Glanders has been estimated to be ~50% despite aggressive treatment.[2, 6, 13, 30, 33]

Pulmonary Glanders may be the result of inhalation of B. mallei or through the hemato-genous spread (dissemination) from other forms of Glanders infection. The onset of this form of infection is generally acute and characterized by pulmonary abscesses, pleuritis, pleural effusion and extensive pneumonia. The symptoms are high fever (>38.9° C or >102° F), chills, fatigue, severe headaches, myalgias, rigors, diaphoresis (night sweats), coughing, dyspnea, hemoptysis, tachypnea, tachycardia, nausea, weight loss, dizziness, mucosal eruptions, mucopurulent sputum, gastrointestinal signs and pleuritic chest pains. Patients suffering from the pneumonic form will produce pustular skin lesions which may resemble smallpox eruptions. If the upper respiratory tract is involved, nasal exudates and cervical or mediastinal lymphadenopathy are often observed. Ulcers and nodules are often observed in the nose, while abscesses in the skin may also appear. If left untreated, the mortality rate for the pulmonary form of Glanders is ~90 to 95%. However, even with proper treatment, the mortality rate has been estimated to be ~40% (Table 4).[2, 6, 13, 15, 30, 31, 33]

Table 4: An overview of the clinical symptoms of pulmonary Glanders

Symptoms	+	++	+++
High fever			■
Chills			■
Fatigue			■
Severe headaches			■
Myalgias			■
Rigors			■
Diaphoresis			■
Coughing			■
Dyspnoea			■
Hemoptysis			■
Tachypnea			■
Tachycardia			■
Nausea			■
Weight loss			■
Dizziness			■
Mucosal eruptions			■
Mucopurulent sputum			■
Gastrointestinal signs			■
Pleuritic chest pain			■
Pulmonary abscesses			■
Pleuritis			■
Pleural effusion			■
Extensive pneumonia			■
Pustular skin lesions		■	
Nasal exudates		■	
Cervical lymphadenopathy		■	
Mediastinal lymphadenopathy		■	
Ulcers of the nose		■	
Nodules of the nose		■	
Abscesses in the skin		■	

+ Rare ++ Common +++ Frequent

Table 5: An overview of the clinical symptoms of septicemic Glanders

Symptoms	+	++	+++
Fever			■
Chills			■
Headaches			■
Myalgias			■
Acute pleuritic chest pains		■	
Lymphadenopathy		■	
Cellulitis		■	
Cyanosis		■	
Jaundice		■	
Photophobia		■	
Diarrhea		■	
Pustular rash		■	
Papular rash		■	
Granulomatous lesions		■	
Necrotizing lesions		■	
Tachycardia		■	
Generalized erythroderma		■	
Thrombosis & embolisms		■	
Mild hepatomegaly		■	
Mild spenomegaly		■	

+ Rare ++ Common +++ Frequent

The septicemic form of the disease is the result of *B. mallei* invading the bloodstream and may result from any form of Glanders infection. The symptoms for the septicemic form of of Glanders are fever, chills, myalgia, headaches and pleuritic chest pains which generally develop acutely. Other symptoms include lymphadenopathy, cellulitis, cyanosis, jaundice, photophobia, diarrhea, pustular or papular rash may also be observed. In addition, granulomatous or necrotizing lesions are also commonly seen. Furthermore, patients suffering from the septicemic form of the disease may also develop tachycardia, generalized erythroderma, jaundice, mild hepatomegaly or spenomegaly. It has been reported that *B. mallei* causes damage and subsequently the death of the endothelial cells of blood vessels. As the dead or dying cells detach, the endothelial lining is predisposed to thrombosis, resulting in embolisms. If left untreated, multi-organ failure is common and death generally occurs within 24 to 48 hours after the onset of the symptoms. It has been reported that without treatment, the mortality rate for the septicemic form of Glanders is greater than ~95%. Even with proper antibacterial treatment the mortality rate is still nearly 50%. (Table 5). [2, 6, 13, 16, 33]

DETECTION

Definitive diagnosis of Glanders is accomplished through the isolation and positive identification of *B. mallei* bacilli. *B. mallei* can be isolated from lesions, sputum, blood or urine, and is easily cultivated on basic nutrient media, including blood agar, Loeffler's serum agar, glycerin-potato agar, chocolate agar or meat nutrient agar between the temperature ranges of 37° to 43° C (98.6°-109.4° F). It is necessary to note that these bacteria are slow growing. Nonetheless, their growth can be accelerated by using 1 to 5% glucose and glycerol in addition to the broth or agar which will bring the incubation to 48 hours. [2, 6, 13]

B. mallei colonies are typically 1 mm in width, white (which turns yellow with age) or semi-translucent and viscid when grown on blood agar or Loeffler's serum agar. After 72 hours of culture, these colonies have a clear honey-like layer. This clear honey-like layer will darken to brownish or reddish-brown in color when grown on glycerin-potato agar. Subsequently, *B. mallei* may be stained with methylene blue, Wright's stain, Gram stain or Giemsa. Organisms isolated from clinical samples will appear as rods, however, bacteria from older cultures may appear pleomorphic (Figure 2.3-4). [2, 6, 13]

Dr. T. Parker
A. Marsh
CDC

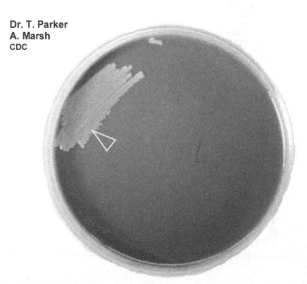

Figure 2.3-4: *B. mallei* grown on chocolate agar for 48 hours at a temperature of 37°C (arrow)

Distinguishing *B. mallei* and *B. pseudomallei* has always been problematic, since these two species are very closely related, with very similar phenotypic and genotypic characteristics. Automated bacterial identification systems do not always correctly identify *B. mallei*, therefore, various more specific assays have been developed.[13] For example, a polymerase chain reaction (PCR) procedure for the discrimination of *B. mallei* and *B. pseudomallei*. This procedure is based on the nucleotide difference at T 2143 C (T versus C at position 2143) between *B. mallei* and *B. pseudomallei*, found within the 23S rDNA sequences.[34] Other genetic techniques have also been developed. For example, PCR-restriction fragment length polymorphism (PCR-RFLP) has been used and compared the distinctive *Sau3A*I-digested genomic DNA fragments of *B. mallei* and *B. pseudomallei*.[35] Additionally, genomic comparisons made by using pulsed-field gel electrophoresis (PFGE) can show the differences between the species.[36] Sequencing the 1.5 kb 16S rRNA gene of *B. pseudomallei* and *B. mallei* isolates[37] or by screening 23 loci from an established 32-marker multiple locus variable number tandem repeat (VNTR) polymorphism may be used to distinguish between the two organisms.[38, 39] Also, multilocus sequence typing (MLST) has been used to distinguish the organisms. For example, Godoy *et al.* (2003), demonstrated that alleles at six of the seven loci in *B. mallei* were also present within *B. pseudomallei* isolates.[40]

Serological tests including agglutination, compliment fixation test (CFT), mullein testing, indirect hemagglitination, enzyme-linked immunosorbent assays (ELISAs) and immunofluorescence can be used to identify *Burkholderia* spp. However, there are no specific serologic tests for human Glanders, although attempts have been made to adapt animal Glanders tests for human subjects. For example, agglutination and compliment fixation are not consistent or timely in humans. The agglutination test, in particular, may be difficult to interpret because of its high background titers of up to ~1:320 to 1:640 units.[2] The mullein test is the most commonly used test for the diagnosis of Glanders in animals. This test contains endotoxins and exotoxins produced by *B. mallei* where upon injection, infected subjects will demonstrate an allergic reaction to the inoculation. Development of a human mullein skin test has been attempted, however, the positive results were delayed for several weeks post-infection, rendering the test of little or no diagnostic value.[41] CFT are more specific but less sensitive and may require up to 40 days for sero conversion, thereby, making it useless in a clinical situation. US Army Medical Research Institute of Infectious Diseases (USAMRID) has developed an ELISA test for human *B. mallei* infections and it is effective in distinguishing human Glanders infections from other diseases such as anthrax, brucellosis and tularemia. However, due to the similarities between the species, *B. mallei* and *B. pseudomallei* cannot be differentiated with this test.[2, 6 13, 33]

TREATMENT

Although human cases of Glanders are rare and there is a limited amount of information in regards to the treatment of the disease, antimicrobial agents are the preferred initial treatment. In several reports, *B. mallei* has been shown to be highly susceptible to cefotoxime, ceftazidime, cipro-floxacin, amoxicillin-clavulanate, imipenem, meropenem, trimethoprim-sulfamethoxazole (TMP-SMZ), streptomycin, gentamicin, doxy-cycline and tetracyclines.[8, 42, 43, 44, 45] Resistance to chloramphenicol has been reported.[2]

For localized infections, the initial treatment recommended is for an 8 week course of chloramphenicol followed by 60 to 150 days course of oral amoxicillin-clavulanate, doxycycline, tetracycline or TMP-SMZ.[2] In severe cases of Glanders, patients will require aggressive supportive care including fluid replenishment, vasopressors and management of coagulopathy.

Table 6a: Medication and side effects of various treatment for Glanders

Medications	Mechanism of Action	Side Effects	Recommended Dosage
Amoxicillin-clavulanate	Inhibits bacterial cell wall synthesis	Fever, chills, body aches, flu symptoms, sore throat, headache, severe blistering, peeling, skin rash, nausea, vomiting, stomach pain, anorexia, jaundice, dark urine, diarrhea (watery or bloody), easy bruising/bleeding, weakness, agitation, confusion, seizure, vaginal itching/ discharge	60 mg/kg/day in 3 divided doses
Cefotoxime	Inhibits bacterial cell wall synthesis	Fever, headache, stomach pain/cramps, nausea, vomiting, mild-severe diarrhea (watery and bloody), rash, hives, itching, respiration difficulties, tightness in the chest, swelling (mouth, face, lips, or tongue), oliguria, hoarseness, arrhythmia, injection site inflammation, blisters, seizures, vaginal irritation/discharge, white patches in mouth, jaundice	1-2 grams every 8 hours IM or IV
Ceftazidime	Inhibits bacterial cell wall synthesis	Fever, headache, severe diarrhea (watery or bloody), nausea, vomiting, stomach pain, numbness, rash, hives, itching, difficulty breathing, tightness in the chest, swelling (mouth, face, lips, or tongue), hoarseness, abnormal muscle movements, oliguria, seizures, vaginal irritation/discharge, vein inflammation, white patches in the mouth, jaundice	120 mg/kg/day in 3 divided doses
Ciprofloxacin	Inhibits the function of DNA gyrase	Nausea, headache, diarrhea, liver function tests abnormal, vomiting, rash, abdominal pain/discomfort, foot pain, pain in extremities, injection site reaction	40 mg/kg body weight
Clavulanate	β-lactamase inhibitor	In conjunction with Amoxicillin (Augmentin): headache, low fever, diarrhea, gas, stomach pain, nausea, vomiting, dark colored urine, fever, confusion, easy bruising, bleeding, skin rash, bruising, severe tingling, numbness, pain, muscle weakness, agitation, confusion, seizure (convulsions), loss of appetite, dark urine, clay-colored stools, jaundice, sore throat, blistering, peeling rash, vaginal yeast infection (itching or discharge)	60 mg/kg/day
Doxycycline	Inhibits protein synthesis	Nausea, diarrhea, bloody stools, severe stomach cramps, indigestion, heartburn, vomiting, photosensitivity, loss of appetite, dysphagia, headaches, blurred vision, rash, joint pain, fever, feeling tired	100 mg b.i.d.

Table 6b: Medication and side effects of various treatment for Glanders

Medications	Mechanism of Action	Side Effects	Recommended Dosage
Gentamicin	Inhibits protein synthesis	Shortness of breath, increased thirst, loss of appetite, closing of the throat, hives, swellings (lips, face, or tongue), rash, fainting, lack of urine, decreased hearing, ringing in the ears, dizziness, clumsiness, unsteadiness, numbness, skin tingling, muscle twitching, seizures, diarrhea, abdominal cramps, nausea, vomiting	Not reported
Imipenem	Cell wall synthesis inhibitor	Rapid heartbeats, diarrhea, nausea, vomiting, nausea, stomach pain, heartburn, sore throat, confusion, tremors, hallucinations, seizure, headache, fainting, fever, chills, body aches, flu symptoms	60 mg/kg/day in 4 divided doses
Meropenem	Cell wall synthesis inhibitor	Difficulty breathing, headaches, closing of the throat, swelling (lips, tongue, or face), hives, skin rash, seizures, severe diarrhea, constipation, nausea, vomiting, unusual tiredness or weakness, unusual bleeding or bruising	75 mg/kg/day in 3 divided doses
Streptomycin	Inhibits protein synthesis	Fever, swelling, rash, hives, difficulty breathing, tightness in the chest, swellings (mouth, face, lips, or tongue), decreased urination, dizziness, headache, hearing loss, hives, lightheadedness, loss of balance, muscle weakness, nausea, numbness, tingling, ringing or roaring in the ears, skin rash, vaginal irritation/discharge, vomiting	Not reported
Tetracycline	Inhibits protein synthesis	Fever, chills, lingua villosa, blurred vision, diarrhea, nausea, vomiting sore throat, stomach pain, loss of appetite, difficulty swallowing, difficulty breathing, fever, headache, hives, hoarseness, indigestion, inflammation of tongue, swellings (mouth, face, lips, or tongue), joint pain, sores in the mouth, rash, sensitivity to sunlight, swelling and itching of the rectum, rash, hives, itching, tightness in the chest, vaginal irritation/ discharge	40 mg/kg/day divided TID
Trimethoprim /sulfamethoxazole	Inhibit successive steps in the folate synthesis pathway in bacteria	Appetite loss, nausea, vomiting, severe diarrhea, rash, hives, itching, difficulty breathing, severe or persistent cough, swellings (mouth, face, lips, or tongue), skin irritation (blistering, peeling, red, or swollen skin), bloody stools, chest pain, chills, fever, sore throat, decreased urination, depression, hallucinations, joint or muscle pain, seizures, headache, vaginal irritation/discharge	TMP 4 mg/kg/dose and SMX 20 mg/kg/dose divided BID

Table 7: Differential diagnosis of localized (skin) Glanders. Please note that the abbreviation TB represents tuberculosis

Symptoms	Glanders	Smallpox	Melioidosis	Plague	Typhoid	TB	Syphilis
Low-grade fever	■	■	■	■	■	■	■
Chills	■	■				■	
Fatigue	■	■				■	
Severe headaches	■				■		
Generalized myalgias	■						■
Malaise	■					■	
Dizziness	■						
Nausea	■			■			
Vomiting	■			■			
Diarrhea	■			■			
Sore throat	■		■				■
Blisters	■						
Pus-forming nodules	■						
Ulcerate abscesses	■	■				■	
Diaphoresis	■					■	
Tachypnea	■						
Chest pains	■		■				
Abdominal pains	■	■					
Splenomegaly	■						■
Altered mental states	■			■	■		

Large abscesses on patients need to be drained when possible. Initial antimicrobial treatment of the severe form of the disease, including septicemia, should use intravenous injections of ceftazidime, imipenem and meropenem for two weeks. Subsequently an additional ~20-25 weeks of oral antibiotics such as ciprofloxacin, doxycycline in combination with TMP-SMZ (100 mg po b.i.d. and 4mg/kg/day in 2 divided doses respectively) or amoxicillin-clavulanate should be utilized to complete the treatment.[2, 46] For the treatment of the pulmonary form, antibiotics such as imipenem, meropenem or a combination of ceftazidime and doxycycline should be used for a period of 6 to 12 months.[2] Please examine Tables 6a and 6b for more information in regards to the antibiotic effective in treating this disease.

DIFFERENTIAL DIAGNOSIS

Due to the wide range of bodily regions/organs involved and numerous symptomatic displays, human Glanders may be easily confused with a variety of other diseases with similar symptoms. Therefore, laboratory diagnosis is essential for positively

Table 8: Differential diagnosis of localized (ocular involvement) and (nasal/respiratory) Glanders. Please note that the abbreviation TB represents tuberculosis

Symptoms	Glanders	Smallpox	Melioidosis	Plague	Typhoid	TB	Syphilis
Excessive lacrimation	■						
Muco-conjunct. discharge	■						
Blurred vision	■						
Photophobia	■						
Lymphadenopathy	■			■		■	
Inflamed and swollen nose	■						
Copious nasal discharges	■						
Fistulae & tissue destruction	■						
Tracheitis	■	■					
Bronchitis	■			■		■	
Coughing	■		■			■	
Muco. sputum production	■	■	■			■	
Lymphangitis	■						■
Regional lymphadenopathy	■			■			■

Table 9: Differential diagnosis of pulmonary Glanders. Please note that the abbreviation TB represents tuberculosis

Symptoms	Glanders	Smallpox	Melioidosis	Plague	Typhoid	TB	Syphilis
Fever	■	■		■	■	■	■
Chills	■	■		■	■		
Fatigue	■					■	
Severe headaches	■						■
Myalgias	■	■		■	■		
Rigors	■						
Diaphoresis	■	■					
Coughing	■					■	
Dyspnea	■					■	
Hemoptysis	■					■	
Tachypnea	■						
Tachycardia	■						
Nausea	■		■				
Weight loss	■					■	■
Dizziness	■						
Mucosal eruptions	■	■					
Mucopurulent sputum	■		■			■	
Gastrointestinal signs	■						
Pleuritic chest pain	■		■				
Pulmonary abscesses	■						
Pleuritis	■	■					
Pleural effusion	■					■	
Extensive pneumonia	■					■	■
Putular skin lesions	■	■		■			
Nasal exudates	■		■				
Cervical lymphadenopathy	■	■		■		■	
Media. lymphadenopathy	■	■				■	■
Ulcers/nodules of the nose	■						
Abscesses in the skin	■						

identifying *B. mallei* as the causative agent. For example, the diffused pustular rashes could be mistakenly diagnosed with melioidosis or smallpox. In addition, the pulmonary symptoms of Glanders could be mistaken for melioidosis, smallpox, or the plague. Differential diagnosis of Glanders should include smallpox, melioidosis, plague, typhoid fever, tuberculosis, syphilis, erysipelas, lymphangitis, pyemia, and yaws.[47] Please examine Tables 7 to 10 for more information.

References

1. Gorbach S.L., Bartlett J.G., Blacklow N.R. Infectious Diseases. Third Edition. Philadelphia: Lippincott, Williams and Wilkins. 1992. pp. 1294
2. Bossi P., Tegnell A., Baka A., van Loock F., Hendriks J., Werner A., Maidgof H., Gouvras G. Bichat Guidelines for the Clinical Managemnet of Glanders and Meliodosis and Bioterrorism-related Glanders and Meliodosis. Eurosurveillance, 2004. 9: pp. 1-6
3. Martin J.W., Christopher G.W., Eitzen E.M. History of Biological Weapons: from Poisoned Darts to Intentional Epidemics. Medical Aspects of Biological Warfare. Chapter 1. Washington D.C.: The Surgeon General United States Army Medical Department Medical Center and School Borden Institute. 2007. pp. 1-20
4. Wheelis M. First Shots Fired in Biological Warfare. Nature, 1998. 395: pp. 213
5. Carus W.S. Bioterrorism and Biocrimes. The Illicit use of Biological Agents Since 1900. Amsterdam: Fredonia Books. 2002. pp. 69-70
6. Gregory B.C., Waag D.M. Glanders. Aspects of Biological Warfare. Chapter 6. Washington D.C.: The Surgeon General United States Army Medical Department Medical Center and School Borden Institute. 2007. pp. 121-146
7. Riedel S. Biological Warfare and Bioterrorism: a Historical Review. Baylor University Medical Center Proceedings, 2004. 17: pp. 400-406
8. Center for Disease Control and Prevention. Laboratory-acquired Human Glanders – Maryland, May 2000. Morbidity and Mortality Weekly Report, 2000. 49: pp. 532-535
9. Srinivasan A., Kraus C.N., DeShazer D., Becker P.M., Dick J.D., Spacek L., Bartlett J.G., Byrne R., Thomas D.L. Glanders in a Military Research Microbiologist. The New England Journal of Medicine, 2001. 345: pp. 256-258
10. Rotz L.D., Khan A.S., Lillibridge S.R., Ostroff S.M., Hughes J.M. Public Health Assessment of Potential Biological Terrorism Agents. Emerging Infectious Diseases, 2002. 8: pp. 225-230
11. Horn J.K. Bacterial Agents Used for Bioterrorism. Surgical Infections, 2003. 4: pp. 281-287
12. Sanford J.P. Pseudomonas Species (Including Melioidosis and Glanders). Principle and Practice of Infectious Diseases. Third Edition. New York: Churchill Livingstone. 1990. pp. 1692-1696
13. The Center for Food Security & Public Health. Iowa State University. Glanders. Revised August 31, 2007.Retrieved December 24, 2009. Website: http://www.cfsph. iastate.edu/Factsheets/pdfs/Glanders.pdf
14. Nierman W.C., DeShazer D., Kim H.S., Tettelin H., Nelson K.E., Feldblyum T., Ulrich R.L., Ronning C.M., Brinkac L.M., Daugherty S.C., Davidson T.D., Deboy R.T., Dimitrov G., Dodson R., Durkin A.S., Gwinn M.L., Haft D.H., Khouri H., Kolonay J.F., Madupu R., Mohammoud Y., Nelson W.C., Radune D., Romero C.M., Sarria S., Selengut J., Shamblin C., Sullivan S.A., White O., Yu Y., Zafar N., Zhou L., Fraser C.M. Structural Flexibility in

Table 10: Differential diagnosis of septicemic Glanders. Please note that the abbreviation TB represents tuberculosis

Symptoms	Glanders	Smallpox	Melioidosis	Plague	Typhoid	TB	Syphilis
Fever	■	■	■	■	■	■	■
Chills	■	■		■	■		
Headaches	■	■	■	■	■		■
Myalgias	■		■				
Pleuritic chest pains	■	■		■		■	
Lymphadenopathy	■			■			
Cellulitis	■						
Cyanosis	■						
Jaundice	■						
Photophobia	■						
Diarrhea				■	■		
Pustular rash	■	■					■
Papular rash	■				■		■
Granulomatous lesions	■						■
Necrotizing lesions	■	■					
Tachycardia				■			
Generalized erythroderma	■						
Jaundice	■						
Mild hepatomegaly	■						■
Mild spenomegaly	■				■		■
Septicemia	■		■	■			

the Burkholderia mallei Genome. Proceedings of the National Academy of Sciences, 2004. 101: pp. 14246-14251

15. Larsen J.C., Johnson N.H. Pathogenesis of Burkholderia pseudomallei and Burkholderia mallei. Military Medicine, 2009. 174: pp. 647-651

16. Whitlock G.C., Estes D.M., Torres A.G. Glanders: Off to the Races with Burkholderia mallei. Federation of European Microbiological Societies (FEMS) Microbiology Letters, 2007. 277: pp. 115-122

17. Fritz D.L., Vogel P., Brown D.R. Waag D.M. The Hamster Model of Intraperitoneal Burkholderia mallei (Glanders). Veterinary Pathology, 1999. 36: pp. 276-291

18. Fritz D.L., Vogel P., Brown D.R., DeShazer D., Waag D.M. Mouse Model of Sublethal and Lethal Intraperitoneal Glanders (Burkholderia mallei). Veterinary Pathology, 2000. 37: pp. 626-636

19. DeShazer D., Waag D.M., Fritz D.L., Woods D.E. Identification of Burkholderia mallei polysaccharoide Gene Cluster by Subtractive Hybridization and Demonstrating that the Encoded Capsule is an Essential Virulence Determinant. Microbial Pathogen, 2001. 30: pp. 253-269

20. Alexander C., Rietschel E.T. Bacterial Lipopolysaccharides and Innate Immunity. Journal of Endotoxin Research, 2001. 7: pp. 167-202

21. Trent M.S. Biosynthesis, Transport, and Modification of Lipid A. Biochemistry and Cell Biology, 2004. 82: pp. 71-86

22. Burtnick M.N., Brett P.J., Woods D.E. Molecular and Physical Characterization of Burjolderia mallei O antigens. The Journal of Bacteriology, 2002. 184: pp. 849-852

23. DeShazer D., Brett P.J., Woods D.E. The Type II O-antigenic Polysaccharide moiety of Burkholderia pseudomallei lipopolysaccharide is required for Serum Resistance and Virulence. Molecular Microbiology, 1998. 30: pp. 1081-1100

24. Brett P.J., Burtnick M.N., Snyder D.S., Shannon J.G., Azadi P., Gherardini F.C. Burkholderia mallei Expresses a Unique Lipopolysaccharide Mixture that is a Potent Activator of Human Toll-like Receptor 4 Complexes. Molecular Microbiology, 2007. 63: pp. 379-390

25. Ulrich R.L., DeShazer D. Type III Secretion: a Virulence Factor Delivery System Essential for the Pathogenicity of Burkholderia mallei. Infectioin and Immunity, 2004. 72: pp. 1150-1154

26. Ribot W.J., Ulrich R.L. The Animal Pathogen-like Type III Secretion System is Required for the Intracellular Survival of Burkholderia mallei within J774.2 Macrophages. Infection and Immunity, 2006. 74: pp. 4349-4353

27. Ulrich R.L., DeShazer D., Hines H.B., Jeddeloh J.A. Quorum Sensing: a Transcriptional Regulatory System Involved in the Pathogenicity of Burkholderia mallei. Infection and Immunity, 2004. 72: pp. 6589-6596

28. Henderson I.R., Navarro-Garcia F., Desvaux M., Fernandez R.C., Ala'Aldeen D. Type V Protein Secretion Pathway: Autotransporter Story. Microbiology and Molecular Biology Reviews, 2004. 68: pp. 692-744

29. Stevens J.M., Ulrich R.L., Taylor L.A., Wood M.W., DeShazer D., Stevens M.P., Galyov E.E. Actin-binding Proteins from Burkholderia mallei and Burholderia thailandensis can Functionally Compensate foir the Actin-based Motility Defect of Burkholderia pseudomallei bimA Mutant. The Journal of Bacteriology, 2005. 187: pp. 7857-7862

30. Van Zandt K.E., Greer M.T., Gelhaus H.C. Glanders: an overview of infection in humans. Orphanet Journal of Rare Diseases, 2013. 8: pp. 131-137

31. Lever M.S., Nelson M., Ireland P.I., Stagg A.J., Beedham R.J., Hall G.A., Knight G., Titball R.W. Experimental Aerogenic Burkholderia mallei (Glanders) Infection in the BALB/c Mouse. Journal of Medical Microbiology, 2003. 52: pp. 1109-1115

32. Guerrant R.L., Walker D.H., Weller P.F. Tropical Infectious Diseases – Principles, Pathogens & Practice. Volume 2. Philadelphia: Churchill Livingstone Elsevier. 2006. pp. 1575

33. Gilad J., Harary I., Dushnitsky T., Schwartz D., Amsalem Y. Burkholderia mallei and Burkholderia pseudomallei as Bioterrorism Agents: National Aspects of Emergency Preparedness. Israeli Medical Association Journal, 2007. 9: pp. 499-503

34. Bauernfeind A., Roller C., Meyer D., Jungwirth R., Schneider I. Molecular Procedure for Rapid Detection of Burkholderia mallei and Burkholderia pseudomallei. Journal of Clinical Microbiology, 1998. 36: pp. 2737-2741

35. Tanpiboonsak S., Paemanee A., Bunyarataphan S., Tungpradabkul S. PCR-RFLP Based Differentiation of Burkholderia mallei and Burkholderia pseudomallei. Molecular and Cellular Probes, 2004. 18: pp. 97-101

36. Winstanley C., Hales B.A., Corkill J.E., Gallagher M.J., Hart C.A. Flagellin Gene Variation between Clinical and Environmental Isolates of Burkholderia pseudomallei Contrasts With the Invariance Among Clinical Isolates. Journal of Medical Microbiology, 1998. 47: pp. 689-694

37. Gee J.E., Sacchi C.T., Glass M.B., De B.K., Weyant R.S., Levett P.N., Whitney A.M., Hoffmaster A.R., Popovic T. Use of 16S rRNA Sequencing for Rapid Identification and Differentiation of Burkholderia pseudomallei and B. mallei. Journal of Clinical Microbiology, 2003. 41: pp. 4647-4654

38. U'Ren J.M., Schupp J.M., Pearson T., Hornstra H., Friedman C.L., Smith K.L., Daugherty R.R.L., Rhoton S.D., Leadem B., Georgia S., Cardon M., Huynh L.Y., DeShazer D., Harvey S.P., Robison R., Gal D., Mayo M.J., Wagner D., Currie B.T., Keim P. Tandem Repeat Regions within the Burkholderia pseudomallei Genome and Their Application for High Resolution Genotyping. BioMed Central Microbiology, 2007. ;7: pp. 1-20

39. Hornstra H., Pearson T., Georgia S., Liguori A., Dale J., Price E., O'Neill M., SeShazer D., Muhammad G., Saqib M., Naureen A., Keim P. Molecular Epidemiology of Glanders, Pakistan. Emerging Infectious Diseases, 2009. 15: pp. 2036-2039

40. Godoy D., Randel G., Simpson A.J., Aanensen D.M., Pitt T.L., Kinoshita R., Spratt B.G. Multilocus Sequence Typing and Evolutionary Relationships among the Causative Agents of Melioidosis and Glanders, Burkholderia pseudomallei and Burkholderia mallei. Journal of Clinical Microbiology, 2003. 41: pp. 2068-2079

41. Redfearn M.S., Palleroni N.J. Glanders and Melioidosis. Disease Transmitted from Animals to Man. Springfield: Charles C. Thomas. 1975. pp. 110-128

42. Kenny D.J., Russell P., Rogers D., Eley S., Titball R. In Vitro Susceptibilities of Burkholderia mallei in Comparison to those of other Pathogenic Burkholderia spp. Antimicrobial Agents and Chemotherapy, 1999. 43: pp. 2773-2775

43. Russell P., Eley S.M., Ellis J., Green M., Bell D.L., Kenny D.J., Titball R.W. Comparison of Efficacy of Ciprofloxacin and Doxycycline Against Experimental Melioidosis and Glanders. Journal of Antimicrobial Chemotherapy, 2000. 45: 813-818

44. Heine H.S., England M.J., Waag D.M., Byrne W.R. In Vitro Antibiotic Susceptibilities of Burholderia mallei (Caustic Agent of Glanders) Determined by Broth Microdilution and E-test. Antimicrobial Agents and Chemotherapy, 2001. 45: pp. 2119-2121

45. Thibault F.M., Hernandez E., Vidal D.R., Girardet M., Cavallo I.D. Antibiotic Susceptibility of 65 Isolates of Burkholderia pseudomallei and Burkholderia mallei to 35 Antimicrobial Agents. Journal of Antimicrobial Chemotherapy, 2004. 54: pp. 1134-1138

46. Darling R.G., Woods, J.B. USAMRIID's Medical Management of Biological Casulties Handbook. Fifth Edition. Fort Detrick: US Army Medical Research Institute of Infectious Diseases, 2004. pp. 32-39

47. J.H. McIsaac. Hospital Preparation for Bioterror. A Medical and Biomedical System Approach. Burlington: Academic Press. 2006. pp. 57

Photo Bibliography

Figure 2.3-2: Scanning electronmicrograph (SEM) of *Burkholderia spp.* This electronphotomicrograph was taken by Dr. Jim Tiedje of Michigan State University. This work was performed under the auspices of the US Department of Energy's Office of Science, Biological and Environmental Research Program, and by the University of California, Lawrence Berkeley National Laboratory under contract No. DE-AC02-05CH11231, Lawrence Livermore National Laboratory under Contract No. DE-AC52-07NA27344, and Los Alamos National Laboratory under contract No. DE-AC02-06NA25396. Public domain photo

Figure 2.3-3: *B. mallei* infection diagram. The human anatomical illustration was created by Dr. Alexander J. da Silva and Melanie Moser in 2003. The illustration was released by the CDC. Public domain graphics

Figure 2.3-4: *B. mallei* grown on chocolate agar for 48 hours at a temperature of 37°C. *B. mallei* is the caustic agent that causes the the serious zoonotic disease known as Glanders. The photograph (highly zoomed) was taken by Todd Parke, Audra Marsh in 2010 and released by the CDC. Public domain photo

Burkholderia pseudomallei are small (0.4 to 0.6 µm in width and 2 to 5 µm in length), mobile (flagellated), oxidase-positive, aerobic, non-sporulating, Gram-negative, saprotrophic, facultative intracellular pathogenic bacillus shaped bacteria. They are responsible for the disease called melioidosis in humans.[1, 2, 3] *B. pseudomallei* was previously classified in various genera, such as *Malleomyces, Pfeifferella, Actinobacillus, Bacillus* and *Pseudomonas*. In 1992, this organism was finally reclassified as *Burkholderia*, along with other organisms of the group II *Pseudomonas* based on their 16S ribosomal RNA (rRNA) sequences, DNA-DNA homology, cellular lipid and fatty acid composition, as well as, their phenotypic characteristics (Figure 2.4-1).[4]

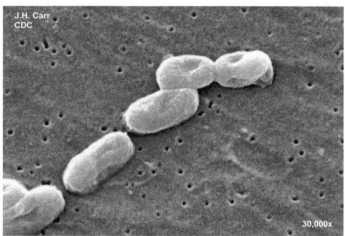

Figure 2.4-1: Scanning electron photomicrograph of *Burkholderia pseudomallei*

Melioidosis, also known as Witmore Disease, was first discovered in 1911 by Alfred Witmore and his assistant C.S. Krishnaswami. The authors described the ailment as a Glanders-like disease among morphine addicts in Rangoon, Burma. But during the latter half of the 20th century this disease has emerged as a major health concern in southeastern Asian and northern Australia.[5, 6] For example, in north-eastern Thailand and the Northern Territory of Australia, melioidosis is the most common cause of fatal bacteremic pneumonia and septicemia during the monsoon season.[7, 8]

B. pseudomallei has been classified as a Category B biological weapon by the Center of Disease Control (CDC). This bacterium was studied by the United States as a potential biological weapon during the 1950's, but was never weaponized. Nonetheless, according to Alibek (1999), this bacterial agent has been developed and stockpiled by the Soviet Union and is categorized as L6 bacterial biological weapon in the Soviet arsenal.[9, 10] Therefore, within the confines of this text, *B. pseudomallei* will be grouped among the Category A biological weapons.

B. pseudomallei is readily isolated from surface water and soil, particularly in irrigated areas such as rice paddies, within its endemic regions, southeastern Asia and northern Australia.[11, 12] It is believed that this bacillus persists inside the clay layers during the dry season only to reappear during the rainy season, although the mechanism of how this occurs is not presently understood. In addition, *B. pseudomallei* is highly resilient and able to endure prolonged nutrient deficiency, for up to 10 years. For example, reports have indicated that *B. pseudomallei* can survive in double

distilled water for up to 3 years. Additionally, this microbe has a high tolerance for antiseptic solutions, detergents, alkali and acidic environments (pH 4 >70 days), dehydration (<10% water for ~70 days), many antibiotics, and a wide range of temperatures (37°-42° C) (Figure 2.4-2). However, *B. pseudomallei* cannot survive exposure to UV radiation.[13, 14, 15, 16, 17, 18, 19]

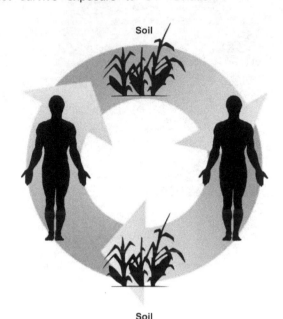

Figure 2.4-2: Sylvatic cycle of *B. pseudomallei*

B. pseudomallei infections involve various route of transmission, although human-to-human transmissions are occasionally reported. These opportunistic bacteria can be transmitted to humans through direct contact with contaminated soil via inoculation through the epidermis (e.g. mucous membrane of the nasal, oral and conjunctiva), contamination of wounds and/or through ingestion of the bacteria. Additionally, *B. pseudomallei* can be transmitted through contaminated water, as well as, the inhalation of aerosolized microbes. In endemic areas, especially within the farming and rice growing communities, a disproportionate melioidosis infection of males in comparison to females exists (~4:1 ratio). This discrepancy is most likely the result of occupational exposure, rather than gender differences.[2, 10, 12, 13, 20] Sexual transmission has also been documented. Although uncommon in most regions of the world, this form of transmission does account for ~37% of the incidences of lower genitourinary tract infections in Aboriginals of Australia[1] (Figure 2.4-3).[12, 13, 21]

Melioidosis transmission via the respiratory tract was common during the Vietnam War, where a high percentage of helicopter winch men suffered from the disease. It is postulated that the dust produced by the helicopter blades inadvertently aerosolized the microbe, thereby leading to its subsequent inhalation and innoculation.[22] Being an extremely resilient microbe, *B. pseudomallei* can remain dormant in patients long after the initial exposure. For instance, a case of septicemic melioidosis was reported ~29 years after the presumed exposure, while a case of cutaneous melioidosis appeared after a presumed dormancy period of 62 years (Figure 2.4-4).[23, 24]

The genome of *B. pseudomallei* is relatively large measuring at ~7.24 Mb and it is divided between 2 chromosomes: Large (L) chromosome 4.07 Mb and small (S) chromosome 3.17 Mb, with 68% G+C nucleotide content. The L chromosome encodes functions associated with central metabolism and cell growth, while the S chromosome encodes accessory functions related to adaptation and survival. It has been estimated that the genome of *B. pseudomallei* stores ~5855 coding sequences, however, a large proportion of *B. pseudomallei* genes are still poorly interpreted.[25]

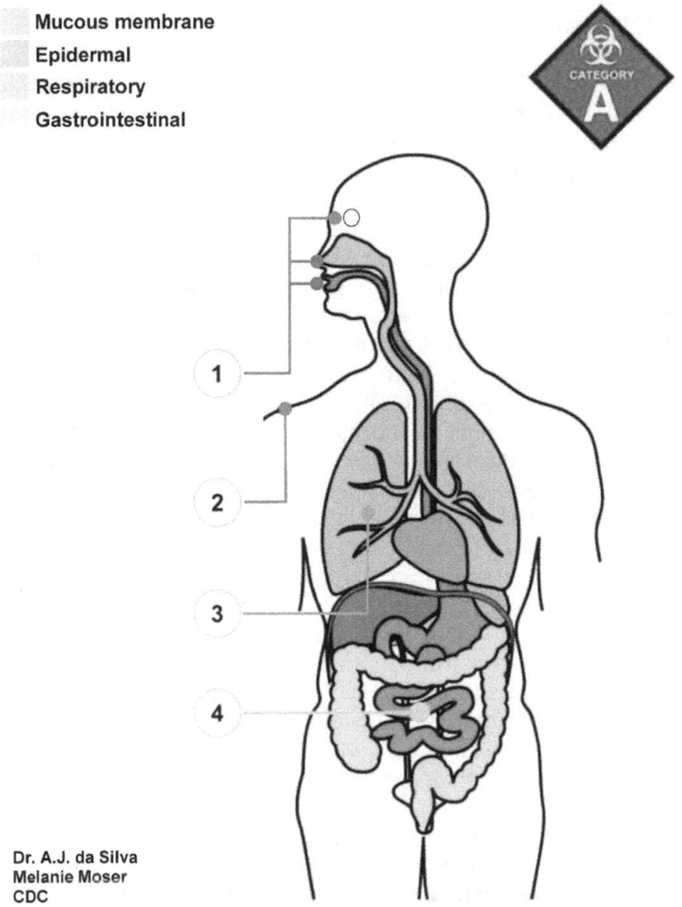

Mucous membrane
Epidermal
Respiratory
Gastrointestinal

Figure 2.4-3: *B. pseudomallei* infection diagram. ① *B. pseudomallei* spores could be introduced via oral, nasal or mucous membrane. ② *B. pseudomallei* spores are introduced via abrasion or cuts on the epidermis. ③ *B. pseudomallei* spores could be introduced via respiratory tract. ④ *B. pseudomallei* spores could be introducedvia gastrointestinal tract

An unusual feature of this microbe's genome is the existence of genomic islands (GIs) which contain regions of mobile genetic elements. These mobile genetic elements are comprised of insertion sequence elements, genetic information acquired from bacteriophages through transduction and/or plasmids acquired through conjugation from other bacteria. Altogether, GIs comprise ~6.1% of the entire genome and they are believed to represent the driving force in the evolution of *B. pseudomallei* virulence.[25] Using whole-genome microarrays, Sim *et al.* (2008) examined the genetic patterns of 94 South East Asian *B. pseudomallei* strains isolated from a variety of sources. These researchers demonstrated that 86% of the genome from the different strains showed commonality towards the *B. pseudomallei* K96243 reference genome. These similar genes comprise the 'core genome', which are involved in essential bacterial functions such as metabolism and protein translations etc. In contrast, 14% of the genome demonstrated notable variability among the isolates. It has been noted that the variability arises within the accessory genome which is composed of GIs, paralogous

genes and alterations of the genetic codes due to insertions and deletions, and three distinct lipopolysaccharide (LPS) related gene clusters.[26]

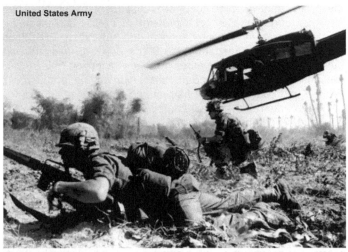

Figure 2.4-4: **Air mobile assault by US troops during the Vietnam War. It is believed that the dust produced by the helicopter blades inadvertently aerosolized the microbe, leading to its subsequent transmission to the troops**

Numerous reports have shown that *B. pseudomallei* are capable of secreting numerous soluble factors through the type II general secretory pathways. These secreted products include proteases such as serine metalloprotease (MprA) which has been suggested to be a possible virulence factor. Chin *et al.* (2007) reported that MprA are capable of causing extensive damage to mammalian physiological proteins thereby preventing their role in thwarting the damaging effects of bacterially secreted proteases.[27] Additionally, *B. pseudomallei* are also capable of secreting phospholipase C, hemolysin, lipase, lecithinase, as well as, cytotoxic exolipid, which is known to cause necrosis, hemolysis and cytolysis of the host tissues.[28] In 2011, Cruz-Migoni *et al.* reported the discovery of a potent toxin called *Burkholderia* lethal factor 1 (BLF1). BLF1 is known to interfere with the protein translation elongation factor eIF4A and can act as a potent cytotoxin in eukaryotic cells.[29]

Quorum sensing (QS) is a cell-density-dependent communication system utilized by various bacteria to regulate biofilm formation, antibiotic synthesis and the expression of virulence factors. In many species of Gram-negative bacteria, QS is mediated by *N*-acyl-homoserine lactones (AHLs). In 2004, Ulrich *et al.* reported that *B. pseudomallei* LuxI proteins are responsible for AHL biosynthesis. LuxR, on the other hand, is a type of transcriptional regulator, which, in association with AHL, promotes gene repression or expression.[30] The extracellular secretion of QS AHLs is highly dependent on the *B. pseudomallei* BpeAB-OprB efflux pump. It has been reported that this efflux pump is capable of aiding the microbe to proceed with optimal production of siderophores and phospholipase C, biofilm formation, as well as, conferring antimicrobial resistance to amino glycosides and macrolides.[31]

Type III secretion system (TTSS) is ancestrally related to flagella and is an essential part of the Gram-negative bacteria's protein secretion systems. TTSS is a membrane spanning needle that facilitates the injection of bacteria produced effectors proteins into the cytosol of the target-cell. *B. pseudomallei* possess three TTSS gene clusters, designated TTSS1, TTSS2, and TTSS3, existing on the S chromosome. The *bpscN* gene encodes both TTSS1 effector proteins and TTSS-associated ATPase. Research has shown that this TTSS1 gene cluster is absent from the related *Burkholderia* species, such as *B. mallei*. In 2011, D'Cruze *et al.* reported that through ATP hydrolysis, the TTSS-associated ATPase is believed to enable the initial docking of the TTSS substrates to the secretion apparatus and provide the proton motive force for their subsequent expulsion. Their findings suggest that effector proteins of TTSS1 are critical for *B. pseudomallei* intracellular survival and replication. TTSS2, on the other hand, is present in both *B. mallei* and *B. thailandensis* but its exact function requires further elucidation.[32, 33] TTSS3 resembles those found on *Salmonella typhimurium* and *Shigella flexneri* and codes for proteins required for the synthesis of the secretion apparatus, as well as, the effector proteins.[34] Stevens *et al.* (2002) demonstrated that *B. pseudomallei* TTSS3 mutants showed impaired intracellular survival. For example, these mutants are incapable of escaping from endocytic vacuoles, replicate or form actin tails within 8 hours after infection of J774.2 macrophage cells.[35]

In addition to TTSS, *B. pseudomallei* also possesses six copies of type VI secretion systems (T6SSs). T6SS-1 has been shown to be critical for virulence for *B. pseudomallei* in a hamster infection model and is essential for intracellular growth of the bacteria, actin polymerization, as well as, the formation of multinucleated giant cells (MNGCs) *in vitro*.[36] In 2010, Schwarz *et al.* found that T6SS-5 plays a critical role in the virulence of the organism in a murine melioidosis model. The authors postulated that T6SS-5 evolved to target simple eukaryotes in the environment and allowed the bacteria to transition into an obligate pathogen.[37] Unfortunately, until now, the exact functions of the remaining 4 T6SS secretion systems are still unknown.

B. pseudomallei produce various factors such as cytotoxic exolipid, proteases, lecithinase, lipase, hemolysins, catalase, peroxidase, superoxide dismutase and water-soluble siderophore, which contribute to its intracellular survival within a phagocytic and/or nonphagocytic host cell. This organism is resistant to complement lysosomal defensins (HNP-1) and cationic peptide protamine. *B. pseudomallei* has been known to survive and/or remain dormant intracellularly within phagocytes, such as neutrophils and macrophages (Figure 2.4-5).[13, 37, 38]

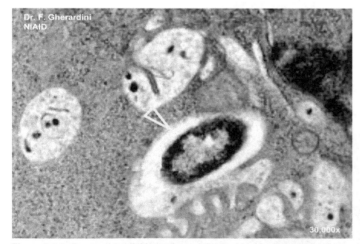

Figure 2.4-5: *B. pseudomallei* (arrow) surviving inside a human macrophage

The O-antigenic polysaccharide moiety of the lipopolysaccharide (LPS), found within the capsule of *B. pseudomallei*, interferes with the expression of inducible nitric oxide synthase (iNOS) within macrophages, inhibiting its destruction. It has been reported that the failure to induce iNOS expression may result from the bacterium's inability to activate beta interferon (IFN-β) production resulting in the lack of expression of Y701-STAT-1

phosphorylation and IFN-regulatory factor 1 (IRF-1).[39, 40, 41, 42] Nonetheless, the exact mechanism in which *B. pseudomallei* escapes innate immunoresponse within infected individuals has yet to be elucidated. *B. pseudomallei* is capable of multiplying within the phagosomes and eventually causes lysis of the host cell. Once the bacteria escapes from a membrane-bound phagosome into the cytoplasm, it induces cell-to-cell fusion resulting in the formation of a multinucleated giant cell. The formation of this unique multinucleated giant cell may facilitate the spread of the bacteria within the host.[37, 43, 44]

SYMPTOMS

As stated by Poe *et al.* (1971), melioidosis is the "remarkable imitator", because the clinical manifestation of the disease possesses variable presentations and is hard to categorize.[45] Melioidosis may appear as mild or subclinical infections, localized illness, latent infections, acute or chronic suppurative infections, in addition to the often fatal septicemia. *B. pseudomallei* infections generally take one of the three common courses: ① rapidly progressing septicemic melioidosis with or without pneumonia, ② a localized soft tissue infection or ③ subclinical infection with a delayed conversion to a clinically recognizable disease. It has been reported that melioidosis can progress from one form to another and possibly turn fatal, often in immunocompromised individuals. Additionally, patients with non-related medical issues have a higher instance of developing melioidosis. For example, up to 60% of patients diagnosed with Type 2 diabetes may develop melioidosis if exposed to *B. pseudomallei*. Other medical conditions such as thalassaemia, renal impairment or failure, chronic lung disease, splenectomy, systemic lupus, erythematosis and cystic fibrosis may increase the chance of patients developing melioidosis, if exposed to these infectious microbes. Five reported cases of pediatric patients in Thailand suffering from dengue hemorrhagic fever have developed melioidosis, signifying the opportunistic nature of *B. pseudomallei*. Interestingly, HIV infections do not appear to be a major risk factor for patients contracting melioidosis.[13, 46, 47, 48]

The incubation period of naturally acquired melioidosis varies greatly. For example, in naturally occurring infections, the incubation period after exposure to high amounts of *B. pseudomallei* may be as short as 24 hours or as long as two months. However, the weaponized form of aerosolized *B. pseudomallei* has been reported to have an incubation period of 10 to 14 days.[12, 23, 24, 49, 50]

Mild and Subclinical Infections

Melioidosis is uncommon in endemic areas, such as Thailand, however, a random serological study with 1000 selected children demonstrated that 12% of the infants, between 1-6 months, had antibodies against *B. pseudomallei*. The seroprevalence rose at a conversion rate of 24% per year and by the age of 4, 80% of children possess antibodies against this microbe.

Table 1: An overview of the clinical symptoms of mild and subclinical melioidosis

Symptoms	+	++	+++
Fever			▪
Chills			▪
Headaches			▪
Myalgia			▪
Fatigue			▪
Cough			▪
Rhinorrhea		▪	

+ Rare ++ Common +++ Frequent

It is suspected that environmental exposure to this microbe begins soon after the child becomes mobile. These mild and subclinical infections are either asymptomatic or display mild flu-like symptoms. It is believed that in these cases, the immune system is responsible for suppressing the infection (Table 1).[12, 46, 51]

Localized Infections

Localized melioidosis infections generally occur at the site of initial inoculation. For example, in the skin, the infections appear as ulcers and nodules with gray/white coloration and may be surrounded by inflammation. Regional lymph-adenopathy and lymphangitis are frequently associated with the cutaneous form of the infection. Additionally, fever and muscle tender-ness is also present. The cutaneous form of infection can rapidly progress into the acute septicemia or other forms of acute infection.[46, 49]

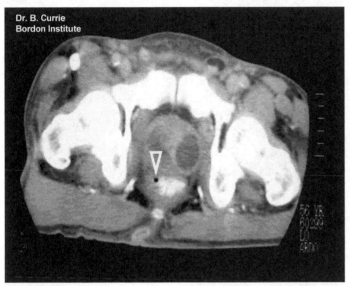

Figure 2.4-6: Computed tomography scan showing prostatic abscess (arrow)

Other localized melioidosis symptoms may include infections of the genitourinary tract or appear as prostatic abscesses (Figure 2.4-6). This form of localized infection is often seen in patients in Australia (18%), while less commonly observed in Thailand. In contrast, suppurative parotiditis is frequently seen in ~30-40% of the pediatric cases and in small numbers of adults in Thailand, while this form of melioidosis is rarely observed in Australia.[13, 49]

Other less common representations of melioidosis can be seen when the microbes infect the eyes. Corneal ulcerations tend to result from trauma and subsequently become infected with *B. pseudomallei*. Infections generally occur on the eye lids and spread progressively to the eyes, producing panoph-thalmitis and resulting in regional lymphadenopathy (Table 2).[52]

Table 2: An overview of the clinical symptoms of Localized melioidosis

Symptoms	+	++	+++
Fever			▪
Myalgia			▪
Ulcers			▪
Nodules			▪
Cellulitis			▪
Lymphadenopathy		▪	
Lymphangitis			▪
Corneal ulcerations			▪

+ Rare ++ Common +++ Frequent

Latent Infections

The incubation period for melioidosis may have long periods of latency, up to 62 years, before the first clinical signs are apparent. It is suspected that this infection appears when the immunity of the patients is suppressed. For example, relapse of this disease generally occurs during times of stress, other acute infections, medical conditions, burns, trauma and/or other malignancies. These recrudescent melioidosis infections have earned the nickname of 'Vietnamese Time Bomb' by veterans of the Vietnam War. Unfortunately, the mechanism of the latent infections, as well as, the proportion of seropositive patients who harbor this latent infection, is presently unknown.[12, 24, 49, 53]

SYSTEMIC INVOLVEMENT

Respiratory Infections

Melioidosis infection of the respiratory tract is the most common form of infection, appearing in about 50% of all cases. Clinically, this form of melioidosis can produce infections ranging from mild bronchitis to severe pneumonia (Figure 2.4-7).

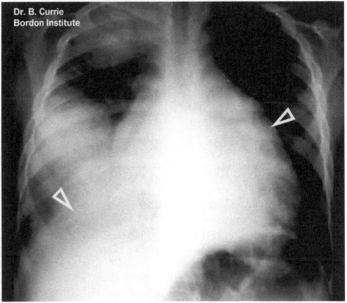

Figure 2.4-7: Chest radiograph demonstrating a severe multilobar pneumonia (arrows)

Respiratory melioidosis may present itself as acute or display symptoms that mimic tuberculosis. It is believed that the respiratory form of melioidosis is transmitted through two possible routes. The first manner by which *B. pseudomallei* are introduced is through hematogenous spread to the lungs following inoculation. In this scenario, the clinician often finds that the radiographic assessment of pneumonia often follows the initial introduction of the microbe from other areas of the body (e.g. cutaneous). The second manner by which the bacteria are introduced is direct inhalation. Evidence of this direct route of infection is demonstrated by the high percentage of helicopter winch men who suffered from respiratory melioidosis during the Vietnam War. It is thought that the dust produced by the helicopter blades inadvertently aerosolized the microbe and led to its subsequent transmission.[22, 48] Further evidence of direct respiratory infection by *B. pseudomallei* is presented by a 12-year retrospective study of 318 culture-confirmed cases of melioidosis in Northern Territories of Australia, where a marked association of cases of pneumonia with rainfall was seen.[54]

Signs of the infection generally follow the path the microbes traveled. For instance, ulcerative lesions and nodules are commonly found in the nose. Signs of respiratory infection may appear suddenly or occur after a prodromal phase, characterized by headaches, weight loss, pharyngitis, anorexia, dyspnoea and generalized myalgia. Symptoms of melioidosis of the respiratory tract include fever, coughing, excessive sputum production, pleuritic chest pain and hemoptysis. If left untreated or undertreated, the condition may deteriorate into pneumothroax, empyema, pericaditis or septicemia. The mortality rate for respiratory infections has been reported to be as high as 40 to 55% (Table 3).[1, 13, 49]

Table 3: An overview of the clinical symptoms of respiratory melioidosis

Symptoms	+	++	+++
Fever			■
Coughing			■
Sputum production			■
Pleuritic chest pain			■
Hemoptysis			■
Headaches			■
Weight loss			■
Pharyngitis			■
Anorexia			■
Dyspnoea			■
Generalized myalgia			■
Ulcerative lesions			■
Pneumothroax	■		
Empyema	■		
Pericaditis	■		
Septicemia	■		

+ Rare ++ Common +++ Frequent

Septicemia

Septicemia is the most serious form of melioidosis, appearing most often in patients suffering from other medical conditions, such as diabetes, cancer and kidney failure. As reported by the Infectious Disease Association of Thailand, 345 cases of septicemia are generally found within 2000-3000 cases of melioidosis. These cases can be divided into two categories. The first, disseminated septicemia, occurs in 45% of cases, with 87% mortality rates. The second, known as localized septicemia, occurs in 42% of cases and has a mortality rate of 9%. Nondisseminated septicemia occurs in 12% of cases, with a 17% mortality rate and a rarely occurring transient bacteremia, occurring in 0.3% of cases.[55] The initial signs of septicemia are generally acute and involves fever, rigor, confusion, stupor, jaundice, diarrhea, and signs of sepsis. Nonetheless, in a few cases, septicemia developed gradually with symptoms of fluctuating fever associated with severe weight loss.[12, 49, 55]

Septicemic melioidosis includes symptoms of high fever, severe headache, disorientation, pharyngitis, upper abdominal pain, diarrhea, jaundice, tachypnoea, tachycardia, skin flushing, tenderness of muscles and arthritis. Additionally, anemia, neutrophil leukocytosis, coagulopathy and signs of renal and hepatic impairment may also be detected. Furthermore, skin lesions may also appear in the form of erythematous papules to violaceous abscesses.[1, 12, 13, 49]

Patients who develop the above symptoms generally deteriorate rapidly and develop metastatic abscesses in the lungs, spleen and liver as well as metabolic acidosis (Figure 2.4-8). Respiratory signs, including dyspnea, may be seen in some cases. Septicemic melioidosis may deteriorate into neurological melioidosis, which may include peripheral motor nerve weakness (mimicking

Guillain-Barré Syndrome), encephalomyelitis characterized by brain stem encephalitis, aseptic meningitis and respiratory failure.

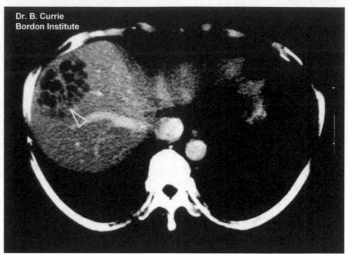

Figure 2.4-8: Computed tomography scan showing multiloculated liver abscess (arrow)

Table 4: An overview of the clinical symptoms of septicemic melioidosis. The term metastatic (Met.) is abbreviated in the table below

Symptoms	+	++	+++
Fever			■
Rigors			■
Confusion/ disorientation			■
Stupor			■
Jaundice			■
Diarrhea			■
Signs of sepsis			■
Severe headache			■
Pharyngitis			■
Upper abdominal pain			■
Tachypnoea			■
Tachycardia			■
Flushing of the skin			■
Tenderness of muscles			■
Arthritis			■
Anemia		■	
Neutrophil leukocytosis		■	
Coagulopathy		■	
Renal impairment		■	
Hepatic impairment		■	
Erythematous papules		■	
Violaceous abscesses		■	
Meta. abscesses – lung		■	
Meta. abscesses – spleen		■	
Meta. abscesses – liver		■	
Metabolic acidosis		■	
Dyspnea		■	
Fluctuating fever	■		
Severe weight loss	■		
Motor nerve weakness	■		
Encephalomyelitis	■		
Aseptic meningitis	■		
Respiratory failure	■		
Septic shock	■		

+ Rare ++ Common +++ Frequent

In cases of neurological melioidosis, evidence of direct infection with *B. pseudomallei* is rarely seen and it is thought that this condition is the result of an exotoxin-induced neurological syndrome. Septic shock is common and if left untreated the mortality rate approaches 95% within 48 hours.[12, 13, 49, 56]

Of the few patients that manage to survive septic shock, multiple septic foci, resulting from bacterial dissemination became prominent on all tissues affected by the infection. Nonetheless, the most common foci involve the lungs, liver, prostate, spleen and skin. Chest radiographs demonstrate widespread nodular shadowing in 60 to 80% of patients, mimicking tuberculosis, while multiple spleen and liver abscesses are also commonly observed (Figure 2.8-8). Secondary lesions may also appear in various organs, such as kidneys, bones, joints and the brain. Additionally, in 10 to 20% of patients, cutaneous pustules and subcutaneous abscesses are also seen (Table 4).[12, 49, 57]

DETECTION

Being the "remarkable imitator," the diagnosis of melioidosis on clinical grounds is difficult.[43] Therefore, it is essential to use specific laboratory tests that isolate and detect B. pseudomallei using clinical specimens such as blood, liver/splenic pus, parotid pus, sputum, urine, throat and rectal swabs, as well as, tissue or wound exudates. In addition, bacteria can also be isolated from joint, pericardial, pleural and peritoneal fluid. [12, 50, 55, 57] Microscopy of a Gram-stained B. pseudomallei will appear as short Gram-negative bacilli, with bipolar or irregular staining in young cultures. Nonetheless, this form of identification has low specificity and may be easily confused with other Gram-negative organisms.[12]

Dr. T. Parker
A. Marsh
CDC

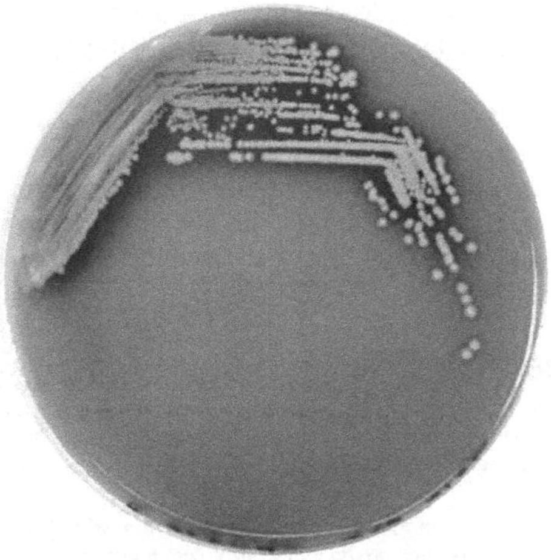

Figure 2.4-9: A photograph of the colonial morphology displayed by Gram-negative B. pseudomallei bacteria grown on sheep's blood agar for a 48 hour at a temperature of 37°C

Culture of B. pseudomallei is considered the 'gold standard' for diagnostic testing, however, this form of examination is often time consuming and may take 24 to 48 hours from specimen plating,

to bacterial growth and finally to the presumptive identification of the microbe.[58] B. pseudomallei can be grown with most routine laboratory media such as blood, McConkey or cystine-lactose-electrolyte deficient (CLED) agars, or routine blood culture broth. For example, the characteristic colonial morphology is generally detected in blood culture within 48 hours (Figure 2.4-9).[12, 50, 55, 57] Nonetheless, by using selective media such as Ashdown's medium, a crystal violet and gentamicin-containing medium, B. pseudomallei can be selectively grown, increasing the sensitivity of the culture in comparison with other forms of media.[47]

Mature colonies of the bacteria have a wrinkled appearance, mixed in with some smooth forms, especially when grown in a glycerol containing medium, and some strains isolated from human sputum samples have displayed mucoid colonies. It has been reported that B. pseudomallei colonies have a characteristic putrid and earthy odor, but direct inhalation of bacterial samples is not recommended and dangerous due to the high risk of infection.[48, 50]

Direct immunofluorescence is a rapid and rather effective method for detecting B. pseudomallei. This exam demonstrates a 66% sensitivity, in comparison with cultured B. pseudomallei, in patients suffering from melioidosis. Nonetheless, the availability of the materials required may be limited to certain endemic regions.[58, 60] Other techniques have been developed to rapidly identify the B. pseudomallei antigens in both plate and broth cultures through the use of monoclonal antibodies. One example is latex agglutination, where specific monoclonal antibodies are used to identify the lipopoly-saccharides (LPSs) of B. pseudomallei. In the study conducted by Dharakul et al. (1994), the field evaluation of the Bps-L1 latex agglutination test kit demonstrated a sensitivity and specificity of 100%.[61]

Serological tests have also been useful in detecting B. pseudomallei, however the utility of this technique is limited when examining patients in endemic areas, where much of the population has already developed antibodies for the pathogen. Nonetheless, the measurement of high single titers of antibodies where in conjunction with the values associated with clinical signs, could be suggestive of melioidosis. Serological screens that have been developed include agglutination, indirect hemagglutination (detecting IgM antibodies to crude heat-stable antigens), dot immunoassay, western blotting and the immunochromatographic test. Other serological tests including indirect immune-fluorescence, for IgM have also been used for B. pseudomallei identification. Enzyme-linked immunosorbant assays (ELISAs) targeting IgG antibodies for exotoxins and other B. pseudomallei cellular components can also be used to obtain a positive identity. [50, 62, 63, 64]

Polymerase Chain Reaction (PCR) assays have been

Table 5: Therapeutic intravenous regiment for adults suffering from melioidosis

	Doxycycline	Chloramphenicol	Ceftazidime	Imipenem	Meropenem	TMP/SMZ	G-CSF
1			120 mg/kg/day				
2				50 mg/kg/day			
3					50 mg/kg/day		
4			120 mg/kg/day			10 & 50 mg/kg/d	
5				50 mg/kg/day		10 & 50 mg/kg/d	
6					50 mg/kg/day	10 & 50 mg/kg/d	
7					50 mg/kg/day	10 & 50 mg/kg/d	300 µg
8	4 mg/kg/day	100 mg/kg/day				10 & 50 mg/kg/d	
9			2 g/6 hrs 8g/day			320 mg/1600 mg	
10				1g/6 hrs		320 mg/1600 mg	
11					1g/8 hrs	320 mg/1600 mg	

Table 6: Recommended oral treatment to prevent melioidosis relapse

	Doxycycline	Chloramphenicol	Amoxicillin	Clavulanate	TMP/SMZ
1	4 mg/kg/day	40 mg/kg/day			10/50 mg/kg/day
2	4 mg/kg/day				8mg/40mg/kg/day
3			60mg/day	15 mg/kg/day	

developed to distinguish the genetic sequences of *B. mallei*, *B. pseudomallei*, as well as, other closely related species. For example, laboratory techniques such as PCR-restriction fragment length polymorphism (through Southern blot hybridization) utilize the *Sau3A*l-digested genomic DNA patterns of *B. mallei* and *B. pseudomallei* for comparison.[65, 66] The 16s rRNA sequencing and pulse-field gel electrophoresis have also been used to distinguish *B. pseudomallei* from other closely related species.[67] Additionally, techniques such as variable number tandem repeat polymorphism and multilocus sequence typing (MLST) have also been developed by researchers to detect the microbe in question.[50]

TREATMENT

B. pseudomallei, the causative agent of melioidosis, is intrinsically resistant to various antibiotics, such as aminoglycosides, first and second generation cephalosporins, rifamycins, nonureidopenicillin and gentamicin. In addition, *B. pseudomallei* also demonstrate insensitivities to quinolones and macrolides, limiting therapeutic options to treat this disease.[68, 69] Nonetheless, even with the inherent handicap for the treatment of melioidosis, effective medications and treatment regiments have been developed. The treatment regiment for melioidosis generally consists of two phases: ① an acute treatment phase aimed at reducing mortality and ② an eradication phase aimed at reducing the risk of relapse.

The conventional therapy for treating the acute phase of melioidosis involves antimicrobial agents like chloramphenicol,

doxycycline, trimethoprim and sulphamethoxazole (co-trimoxazole TMP/SMZ). However, newer β-lactam agents, such as ceftazidime (120 mg/kg/day), imipenem (50 mg/kg/day), meropenem (50 mg/kg/day) and cefoperazone-sulbactam (with or without the simultaneous treatment of co-trimoxazole), administered for 2 to 4 weeks have been effectively used to reduce mortality rates.[12] For example, ceftazidime intravenously administered at 120 mg/kg/day has been shown to the reduce the mortality rate from 74% to 37%, in comparison to the conventional therapy.[70] In addition, clinical trials have demonstrated that by administering granulocyte colony stimulating factor (G-CSF – 300 µg) in conjunction with meropenem and co-trimoxazole, has effectively reduced melioidosis septic shock from 95% to 10%.[71] Unfortunately, in certain endemic areas, the cost of the newer antibiotics may be prohibitive. Due to financial limitations, it is common that practitioners in these areas continue to use inferior antimicrobial agents, such as chloramphenicol succinate (100 mg/kg/day), doxycycline (4 mg/kg/day) and co-trimoxazole (TMP/SMZ: trimethoprim 10 mg/kg/day and sulfamethoxazole 50 mg/kg/day), with expected inferior outcomes.[12] Please examine Tables 5 and 6 for the recommended treatment regiment for the acute form of melioidosis and recommended doses for preventions of melioidosis relaps respectively. Please also examine Tables 7 for characteristics of the various medications.

Following conventional therapy for treating the acute phase of melioidosis includes a prolonged oral antibiotic treatment for ~12 to 20 weeks, in order to prevent relapse. It has been estimated that ~13 to 23% of patients relapse after initial treatment for the acute form of the disease.[72, 73] The recommended treatment to lower

Table 7: Medication side effects of various treatment for melioidosis

Medications	Mechanism of Action	Side Effects
Amoxicillin/Ampicillin	Inhibits bacterial cell wall synthesis	Fever, chills, body aches, flu symptoms, headache, nausea, vomiting, stomach pain, diarrhea (watery or bloody), loss of appetite, sore throat, severe blistering, peeling, and red skin rash, dark urine, jaundice, easy bruising or bleeding, unusual weakness, agitation, confusion, seizure, vaginal itching or discharge
Ceftazidime	Inhibits bacterial cell wall synthesis	Fever, headache, nausea, stomach pain, vomiting, severe diarrhea (watery or bloody), numbness, tingling of skin, rash, hives, itching, difficulty breathing, tightness in the chest, swelling (mouth, face, lips, or tongue), hoarseness, abnormal muscle movements, decreased urination, seizures, vaginal irritation or discharge, vein inflammation, white patches in the mouth jaundice
Chloramphenicol	Inhibits protein synthesis	Headache, nausea, vomiting, diarrhea, abdominal pain, fever, fatigue, sore throat, unusual bleeding or bruising, bloating, vision changes, eye pain, rash, itching, swelling, dizziness, trouble breathing and tingling of the hands or feet.
Clavulanate	β-lactamase inhibitor	In conjunction with Amoxicillin (Augmentin): diarrhea, gas, stomach pain, nausea, vomiting, jaundice, dark colored urine, fever, headache, confusion, easy bruising, bleeding, skin rash, bruising, severe tingling, numbness, pain, muscle weakness, agitation, confusion, seizure (convulsions), loss of appetite, dark urine, sore throat, blistering and peeling rash, vaginal yeast infection (itching or discharge)
Doxycycline	Inhibits protein synthesis	Nausea, diarrhea, bloody stools, severe stomach cramps, indigestion, heartburn, vomiting, photosensitivity, loss of appetite, dysphagia, headaches, blurred vision, rash, joint pain, fever, feeling tired
Imipenem	Cell wall synthesis inhibitor	Rapid heartbeats, diarrhea, sore throat, nausea, vomiting, nausea, stomach pain, heartburn, stomach pain, confusion, tremors, hallucinations, seizure, headache, fainting, fever, chills, body aches, flu symptoms
Meropenem	Cell wall synthesis inhibitor	Difficulty breathing, headaches, closing of the throat, swelling (lips, tongue, or face), hives, skin rash, seizures, severe diarrhea, constipation, nausea, vomiting, unusual tiredness or weakness, unusual bleeding or bruising
Trimethoprim/ Sulfamethoxazole	Inhibit successive steps in the folate synthesis pathway in bacteria	Appetite loss, nausea, vomiting, rash, hives, itching, difficulty breathing, shortness of breath, severe or persistent cough, swellings (mouth, face, lips, or tongue), skin irritation (blistering, peeling, red, or swollen skin), bloody stools, severe diarrhea, nausea, vomiting, chest pain, chills, fever, sore throat, decreased urination, depression, hallucinations, joint or muscle pain, seizures, headache, vaginal irritation or discharge

Table 8: Differential diagnosis of melioidosis

Symptoms	Melioidosis	Glanders	Influenza	Brucellosis	TB	Plague	DF
Fever	■	■	■	■	■	■	■
Fluctuating fever	■			■			■
Chills	■	■		■	■	■	■
Fatigue	■	■	■	■	■		■
Severe headaches	■	■	■	■	■		
Myalgias	■	■	■	■	■		■
Rigors	■						
Arthritis				■	■		■
Cough				■	■	■	
Rhinorrhea	■						
Ulcerative lesions	■			■			
Nodules	■				■		
Cellulitis	■				■		
Lymphadenopathy				■	■	■	■
Lymphangitis				■	■	■	
Sputum production	■				■		
Pleuritic chest pain	■			■	■	■	
Hemoptysis	■				■		
Weight loss	■		■	■	■		
Pharyngitis	■		■			■	
Anorexia	■	■	■		■		
Dyspnoea	■	■			■		
Pneumothroax	■						
Empyema	■						
Pericaditis	■				■		
Jaundice	■	■					
Diarrhea	■					■	■
Anemia	■			■			
Upper abdominal pain	■	■		■		■	
Tachypnoea	■	■					
Tachycardia	■				■	■	■
Flushing of the skin	■						
Neutrophil leukocytosis	■					■	
Coagulopathy	■				■	■	■
Renal impairment	■					■	
Hepatic impairment	■					■	
Erythematous papules	■				■		
Violaceous abscesses	■						
Meta. abscesses – lung	■	■			■		
Meta. abscesses – spleen	■						
Meta. abscesses – liver	■						
Metabolic acidosis	■				■		
Dyspnea	■				■		
Confusion/ disorientation	■	■			■	■	
Stupor	■				■		
Motor nerve weakness	■						
Encephalomyelitis	■				■		
Aseptic meningitis	■				■		
Respiratory failure	■				■	■	
Septic shock	■				■	■	

the rate of relapse for adults is a combination of chloramphenicol succinate (40 mg/kg/day), doxycycline (4 mg/kg/day) and co-trimoxazole (trimethoprim 10 mg/kg/day and sulfamethoxazole 50 mg/kg/day), which has been reported to have reduced the relapse rate of melioidosis to ~4%.[74] Nonetheless, this treatment regiment frequently causes severe side-effects, hindering patient compliance.[55] Another regiment recommended is a high-dosage of TMP/SMZ (8mg/40mg/kg up to 320mg/1600 mg) in conjunction with doxycycline (4 mg/kg/day) which is better tolerated by patients, thereby increasing compliance. For children and/or pregnant women, a combination treatment of amoxicillin (60 mg/day) and clavulanate acid (15 mg/kg/day), have also reportedly reduced the rate of relapse.[12, 55, 74, 75] Please examine Table 5 for the recommended treatment regiment to prevent melioidosis

relapse, and Table 6 for characteristics of the various medications utilized.

Currently, there is no *B. pseudomallei* vaccine approved or available for human use. However, experimental vaccines, such as live attenuated vaccines, heterologous vaccines, acellular vaccines and subunit vaccines using rodent models have been developed.[76]

DIFFERENTIAL DIAGNOSIS

The differential diagnosis of melioidosis based on clinical grounds is challenging and most often requires the assistance of laboratory analysis. Known as the 'remarkable imitator', the differential diagnosis of the melioidosis will include numerous symptomatically similar illnesses based upon the various presentation of the disease.[45] Nonetheless, it is important to note that melioidosis is clinically and pathologically similar to Glanders and that careful laboratory diagnosis should be performed to distinguish the diseases.

The differential diagnosis for mild and subclinical melioidosis infections are indistinguishable than an individual displaying mild flu-like symptoms which includes fever, chills, headaches, myalgia, fatigue, cough and rhinorrhea (which is most common in children).

Differential diagnosis for localized infections is equally difficult to differentially diagnose due to the many different presentation of the disease. Most often the initial symptom of localized melioidosis will include ulcers and nodules (with gray/white coloration and maybe surrounded by inflammation) which are indistinguishable from a simple insect bite to lupus. Other symptoms such as lymphadenopathy, lymphangitis, fever and myalgias could be symptomatic presentations of myriad of diseases that include brucellosis, mononucleosis, cellulitis, lymphatic obstruction and *Staphylococcus* infection. Other localized melioidosis symptoms may include prostatic abscesses, which can be difficult to differentiate from Coliform infection that frequently involves ubiquitous, Gram-negative bacteria such as *Escherichia coli* (*E. coli*), and suppurative parotiditis, which are also commonly caused by mumps (caused by *Rubulavirus*), *cytomegalo-virus* infection, influenza, and bacterial infection caused by *Staphylococcus aureus*.[13, 46, 49]

Melioidosis infection of the respiratory tract can produce infections ranging from mild bronchitis to severe pneumonia. Most often, respiratory melioidosis may present symptoms that mimic tuberculosis (TB). The differential diagnosis for septicemic melioidosis should include disease that mimics enteric fevers such as bartonellosis (Bart), plague, leptospirosis (Lepto), hepatitis, relapsing fever, and dengue fever (DF), to name a few (Table 8).[3]

References

1. Fernando R.L., Fernando S.E., Leong S.Y. Tropical Infectious Diseases – Epidemiology, Investigation, Diagnosis & Management. London: Greenwich Medical Media. 2001. pp. 245-249
2. Murray P.R., Rosenthal K.S., Kobayashi G.S., Pfaller M.A. Medical Microbiology. Fourth Edition. St. Louis: Mosby College Publishing, 2002. pp. 302-303
3. Kwan-Gett T.S.C., Kemp C., Kovarik C. Infectious and Tropical Diseases. St. Louis: Elsevier Mosby. 2006. pp. 381-387
4. Yabuuchi E., Kosako Y., Oyaizu H., Yano I., Hotta H., Hashimoto Y., Ezaki T., Arakawa M. Proposal of Burkholderia gen. nov. and Transfer of Seven Species of the Genus Pseudomonas Homology Group II to the New Genus, with the Type Species Burkholderia cepacia (Palleroni and Holmes 1981) Comb. Nov. Microbiology and Immunology, 1992. 36: pp. 1251-1275
5. Wutmore A., Krishnaswami C.S. An Account of the Discovery of a Hitherto Underscribed Infective Disease Occurring Among the Population of Rangoon. Indian Medical Gazette, 1912. 47: pp. 262-267
6. Witmore A. An Account of Glanders-like Disease Occurring in Rangoon. Journal of Hygiene, 13: pp. 1-34
7. Currie B.J. Melioidosis and the Monsoon in Tropical Australia. Communicable Diseases Intelligence, 1996. 20: pp. 63
8. Chaowagul W., White N.J., Dance D.A., Wattanagoon Y., Naigowit P., Davis T.M., Looareesuwan S., Pitakwatchara N. Melioidosis: a Majory Cause of Community-aquired Septicemia in Northeastern Thailand. Journal of Infectious Diseases, 1989. 159: pp. 890-899
9. Alibek K. Biohazard. New York: Dell Publishing. 1999. pp. 20
10. Darling R.G., Woods, J.B. USAMRIID's Medical Management of Biological Casulties Handbook. Fifth Edition. Fort Detrick: US Army Medical Research Institute of Infectious Diseases, 2004. pp. 32-39
11. Strauss J.M., Groves M.G., Mariappan M., Ellison DW. Melioidosis in Malaysia. II. Distribution of Pseudomonas pseudomallei in Soil and Surface Water. American Journal of Tropical Medicine and Hygiene, 1969. 18: pp. 698-702
12. Guerrant R.L., Walker D.H., Weller P.F. Tropical Infectious Diseases – Principles, Pathogens & Practice. Volume 1. Philadelphia: Churchill Livingstone Elsevier. 2006. pp. 381-388
13. Cheng A.C., Currie B.J. Melioidosis: Epidemiology, Pathophysiology, and Management. Clinical Microbiology Reviews, 2005. pp. 383-416
14. Wuthiekanun V., Smith M.D., White N.J. Survival of Burkholderia pseudomallei in the Absence of Nutrients. Transactions of the Royal Society of Tropical Medicine and Hygiene, 1995. pp. 491

15. Gal D., Mayo M., Smith-Vaughan H., Dasari P., McKinnon M., Jacups S.P., Urquhart A.I., Hassell M., Currie B.J. Contamination of Hand Wash Detergent Linked to Occupationally Acquired Melioidosis. American Journal of Tropical Medicine and Hygiene, 71: pp. 360-362
16. Dejsirilert S., Kondo E., Chiewsilp D., Kanai K. Growth and Survival of Pseudomonas pseudomallei in Acidic Environments. Japanese Journal of Medical Science and Biology, 1991. 44: pp. 63-74
17. Chen Y.S., Chen S.C., Kao C.M., Chen Y.L. Effects of Soil pH Temperature and Water Content on the Growth of Pseudomonas pseudomallei. Folia Microbiologica. 48: pp. 253-256
18. Moore R.A., Tuanyok A., Woods D.E. Survival of Burkholderia pseudomallei in Water. BioMed Central Research Notes, 2008. 1: 11-16
19. Tong S., Yang S., Lu Z., He W. Laboratory investigation of ecological factors influencing the environmental presence of Burkholderia pseudomallei. Microbiology and Immunology, 1996.40: pp. 451–453.
20. Limmathurotsakul D., Wongsuvan G., Aanensen D., Ngamwilai S., Saiprom N., Rongkard P., Thaipadungpanit J., Kanoksil M., Chantratita N., Day N.P.J., Peacock S.J. Melioidosis Caused by Burkholderia pseudomallei in Drinking Water, Thailand, 2012. Emerging Infectious Diseases, 2014. 20: pp. 265-268
21. Currie B.J., Mayo M., Anstey N.M., Donohoe P., Haase A., Kemp D.J. A Cluster of Melioidosis Cases from an Endemic Region is Clonal and is linked to the Water Supply Using Molecular Typing of Burkholderia pseudomallei Isolates. American Journal of Tropical Medicine and Hygiene, 2001. 65: pp. 177-179
22. Howe C.A., Sampath A., Spotnitz M. The Pseudomallei Group: a Review. Journal of Infectious Diseases, 1971. 124: pp. 598-606
23. Chodimella U., Hoppes W.L., Whalen S., Ognibene A.J., Rutecki G.W. Septicemia and Supporation in a Vietnam Veteran. Hospital Practice, 1997. 32: pp. 219-221
24. Ngauy V., Lemeshev Y., Sadkowski L., Crawford G. Cutaneous Melioidosis in a Man Who was taken as a Prisoner of War by the Japanese During World War II. Journal of Clinical Microbiology, 2005. 43: pp. 970-972
25. Holden M.T., Titball R.W., Peacock S.J., Cerdeno-Tarraga A.M., Atkins T., Crossman L.C., Pitt T., Churcher C., Mungall K., Bentley S.D.,Sebaihia M., Thomson N.R., Bason N.,Beacham I.R., Brooks K., Brown K.A., Brown N.F., Challis G.L., Cherevach I., Chillingworth T., Cronin A., Crossett B., Davis P., DeShazerD., Feltwell T., Fraser A., Hance Z., Hauser H.,Holroyd S., Jagels K., Keith K.E., Maddison M., Moule S., Price C., Quail M.A.,Rabbinowitsch E., Rutherford K., Sanders M.,Simmonds M., Songsivilai S., Stevens K.,Tumapa S., Vesaratchavest M., Whitehead S.,Yeats C., Barrell B.G., Oyston P.C., Parkhill J. 2004. Genomic plasticity of the causative agent of melioidosis, Burkholderia pseudomallei. Proceedings of the National Academy of Sciences of the United States of America, 2004. 101: pp. 14240–14245
26. Sim S.H., Yu Y., Lin C.H., Karuturi R.K., Wuthiekanun V., Tuanyok A., Chua H.H., Ong C., Paramalingam S.S., Tan G., Tang L., Lau G., Ooi E.E., Woods D., Feil E., Peacock S.J., Tan P. The core and accessory genomes of Burkholderia pseudomallei: implications for human melioidosis. Public Library of Science (PLoS), 2008. 4: pp. e1000178
27. Chin C.Y., Othman R., Nathan S. The Burkholderia pseudomallei serine protease MprA is autoproteolytically activated to produce a highly stable enzyme. Enzyme and Microbial Technology, 2007. 40: pp. 373–377
28. Ashdown L.R., Koehler J.M. Production of hemolysin and other extracellular enzymes by clinical isolates of Pseudomonas pseudomallei. Journal of Clinical Microbiology, 1990. 28: pp. 2331–2334
29. Cruz-Migoni A., Hautbergue G.M., Artymiuk P.J., Baker P.J., Bokori-Brown M., Chang C.T., Dickman M.J., Essex-Lopresti A., Harding S.V., Mahadi N.M., Marshall L.E., Mobbs G.W., Mohamed R., Nathan S., Ngugi S.A., Ong C., Ooi W.F., Partridge L.J., Phillips H.L., Raih M.F., Ruzheinikov S., Sarkar-Tyson M., Sedelnikova S.E., Smither S.J., Tan P., Titball R.W., Wilson S.A., Rice D.W. 2011. A Burkholderia pseudomallei toxin inhibits helicase activity of translation factor eIF4A.Science, 2011. 334: pp. 821–824
30. Ulrich R.L., DeShazer D., Brueggemann E.E., Hines H.B., Oyston P.C., Jeddeloh J.A. Role of quorum sensing in the pathogenicity of Burkholderia pseudomallei. Journal of Medical Microbiology, 2004. 53: pp. 1053-1064
31. Chan Y.Y., Bian H.S., Tan T.M., Mattmann M.E.,Geske G.D., Igarashi J., Hatano T., Suga H., Blackwell H.E., Chua K.L. Control of quorum sensing by a Burkholderia pseudomallei multidrug efflux pump. Journal of Bacteriology, 2007. 189: pp. 4320–4324
32. D'Cruze T., Gong L., Treerat P., Ramm G., Boyce J.D., Prescott M., Adler B., Devenish R.J. Role for the Burkholderia pseudomallei Type Three Secretion System Cluster 1 bpscN Gene in Virulence. Infection and Immunity, 2011. 79: pp. 3659-3664
33. Lee S., Nathan S. Burkholderia pseudomallei: an update on disease, virulence and host interactions. Malaysian Applied Biology Journal, 2013. 42: pp. 1-14
34. Stevens M.P., Wood M.W., Taylor L.A., Monaghan P., Hawes P., Jones P.W., Wallis T.S., Galyov E.E. An Inv/Mxi-Spalike type III protein secretion system in Burkholderia pseudomallei modulates intracellular behaviour of the pathogen. Molecular Microbiology, 2002. 46: pp. 649–659
35. Chen Y., Wong J., Sun G.W., Liu Y., Tan G-Y. G., Gan Y-H. Regulation of Type VI Secretion System during Burkholderia pseudomallei Infection. Infection and Immunity, 2011. 79: pp. 3064–3073
36. Schwarz S., West T.E., Boyer F., Chiang W-C., Carl M.A., Hood R.D., Rohmer L., Tolker-Nielsen T., Skerrett S.J., Mougous J.D. Burkholderia Type VI Secretion Systems Have Distinct Roles in Eukaryotic and Bacterial Cell Interactions. Public Library of Science (PLoS) Pathogens, 2010. 6: pp. e1001068
37. Jones A.L., Beveridge T.J., Woods D.E. Intracellular Survival of Burholderia pseudomallei. Infection and Immunity, 1996. 64: pp. 782-790
38. White N.J. Melioidosis. Lancet, 2003. 361: pp. 1715-1722
39. Steinmetz I., Rohde M., Brenneke B. Purification and Characterization of an Exopolysaccharide of Burkholderia (Pseudomonas) pseudomallei. Infection and Immunity, 1995. 63: pp. 3959-3965
40. Arjcharoen S., Wikraiphat C., Pudla M., Limposuwan K., Woods D.E., Sirisinha S., Utaisincharoen P. Fate of a Burkholderia pseudomallei Lipopolysaccharide Mutant in the Mouse Macrophage Cell Line RAW 264.7: Possible Role for the O-Antigenic Polysaccharide Moiety of Lipopolysaccharide in Internalization and Intracellular Survival. Infection and Immunity, 2007. 75: pp. 4298-4304
41. Utaisincharoen P., Anuntagool N., Limposuwan K., Chaisuriya P., Sirisinha S. Involvement of Beta Interferon in Enhancing Inducible Nitric Oxide Synthase Production and Antimicrobial Activity of Burkholderia pseudomallei-Infected Macrophages. Infection and Immunity, 2003. 71: pp. 3053-3057.
42. Ekchariyawat P., Pudla S., Limposuwan K., Arjcharoen S., Sirisinha S., Utaisincharoen P. Burkholderia pseudomallei-Induced Expression of Suppressor of Cytokine Signaling 3 (SOCS3) and Cytokine-Inducible Src Homology 2-Containing Protein (CIS) in Mouse Macrophages: a Possible Mechanism for Suppression of the Response to Gamma Interferon Stimulation. Infection and Immunity, 2005. 73: pp. 7332-7339.
43. Harley V. S., Dance D. A. B., Drasar B.J., Tovey G. Effects of Burkholderia pseudomallei and Other Burkholderia Species on Eukaryotic Cells in Tissue Culture. Microbios, 1998. 96: pp. 71-93.

44. Kespichayawattana W., Rattanachetkul S., Wanun T., Utaisincharoen P., Sirisinha S. 2000. Burkholderia pseudomallei Induces Cell Fusion and Actin-Associated Membrane Protrusion: a Possible Mechanism for Cell-to-Cell Spreading. Infection and Immunity, 2000. 68: pp. 5377-5384

45. Poe R.H., Vassallo C.L., Domm B.M. Melioidosis: The Remarkable Imitator. American Review of Respiratory Diseases, 1971. 104: pp. 427-431

46. Pongrithsukda V., Simakachorn N., Pimda J. Childhood Melioidosis in Northeastern Thailand. The Southeast Asian Journal of Tropical Medicine and Public Health, 1988. 19: pp. 309-316

47. Ashdown L.R., Duffy V.A., Douglas R.A. Melioidosis. Medical Journal of Australia, 1980. 5: pp. 314–316

48. Inglis T.J.J., Sagripanti J-L. Environmental Factors that Affect the Survival and Persistence of Burkholderia pseudomallei. Minireview. Applied and Environmental Microbiology, 2006. 72: pp. 6865-6875

49. Loveleena, Chaudhry R., Dhawan B. Melioidosis; the Remarkable Imitator: Recent Perspectives. The Journal of the Association of Physicians of India, 2004. 52: pp. 417-420

50. The Center for Food Security & Public Health. Iowa State University. Melioidosis. Revised November 30, 2007. Retrieved October 15, 2009. Website: www.cfsph. iastate.edu/Factsheets/pdfs/Melioidosis.pdf

51. Kanaphun P., Thirawattanasuk N., Suputtamongkol Y. Naigowit P., Dance D.A., Smith M.D., White N.J. Serology and Carriage of Pseudomonas pseudomallei: a Prospective Study in 1000 Hospitalized Children in Northeast Thailand. The Journal of Infectious Disease, 1993. 167: pp. 230-233

52. Ostler H.B., Maibach H.I., Hoke A.W., Schwab I.R. Diseases of the Eyes and Skin: A Color Atlas. Philadelphia: Lippincott, Williams and Wilkins. 2004. pp. 247-248

53. Goshorn R.K. Recrudescent Pulmonary Melioidosis. A Case Report Involving the So-Called "Vietnamese Time Bomb." Indiana Medicine, 1987. 80: pp. 247-249

54. Currie B.J., Jacups S.P. Intensity of Rainfall and Severity of Melioidosis, Australia. Emerging Infectious Diseases, 2003. 9: pp. 1538-1542

55. Vietri N.J., Deshazer D. Melioidosis. Medical Aspects of Biological Warfare. Chapter 7. Washington D.C.: The Surgeon General United States Army Medical Department Medical Center and School Borden Institute. 2007. pp. 147-166

56. Woods M.L., Currie B.J., Howard D.M., Tierney A., Watson A., Anstey N.M., Philpott J., Asche V., Withnall K. Neurological Melioidosis: Seven Cases from the Northern Territory of Australia. Clinical Infectious Diseases, 1992. 15: pp. 163-169

57. Ereno I.L., Mariano N., Reyes J., Amando C. Melioidosis: a Case Report. Philippine Journal of Microbiology and Infectious Diseases, 2002. 31: pp. 125-133

58. Wuthiekanun V., Desakorn V., Wongsuvan G., Amornchai P., Cheng A.C., Maharjan B., Limmathurotsakul D., Chierakul W., White N.J., Day N.P.J., Peacock S.J. Rapid Immunofluorscence Microscopy for Diagnosis of Melioidosis. Clinical and Diagnostic Laboratory Immunology, 2005. 12: pp. 555-556

59. Ashdown L.R. An Improved Screening Technique for Isolation of Pseudomonas pseudomallei from Clinical Specimens. Pathology, 1979. 11: pp. 293-297

60. Walsh A.L., Smith M.D., Wuthiekanun V. Suputtamongkol Y., Desakorn V., Chaowagul W., White N.J. Immunofluorescence Microscopy for the Rapid Diagnosis of Melioidosis. Journal of Clinical Pathology, 1994. 47: pp. 377-379

61. Dharaqkul T., Songsivilai S., Smithikarn S., Thepthai C., Leelaporn A. Rapid Identification of Burkholderia pseudomallei in Blood Cultures by Latex Agglutination using Lipopolysaccharide-specific Monoclonal Antibody. American Journal of Tropical Medicine and Hygiene, 1999. 61: pp. 658-662

62. Ashdown L.R. Indirect Haemagglutination Test for Melioidosis. The Medical Journal of Australia, 1987. 147: pp. 364-365

63. Ashdown L.R. Relationship and Significance of Specific Immunoglobulin M Antibody Response in Clinical and Subclinical Melioidosis. Journal of Clinical Microbiology, 1981. 14: pp. 361-364

64. Khupulsup K., Petchclai B. Application of Indirect Hemagglutination Test and Indirect Fluorescent Antibody Test for IgM Antibody for Diagnosis of Melioidosis in Thailand. American Journal of Tropical Medicine and Hygiene, 1986. 35: pp. 366-369

65. Tanpiboonsak S., Paemanee A., Sasinee Bunyarataphan S., Tungpradabkul S. PCR-RFLP Based Differentiation of Burkholderia mallei and Burkholderia pseudomallei. Molecular and Cellular Probes, 2004. 18: pp. 97-101

66. Dharakul T., Songsivilai S., Viriyachitra S., Luangwedchakarn V., Tassaneetritap B., Chaowagul W. Detection of Burkholderia pseudomallei DNA in Patients with Septicemic Melioidosis. Journal of Clinical Microbiology, 1996. 34: 609–614

67. Gee J.E., Sacchi C.T., Glass M.B., De B.K., Weyant R.S., Levett P.N., Whitney A.M., Hoffmaster A.R., Popovic T. Use of 16S rRNA Gene Sequencing for Rapid Identification and Differentiation of Burkholderia pseudomallei and B. mallei. Journal of Clinical Microbiology, 2003. 41: pp. 4647-4654

68. Thibault F.M., Hernandez E., Vidal D.R., Girardet M., Cavallo J.D. Antibioic Susceptibility of 65 isolates of Burkholderia pseudomallei and Burkholderia mallei to 35 Antimicrobial Agents. Journal of Antimicrobial Chemotherapy, 2004. 54: pp. 1134-1138

69. Cheng A.C., Fisher D.A., Anstey N.M., Stephens D.P., Jacups S.P., Currie B.J. Outcomes of Patients with Melioidosis Treated with Meropenem. Antimicrobial Agents and Chemotherapy, 2004. 48: pp. 1763-1765

70. White N.J., Dance D.A., Chaowagul W., Wattanagoon Y., Wuthiekanun V., Pitakwatchara N. Halving of Mortality of Severe Melioidosis by ceftazidime. Lancet, 1989. 2: pp. 697-701

71. Cheng A.C., Stephens D.P., Anstey N.M., Currie B.J. Adjunctive Granulocyte Colony-Stimulating Factor for Treatment of Septic Shock due to Melioidosis. Clinical Infectious Diseases, 2004. 38: pp. 32-37

72. Chaowagul W., Suputtamongkol Y., Dance D.A., Rajchanuvong A., Pattara-arechachai J., White N.J. Relapse in Melioidosis: Incidence and Risk Factors. The Journal of Infectious Disease, 1993. 168: pp. 1181-1185

73. Currie B.J., Fisher D.A., Anstey N.M., Jacups S. Melioidosis: Acute and Chronic Disease, Relapse and Re-activation. Transactions of the Royal Society of Tropical Medicine and Hygiene, 2000. 94: pp. 301-304

74. Rajchanuvong A., Chaowagul W., Suputtamongkol Y., Smith M.D., Dance D.A.B., White N.J. A Prospective of Co-amoxiclav and the Combination of Chloramphenicol, doxycycline, and Co-trimoxazole for the Oral Maintenance Treatment of Melioidosis. Transactions of the Royal Society of Tropical Medicine and Hygiene, 1995. 89: pp. 546-549

75. Chetchotisakd P., Chaowagul W., Mootsikapun P., Budhsarawong D., Thinkamrop B. Maintenance Therapy of Melioidosis with Ciprofloxacin plus Azithromycin Compared with Co-trimoxazole plus Doxycycline. American Journal of Tropical Medicine and Hygiene, 2001. 64: pp. 24-27

76. Warawa J., Woods D.E. Melioidosis Vaccines. Expert Reviews of Vaccines, 2002. 1: pp. 477-482

Photo Bibliography

Figure 2.4-1: Scanning electron photomicrograph of Burkholderia pseudomallei. Photomicrograph was taken by Janice Haney Carr and released by the CDC. Public domain photo

Figure 2.4-3: B. pseudomallei infection diagram. The human anatomical illustration is created by Dr. Alexander J. da Silva and Melanie Moser in 2003. The illustration is released by the CDC. Public domain graphics

Figure 2.4-4: Air mobile assault by US troops during the Vietnam War. It is believed that the dust produced by the helicopter blades inadvertently aerosolized the microbe thereby leading to its subsequent transmission. This photo was released by the United States Army. Public domain photo

Figure 2.4-5: B. pseudomallei surviving inside a human macrophage. This transmission electron micrograph was taken by Dr. Frank Gherardini and released by the National Institute of Allergy and Infectious Diseases. Public domain photo

Figure 2.4-6: Computed tomography scan showing prostatic abscess. This photograph was taken by Dr. Bart Currie of the Royal Darwin Hospital, Australia and released by the United States Army Medical Department, Borden Institute. Public domain photo

Figure 2.4-7: Chest radiograph demonstrating a severe multilobar pneumonia. This radiograph was taken by Dr. Bart Currie of the Royal Darwin Hospital, Australia and released by the United States Army Medical Department, Borden Institute. Public domain photo

Figure 2.4-8: Computed tomography scan showing multiloculated liver abscess. This photograph was taken by Dr. Bart Currie of the Royal Darwin Hospital, Australia and released by the United States Army Medical Department, Borden Institute. Public domain photo

Figure 2.4-9: A photograph of the colonial morphology displayed by Gram-negative B. pseudomallei bacteria grown on sheep's blood agar for a 48 hour at a temperature of 37°C. The photograph was taken by Dr. Todd Parker, Audra Marsh in 2010 and released by the CDC

Clostridium botulinum is a spore forming, obligate anaerobe, Gram-positive bacilli (0.5 to 2.0 μm in width and 1.6-22.0 μm in length) and is the etiologic agent of botulism (Figure 2.5-1).[1] *C. botulinum* consists of 4 genetically diverse groups that would be considered different species, except for their common characteristic of producing botulinum neurotoxins (BoNT).[2] BoNT is the most toxic substance known to man and is estimated to have a median lethal dose (LD_{50}) of 0.5 to 5.0 ng/kg in mice and ~1 ng/kg in humans.[3] The Center for Disease Control (CDC) has categorized *C. botulinum* and its neurotoxins as a Category A biological warfare agent because it possesses the greatest potential for mass dissemination, as well as, mass casualties.[4]

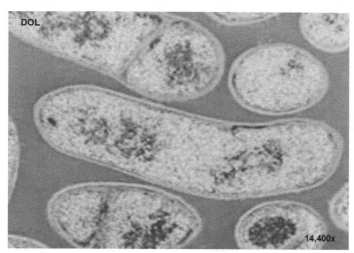

Figure 2.5-1: Electron photomicrograph of *Clostridium botulinum*

The history of the development and use of BoNTs as a biological weapons began in 1937, during the Japanese occupation of Manchuria. The Japanese biological warfare command, Unit 731, headed by General Shiro Ishii developed and manufactured numerous biological warfare agents including lethal cultures of *C. botulinum* and experimented on prisoners of war with them.[5] During World War II, the concerns over the weaponization of botulinum neurotoxin by Germany as a cross-channel weapon against invading Allied forces prompted the United States, Great Britain and Canada to initiate a biological warfare programs of their own with their primary focus on *B. anthracis* (discussed in chapter 2.1) and *C. botulinum* neurotoxins which the Allies termed *Agent X*.[6, 7, 8] The fear of weaponized BoNT prompted the US to prepare over one million doses of formalin-inactivated botulinum toxoid vaccine for the Allied troops in preparation for the D-Day invasion. However, for reasons not expanded upon in the official history, the invading Allied troops were never vaccinated.[8, 9]

The offensive production of biological weapons by the United States was terminated between the years of 1969 and 1970 via executive order from President Richard Nixon. By April 10th, 1972 the United States became one of the signatories of the Convention on the Prohibition of the Development, Production and Stockpiling of Bacteriological (Biological) and Toxin Weapons and on their Destruction, along with the Soviet Union, and many other nations, such as, Iraq.[10] Although the United States abided by the treaty and proceeded with the decommission and destruction of the entire stock of biological warfare agents, the Soviet Union and Iraq regarded the disarmament agreement as a 'worthless piece of paper.' In response to the treaty, both Soviet Union and Iraq actually expanded their offensive biological warfare

programs.[11] For instance, the Soviet Union stockpiled and tested the effectiveness of BoNT up to the 1990's, along with numerous other biological agents, at Aralsk-7 on Vozrozhdeniye Island in the Aral Sea.[9, 11]

After the first Persian Gulf War in 1991, Iraq admitted to the inspection team from the United Nations, that they had produced 4900 gallons of concentrated BoNT for use in specifically designed missiles and bombs.[12, 13] It is interesting to note, that Iraq under the leadership of Saddam Hussein, weaponized more BoNT than any other biological warfare agent (Figure 2.5-2).[9] In addition to state sponsored biological warfare programs, BoNT has also been used in terrorist attacks on civilian populations. For example, Aum Shinrikyo, a Japanese cult responsible for the deadly 1995 Tokyo subway sarin gas attack, also produced and attempted to disseminate botulinium neurotoxin. On at least three occasions between 1990 and 1995, the cult attempted botulinum assaults on Tokyo subway stations; fortunately the attempts failed to produce any casulties.[14]

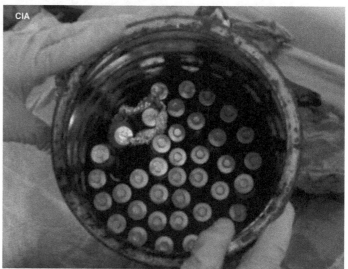

Figure 2.5-2: 97 vials of live *C. botulinum* bacilli from which biological weapons could be produced. These vials were found hidden in the home of an Iraqi biological weapon scientist in 2002 during an United Nations Special Commission (UNSCOM) weapons inspection

C. botulinum bacteria are ubiquitous, they are widely distributed in soil, marine sediments and even in the intestinal tract of domestic grazing animals, where they generally pose no threat. Nonetheless, under appropriate anaerobic conditions (environmental or laboratory), the endospores of these organisms can germinate into vegetative cells that produce BoNT.[12, 15, 16]

C. botulinum is known to produce seven antigenically distinct neurotoxins. These neurotoxins are structurally similar and have been designated by the letters A through G: serotypes A, B, C (C_1, C_2), D, E, F, G. It is also known that the unique strain *C. baratii* produces only neurotoxin F, while *C. butyricum* produces only neurotoxin E.[12, 17, 18, 19] The toxin types are defined by their lack of cross-neutralization when antitoxins are applied. For example, anti-A antitoxin does not neutralize neurotoxins B thru G.[9] Most human botulism is caused by neurotoxin A, B, and E, and only occasional cases can be attributed to neurotoxin F. Neurotoxins C and D may potentially cause botulism in humans but are known to instigate this disease in mammals. As mentioned previously, neurotoxin E causes botulism in humans, but will also instigate

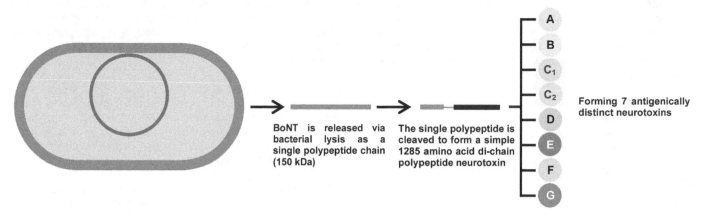

Figure 2.5-3: *C. botulinum,* producing 8 antigenically distinct neurotoxins (A-G). Please note that C_1 and C_2 are classified as neurotoxin C

botulism in fish. Finally, neurotoxin G has not been shown to cause neuroparalytic disease in humans but has been associated with sudden death with five cases in Switzerland. Neurotoxin G is produced by *Clostridium argentinense,* which was discovered in 1969 (Figure 2.5-3).[8, 12, 20]

There are four groups of botulin toxin producing *Clostridium* spp. Group I are proteolytic organisms producing A, B, or F neurotoxins. The optimal growth temperature for Group I organisms is 35°-40° C. Group II are non-proteolytic organisms producing B, E, or F neurotoxins. The optimal growth temperature for Group I organisms is 18° to 25° C. Group III organisms span from slightly proteolytic to non-proteolytic. These organisms produce C or D neurotoxins and grow optimally at 25°-45° C. Finally, Group IV organisms are proteolytic and they produce G neurotoxin. The optimal growth temperature for Group IV organisms is 35 to 40° C.[20]

In addition to being antigenically distinct, the seven botulinum neurotoxins have different toxicities and lengths of persistence in nerve cells.[21, 22] Nonetheless, all BoNT serotypes act to inhibit acetylcholine (Ach) release. Although they have different intracellular protein targets, they exhibit different periods of effects and have different potencies.[21]

Table 1: *C. botulinum* subgroups and the toxins that they produce. Please note that C_1 and C_2 are classified under neurotoxin C

Groups	A	B	C_1	C_2	D	E	F	G
I	■	■					■	
II		■				■	■	
III			■	■	■			
IV								■

In general, botulinum neurotoxins are synthesized as a single polypeptide chain (150 kDa) and are released from the organism via cell lysis. Subsequently, bacterial or tissue proteases cleave the toxins at a protease sensitive loop location within the structure of the toxin, and generate a simple 1285 amino acid di-chain polypeptide, consisting of 100 kDa heavy chain. The heavy chain is composed of a 50 kDa amino terminal H_N domain and a 50 kDa carboxy-terminal H_C domain jointed by a single interchain disulfide bond to 50 kDa zinc containing endopeptidase light chains (L domain is an example of zinc metalloprotease). This neurotoxin has a three dimensional structure of 3.3A resolution (Figure 2.5-4).[9, 23, 24, 25, 26] The lone exception to the overall molecular structure of BoNT is neurotoxin C_2. BoNT-C_2 is constructed with two separate protein components (C_2I and C_2II) that are not joined by a disulfide bond. BoNT-C_2II (~80 kDa) is involved in the transport of the enzymatic component into the cytosol of the

targeted cell via a raft-dependent mechanism. BoNT-C_2I (~49 kDa) is the enzymatically active subunit composed of ADP-ribosyltransferase.[27, 28, 29]

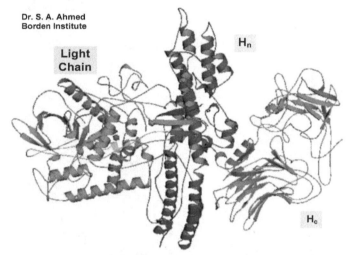

Figure 2.5-4: Computer generated image of botulinum neurotoxin A is composed of a ~50 kDa light chain (red) and an ~100 kDa heavy chain linked by a single disulfide bond. The heavy chain contains two functional ~50 kDa domains: a C-terminal ganglioside binding domain (H_C-purple), and an N-terminal translocation domain (H_n-blue). A belt portion of H_n (green) wraps around the light chain

BoNTs can gain entry into the human body via the respiratory tract, gastrointestinal tract and wounds (Figure 2.5-5). Once they are absorbed within the body, they proceed into the circulatory system and are transported to the peripheral cholinergic synapses at the neuromuscular junctions and sympathetic autonomic junctions. At the neuromuscular junctions, the H_C chains of the neurotoxin mediate binding to the high affinity presynaptic receptors (e.g. polysialoganglioside) and are subsequently incorporated into endocytic vesicles containing an ATPase proton pump. The ensuing acidification of the vesicular lumen (lowers to ~pH 4.5) alters the structure of the toxin, where the H_N domain is incorporated into the membrane and the L domain is translocated into the cytosol of the affected cholinergic nerve cell. Once inside the targeted nerve cell, the zinc containing endopeptidase light chain (L domain) of the neurotoxin targets and blocks Achylcholine-containing vesicles from fusing with the terminal membrane of the neuron.[8, 9, 12, 30] For example, there are three proteins that are involved in cellular exocytosis: synaptosomal-associated protein-25 (SNAP-25), synaptobrevin 2 (VAMP2) and syntaxin 1A, which belong to a family of Q-SNARE proteins that are involved in exocytosis. The

179

disruption of any one of the three proteins will prevent vesicle docking and subsequent nerve impulse transmission. The zinc metalloprotease (L domain) of BoNT-A cleaves 9 amino acids from the c-terminus of SNAP-25, while BoNT-E cleaves 26 amino acids from the c-terminus of SNAP-25. Other BoNT serotypes-B, -D, -F and -G target and cleave VAMP 2. BoNT-C$_1$ is known for its dual function: cleaving SNAP-25, as well as, syntaxin 1A. It has been reported that BoNT-C$_1$ also blocks other co-transmitter releases resulting in neuromuscular paralysis. BoNT-C$_2$, on the other hand, possesses a different course of action within the host cell. For example, once released into the cytosol through the actions of C$_2$II, C$_2$I proceeds through ADP-ribosylation of monomeric G-actins at the molecular position of arginine 177. The actions of C$_2$I effectively prohibits the polymerization of G-actin and largely interrupts ATP binding and ATPase activity. Because of the enzymatic actions of C$_2$I, the actin cytoskeleton structure of the targeted cell will break down, leading to cellular rounding and cell death (Table 2).[9, 12, 27, 28, 29, 31, 32, 33, 34, 35, 36]

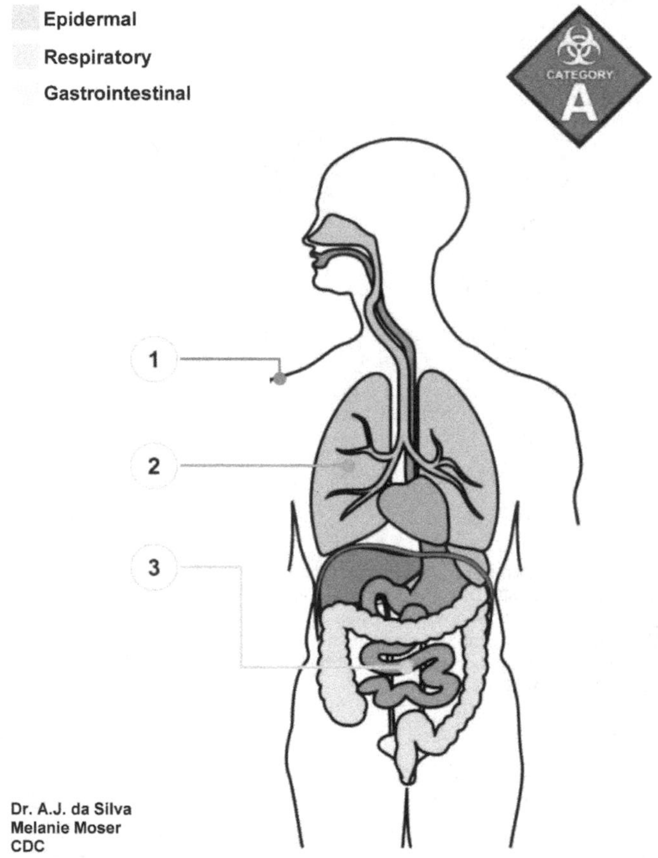

Epidermal

Respiratory

Gastrointestinal

1

2

3

Dr. A.J. da Silva
Melanie Moser
CDC

Figure 2.5-5: A diagram demonstrating the possible routes of infection for BoNT. ① BoNT can be introduced via epidermal cuts/ abrasion. ② BoNT can be introduced via respiratory tract. ③ BoNT can be introduced via gastrointestinal tract

The direct BoNT effect on the central nervous system (CNS) occurs via retrograde axonal transport, since the size of the toxin (150 kDa) is too large to penetrate the blood brain barrier. Nonetheless, it has been reported that retrograde axonal transport is so slow, that the BoNT may be inactivated before it reaches the CNS.[36]

The exact lethal dose of BoNT for humans is not known but can be extrapolated from data obtained from various animal models. For example, the lethal dose for BoNT type A for an individual weighing 70 kg (154.3 pounds) is calculated to be 0.09 to 0.15 μg intravenously or intramuscularly, 0.70 to 0.90 μg through the respiratory tract and 70 μg through the digestive tract.[9, 21]

Although BoNT is regarded as the most toxic substance known to man, it is also the first microbial protein administered by injection as a therapeutic agent in humans.[8, 37] The credit for pioneering BoNT's clinical applications goes to Dr. Alan Scott who investigated BoNT serotype A as a treatment for strabismus. Scott discovered that an injection of a few picograms (1 trillionth 10^{-12} of a gram) would induce paralysis to the targeted muscles.[38] Some of the clinical applications of BoNT include blepharospasm, periocular muscle contractions, cervical dystonia, dynamic equinus foot deformity, hemifacial spasm, hyperhidrosis, strabismus, post stroke spasticity and improvement of glabellar lines. Presently, BoNT serotype A is packaged and sold under the brand names of Botox®, Dysport® and Xeomin®, while BoNT serotype B is approved for therapeutic use, and is market as Myobloc® and Neurobloc®.[33, 37]

SYMPTOMS

If left untreated, botulism is frequently fatal. The duration until the onset of symptoms, as well as, the severity of the illness depends on the amount and the serotype of BoNT that was introduced.[4] For example, BoNT-A generally displays initial symptoms 0-7 days and results in a more severe disease. BoNT-A is often associated with bulbar and skeletal muscle impairment, therefore, patients generally require the aid of mechanical ventilation for approximately two weeks to seven months. Patients exposed to BoNT-B typically begin to display symptoms between 0 to 5 days, while exposure to BoNT-E will result in a shorter incubation period estimated to be 0 to 2 days. It has been reported that patients who come into contact with BoNT-B or -E, generally display signs of autonomic dysfunction, including symptoms of internal ophthalmoplegia, non-reactive dilated pupils (mydriasis) and dry mouth.[12, 20, 39, 40] Overall, the estimated incubation period is between 12 to 72 hours, with a median of ~24 hours for all BoNT serotypes.[12, 41]

Regardless of the route of introduction, this family of neurotoxins produces similar neurological signs that we recognize as botulism. Individuals with foodborne botulism often display initial gastrointestinal symptoms of nausea, vomiting, abdominal cramps, pains and diarrhea before signs of neurological distress appear. Alternatively, individuals that acquire botulism

Table 2: Summary of BoNT enzymatic actions within the targeted cells

Neurotoxin Type	Target	Cytosol Substrate	Cleavage site
A	Human	SNAP-25	Gln 197-Arg198
B	Human	VAMP 2	Gln76-phe77
C$_1$	Mammals	SNAP-25, syntaxin 1A	Arg198-Ala199; Lys253-Ala254
C$_2$	Mammals	ADP-ribosylation of G-actins	Arg177
D	Mammals	VAMP 2	Lys59-Leu60
E	Human, fish	SNAP-25	Arg180-Lle181
F	Human	VAMP 2	Gln58-Lys59
G	Human	VAMP 2	Ala81-Ala82

through the respiratory tract or from wounds will not exhibit any gastrointestinal symptoms, but will immediately display indications of neurological dysfunctions.[42]

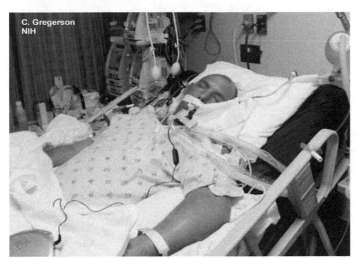

Figure 2.5-6: Utilization of mechanical ventilation for a patient suffering from respiratory failure

Table 3: An overview of the clinical symptoms of BoNT poisoning

Symptoms	+	++	+++
Nausea			■
Vomiting			■
Abdominal cramps/pains			■
Diarrhea			■
Dryness of the mouth			■
Blurred vision			■
Nystagmus			■
Ptosis			■
Diplopia			■
Ophthalmoplegia			■
Photophobia			■
Dysarthria			■
Dysphonia			■
Dysphagia			■
Descending paralysis			■
Acute flaccid paralysis			■
Extremity weaknesses		■	
Fatigue		■	
Respiratory Difficulties		■	
Respiratory failure		■	
Dizziness		■	
Sore throat		■	
Mucous plug (throat)		■	
Difficulties in swallowing		■	
Constipation		■	
Internal ophthalmoplegia		■	
Mydriasis		■	

+ Rare ++ Common +++ Frequent

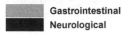
Gastrointestinal
Neurological

Initial neurological indications generally involve the cranial nerves with patients displaying dryness of the mouth, blurred vision, nystagmus, ptosis, diplopia, ophthalmoplegia and photophobia. Additional symptoms of secondary to fixed pupillary dilation with palsies of oculomotor nerve (III), trochlear nerve (IV) and abducens nerve (VI).[20] These initial symptoms, are followed by signs of bulbar nerve dysfunction, where patients will display signs of dysarthria, dysphonia and dysphagia.[8, 42, 43, 44] Soon after, patients will display muscular dysfunction in the form of asthenia. For example, signs of muscle weakness will initiate among the muscles controlling head movements, muscles of the upper extremities, respiratory muscles and finally muscles of the lower extremities. The signs of muscle weakness of the extremities usually proceed symmetrically in a proximal to distal fashion (e.g. symmetric descending paralysis), although on occasion asymmetric extremity weaknesses could also be observed. The onset of acute flaccid paralysis generally occurs 18-36 hours after exposure (range: 6 hours to 8 days). Weaknesses in the muscles of the respiratory tract generally lead to respiratory failure, which will require the use of mechanical ventilation. Ventilation support is generally needed for 2 to 8 weeks (Figure 2.5-6). Recovery of patients generally follows the generation of new neuromuscular connections.[8, 12, 39, 42, 45] Other commonly reported symptoms involved in BoNT induced neurological dysfunctions are fatigue, dizziness, sore throat, mucous plug in the throat, dry mouth, difficulty in swallowing and constipation. Fatalities generally result from respiratory failure and/or secondary infection that require prolonged mechanical ventilation (Table 3).[8, 12, 39, 42, 43]

Symptoms associated with infant botulism always seem to develop suddenly. One possible reason for this sudden onset may be the inability of infants to verbalize their complaints in regards to the early effects of botulism.[42] Signs of infant botulism include poor feeding, diminished suckling, difficulties swallowing, reduced crying capability, hypotonia, pooled oral secretions, constipation (~3 to 4 days without defecation), weakness of the muscles of the neck and peripheries, resulting in the description "floppy babies" (Figure 2.5-7).

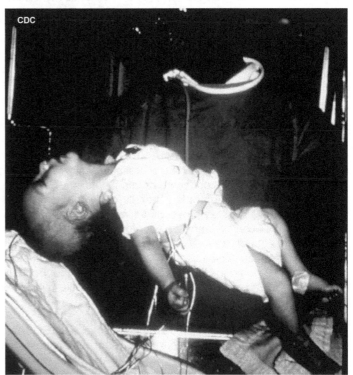

Figure 2.5-7: Six month old infant suffering from botulism. Please note the loss of muscle tone, especially in the region of the head and neck

Other symptoms may include loss of facial expression, ptosis, ophthalmoplegia, extraocular muscle paralysis, dilated pupils (mydriasis), dry mouth, neurogenic bladder and depression of deep tendon reflex; however, these symptoms have been associated more with BoNT serotype B, than with serotype A.[42, 43, 46, 47, 48] Weaknesses in the muscles of the respiratory tract are also commonly observed, which will generally lead to respiratory failure and require the use of mechanical ventilation. With proper diagnosis and treatment, infant botulism fatalities are extremely rare (less than 2%) (Table 4).[42]

Table 4: An overview of the clinical symptoms of infant BoNT poisoning. The abbreviated term 'extra' stands for extraocular and 'depress' means depression

Symptoms	+	++	+++
Poor feeding			▪
Diminished suckling			▪
Difficulties swallowing			▪
Reduce crying			▪
Hypotonia			▪
Pooled oral secretions			▪
Constipation			▪
Muscle weakness (neck)			▪
Muscle weakness (gen.)			▪
Loss of facial expression		▪	
Ptosis		▪	
Ophthalmoplegia		▪	
Extra. muscle paralysis		▪	
Mydriasis		▪	
Dry mouth		▪	
Neurogenic		▪	
Bladder		▪	
Deep tendon reflex depr.		▪	
Weak respiratory muscle		▪	

+ Rare ++ Common +++ Frequent

DETECTION

In general, botulism can be tentatively diagnosed by clinical symptoms through the process of eliminating other potential neurological ailments. Because of the importance of immediate and early treatment, botulism must be initially diagnosed on the basis of history and physical examination findings.[20] Definitive diagnosis of botulism requires identification of the toxin from the sera, feces, blood, vomit, gastric aspirates, respiratory secretions or in the case of possible foodborne poisoning, examining the samples of food may prove useful. Nonetheless, the availability of properly equipped and qualified laboratories may prove to be a limitation.[49]

Feces, in general, are the most reliable sample for the identification of BoNT in foodborne or infant botulism. Since, the amount of BoNT is minute it is generally not detected in blood samples of adults but may prove useful in detecting neurotoxins in infants. BoNT can be identified via mouse inoculation studies (e.g. mouse neutralization test), where mice are injected with specimen samples suspected to contain BoNT. This mouse bioassay can detect as little as 0.03 ng of BoNT and if BoNT is present, the injected mice will usually die from botulism within 6 to 96 hours.[9, 12, 49, 50]

Toxin assays, such as enzyme linked immunoassays (ELISAs), or electrochemilumine-scent tests (ECL) can demonstrate the presence of BoNT from collected specimens. For example, BoNT can be detected in ~37% of sera, ~23% fecal samples, and in ~5% of gastric aspirates. The sooner the samples from patients can be tested, the more likely a positive test result will be obtained.[12, 41] Serology is not useful in detecting BoNT, since the minute amount of neurotoxin present rarely promotes antibody development (Figure 2.5-8).[49]

Positive identification of BoNT introduced into a patient via the respiratory route may be difficult, since the neurotoxin may not be identifiable using serum or stool samples. Positive identification of BoNT may be obtained through nasal swabs, up to 24 hours post-exposure via ELISA or polymerase chain reaction test.[8, 12, 51, 52]

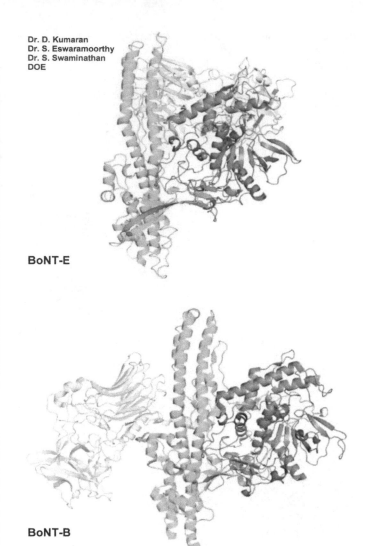

Dr. D. Kumaran
Dr. S. Eswaramoorthy
Dr. S. Swaminathan
DOE

BoNT-E

BoNT-B

Figure 2.5-8: Computer-generated molecular structure of botulinum neruotoxin subtypes E and B

TREATMENT

Supportive therapy is still the mainstay of botulism. Patients suffering from botulism generally require parenteral nutrition via an enteral tube, since acute flaccid paralysis may have incapacitated the patient's ability to ingest or swallow. Mechanical ventilation may also be required due to respiratory difficulties and/ or failure. In addition, magnesium containing cathartic agents should not be used due to the theoretical concern that increased magnesium levels may enhance the action of BoNT.[9, 45]

Passive immunization of BoNT equine antitoxin needs to be administered as early as possible following the positive identification of the neurotoxin. Currently, the only available treatment for botulism is the CDC-sponsored, Food and Drug Administration (FDA) Investigational New Drug (IND) protocol heptavalent botulinum antitoxin (H-BAT) manufactured by Cangene Corporation. H-BAT replaces a licensed bivalent botulinum antitoxin AB and an investigational monovalent botulinum antitoxin E (BAT-AB and BAT-E) manufactured by Sanofi Pasteur®. The licence for BAT-AB and BAT-E expired in 2010 and was not renewed.[9, 12, 40, 45, 53, 54, 55]

H-BAT contains equine-derived immune globulin (<2% intact immunoglobulin G (IgG) and ≥90% Fab and F(ab')2 immunoglobulin fragments) to all seven serotypes of BoNT. Each single use vial contains a minimal potency value of 4,500 Units

(U) for serotype A antitoxin, 3,300 U for serotype B antitoxin, 3,000 U for both serotype C and F antitoxin, 600 U serotype D antitoxin, 5,100 U for serotype E antitoxin, and 600 U serotype G antitoxin. H-BAT is administered through slow intravenous infusion after dilution 1:10 in normal saline solution (Table 5).[55, 56] Although the dosage for infant botulism is listed in Table 5, H-BAT is not recommended due to the fear of a hypersensitivity reaction (anaphylaxis).[57] In 2003, the FDA approved a human derived botulism immunoglobulin, known as BabyBIG®, for the treatment of infant botulism. BabyBIG®, produced by Baxter Healthcare Corporation and Cangene Corporation, contains neutralizing antibodies for BoNT serotypes A and B, derived from the pooled plasma of human subjects immunized with botulinum toxoid.[12, 45, 54, 56] The administration of BabyBIG® should begin slowly at 0.5 mL per kg body weight per hour (25 mg/kg/h). If no adverse reaction towards the antitoxin occurs after 15 minutes, the infusion rate to the patient may be increased to 1.0 mL/kg/h (50 mg/kg/h).[58, 59]

Table 5: Recommended dosage for H-BAT. Please note that ① represents starting infusion arte (first 30 minutes), ② represents incremetal infusion rate if tolerated (every 30 minutes) and ③ represents maximum infusion rate

	Dose	1	2	3
A	1 vial	0.5 mL/min	2x rate	2 mL/min
B	20-100% A dose	0.01 mL/kg/min	0.01 mL/kg/min	0.03 mL/kg/min
C	10% A dose	0.01 mL/kg/min	0.01 mL/kg/min	0.03 mL/kg/min

A Adults (≥ 17 years)
B Pediatric (1 to < 17 years)
C Infants (< 1 year)

Due to the insignificant rate of botulism in the U.S., vaccination of the general public is presently deemed unnecessary. Nonetheless, a vaccine was developed by the U.S. Army Medical Research and Material Command (MRMC), at Fort Detrick, Maryland, during the 1950s. The presently available vaccine is a formalin-fixed toxoid, designed to immunize individuals from BoNT A through E and is listed as Investigational New Drug (IND) under license by the CDC. It is suggested that this vaccine be administered at an interval of 0, 2 and 12 weeks, followed by an annual booster dose. Although this vaccine is listed as an IND, it has been administered to approximately 8000 military service personnel during the first Gulf War between January 23rd and February 28th 1991.[8]

DIFFERENTIAL DIAGNOSIS

On average, most clinicians are unfamiliar with the condition and can easily mistaken botulism for other medical afflictions. For example, differential diagnosis for botulism includes Miller-Fisher variant of Guillain-Barré syndrome (MF-GB), myasthenia gravis (MG), stroke, chemical intoxication (e.g. carbon monoxide, barium carbonate, methyl chloride, methyl alcohol, organic phosphorus compound, atropine), Lambert-Eaton myasthenic syndrome (LEMS) and tick paralysis (TP) such as Lyme disease. Other differential diagnosis can include mushroom poisoning, allergic reaction to antibiotics (e.g. neomycin, streptomysin, kanamycin, gentamicin etc.), shellfish poisoning, poliomyelitis, diphtheria and psychiatric illnesses. In the cases of infant botulism, differential diagnosis may include sepsis (e.g. meningitis), electrolyte-mineral imbalance, metabolic enceph-alopathy, Reye syndrome, Werdnig-Hoffman disease, congenital myopathy and Leigh disease.

Electromyogram (EMG) examination with repetitive nerve stimulation at 20-50 Hz may at times differentiate between causes of acute flaccid paralysis. The EMG readings for patient suffering from botulism will demonstrate normal nerve conduction velocity, normal sensory nerve function, a pattern of small amplitude motor potentials and an incremental response to repetitive nerve stimulation at 50 Hz (Table 6 and 7).[9, 44, 60]

References

1. Murray P.R., Rosenthal K.S., Kobayashi G.S., Pfaller M.A. Medical Microbiology. Fourth Edition. St. Louis: Mosby College Publishing, 2002. pp. 347-353
2. Hatheway C.L., Johnson E.A. Clostridium: the Spore-Bearing Anaerobes. Topley & Wilson's Microbiology and Microbial Infections. 9th Edition. New York: Oxford University Press, 1998. pp. 731-782
3. Cai S., Singh B.R., Dharma S. Botulism siagnostics: from clinical symptoms to in vitro assays. Critical Reviews in Microbiology, 2007. 33: pp. 109-125
4. Kwan-Gett T.S.C., Kemp C., Kovarik C. Infectious and Tropical Diseases. St. Louis:

Table 6: Description of selected conditions that displays similar symptoms as botulism[9]

Differential Conditions	Condition Description	Distinguishing Features
Miller-Fisher Variant	Abnormal muscle coordination, paralysis of the eye muscles, absence of the tendon reflexes, generalized asthenia & respiratory failure. This condition may be preceded by a viral illness	A history of antecedent infection, paresthesias, often ascending paralysis, early areflexia & CSF protein increase. EMG findings will demonstrate abnormal nerve conduction velocity and no facilitation with repetitive nerve stimulation
Myasthenia Gravis	Chronic autoimmune neuromuscular disease & is characterized by varying degrees of skeletal muscles asthenia. Patients suffering from this condition show periods of muscle weakness during activity and improve after periods of rest. This condition is caused by a defect in the transmission of nerve impulses to muscles where antibodies produced by the patient target Ach receptors at the neuromuscular junction	This condition will demonstrate recurrent paralysis & sustained response towards anticholinesterase therapy. EMG findings will demonstrate decrease in muscle action potentials with repetitive nerve stimulation
Stroke	Characterized by the rapid loss of brain functions due to the obstruction of blood supply to the brain	This condition is generally characterized by asymmetric paralysis & abnormal CNS imaging
Chemical Intoxication	Chemicals that may produce symptoms of acute flaccid paralysis are carbon monoxide, barium carbonate, methyl chloride, methyl alcohol, organic phosphorus compounds, atropine, etc.	History of exposure and excessive levels of chemicals within body fluids may distinguish chemical intoxication with botulism
Lambert-Eaton syndrome	This condition occurs due to the lack of Ach released at the neuromuscular junction which results in acute flaccid paralysis. Nonetheless, with repeated contraction, Ach may build up in sufficient levels to produce a brief period of normal contractions in the skeletal muscles.	This condition is generally characterized by increased strength with sustained contractions & evidence of lung carcinoma. Nonetheless the EMG readings may be similar to that of botulism
Tick Paralysis	This condition is caused by a neurotoxin produced by ticks and is transmitted to people via tick bite	Parethesias or the tingling, pricking, or numbness of skin is the general characterization of this condition. In addition, the patient will also experience ascending paralysis. EMG reading will demonstrate abnormal nerve conduction velocity & unresponsivness to repetitive stimulation

Table 7: Differential diagnosis of botulism with selected diseases with similar symptoms. These diseases include Miller-Fisher variant of Guillain-Barré syndrome (MF-GB), myasthenia gravis (MG), stroke, Lambert-Eaton myasthenic syndrome (LEMS), tick paralysis (TP) and Reye syndrome

Symptoms	BoNT	MF-GB	MG	Stroke	LEMS	TP	Reye
Nausea	■	■		■		■	■
Vomiting	■	■		■		■	■
Abdominal cramps/pains	■	■					
Diarrhea	■	■		■		■	
Dryness of the mouth	■	■			■		
Fatigue	■	■	■			■	■
Dizziness	■	■				■	
Sore throat	■						
Constipation	■						
Blurred vision	■		■			■	■
Nystagmus	■		■			■	
Ptosis	■	■	■				
Diplopia	■	■	■			■	■
Mydriasis	■		■				
Ophthalmoplegia	■	■	■			■	
Internal ophthalmoplegia	■	■	■			■	
Photophobia	■						
Dysarthria	■	■	■	■		■	■
Dysphonia	■	■	■			■	■
Dysphagia	■	■	■			■	■
Descending paralysis	■						
Acute flaccid paralysis	■					■	
Extremity weaknesses	■	■	■		■	■	■
Mucous plug in the throat	■						
Difficulties in swallowing	■	■	■			■	
Respiratory difficulties	■	■	■			■	■
Respiratory failure	■	■	■			■	■

Elsevier Mosby. 2006. pp. 106-113

5. Hill E.V. Botulism. In: Summary Report on B.W. Investigations. Memorandum to General Alden C. Waitt, Chief, Chemical Corps, Department of the Army, December 12, 1947. Table D. Archived at The Library of Congress, Washington D.C.

6. Cochrane R.C. Biological Warfare Research in the United States. In: History of the Chemical Warfare Service in World War II (1 July 1940 - 15 August 1945). Volume 2. Historical Section, Plans, Training and Intelligence Division, Office of the Chief, Chemical Corps, United States Department of the Army, 1947. Unclassified. Archived at The United States Army Medical Research Institute of Infectious Diseases, Fort Detrick, Maryland

7. Franz D.R., Parrott C.D., Takafuji E.T. The U.S. Biological Warfare and Biological Defense Programs. Medical Aspects of Chemical and Biological Warfare. Washington D.C. Chapter 19. Office of the Surgeon General Department of the Army, United States of America. 1997. pp. 425-436

8. Middlebrook J.L., Franz D.R. Botulinum Toxins. Medical Aspects of Biological Warfare. Chapter 33. Washington D.C.: The Surgeon General United States Army Medical Department Medical Center and School Borden Institute. 2007. pp. 643-654

9. Arnon S.S., Schechter R., Inglesby T.V., Henderson D.A., Bartlett J.G., Ascher M.S., Eitzen E., Fine A.D., Hauer J., Layton M., Lillibridge S., Osterholm M.T., O'Toole T., Parker G., Perl T.M., Russell P.K., Swerdlow D.L., Tonat K. Botulinum Toxin as a Biological Weapon: Medical and Public Health Management. Journal of the American Medical Association, 2001. 285: pp. 1059-1070

10. Convention on the Prohibition of the Development, Production, and Stockpiling of Bacteriological (Biological) and Toxin Weapons and their Destruction. Retrieved May 11, 2006, from United States Department of the State web site. March 26, 1975. Web site: http://www.state.gov/t/ac/trt/4718.htm

11. Davis C.J. Nuclear Blindness: An Overview of the Biological Weapons Programs of the Former Soviet Union and Iraq. Emerging Infectious Diseases, 1999. 5: pp. 509-512

12. Dembek Z. F., Smith L.A., Rusnak J.M. Botulinum Toxin. Medical Aspects of Biological Warfare. Chapter 16. Washington D.C.: The Surgeon General United States Army Medical Department Medical Center and School Borden Institute. 2007. pp. 337-353

13. Zilinskas R.A. Iraq's Biological Weapons: the Past as Future? Journal of the American Medical Association, 1997. 278: pp. 418-424

14. Sugishima M. Aum Shinrikyo and the Japanese Law on Bioterrorism. Prehospital and Disaster Medicine, 2003. 18: pp. 179-183

15. Smith L.D.S. The Occurrence of Clostridium botulinum and Clostridium tetani in the Soil of the United States. Health Laboratory Science, 1978. 15: pp. 74-80

16. Ward B.Q., Carroll B.J., Garrett E.S., Reese G.B. Survey of U.S. Gulf Coast for the Presence of Clostridium botulinum. Applied Microbiology, 1967. 15: pp. 629-636

17. Hall J.D., McCroskey L.M., Pincomb B.J., Hatheway C.L. Isolation of an Organism Resembling Clostridium baratii which Produces type F Botulinal Toxin from an Infant with Botulism. Journal of Clinical Microbiology, 1985. 21: pp. 654-655

18. Aureli P., Fenicia L., Pasolini B., Gianfranceschi M., McCroskey L.M., Hatheway C.L. Two Cases of Type E Infant Botulism Caused by Neurotoxigenic Clostridium butyricum in Italy. The Journal of Infectious Diseases, 1986. 154: pp. 207-211

19. Raphael B.H., Lautenschlager M., Kalb S.R., de Jong L.I.T., Frace M., Lúquez C., Barr J.R., Fernández R.A., Maslanka S.E. Analysis of a unique Clostridium botulinum strain from the Southern hemisphere producing a novel type E botulinum neurotoxin subtype. BioMedical Center (BMC) Microbiology, 2012. 12: pp. 245

20. Zhang J.C., Sun L., Nie Q.H. Botulism, where are we now? Clinical Toxicology, 2010. 48: pp. 867-879

21. Gill D.M. Bacterial Toxins: a Table of Lethal Amounts. Microbiological Reviews, 1982. 46: pp. 86-94

22. Foran O., Mohammed N., Lisk G.O., Nagwaney S., Lawrence G.W., Johnson E., Smith L., Aoki K.R., Dolly J.O. Evaluation of the Therapeutic Usefulness of Botulinum Neurotoxins B, C1, E, and F Compared with the Long Lasting Type A. Bases for Distinct Durations of Inhibition of Exocytosis in Central Neurons. The Journal of Biological Chemistry, 2003. 278: pp. 1363-1371

23. Aoki K.R., Guyer B. Botulinum Toxin Type A and other Botunlinum Tosin Serotypes: a Comparative Review of Biochemical and Pharmacological Actions. European Journal of Neurology, 2001. 8: pp. 21-29

24. Aoki R. Physiology and Pharmacology of Therapeutic Botulinum Neurotoxins. Hyperhidrosis and Botulinum Toxin in Dermatology. Current Problems in Dermatology, 2002. pp. 107-116

25. Lacy D.B., Tepp W., Cohen A.C., DasGupta B.R., Stevens R.C. Crystal Structure of Botulinum Neurotoxin Type A and Implications for Toxicity. Nature Structural Biology, 1998. 5: pp. 898-902

26. Schiavo G., Rossetto O., Tonello F., Montecucco C. Intracellular Targets and Metalloprotease Activity of Tetanus and Botulism Neurotoxins, Current Topics in Microbiology and Immunology, 1995. 195: pp. 257-274

27. Ohishi I., Iwasaki M., Sakaguchi G. Purification and characterization of two components of botulinum C2 toxin. Infection and Immunity, 1980. 30: pp. 668-673

28. Neumeyer T., Schiffler B., Maier E., Lang A.E., Aktories K., Benz R. Clostridium botulinum C2 toxin. Identification of the binding site for chloroquine and related compounds and influence of the binding site on properties of the C2II channel. The Journal of Biological Chemistry (JBC) Papers, 2007. 283: pp. 3904-3914

29. Pust S., Barth H., Sandvig K. Clostridium botulinum C2 toxin is internalized by clathrin- and Rho-dependent mechanisms. Cellular Microbiology, 2010. 12: pp. 1809-1820

30. Kurazono H., Mochida S., Binz T., Eisel U., Quanz M., Grebenstein O., Wernars K., Poulain B., Tauc L., Niemann H. Minimal Essential Domains Specifying Toxicity of the Light Chains of Tetanus Toxin and Botulinum Neurotoxin Type A. The Journal of Biological Chemistry, 1992. 267: pp. 14721-14729

31. Simpson L.L. Identification of the Major Steps in Botulinum Toxin Action. Annual Review of Pharmacology and Toxicology, 2004. 44: pp. 167-193

32. Barr J.R., Moura H., Boyer A.E., Woolfitt A.R., Kalb S.R., Pavlopoulos A., McWilliams L.G., Schmidt J.G., Martinez R.A., Ashley D.L. Botulinum Neurotoxin Detection and Differentiation by Mass Spectrometry. Emerging Infectious Diseases, 2005. 11: pp. 1578-1583

33. Schiavo G., Matteoli M., Montecucco C. Neurotoxins Affecting Neuroexocytosis. Physiological Reviews, 2000. 80: pp. 717-766

34. Erbguth F.J. From Poison to Remedy: the Chequered History of Botulinum Toxin. Journal of Neural Transmission, 2008. 115: pp. 559-565

35. Dolly J.O., Aoki K.R. The Stucture and Mode of Action of Different Botulinum Toxins. Wuropean Journal of Neurology, 2006. 13: pp. 1-9

36. Dressler D., Saberi F.A. Botulinum Toxin: Mechanisms of Action. European Neurology, 2005. 53: pp. 3-9

37. Carruthers J., Carruthers A. The Evolution of Botulinum Neurotoxins Type A for Cosmetic Applications. Journal of Cosmetic and Laser Therapy, 2007. 9: pp. 186-192

38. Scott A. Development of Botulinum Toxin Therapy. Dermatologic Clinics, 2004. 22: pp. 131-133

39. Hughes J.M., Blumenthal J.R., Merson M.H., Lombard G.L., Dowell V.R. Jr., Gangarosa E.J. Clinical Features of Type A and B Foodborne Botulism. Annals of Internal Medicine, 1981. 95: pp. 442-445

40. Tacket C.O., Shandera W.X., Mann J.M. Hargrett N.T., Blake P.A. Equine Antitoxin use and Other Factors that Predict Outcome in Type A Foodborne Botulism. The American Journal of Medicine, 1984. 76: pp. 794-798

41. Woodruff B.A. Griffin A.M., McCroskey L.M., Smart J.F., Wainwright R.B., Bryant R.G., Hutwagner L.C., Hatheway C.L. Clinical and Laboratory Comparison of Botulism from Toxin Types A, B and E in the Unted States, 1975-1988. The Journal of Infectious

Diseases, 1992. 166: pp. 1281-1286

42. Centers for Disease Control and Prevention National Center for Infectious Diseases of Bacterial and Mycotic Diseases. Botulism in the United States, 189901996. Handbook for Epidemiologists, Clinicians, and Laboratory Workers. Atlanta: Center for Disease Control and Prevention, 1998. pp. 1-42

43. Nantel A.J. International Programme on Chemical Safety Poison Information Monograph 858 Bacteria. Clostridium botulinum. Geneva: World Health Organization, 2000. pp. 1-32

44. Guerrant R.L., Walker D.H., Weller P.F. Tropical Infectious Diseases – Principles, Pathogens & Practice. Volume 1. Philadelphia: Churchill Livingstone Elsevier. 2006. pp. 1573

45. Shapiro R.L., Hatheway C., Swerdlow D.L. Botulism in the United States: a Clinical and Epidemiologic Review. Annals of Internal Medicine, 1998. 129: pp. 221-228

46. Arnon S.S. Infant Botulism. Textbook of Pediatric Infectious Diseases. Philadelphia: W.B. Saunders, 1992. pp. 1095-1102

47. Long S.S. Gajewski J.L., Brown L.W. Gilligan P.H. Clinical, Laboratory, and Environmental Features of Infant Botulism in Southeastern Pennsylvania. Pediatrics, 1985. 75: pp. 935-941

48. Wilson R., Morris J.G. Jr, Snyder J.D., Feldman RA. Clinical Characteristics of Infant Botulism in the United States: A Study of the Non-California Cases. The Pediatric Infectious Disease Journal, 1982. 1: pp. 148-150

49. The Center for Food Security & Public Health. Iowa State University. Botulism. Revised June 2010. Retrieved December 12, 2014. Website: http://www.cfsph.iastate.edu/ Factsheets/pdfs/ botulism.pdf

50. Schantz E.J., Johnson E.A. Properties and use of Botulinum Toxin and Other Microbial Neurotoxins in Medicine. Microbiological Reviews, 1992. 56: pp. 80-99

51. Heymann D.L. Control of Communicable Diseases in Man. 18th Edition. Washington D.C.: American Public Health Association, 2004. pp. 69-75

52. Chao H.Y., Wang Y.C., Tang S.S., Liu H.W. A Highly Sensitive Immunopolymerase Chain Reaction Assay for Clostridium botulinum Neurotoxin Type A. Toxicon, 2004. 43: pp. 27-34

53. Drug Services: Formulary. Centers for Disease Control and Prevention. February 6, 2009. Retrieved November 5, 2009. Website: http://www.cdc.gov/ncidod/srp/ drugs/formulary. html

54. Black R., Gunn R. Hypersensitivity Reactions Associated with Botulinal Antitoxin. The American Journal of Medicine, 1980. 69: pp. 567-570

55. Investigational Heptavalent Botulinum Antitoxin (HBAT) to Replace Licensed Botulinum Antitoxin AB and Investigational Botulinum Antitoxin E. Morbidity and Mortality Weekly Report (MMWR), 2010. 59: pp. 299

56. BAT, Botulism Antitoxin Heptavalent (A, B, C, D, E, F, G). Food and Drug Administration. Revised March 2013. Retrieved December 11, 2014. Website: http://www.fda. gov/downloads/BiologicsBlood   Vaccines/BloodBloodProducts/ApprovedProducts/ LicensedProductsBLAs/FractionatedPlasmaProducts/UCM345147.pdf

57. McLaughlin J., Funk B. New Recommendation for Use of Heptavalent Botulinum Antotoxin (H-BAT). State of Alaska Epidemiology Bulletin. Revised March 3, 2010. Retrieved December 12, 2014. Website: http://www. epi.hss.state.ak.us /bulletins/docs/b2010_05. pdf

58. Arnon S.S., Schechter R., Maslanka S.E., Jewell N.P., Hatheway C.L. Human botulism immune globulin for the treatment of infant botulism. The New England Journal of Medicine, 2006. 354: pp. 462-471

59. BabyBIG [Botulism Immune Globulin Intravenous (Human) (BIG-IV)] Lyophilized Powder for Reconstitution and Injection Initial U.S. Approval: 2003. Revised October 2011. Retrieved December 12, 2014. Website: http://www.fda.gov/downloads/BiologicsBlood Vaccines/BloodBloodProducts/ApprovedProducts/LicensedProductsBLAs/ FractionatedPlasmaProducts/UCM117160.pdf

60. Botulism: Diagnosis & Laboratory Guidance for Clinicians. Centers for Disease Control and Prevention. Revised October 6, 2006. Retrieved December 14, 2011. Website: http:// www.bt.cdc. gov/agent/botulism/clinicians/diagnosis.asp

Photo Bibliography

Figure 2.5-1: Transmission electron photomicrograph of *Clostridium botulinum*. This electron photomicrograph was taken at a magnification of 14,400 and was released by the United States Department of Labor Occupational Safety and Health Administration (OSHA). Public domain Photo

Figure 2.5-2: Photograph of 97 vials of *Clostridium botulinum* bacilli from which biological weapons could be produced. These vials were found hidden in the home of an Iraqi biological weapon scientist in 2002 during an United Nations Special Commission (UNSCOM) weapons inspection. The photograph was released within the Central Intelligence Agency's Statement on the Interim Progress Report on the Activities of the Iraq Survey Group. The report was given on October 2, 2003 by David Kay, the head of the Iraqi Survey Group to the House Permanent Select Committee on Intelligence, the House Committee on Appropriations, Subcommittee on Defense, and the Senate Select Committee on Intelligence. Public domain photo

Figure 2.5-4: Computer generated image of botulinum neurotoxin A is composed of an ~50 kDa light chain (a zinc-dependent endopeptidase shown in red) and an ~100 kDa heavy chain linked by a single disulfide bond. The heavy chain contains two functional ~50 kDa domains: a C-terminal ganglioside binding domain (H_c-purple), and an N-terminal translocation domain (H_n-blue). Abelt portion of Hn (green) wraps around the light chain. The computer image is created by Dr. S. Ashraf Ahmed, Integrated Toxicology Division, US Army Medical Research Institute of Infectious Diseases, Fort Detrick, Maryland and released by United States Army Medical Department, Borden Institute. Public domain photo

Figure 2.5-5: *C.botulinum* infection diagram. The human anatomical illustration was created by Dr. Alexander J. da Silva and Melanie Moser in 2003. The illustration is released by the CDC. Public domain graphics

Figure 2.5-6: Utilization of mechanical ventilation for a patient suffering from respiratory failure. The photograph was taken by Chris Gregerson and released by the National Institute of Health. Public domain photo

Figure 2.5-7: Six month old infant suffering from botulism. Please note the loss of muscle tone, especially in the region of the head and neck. Picture was taken and released by the CDC. Public domain photo

Figure 2.5-8: Computer-generated molecular structure of botulinum neruotoxin subtypes E and B. The molecular graphics was developed by Drs. Desigan Kumaran, Subramaniam Eswaramoorthy and Subramanyam Swaminathan. The graphics was released in 2008 by the Department of energy. Public domain graphics

Coxiella burnetii is a Gram-negative, obligate intracellular coccobacillus, approximately 0.2 to 0.4 μm wide and 0.4 to 1.0 μm long, and is the causative agent of the zoonotic disease Q-fever (Figure 2.6-1).[1, 2] The term Q-fever or 'query fever' was first proposed in 1937 by Edward Holbrook Derrick to describe the illness suffered by meat workers in Brisbane, Australia, although at this time the caustic agent has yet to be isolated.[3] During this same time, working independently from Derrick, Herald Rea Cox and Gordon Davis of the Rocky Mountain Laboratory in Hamilton, Montana, succeeded in isolating the infectious agent in embyonated eggs, which they termed *Rickettsia burnetii*.[4, 5] It wasn't until 1938 that this bacterium was renamed *Coxiella burnetii*. Presently, *Coxiella burnetii* is listed as a Category B biological weapon by the Center for Disease Control and prevention and has been successfully weaponized by the United States, Soviet Union, as well as, numerous other countries.[6]

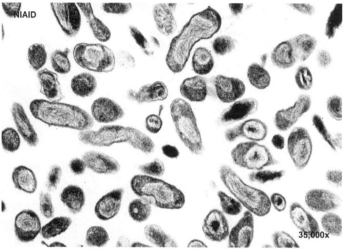

Figure 2.6-1: Transmission electronmicrograph (TEM) of numerous *C. burnetii* coccobacilli

During the early stages of research into *C. burnetii*, it was discovered that the natural reservoir of this bacterium is bandicoots (*Isoodontorus* and *Isoodono besulus*), which are omnivorous terrestrial marsupials found in Australia. *Haemaphysalis humerosa*, a tick known to be an ecoparasite of the marsupials, is believed to be the vector. In the United States, the tick species *Dermacentor andersoni* and *Ornithodorus tunicate*, are the vectors for *C. burnetii*.[7] Presently, cattle, sheep, and less frequently goats, along with a variety of other domesticated animals (including domesticated pets) are the primary reservoirs of *C. burnetii* around the globe. In general, the bacteria do not produce any clinical symptoms in these animals. Nonetheless, these coccobacilli have been discovered in the milk, urine, and feces of animals, which may result in the spread of the bacteria via the gastrointestinal tract (Figure 2.6-2).[2, 5]

Research on the military application of *C. burnetii* as an incapacitating agent began prior to World War II by the Soviet Union. As stated by Alibek (1999), an outbreak of Q-fever among German soldiers in the Crimea may have been caused by the purposeful dissemination of the bacterial agent by the Soviet Military.[8] Military use of *C. burnetii* continued in the mid 1950's and 1960's. The United States Military experimented with *C. burnetii* infections in soldiers. In experimental aerosolized *C. burnetii* trials at Dugway Proving Grounds in Utah, it was discovered that *C. burnetii* had an exceptional

infectivity among the volunteers. It was shown that inhalation of a single bacterium in susceptible personnel may result in Q-fever within 40 days post-exposure.[9] In a 1970 report by the World Health Organization (WHO), it was estimated that if 50 kg of *C. burnetii* was released upwind of a city of 500,000, the disease caused by the bacteria could incapacitate 125,000 and cause approximately 150 deaths (Figure 2.6-3).[10]

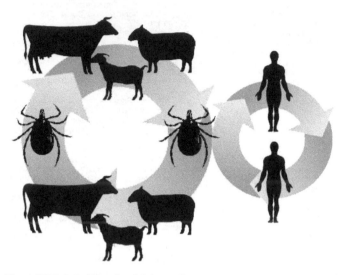

Figure 2.6-2: Sylvatic cycle of *C. burnetii*

C. burnetii can be manipulated into spore-like forms, also referred to as small cell variants (SCV), and stored as an aerosol or as a dry powder at a wide range of temperatures (-52° to 40° C) and environments. For example, SCVs have been reported to survive 586 days in tick feces at room temperature, longer than 160 days in water, 30 to 40 days in dried cheese made from contaminated milk and up to 150 days in soil.[11] It has been suggested that the environmental stability of this coccobacillus could be attributed to its ability to transition between SCV to the metabolic-active form called the large cell variant (LCV).[12]

If infection takes place via the respiratory route, the alveolar macrophages are the primary cells infected by *C. burnetii*. To a lesser extent, during later phases of infection, Kupffer cells in the liver are also susceptible and may be infected via the blood stream and/or the digestive system with the pathogen.[5]

C. burnetii SCV, as with numerous other intracellular parasites, must gain entry into professional phagocytic cells, as well as non-phagocytic cells such as epithelial and endothelial cells. The manner by which they gain entry is subdivided into phase I and II. During phase I, *C. burnetii* SCV blocks entry via CR3 receptors, an adhesion-promoting leukocyte surface membrane heterodimer, and binds to human monocytes through the leukocyte response integrin $\alpha_V\beta_3$ (LRI). Once bounded, the SCV enters the macrophage through RAC1-dependent phagocytosis, which requires the formation of a motile cell surface that contains a meshwork of newly polymerized actin filaments also known as cell ruffling. It is interesting to note that $\alpha_V\beta_3$ integrin is generally involved in the removal of apoptotic cells through phagocytosis, and *C. burnetii* SCV's ability to use this membrane receptor allows it to avoid triggering an inflammation response. Presently, the identity of the bacterial ligand that triggers RAC1-dependent phagocytosis is unknown but likely candidates are membrane-associated proteins that possess integrin binding domain arginine-glycine-aspartic acid (RGD).[13] In contrast, during phase II, *C. burnetii* SCV engages the CR3 receptors and are readily internalized in the phagocytes but are quickly killed via the phagolysosomal pathway.[14]

Respiratory

Gastrointestinal

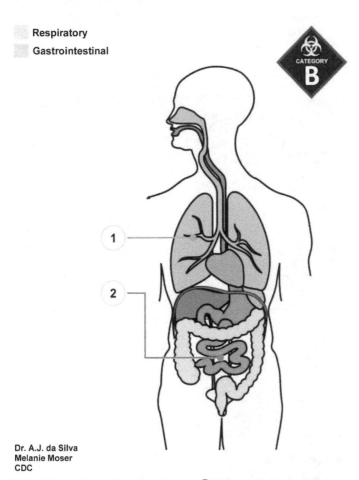

Dr. A.J. da Silva
Melanie Moser
CDC

Figure 2.6-3: *C. brunetii* infection diagram. ① *C. burnetii* could be introduced via respiratory tract. ② *C. burnetii* could be introduced via gastrointestinal

After internalization of *C. burnetii* SCV through phase I mechanism, the bacterium appears within a coccobacillus-dedicated phagosome called *Coxilla*-containing vacuole (CCV). Immediately after its formation, the nascent CCV will begin recruiting the GTPase activating proteins RAB5 and early-endosomal marker protein EEA1 approximately five minutes after internalization. In keeping with the normal characteristic of phagosomal development, the CCV will acidify to ~pH 5.4. During this time, CCV will recruit autophagosomal markers called microtubule-associated protein light-chain 3 (LC3) via a process that is dependent on bacterial protein synthesis.[15] Within 40-60 minutes after internalization, nascent CCV continue to develop through fusion and fission events with early endosomes and then late endosomes. Concurrently, RAB5 and EEA1 are removed from the surface of the vacuole and in their place, RAB7, lysosome-associated membrane glycoprotein 1 (LAMP1) and vacuolar ATPase are recruited by the CCV. The recruitment of vacuolar ATPase, which pumps protons into the maturing phagosome, will allow the further acidification of the CCV to ~pH 5.[16]

At approximately two hours post-infection, the acidification of the CCV will continue until the internal environment reaches ~pH 4.5. In concurrence with the increased acidity, lysosomal enzymes will begin to accumulate within the CCV. Unlike most intracellular pathogens that subvert the endosomal cascade and

the maturation of the phagosome to avoid fusion with lysosomes, *C. burnetii* allows lysosomal enzymes, such as cathepsin D and lysosomal acid phosphatase, to accumulate within the CCV. Nonetheless, this accumulation of lysosomal enzymes occurs ~2 hours post-infection which is in contrast to ~15 minutes via normal phagocytosis process.[17] It is believed that this delay in the accumulation of lysosomal enzymes allows the conversion of the bacteria from SCVs to the metabolically active LCVs. It has been estimated that the conversion of the SCV to LCV is ~80% an hour post-infection and reaches 100% by 16th hour post-infection.[12, 18, 19]

Between 8 to 48 hours post infection, the CCV expands to occupy an increasingly dominant portion of the cytoplasmic space of the host cell. This large CCV is created via the homotypic fusion of multiple smaller CCVs and can continue to expand through heterotypic fusion with other host cellular vesicles (e.g. lysosomal, autophagic, endocytic vesicles).[20] The process of CCV expansion is dependent upon the recruitment of both RHO GTPase and RAB1B to the CCV membrane, as well as, bacterial protein synthesis. It is postulated that the RHO GTPase is involved in the maintenance of the enlarged CCV, while the recruitment of RAB1B from the host cellular endoplasmic reticulum may enable the acquisition of additional membranes to create this spacious CCV.[12]

Approximately six days post-infection, now matured CCV will appear heavily laden with LCV, although some are differentiating back into SCV. This matured CCV possesses a pH ~4.5-5 and retains its fusogenic capacity. Astonishingly, during this time of massive CCV expansion, the stability of host cell's genome remains unchanged, while its viability appears unaffected. It is believed that the viability of the host cell is maintained by intracellular parasite in two manners. First, *C. burnetii* inhibits apoptotic signaling pathways, while inducing pro-survival factors. Researchers suggest that the anti-apoptotic activity of *C. burnetii* could be the result of the interaction between two proteins found within the membrane of the CCV: beclin 1 (BECN1), an autophagy initiation protein, and B-cell lymphoma 2 (BCL2), an anti-apoptotic protein. The interactions between the two proteins prevent the release of cytochrome *c* from the mitochondria, whereby inhibiting apoptosis.[19, 20, 21] Secondly, *C. burnetii* triggers the anti-apoptotic actions through the activation of pro-survival signaling proteins mitogen-activated protein kinase 1 and 3 (MAPK1, 3), as well as, the AKT family of serine-threonine kinases (e.g. Akt1/PKBα, Akt2/PKBβ, and Akt3/PKBγ).[12, 22]

The ability for *C. burnetii* to prevent apoptosis of the host cell is beneficial for the persistence of the infection. It has been suggested that the anti-apoptotic behavior of *C. burnetii* will allow this bacterium to continue its replication within the host cell, along with allowing the host cell to continue its cellular division. For example, evidence suggests that during cytokinesis of the host cell, the mature CCV only segregates into one of the daughter cells, leaving the others unaffected. Through this lifecycle strategy, *C. burnetii* leaves available host cells to infect, thereby promoting chronic infections.[12, 23]

SYMPTOMS

Approximately 60% of *C. burnetii* infections do not result in the development of Q-fever. Only 40% of infections result in symptoms of the disease. Q-fever may take on two different forms of infection: acute and chronic.[5] In acute Q-fever infections, the incubation period may last between 2-3 weeks. In the majority of patients, initial symptoms are abrupt and begin with severe fever (39 to 40°C; 102.2 to 104°F). If the patient is immediately treated by clinicians, the fever generally lasts 2 to 4 days and within 5 to 14 days the fever subsides. However, in untreated patients, the fever may last anywhere from 5 to 57 days.[24] Fatigue, sore throat, chills, headaches and confusion are also common symptoms of Q-fever. In some cases, myalgia, sweats, nausea, vomiting, dry nonproductive cough, scant mucoid sputum, weight loss, retro-orbital pains, abdominal pains and chest pains are also present. On rare occasions, some patients may exhibit symptoms of diarrhea, skin rash, myocarditis, pericarditis, meningoencephalitis, hemolytic anemia, mediastinal lymphadenopathy, erythema nodosum, throiditis, pancreatitis, mesenteric paniculitis, epididymitis, orchitis, priapism, abnormal secretion of antidiuretic hormone, optic neuritis, Guillain-Barré syndrome and extrapyramidal neurological disease.[2, 10, 25, 26] Other manifestations as a result of acute *C. burnetii* infection are atypical pneumonia, due to secondary infections by *Mycoplasma pneumonia* or *Chlamydia pneumonia*, which are generally diagnosed via X-rays. On rare occasion, patients suffering from Q-fever develop pneumonia which results in acute respiratory distress (Figure 2.6-4).[27]

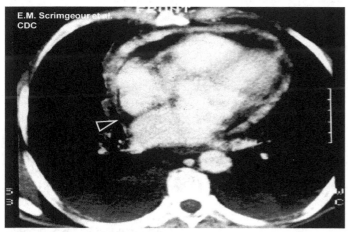

Figure 2.6-4: X-ray picture demonstraing Q-fever pneumonia (arrow)

Other frequent presentation of acute Q-fever is hepatitis.[28, 29, 30] Diagnosis of Q-fever induced hepatitis generally results from laboratory examinations showing raised levels of hepatic enzymes, such as aspartate aminotransferase (AST), alanine aminotrans-ferase (ALT) and alkaline phosphatase. Clinical signs of hepatomegaly may be one of the symptoms; however, patients generally do not suffer from jaundice. It is known that death resulting from acute Q-fever is extremely rare (Table1).[5]

Chronic Q-fever, defined as an infection lasting more than six months, endocarditis may be present in as many as 70% of all cases, [2, 31, 32, 33] although, if promptly treated, the mortality from chronic Q-fever endocarditis is less than 10%.[5] Approximately 68% of patients suffering from chronic Q-fever endocarditis may exhibit low grade fever, malaise, weakness, fatigue, weightloss, anorexia, chills, and night sweats. Typically chronic Q-fever endocarditis occurs in patients with pre-existing cardiac valve defects (~90% of patients suffering from this condition have aortic or mitral valve problems), which may be congenital, rheumatic, degenerative or result from previous syphilis infections.[10, 34]

Patients who are immunosuppressed (e.g. HIV infections), suffering from cancer (e.g. lymphoma), chronic renal insufficiencies, as well as, those who have undergone organ transplantation or are pregnant are more commonly observed to have chronic Q-fever endocarditis. Approximately 67% of patients suffering from cardiac symptoms resulting in heart failure have previously suffered from valvulopathy, dyspnea, acute pulmonary edema and/or angina and heart palpitations. Thoracic examinations using X-rays may demonstrate cardiomegaly, while electrocardio-graphy may show arrhythmias and ventricular hypertrophy.[5] Other symptoms associated with chronic Q-fever endocarditis include digital clubbing (~37% of patients), purpuric rash (generally found on the extremities and mucosa in ~19% of the patients),[10, 34] as well as, splenomegaly and hepatomegaly (~55% and 56% of the patients respectively).[25, 34]

Table 1: An overview of the clinical symptoms of acute Q-fever. Please note that the abbreviation 'media' is referring to mediastinal

Symptoms	+	++	+++
Severe fever			■
Fatigue			■
Sore throat			■
Chills			■
Headaches			■
Confusion			■
Myalgia		■	
Sweats		■	
Nausea		■	
Vomiting		■	
Dry nonproductive cough		■	
Scant mucoid sputum		■	
Weight loss		■	
Retro-orbital pains		■	
Abdominal pains		■	
Chest pains		■	
Diarrhea	■		
Skin rash	■		
Myocarditis	■		
Pericarditis	■		
Meningoencephalitis	■		
Hemolytic anemia	■		
Media. lymphadenopathy	■		
Erythema nodosum	■		
Thyroiditis	■		
Pancreatitis	■		
Mesenteric paniculitis	■		
Epididymitis	■		
Orchitis	■		
Priapism	■		
Abnormal ADH secretion	■		
Optic neuritis	■		
Guillain-Barré syndrome	■		
Extrapyramid neuro.	■		
Atypical pneumonia	■		
Hepatomegaly	■		

+ Rare ++ Common +++ Frequent

In the remaining ~30% of cases, chronic Q-fever that does not involve endocarditis, vascular infections related to aneurysms and vascular graphs were seen in male patients age 65 ± 11.5 years.[36, 37, 38] Cases of osteoarticular infections involving osteomyelitis, osteoarthritis, and aortic graph infections with contiguous spinal osteomyelitis have also been reported (Figure 2.3-4).[39, 40, 41]

Rare cases of chronic Q-fever induced chronic hepatitis, that do not involve endocarditis or chronic pulmonary infections (pulmonary fibrosis or pseudotumors), have also been reported.[42, 43, 44] Finally, chronic fatigue syndrome has been observed in patients convalescing from chronic Q-fever. These patients show symptoms of prolonged fatigue, arthralgia, myalgia, muscle fasciculation, blurred vision, sweats and enlarged painful lymph nodes (Table 2).[5, 45, 46]

Table 2: An overview of the clinical symptoms of chronic Q-fever

Symptoms	+	++	+++
Endocarditis			■
Low grade fever			■
Malaise			■
Weakness			■
Fatigue			■
Weight loss			■
Anorexia			■
Chills			■
Night sweats			■
Heart failure		■	
Splenpmegaly		■	
Hepatomegaly		■	
Cardiomegaly		■	
Arrhythmia		■	
Ventricular hypertrophy		■	
Digital clubbing	■		
Purpuric rash	■		
Osteoarticular infections	■		
Osteomyelitis	■		
Osteoarthritis	■		
Spinal osteomyelitis	■		
Chronic hepatitis	■		
Pulmonary fibrosis	■		
Pseudotumors	■		
Chronic fatigue syn.	■		
Arthralgia	■		
Myalgia	■		
Muscle fasciculation	■		
Blurred vision	■		
Sweats	■		
Enlarged lymph nodes	■		
Painful lymph nodes	■		

+ Rare   ++ Common   +++ Frequent

■ Q-fever endocarditis
■ Non-endocarditis Q-fever

DETECTION

C. burnetii is a highly infectious agent and mishandling may result in the contamination of the laboratory and workers. Presently, accurate detection of the *C. burnetii* requires the availability of a level 3 biosafety laboratory.[5]

Biopsy samples can be tested if they are fresh or after formalin fixation. A number of detection methods have been developed, such as immunoperoxidase techniques, enzyme linked immunoassay (ELISA) and/or enzyme linked immunofilter assay (ELIFA), as well as, immunofluorescence techniques using either polyclonal or monoclonal antibodies.[47, 48, 49] Serological testing for IgG, IgM and IgA antibodies to *C. burnettii* remain the most common methods for Q-fever diagnosis. Generally, antibodies against the bacteria are detected 2 to 3 weeks after the onset of disease and also allows for the differentiation of acute versus chronic Q-fever infections. It is worthy to note that *C. burnetii* exists in two antigenic phases: phase I and II, as indicated in the previous section. These phases are important in diagnosing acute versus chronic Q-fever. For example, in acute Q-fever, the antibody titers in phase II are generally higher in comparison to those found in phase I. In chronic Q-fever, the reverse is true, where the antibody titers in phase I are higher in comparison to phase II. The types of antibodies found in the specific phases are another manner by which acute and chronic Q-fever can be differentiated. For example, in acute Q-fever, patients will develop IgG antibodies in phase II and IgM antibodies in both phase I and II. In chronic Q-fever endocarditis, patients will develop IgG and IgA in phase I of the infection. Serological methods that have been used includes microagglutination, complement fixation, radioimmunoassay, indirect fluorescent antibody (IFA) technique, indirect hemolysis examination, enzyme linked immunoassay (ELISA) and/or enzyme linked immunofilter assay (ELIFA), dot immunoblotting and Western blotting.[2, 50, 51, 52, 53, 54, 55, 56, 57, 58, 59, 60, 61, 62]

Isolation of *C. Burnettii* via culture is another way by which these bacteria are identified and analyzed. Generally, clinical specimens are injected intraperitoneally into guinea pigs and the animals are permitted to become febrile. Within 5 to 8 days, these guinea pigs are sacrificed and their spleen extracts are used for bacterial isolation. Numerous human cell lines may be used for *in vitro* cultures. For example, human embryonic lung fibroblasts (HELA cells), blood, cerebrospinal fluid, bone marrow, cardiac valve, vascular aneurysm, vascular graft, bone biopsy, liver biopsy, milk, placenta and fetal tissues are all suitable for culturing *C. burnettii* bacteria.[5, 63, 64, 65]

By using polymerase chain reaction (PCR), *C. burnetii* 16S rDNA, *sodB* and *gltA* could be amplified and detected in frozen samples and paraffin embedded tissues. In addition, this PCR-based technique was used to detect *C. burnetii* DNA within the supernatants of infected cultures making it more accurate and faster than the traditional methods.[5, 66, 67]

TREATMENT

The prognosis for acute Q-fever is excellent. As indicated in previous sections, the mortality rate is extremely low. In general, acute Q-fever is treated with a 10 day course of doxycycline,

Table 3a: Medication dosage, side effects of various treatments for acute Q-fever

Medication	Mechanism of Action	Side Effects	Recommended Dosage
Doxycycline	Inhibits protein synthesis	Nausea, diarrhea, bloody stools, severe stomach cramps, indigestion, heartburn, vomiting, photosensitivity, loss of appetite, dysphagia, headaches, blurred vision, rash, joint pain, fever, feeling tired	Adults: 100 mg every 12 h; Children under 45 kg (100 lbs): 2.2 mg/kg body weight 2x/d. Patients should be treated for at least 3 days after the fever subsides and until there is evidence of clinical improvement. Standard duration of treatment is 2-3 weeks
Tetracycline	Inhibits protein synthesis	Fever, chills, headache, blurred vision, fever, hives, diarrhea, nausea, vomiting, dysphagia & breathing, hoarseness, indigestion, lingua villosa, inflammation of tongue, swellings (mouth, face, lips, or tongue), joint pain, loss of appetite, mouth sores, rash, itching, photophobia, sore throat, stomach pain, swelling and itching of the rectum, tightness in the chest, vaginal irritation or discharge	Adults: 1-2 g/d PO given in 2-4 divided doses. Do not provide tetracycline to children under the age of 8. Children < age 8 The usual dose is 6.25 to 12.5 mg/kg of body weight every six hours; or 12.5 to 25 mg/kg of body weight every twelve hours
Ciprofloxacin (Cipro)	Inhibits the function of DNA gyrase	Nausea, diarrhea, abnormal liver function tests, vomiting, rash, headache, abdominal pain/discomfort, foot pain, pain in extremities, injection site reaction	Adult: 250-750 mg bid. Child: 5-15 mg/kg bid

Table 3b – Medication dosage, side effects of various treatments for acute Q-fever

Medication	Mechanism of Action	Side Effects	Recommended Dosage
Levofloxacin	Inhibits the function of DNA gyrase	Nausea, stomach upset, loss of appetite, diarrhea, abdominal pains, cramping, drowsiness, dizziness, headache, insomnia, joint/muscle/tendon pain, swelling, tendonitis, hypersensitivity to sunlight, rash itching, swelling, chest pain, change in the amount of urine, dark urine, easy bruising/bleeding, dizziness, fainting, fast/irregular heartbeat, difficult breathing, mental/mood changes, severe depression, nausea, vomiting, pharyn-gitis, fever, seizures, fatigue, yellowing eyes and skin	Adult: 250-750 mg. Patients should be treated for at least 3 days after the fever subsides and until there is evidence of clinical improvement. Standard duration of treatment is ~60 d. Children: >50 kg and > 6 months of age 500 mg every 24 hr for ~60 d and children < 50 kg and >6 months of age 8 mg/kg (not exceeding 250 mg per dose) every 12 h for ~60 d
Moxifloxacin	Inhibits the function of DNA gyrase	Tendinitis, tendon rupture, nausea, vomiting, stomach pain, diarrhea (mild or severe), constipation, gas, heartburn, loss of appetite, change in ability to taste food, sores (mouth/tongue), white patches in the mouth, dry mouth, headache, weakness, sweating, vaginal itching or burning, rash, itching, hives, difficulty breathing or swallowing, swelling (face or throat), loss of consciousness, fever, blistering or peeling skin, jaundice-like symptoms, dark urine, exhaustion, muscle/joint pain, pale skin, shortness of breath, unusual bruising or bleeding, fast, pounding or irregular heartbeat, fainting, seizures, dizziness, confusion, nervous-ness, agitation, restlessness, depression, suicidal thoughts, insomnia, nightmares, hallucinations, numbness, burning, tingling and/or weakness in the arms, hands, legs or feet	Adult: 400 mg every 24 hr for the duration of the infection. Dosage indications not available for children
Azithromycin	Inhibits protein synthesis	Rash, hives, itching, skin irritations (peeling, red, swollen, blistered), difficulty breathing, tightness in the chest, swelling (mouth, face, lips, or tongue), unusual hoarseness, bloody or watery stools, changes in hearing, hearing loss, chest pain, eye or vision problems, irregular heartbeat, muscle weakness or pain, inflammation at the injection site, rapid heartbeat, tinnitus, seizure, severe or persistent diarrhea, stomach cramps or pain, jaundice-like symptoms, dark urine, nausea, vomiting, loss of appetite, trouble speaking or swallowing, unusual vaginal itching, odor, or discharge	Adult: 250 mg - 500 mg/d for ~60 d. Children: 5 - 20 mg/kg/ d, once daily for ~60 d.
Erythromycin	Inhibiting protein synthesis	Upset stomach, stomach cramps/pains, diarrhea, vomiting, skin rash, itching, hives, difficulty breathing or swallowing, wheezing, jaundice-like symptoms, dark urine	Adult: 500 mg every 6 hours for the duration of the infection. Children: 50 mg/kg/day orally in divided doses every 6 hours for the duration of the infection
Roxithromycin	Inhibiting protein synthesis	Stomach discomfort and cramp, upper abdominal pain nausea, vomiting, diarrhea, pruritis, urticaria, skin rash, angioedema, purpura, bronchospasm, anaphylaxis, hepatotoxicity, abnormal liver function, jaundice, cholestasis, eosinophilia, fever, dizziness, headache, paraesthesia	Adults: 150 mg twice/d for the duration of the disease. Children: 2.5 - 5.0 mg/kg of body weight for the duration of the disease

Table 4: Medication dosage, side effects of various treatments for chronic Q-fever

Medication	Mechanism of Action	Side Effects	Recommended Dosage
Telithromycin	Inhibiting protein synthesis	Diarrhea, nausea, vomiting, headache, dizziness, fainting, irregular heartbeat (rapid or pounding), hives, rash, itching, difficulty breathing or swallowing, swelling (face, throat, tongue, lips, eyes, hands, feet, ankles, or lower legs), hoarseness	Adult and children 13 years or older: 800 mg taken orally once every 24 h, for the duration of the disease
Clarithromycin	Inhibits protein synthesis	Headache, fever, severe dizziness, diarrhea, nausea, vomiting, stomach upset, abdominal pain, changes in taste, hearing loss, mental/mood changes, fainting, fast/irregular heartbeats, sore throat, rash, itching, swelling, trouble breathing, dark urine, yellowing of eyes or skin	Adult: 500 mg every 12 hr for the duration of the infection. Dosage indications not available for children
Doxycycline /hydroxychloroquine sulfate	Inhibits protein synthesis	Nausea, diarrhea, bloody stools, severe stomach cramps, indigestion, heartburn, vomiting, photosensitivity, loss of appetite, dysphagia, headaches, blurred vision, rash, joint pain, fever, feeling tired	Adults: 100 mg every 12 h; Hydroxychloroquine at 200 mg every 8h for standard duration fo 18 months. Dosage indications not available for children

tetracycline or fluoroquinolone (i.e. ciprofloxacin, levofloxacin and moxifloxacin). Macrolides have also been used to treat this infection; however, there are some strains of *C. burnetii* that are resistant to this compound. Initiation of antibiotic treatment for acute Q-fever is most effective within the first three days of the onset of illness (Table 3a and 3b).[2, 10]

Unlike acute Q-fever, chronic Q fever endo-carditis is much more involved and difficult to treat. In general, chronic Q-fever involves a minimum of three years of treatment; however, some individuals may require a lifelong of regimental treatment. Treating chronic Q-fever often requires the use of multiple drugs. For example, some physicians utilize rifampin and ciprofloxin in combination, while others suggest that doxycycline in combination with hydroxyl-chloroquine sulfate be used (Tables 4).[2, 10] Treatment with tetracycline and quinolone have also been tested and shown to be effective against chronic Q-fever.[68]

DIFFERENTIAL DIAGNOSIS

The symptoms of Q fever are at times vague and could be misdiagnosed with other symptomatically similar diseases. For example, the CDC recommends that physicians carefully evaluate individuals that have recently travelled to foreign countries for Q-fever if they are presented with febrile illness, bacterial (or prokaryotic) pneumonia (*Chlamydia*, *mycoplasmal* pneumonia - BP) and viral pneumonia (VP) and/or hepatitis. The differential diagnosis should include Legionnaire's disease (LD), mononucleosis (Mono), Ornithosis, and tick-borne diseases (e.g. Lyme disease, Tularemia, etc.).[69, 70] Please examine Tables 5 and 6 for the differential diagnosis for acute Q-fever and chronic Q-fever respectively.

References

1. Miller J.D., Shaw E.I., Thompson H.A. Infectious Agents and Pathogenesis - Microorganisms and Bioterrorism. New York, Springer United States of America. 2006. pp. 181-208
2. Q Fever. Center of Disease Control. Revised November 13, 2013. Retrieved December 13, 2014. Website: http://www.cdc.gov/qfever/symptoms/index.html
3. Derrick E.H. "Q" fever, New Fever Entity: Clinical Features, Diagnosis and Laboratory Investigation. The Medical Journal of Australia, 1937. 2: pp. 281-299
4. Cox H.R., Bell E.J. The Cultivation of Rickettsia diaporica in Tissue Culture and in the Tissue of Developing Chicken Embryos. Public Health Reports, 1939. 54: pp. 2171-2175
5. Maurin M., Raoult D. Q Fever. Clinical Microbiology Reviews, 1999. 12: pp. 518-553
6. Stewart C. Weapons of Mass Casualties. Missassauga, Jones and Bartlett Publishers. 2005. pp. 154
7. Fernando R.L., Fernando S.E., Leong S.Y. Tropical Infectious Diseases – Epidemiology, Investigation, Diagnosis & Management. London: Greenwich Medical Media. 2001. pp. 270-271
8. Alibek K. Biohazard. New York: Dell Publishing. 1999. pp. 63-79
9. Weapons of Mass Destruction – An Encyclopedia of Worldwide Policy, Technology and History. Volume 1 Chemical and Biological Weapons. Santa Barbara, American Bibliographic Company – Clio Press. 2004. pp. 235
10. Health Aspects of Chemical and Biological Weapons, Report of a WHO Group of Consultants. Geneva, World Health Organization. 1970. pp. 72
11. Guerrant R.L., Walker D.H., Weller P.F. Tropical Infectious Diseases – Principles, Pathogens & Practice. Volume 1. Philadelphia: Churchill Livingstone Elsevier. 2006. pp. 574-577
12. van Schaik E.J., Chen C., Mertens K., Weber M.M., Samuel J.E. Molecular pathogenesis of the obligate intracellular bacterium Coxiella burnetii. Nature Reviews, 2013. 11: pp.

Table 5: Differential diagnosis of acute Q-fever with selected disease with similar symptoms. These diseases are bacterial pneumonia (BP), viral pneumonia (VP), hepatitis, Legionnaire's disease (LD), mononucleosis (Mono) and tick-borne diseases (TBD)

Symptoms	Q Fever	BP	VP	Hepatitis	LD	Mono	TBD
Severe fever	■	■	■	■	■	■	■
Fatigue	■	■		■	■	■	■
Sore throat	■	■				■	
Chills	■	■			■	■	
Headaches	■	■			■		
Confusion	■						
Myalgia	■	■			■		
Sweats	■	■					
Nausea	■	■					
Vomiting	■						
Dry nonproductive cough	■	■	■				
Scant mucoid sputum	■	■					
Weight loss	■	■					
Retro-orbital pains	■						
Abdominal pains	■	■	■	■	■		
Chest pains	■	■					■
Diarrhea	■	■		■	■		
Skin rash	■	■			■	■	
Myocarditis	■						
Pericarditis	■		■				
Meningoencephalitis	■						■
Hemolytic anemia	■		■				
Media. lymphadenopathy	■				■	■	■
Erythema nodosum	■						
Throiditis	■						
Pancreatitis	■						
Mesenteric panniculitis	■						
Epididymitis	■	■					
Orchitis	■						
Priapism	■						
Abnormal secretion of ADH	■						
Optic neuritis	■						
Guillain-Barré syndrome	■						
Extrapyramid neuro-disease	■						
Atypical pneumonia	■	■			■		■
Hepatomegaly				■		■	

Table 6: Differential diagnosis of chronic Q-fever with selected disease with similar symptoms. These diseases are bacterial pneumonia (BP), viral pneumonia (VP), hepatitis, Legionnaire's disease (LD), mononucleosis (Mono) and tick-borne diseases (TBD)

Symptoms	Q Fever	BP	VP	Hepatitis	LD	Mono	TBD
Endocarditis	■	■					
Low grade fever	■	■	■		■	■	■
Malaise	■	■	■	■	■	■	■
Weakness	■	■	■	■	■	■	■
Fatigue	■	■	■	■	■	■	■
Weight loss	■	■	■	■	■	■	■
Anorexia	■	■	■	■	■	■	■
Chills	■	■	■		■	■	■
Night sweats	■	■					
Heart failure	■	■	■				
Splenomegaly	■			■		■	
Hepatomegaly	■			■		■	
Cardiomegaly	■						
Arrhythmia	■	■					
Ventricular hypertrophy	■						
Digital clubbing							
Purpuric rash	■			■		■	■
Osteoarticular infections	■						
Osteomyelitis	■						
Osteoarthritis	■						
Spinal osteomyelitis	■						
Chronic hepatitis	■			■		■	
Pulmonary fibrosis	■						
Pseudotumors	■						
Chronic fatigue syndrome	■						
Arthralgia	■	■					■
Myalgia	■	■	■		■		■
Muscle fasciculation	■						
Blurred vision	■						
Sweats	■	■	■			■	
Enlarged lymph nodes	■				■	■	■
Painful lymph nodes	■				■	■	■

561- 573

13. Seshadri R., Paulsen I.T., Eisen J.A., Read T.D., Nelson K.E., Nelson W.C., Ward N.L., Tettelin H., Davidsen T.M., Beanan M.J., Deboy R.T., Daugherty S.C., Brinkac L.M., Madupu R., Dodson R.J., Khouri H.M., Lee K.H., Carty H.A., Scanlan D., Heinzen R.A., Thompson H.A., Samuel J.E., Fraser C.M., Heidelberg J.F. Complete genome sequence of the Q-fever pathogen Coxiella burnetii. Proceedings of the National Academy of Sciences of the United States of America, 2003. 100: pp. 5455–5460

14. Mege J.L., Maurin M., Capo C., Raoult D. C. burnetii: the 'Query' Fever Bacterium. A Model of Immune Subversion by a Strictly Intracellular Microorganism. Federation of European Microbiological Societies Microbiology Reviews, 1997. 19: pp. 209-217

15. Beare P.A., Gilk S.D., Larson C.L., Hill J., Stead C.M., Omsland A., Cockrell D.C., Howe D., Voth D.E., Heinzen R.A. Dot/Icm Type IVB Secretion System Requirements for Coxiella burnetii Growth in Human Macrophages. mBIO, 2011. 2: pp. e00175-11

16. Kinchen, J. M., Ravichandran, K. S. Phagosome maturation: going through the acid test. Nature Reviews Molecular Cell Biology, 2008. 9: pp. 781–795

17. Howe, D. & Mallavia, L. P. Coxiella burnetii exhibits morphological change and delays phagolysosomal fusion after internalization by J774A.1 cells. Infection and Immunity, 2000. 68: pp. 3815–3821

18. Romano P. S., Gutierrez M. G., Beron W., Rabinovitch M., Colombo M. I. The autophagic pathway is actively modulated by phase II Coxiella burnetii to efficiently replicate in the host cell. Cellular Microbiology, 2007. 9: pp. 891–909

19. Coleman S. A., Fischer E. R., Howe D., Mead D. J, Heinzen R. A. Temporal analysis of Coxiella burnetii morphological differentiation. Journal of Bacteriology, 2004. 186: pp. 7344–7352

20. Howe D., Melnicâakova J., Barâak I., Heinzen R. A. Fusogenicity of the Coxiella burnetii parasitophorous vacuole. Annals of the New York Academy of Sciences, 2003. 990: pp. 556–562

21. Luhrmann A., Roy C. R. Coxiella burnetii inhibits activation of host cell apoptosis through a mechanism that involves preventing cytochrome c release from mitochondria. Infection and Immunity, 2007. 75: pp. 5282–5289

22. Voth D. E., Heinzen R. A. Sustained activation of Akt and Erk1/2 is required for Coxiella burnetii antiapoptotic activity. Infection and Immunity, 2009. 77: pp. 205–213

23. Roman M. J., Coriz P. D., Baca O. G. A proposed model to explain persistent infection of host cells with Coxiella burnetii. Journal of General Microbiology, 1986. 132: pp. 1415–1422

24. Derrick E.H. The Course of Infection with Coxiella burnetii. The Medical Journal of Australia, 1973. 1: pp. 1051-1057

25. Marrie T.J. Acute Q Fever. Q Fever the Disease, Volume 1. Boca Raton, Chemical Rubber Company Press. 1990. pp. 125-160

26. Fernando R.L., Fernando S.E., Leong S.Y. Tropical Infectious Diseases – Epidemiology, Investigation, Diagnosis & Management. London: Greenwich Medical Media. 2001. pp. 273-277

27. Marrie T.J. Q Fever, 1979-1987 – Nova Scotia. Canada Disease Weekly Report, 1988. 14: pp. 69-70

28. Clark W.H., Lennette E.H., Railsback O.C., Romer M.S. Q Fever Studies in California. VII. Clinical Features in one hundred Eighty Cases. Archives of Internal Medicine, 1951. 88: pp. 155-167

29. Tissot Dupont H., Raoult D., Brouqui P., Janbon F., Peyramond D., Weiller P.J., Chicheportiche C., Nezri M., Poirier R. Epidemiologic Features and Clinical Presentation of Acute Q fever in Hospitalized Patients 323 French Cases. American Journal of Medicine, 1992 93: pp. 427-434

30. Vellend H., Salit I.E., Spence L., McLaughlin B., Carlson J., Palmer N., Van Dreumel A.A., Hodgkinson J.R. Q fever - Ontario. Canada Disease Weekly Report, 1982 8: pp. 171-173

31. Dupuis G., Peter O., Lüthy R., Nicolet J., Peacock M., Burgdorfer W. Serological Diagonosis of Q Fever Endocarditis. European Heart Journal, 1986. 7: pp. 1062-1066

32. Saginur R., Silver S.S., Bonin R., Carlier M., Orizaga M. O-Fever Endocarditis. Canadian Medical Association Journal, 1985. 133: pp. 1228-1230

33. Stein A., Raoult D. Q Fever Endocarditis. European Heart Journal, 16: pp. 19-23

34. Raoult D., Raza A., Marrie T.J. Q Fever Endocarditis and Other Forms of Chronic Q Fever. Q Fever, Volume 1. Boca Raton, Chemical Rubber Company Press. 1990. pp. 179-199

35. Raoult D., Etienne J., Massip P., Iacono S., Prince M.A., Beaurain P., Benichou S., Auvergnat J.C., Mathieu P., Bachet P. Q Fever Endocarditis in the South of France. The Journal of Infectious Disease, 1987. 155: pp. 570-573

36. Brouqui P., Tissot Dupont H., Drancourt M., Berlan Y., Etienne J., Leport C., Goldstein F., Massip P., Micoud M., Bertrand A., Raoult D. Epidemiologic and Clinical Features of Chronic Q Fever: 92 Cases from France (1982-1990). Archives of Internal Medicine, 1993. 153: pp. 642-648

37. Ellis M.E., Smith C.C., Moffat M.A. Chronic and Fatal Q-Fever Infection: a Review of 16 Patients Seen in North-East Scotland (1967-1980). Quarterly Journal of Medicine, 1983. 52: pp. 54-66

38. Fournier P. E., Casalta J.P., Piquet P., Tournigand P., Branchereau A., Raoult D. 1998. Coxiella burnetii Infection of Aneurysms or Vascular Grafts: Report of Seven Cases and Review. Clinical Infectious Disease, 1998. 26: pp. 116-121

39. Cottalorda J., Jouve J.L., Bollini G., Touzet P., Poujol A., Kelberine F., Raoult D. 1995. Osteoarticular Infection due to Coxiella burnetii in Children. Journal of Pediatric Orthopaedics, 1995. 4: pp. 219-221

40. Raoult D., Bollini G., Gallais H. Osteoarticular Infection due to Coxiella burnetii. The Journal of Infectious Disease, 1989. 159: pp. 1159-1160

41. Piquet P., Raoult D., Tranier P., Mercier C.I. Coxiella burnetii Infection of Pseudoaneurysm of an Aortic Bypass Graft with Contiguous Vertebral Osteomyelitis. Journal of Vascular Surgery, 1994. 19: pp. 165-168

42. Yebra M., Marazuela M., Albarran F., Moreno A. 1988. Chronic Q Fever Hepatitis. Reviews of infectious diseases, 1988. 10: pp. 1229-1230

43. Aitken I. D., Bögel K., Cracea E., Edlinger E., Houwers D., Krauss H., Rady M., Rehacek J., Schiefer H.G., Schmeer N., Tarasevich I.V., Tringali G. 1987. Q fever in Europe: Current Aspects of Aetiology, Epidemiology, Human Infection, Diagnosis and Therapy. Infection, 1987. 15: pp. 323-327

44. Janigan D. T., Marrie T.J. An Inflammatory Pseudotumor of the Lung in Q Fever Pneumonia. The New England Journal of Medicine, 1983. 308: pp. 86-87

45. Ayres J. G., Smith E.G., Flint N. 1996. Protracted Fatigue and Debility after Acute Q Fever. Lancet, 1996. 347: pp. 978-979

46. Ayres J. G., Flint N., Smith E.G., Tunnicliffe W.S., Fletcher T.J., Hammond K., Ward D., Marmion B.P. Post-infection Fatigue Syndrome following Q Fever. Quarterly Journal of Medicine, 1998. 91: pp. 105-123

47. Brouqui P., Dumler J.S., Raoult D. Immunohistologic Demonstration of Coxiella burnetii in the Valves of Patients with Q Fever Endocarditis. American Journal of Medicine, 1994. 97: pp. 451-458

48. Thiele D., Karo M., Krauss H. Monoclonal Antibody Based Capture ELISA/ELIFA for Detection of Coxiella burnetii in Clinical Specimens. European Journal of Epidemiology, 1992. 8: pp. 568-574

49. Muhlemann K., Matter L., Meyer B., Schoper K. Isolation of Coxiella burnetii from Heart Valves of Patients Treated for Q Fever Endocarditis. Journal of Clinical Microbiology, 1995. 33: pp. 428-431

50. Kazar J., Brezina R., Schramek S., Palanova A., Tvrda B. 1981. Suitability of the Microaggglutination Test for Detection of Post-infection and Post-vaccination Q fever Antibodies in Human Sera. Acta Virologica, 1981. 25: pp. 235-240

51. Nguyen S. V., Otsuka H., Zhang G.Q., To H., Yamaguchi T., Fukushi H., Noma A., Hirai K. 1996. Rapid Method for Detection of Coxiella burnetii Antibodies using High-density Particle Agglutination. Journal of Clinical Microbiology, 1996. 34: pp. 2947-2951

52. Herr S., Huchzermeyer H.F., Te Brugge L.A., Williamson C.C., Roos J.A. , Schiele G.T. The use of a Single Complement Fixation Test Technique in Bovine Brucellosis, Johne's Disease, Dourine, Equine Piroplasmosis and Q Fever Serology. The Onderstepoort Journal of Veterinary Research, 1985. 52: pp. 279-282

53. Murphy A. M., Field P.R. The Persistence of Complement-fixing Antibodies to Q Fever (Coxiella burnetii) after Infection. The Medical Journal of Australia, 1970. 1: pp. 1148-1150

54. Peter O., Dupuis G., Burgdorfer W., Peacock M. 1985. Evaluation of the Complement Fixation and Indirect Immunofluorescence Tests in the Early Diagnosis of Primary Q Fever. European Journal of Clinical Microbiology and Infectious Diseases, 1985. 4: pp. 394-396

55. Doller G., Doller P.C., Gerth H.J. 1984. Early Diagnosis of Q Fever: Detection of Immunoglobulin M by Radioimmunoassay and Enzyme Immunoassay. European Journal of Clinical Microbiology and Infectious Diseases, 1984. 3: pp. 550-553

56. Field P. R., Hunt J.G., Murphy A.M. 1983. Detection and Persistence of Specific IgM Antibody to Coxiella burnetii by Enzyme-linked Immunosorbent Assay: a Comparison with Immunofluorescence and Complement Fixation Tests. The Journal of Infectious Disease, 1983. 148: pp. 477-487

57. Kovacova E., Gallo J., Schramek S., Kazar J., Brezina R. Coxiella burnetii Antigens for Detection of Q Fever Antibodies by ELISA in Human Sera. Acta virologica,1987. 31: pp. 254-259

58. Peter O., Dupuis G., Bee D., Luthy R., Nicolet J., Burgdorfer W. Enzyme-linked Immunosorbent Assay for Diagnosis of Chronic Q Fever. Journal of Clinical Microbiology, 1988. 26: pp. 1978-1982

59. Uhaa I. J., Fishbein D.B., Olson J.G., Rives C.C., Waag D.M., Williams J.C. Evaluation of Specificity of Indirect Enzyme-linked Immunosorbent Assay for Diagnosis of Human Q Fever. Journal of Clinical Microbiology, 1994. 32: pp. 1560-1565

60. Schmeer N., Muller H.P., Baumgartner W., Wieda J., Krauss H. Enzyme-linked Immunosorbent Fluorescence Assay and High-pressure Liquid Chromatography for Analysis of Humoral Immune Responses to Coxiella burnetii Proteins. Journal of Clinical Microbiology, 1988. 26: pp. 2520-2525

61. Willems H., Thiele D., Glas-Adollah-Baik Kashi M., Krauss H. 1992. Immunoblot Technique for Q Fever.European Journal of Epidemiology, 1992. 8: pp. 103-107

62. Blondeau J. M., Williams J.C., Marrie T.J. 1990. The Immune Response to phase I and II Coxiella burnetii Antigens as Measured by Western Immunoblotting. Annals of the New York Academy of Sciences, 1990. 590: pp. 187-202

63. Gil-Grande R., Aguado J.M., Pastor C., Garcia-Bravo M., Gomez-Pellico C., Soriano F., Noriega A. Conventional Viral Cultures and Shell Vial Assay for Diagnosis of Apparently Culture-negative Coxiella burnetii Endocarditis. European Journal of Clinical Microbiology and Infectious Diseases, 1995. 14: pp. 64-67

64. Raoult D., Vestris G., Enea M. 1990. Isolation of 16 Strains of Coxiella burnetii from Patients by Using a Sensitive Centrifugation Cell Culture System and Establishment of Strains in HELA cells. Journal of Clinical Microbiology, 1990. 28: pp. 2482-2484

65. Musso D., Raoult D. Coxiella burnetii Blood Cultures from Acute and Chronic Q Fever Patients. Journal of Clinical Microbiology, 1995. 33: pp. 3129-3132

66. Stein A., Raoult D. Detection of Coxiella burnetii by DNA Amplification using Polymerase Chain Reaction. Journal of Clinical Microbiology, 1992. 30: pp. 2462-2466

67. Stein A., Raoult D. A Simple Method for Amplification of DNA from Paraffin-embedded Tissues. Nucleic Acids Research, 1992. 20: pp. 5237-5238]

68. Raoult D., Houpikian P., Tissot Dupont H., Riss J.M., Arditi-Djiane J., Brouqui P. Treatment of Q Fever Endocarditis: Comparison of 2 Regimens Containing Doxycycline and Ofloxacin or Hydroxychloroquine. Achieves of Internal Medicine, 1999. 159: pp. 167-73

69. Potential for Q fever infection among travelers returning from Iraq and the Netherlands. Center of Disease Control. Revised May 12, 2010. Retrieved November 19, 2011. http://emergency.cdc.gov/HAN/han00313.asp

70. J.H. McIsaac. Hospital Preparation for Bioterror. A Medical and Biomedical System Approach. Burlington: Academic Press. 2006. pp. 56

Photo Bibliography

Figure 2.6-1: Transmission electronmicrograph (TEM) of *C. burnetii*. This electron photomicrograph was taken and released by Rocky Mountain Laboratories, National Institute of Allergy and Infectious Diseases (NIAID), Department of Health and Human Services. Public domain photo

Figure 2.6-3: *C. burnetii* infection diagram. The human anatomical illustration was created by Dr. Alexander J. da Silva and Melanie Moser in 2003. The illustration is released by the CDC. Public domain graphics

Figure 2.6-4: X-ray picture of Q-fever pneumonia. The X-ray photograph was shown in Scrimgeour E.M., Johnston W.J., Al Dhahry S.H.S., El-Khatim H.S., John V., Musa M. First Report of Q Fever in Oman. Emerging Infectious Diseases, 2000. 6: pp. 74-76. This photograph was released by the CDC. Public domain photo

Belonging to the family Enterobacteriaceae, *Escherichia coli* (*E. coli*), are moderately sized (~0.3 to 1.0 x 1.0 to 6.0 µm), Gram-negative, non-sporulating, facultative anaerobic bacilli that are ubiquitously found in nature and cannot be removed by any conventional decontamination and/or sanitary means.[1, 2] *E. coli* are generally non-pathogenic and are the major constituents of the normal human intestinal flora. It has been estimated that, on average, humans have a density of approximately 10^6 to 10^8 colony-forming units per gram of stool. A great deal of information has been gathered through years of research using this microorganism, as it continues to be an important tool in biological research. Many researchers, in fact, consider this organism as a laboratory pet.[3, 4] Nonetheless, certain strains of *E. coli* can produce enterotoxins, which could result in serious food-borne diseases in humans. For example, *E. coli* strains that could cause diarrhea of varying severity have been divided into six major categories: enterotoxigenic *E. coli* (ETEC), enteroinvasive *E. coli* (EIEC), enteroaggregative *E. coli* (EAEC), diffusely adherent *E. coli* (DAEC), enteropathogenic *E. coli* (EPEC), and enterohemorrhagic *E. coli* (EHEC) (Table 1).

Table 1: Serotypes of pathogenic *E. coli*[5]

Serotype	Symptoms
ETEC	Produces diarrhea resembling mild cholera (e.g. travelers' diarrhea)
EIEC	Produces dysentery that is indistinguishable clinically from shigellosis
EAEC	Persistent diarrhea in children and causing travelers' diarrhea
DAEC	Pathogenicity not conclusively demonstrated
EPEC	Dysentery-like diarrhea with fever; generally associated with infants
EHEC	Watery diarrhea that may progress to bloody diarrhea in 1–3 days

EHEC, also known as 'killer *E.coli*', is subdivided into numerous serotypes such as O26, O45, O91, O103, O111, O113, O121, O104, O145, and O157, to name a few. In particular, O157:H7, also known as the proto-serotype of EHEC, has been listed as a Category B Biological Weapon by the Center for Disease Control and prevention (Figure 2.7-1).[3, 4, 5]

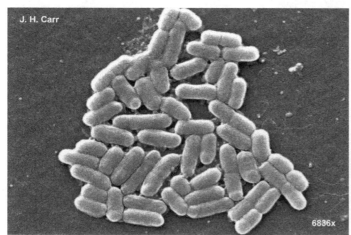

Figure 2.7-1: Scanning electron micrograph (SEM) shows numerous Gram-negative *Escherichia coli* bacteria of the strain O157:H7

Through transduction, O157:H7 managed to acquire new virulence genes, whereby allowing them to encode two verotoxins that cause bloody diarrhea and hemolytic uremic syndrome (HUS). HUS is characterized by three clinical conditions: ① hemorrhagic colitis, ② hemolytic-uremic syndrome and ③ thrombocytopenic-purpura.[6,7]

O157:H7 is generally seen in children ages 1 to 4 and adults over 60 years of age.[8] It is estimated that these bacilli cause over 100,000 infections and approximately 100 deaths in the United States (U.S.) annually.[2, 9] In the U.S., the major source of EHEC O157:H7 is from exposure to contaminated beef cattle. For example, an outbreak of *E. coli* O157:H7 caused 28 infections in July 2002 in Colorado, as well as, in six other states. This outbreak was linked to contaminated ground beef products which resulted from the use of cattle manure as fertilizer (Figure 2.7-2). Seven out of the 28 infected were hospitalized, while five patients developed HUS.[10, 11] Other known events linked to *E. coli* O157:H7 have also been reported. For example, EHEC has been linked to alfalfa sprouts[12], apple cider[13], lettuce[14], parsley[15], raw milk[16], re-contaminated pasteurized milk[17], salami[18], unpasteurized gouda cheese[19] and white radish sprouts.[20] Additionally, cases of waterborne *E. coli* O157:H7 outbreaks have also been reported. For example, during May 2000, an *E. coli* O157:H7 outbreak occurred in the small town of Walkerton (population ~5000) located in Ontario, Canada. This outbreak overwhelmed the local emergency medical services that were not prepared for the inundation of individuals seeking medical attention. The final tally of this outbreak is ~2300 individuals infected, resulting in seven fatalities.[21, 22, 23]

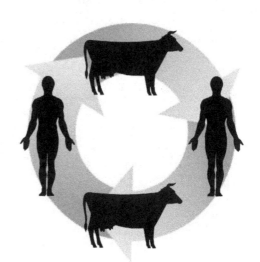

Figure 2.7-2: Transmission cycle of *E. coli* O157:H7

It has been speculated that due to the highly infectious nature of *E. coli* O157:H7, as well as, ease of dispersal, the potential and purposeful release of this bacilli as a form of biological attack is definitely within the realm of possibility.[21, 22] Ingestion of fewer than 100 EHEC bacilli can induce severe symptoms of disease. Once ingested, the bacilli proceed to the intestinal tract where they adhere to the mucosal lining and begin colonization. It is known that EHEC (as well as with EPEC) forms a characteristic histopathologic feature known as 'attaching and effacing' (also termed A/E) lesions in cultured cells and in small and large intestinal tissues. The A/E lesions are characterized by the intimate attachment of the bacilli to the apical surface enterocytes in the intestines, which results in the effacement of the brush border.[24, 25] Because of this effacement, researchers have proposed two possible causes of the symptoms: ① the formation of A/E lesions may severely hamper absorption and promote diarrhea due to the loss of microvilli and/or ② the formation of the A/E lesions may enable the pathogen to modulate the enterocytes signaling processes which result in the development of diarrhea.[26, 27, 28]

All genes necessary for the formation of A/E lesions by EHEC (as well as EPEC) are encoded within the 35 kb chromosomal pathogenicity island known as the locus of enterocyte effacement (LEE).[29] LEE is known to encode type III secretion systems (TTSSs), which allows for the direct injection of effector proteins into host cells.[30] One factor of the LEE that promotes adherence is the product of the gene eaeA, called the outer membrane protein (OMP), also referred to as intimin.[31, 32, 33, 34] The epithelial membrane receptor for intimin, translocated intimin receptor (Tir), is also encoded by LEE and secreted from the bacilli on to the plasma membrane of the enterocyte. Once Tir makes contact with the membrane of the enterocyte, it adopts a hairpin loop conformation and creating an efficient environment for the delivery of effector proteins into the enterocyte.[25, 30, 35]

The binding of intimin to the central extracellular domain of Tir prompts the clustering of the N- and C- terminal cytoplasmic regions and promotes localized actin assembly immediately beneath the plasma membrane of the enterocyte. This noticeable cytoskeletal rearrangement (polymerized and accumulated actin and other host proteins) results in the formation of an actin-rich pedestal.[26, 36, 37] In addition to Tir and intimin, other effector proteins are also created within the pathogenicity island. These effector proteins are EspH, Map, EspF EspG, EspB, EspA, and EspD, which are synthesized within the bacilli and translocated by the TTSS into the cytosol of the enterocytes. For example, EspH, a cytoskeleton modulating protein, is known to down-regulate filopodium formation and promote pedestal formation in cultured HeLa cells.[38] Map effector proteins are known to influence host cytoskeletal processes in laboratory cultured cells, while EspG promotes the formation of pedestals on HeLa cultured cells. EspF, on the other hand, has shown evidence of dampening and subverting the immunoresponse. Experiments have shown that the deletion of the genes associated with EspF cause a marked increase in the activities of the host cytokines, resulting in the accumulation of polymorpho-nuclear leukocytes.[25] EspB is a multifunctional effector protein composed of 312 amino acid residues that can bind to various biomolecules such as α-catenin, $α_1$-antitrypsin and myosin from the host cell, and secreted bacterial effectors such as EspA and EspD. It has been reported that these EspB interactions with target proteins are associated with different events in bacterial infection.[39] For example, EspB and EspD are inserted into the cellular membrane, and together with EspA, these proteins constitute a molecular syringe which channels other effector proteins into the host cell.[40] Additionally, EspB has been reported to inhibit the interaction between myosin and actin within the host cell, which in turn, prevents the formation of microvillus and phagocytosis.[41] Finally, the interactions between EspB with α-catenin are believed to be involved in actin reorganization during bacterial infection, although the precise mechanism of this interaction requires further elucidation.[42]

What distinguishes EHEC O157:H7 from other pathogenic strains of E. coli are the Shiga-like toxins (SLTs) originally found in Shigella dysenteriae type I. EHEC produces two SLTs known as verocytotoxin 1 and 2 (VT1 or VT2 or stx1 or stx2), which are the most virulence characteristic of the bacilli.[32, 43, 44] It is currently believed that the genes available for the EHEC to produce VT1 and VT2 were transduced and lysogenized into the bacilli by lambdoid bacteriophages.[32, 43, 44, 45] VTs are known to cause both local and systemic diseases. For example, the introduction of the toxins locally will block cellular protein synthesis leading to cell death. While in a systemic infection, the toxin will enter the blood stream and bind to receptors located on the endothelial cells of

the kidneys and brain, resulting in HUS.[32, 46]

VT1 and VT2 are AB_5 toxins composed of a single 32 kDa A-subunit in a non-covalent association with a pentamer (5 polypeptides) of B-subunits. Toxin binding is initiated by the B-subunits through their interaction with a membrane glycolipid receptor found commonly on human endothelial cells, known as globotriaosylceramide (Gb_3). It is understood that the binding of B-subunits to Gb_3 initiates clathrin-dependent endocytosis.[47, 48] Once the verotoxins gain access to the cytosol of the endothelial cells, the A-subunit, also an N-glycosidase, catalytically cleaves a single adenine residue from the 28S rRNA component of the eukaryotic ribosome's 60S subunit, thereby inhibiting protein synthesis, which eventually results in cell death and detachment.[48, 49] Once the dead cells detach, the subepithelium is exposed to circulating platelets, initiating the clotting cascade. Additionally, VT1 and VT2 have also shown the ability to induce the expression of neutrophil-specific chemokine interleukin-8, secreted by human intestinal epithelial cells. The secretion of interleukin-8 prompts the process of intestinal inflammation.[46, 47] It has been hypothesized that VT1 and VT2 may enhance the expression of nucleolin on the cell surface thereby promoting the adherence of EHEC. However, this postulation requires further elucidation (Figure 2.7-3).[49]

M. E. Fraser et al.

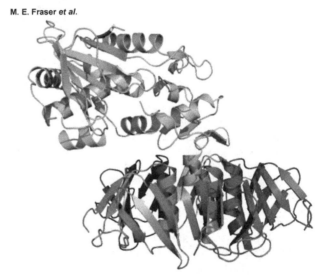

Figure 2.7-3: A 3D structure rendering of shiga toxin. The A subunit (upper left) and B subunit (lower right)

SYMPTOMS

The incubation period of EHEC is approximately 1 to 9 days. Patients infected with O157:H7 may display a wide spectrum of clinical symptoms. These symptoms may include an asymptomatic infection or one with only grossly bloody diarrhea. Nonetheless, approximately 38 to 61% of all EHEC infections result in hemorrhagic colitis, with clinical symptoms including abdominal cramps and diarrhea that progresses from watery to bloody.[50] This condition usually begins with a sudden onset of severe abdominal cramps with little or no fever (>101°F/38.5°C). Within hours of this initial symptom, watery diarrhea will progress within 2 to 8 days into grossly bloody diarrhea, lasting on average 3-8 days.[2, 51, 52, 53] The amount of blood in the stool may be as little as streaks to as much as 0.95 L (~4 cups). In addition, 3 to 30 bowel movements have been reported on the worst day of the diarrhea. During this time, upper gastrointestinal symptoms including nausea and chills may appear. Approximately one-third of patients will have low grade fever, while vomiting may occur in nearly half of the patients.[2, 4, 51, 52, 53, 54] Radiologic and/

or endoscopic examination of these patients will show colonic mucosal edema, erosion and/or hemorrhage. Patients suffering from this condition will also pass stool without the conventional organisms, while fecal leukocytes or lactoferrin are observed in less than 40% of the patients (Table 2).[4, 52, 53] Examine Table 1 for an overview of clinical symptoms of EHEC infection.

Table 2: An overview of the clinical symptoms of EHEC infection

Symptoms	+	++	+++
Abdominal cramps			▪
Diarrhea			▪
Grossly bloody diarrhea			▪
Nausea			▪
Chills			▪
Vomiting			▪
Colonic mucosal edema			▪
Colonic mucosal erosion			▪
Mucosal (colon) hemorr.			▪
Low grade fever		▪	

+ Rare ++ Common +++ Frequent

Uncomplicated *E. coli* O157:H7 infections generally subside in approximately a week, nonetheless for children (~1-4 of age) and elderly adults (~61-91 of age), the condition may proceed into a devastating sequela known as HUS (hemolytic uremic syndrome).[4, 8] HUS occurs in approximately 5-10% of all EHEC cases, although in some studies, 75-95% of children suffering from EHEC developed HUS.[4, 55, 56]

HUS is characterized by microangiopathic hemolytic anemia (anemia with the presence of fragmented erythrocytes and a hemoglobin concentration of <10 g/dL), thrombocytopenia (<100 thousand platelets/mm³) and renal failure (anuria, oliguria or elevated serum creatinine levels: ~1.5 time higher than normal values in age matched controls). HUS generally manifests itself 4-5 days after the onset of the initial bout of diarrhea.[57] Although in rare cases, this condition do appear in adults, HUS mostly appears in infants and children where it leads to acute renal failure.[50, 58, 59] Most patients suffering from HUS have gastrointestinal prodromes where diarrhea (either bloody or non-bloody) is commonly seen. Other symptoms that are also commonly observed are abdominal cramps, vomiting, headaches, oliguria, edema, petechiae, somnolence, hematuria (or proteinuria), fever, lethargy, seizure, pallor and respiratory distress.[51, 57, 60, 61] Liver dysfunctions indicated by the elevation of serum aminotransferases and pancreatitis may also be associated with HUS.[57] Radiographic analysis demonstrates bowel edema, transient segmental narrowing and bowel stenosis, while sigmoidoscopy illustrates rectal ulceration, friable mucosa, pseudomembranes and diffused colitis. In some cases, rectal prolapse, toxic megacolon and ascites have also been reported.[51, 62, 63]

In 30-50% of the patients, central nervous system complications have been reported.[64, 65] Common neurological symptoms include lethargy, seizures or coma during the acute phase of the illness. Postmortem examinations have found evidence of raised cranial pressure along with micro-thrombi and focal areas of infarction in the cerebral cortex.[64, 66, 67, 68, 69, 70] Survivors may experience long-term neurological sequalae, which include generalized chronic seizures, cortical blindness, hemiparesis, concomitant cognitive and behavioral deficits, as well as, developmental delays, psychomotor retardation and mental retardation in children.[64, 66, 67, 69]

The case fatality rate of children suffering from HUS is between 5-10%. Among the elderly patients, the fatality rate is approximately 3-36%. Nonetheless, during a 2003 outbreak of hemorrhagic colitis in a nursing home located in San Mateo County, California, the fatality rate reached 88% (Table 3).[51, 53, 71, 72, 73]

Table 3: An overview of the clinical symptoms of HUS. Please note the following abbreviations: microangiopathic (microangio.), hemolytic (hemo.), and child (C). Note: microangiopathioc hemolytic anemia (MHA); Transient segmental narrowing (TSN); psychomotor retardation (PR)

Symptoms	+	++	+++
Diarrhea (bloody)			▪
Diarrhea (non-bloody)			▪
MHA			▪
Thrombocytopenia			▪
Anuria			▪
Oliguria			▪
Renal failure			▪
Abdominal cramps			▪
Vomiting			▪
Dehydration			▪
Headaches			▪
Edema			▪
Petechiae			▪
Somnolence			▪
Hematuria or proteinuria			▪
Fever			▪
Lethargy			▪
Seizure			▪
Bacteriemia			▪
Pallor			▪
Respiratory distress			▪
Sepsis			▪
Liver dysfunctions		▪	
Bowel edema		▪	
TSN		▪	
Bowel stenosis		▪	
Rectal ulceration		▪	
Friable mucosa		▪	
Pseudomembranes		▪	
Diffused colitis		▪	
Lethargy		▪	
Seizures		▪	
Chronic seizures		▪	
Coma		▪	
Cortical blindness		▪	
Hemiparesis		▪	
Cognitive deficits (C)		▪	
Behavioural deficits (C)		▪	
Development delays (C)		▪	
PR (C)		▪	
Mental retardation (C)		▪	
Rectal prolapse	▪		
Toxic megacolon	▪		
Ascites	▪		

+ Rare ++ Common +++ Frequent

▨ HUS (CNS involvements)
■ HUS

DETECTION

Due to the ubiquitous nature of *E. coli* in human fecal matter, it has always been problematic to identify the virulent strains from the non-virulent strains. Nonetheless, it has been discovered that EHEC O157:H7, unlike most other *E. coli* is slow in fermenting sorbitol, therefore, techniques involving MacConkey agar (an indicator medium) and sorbitol agar (a selective medium) have been developed as screening media to isolate this bacilli serotype. For example, EHEC O157:H7 will be sorbitol-negative (visually clear) after 24 hours of incubation, making a presumptive diagnosis possible. It has been reported that the MacConkey-sorbitol medium is 100% sensitive, 85% specific and 86% accurate for detecting O157:H7 bacilli.[4, 51, 74, 75, 76] Sorbitol-negative colonies can be further serotyped via agglutination by using antisera to both the H7 and O157 antigens, and/or in detecting the presences of verotoxins.[51]

The limitations regarding the use of MacConkey-sorbitol medium is that the rate of positive detection of EHEC decreases with the delay in the collection of stool samples. In a study by Tarr et al. (1990), the rate of positive stool culture ranged from 100% for samples collected within 2 days after the onset of diarrhea to 92% for samples collected between days 3 to 6. The rate of positive detection of EHEC was further reduced for samples collected after the 7th day to approximately 33%.[77]

It has been reported that free verocytotoxins may remain measurable in fecal matter for as long as 4-6 weeks, making it a better candidate (simpler and more sensitive method than culture techniques) for detecting EHEC infections. Therefore, newer methods including genetic probes and immunological techniques have been developed that are designed to detect VT1 and VT2 (SLTs) in fecal matter, although some are less practical for use in clinical situations due to the concerns with radioactive safety and cost effectiveness.[51, 72] For example, VT1 and VT2 producing E. coli could be detected by using DNA hybridization techniques. These in situ methods utilize the nucleotide and fragments of structural genes specific for the verocytotoxins and are very sensitive and specific in that these probes can detect verocytotoxin producing E. coli in as diminutive as 1 in 1200 colonies.[78, 79, 80]

Various monoclonal and polyclonal antibody enzyme-linked immunosorbent assays (ELISA) have also been developed against VT1 and VT2. For example, a particular ELISA, known as Premier EHEC assay developed by Meridian Diagnostics®, has been reported to allow for a timely and cost effective manner for diagnosis, which should be used as a routine screening for enteric pathogens in high-risk individuals, especially children.[81] In addition, an assay called ImmunoCard STAT!®, also developed by Meridian Bioscience®, can be used to rapidly test for EHEC infections. This detection kit has been reported to be an acceptable alternative to Premier EHEC assay.[82] However, a 2013 report by Chui et al. indicated that the performance of ImmunoCard STAT!® is less than satisfactory when copared with real-time PCR methodology in detecting O157:H7 isolates.[83]

Serologic testing to detect antibodies developed against verocytotoxins, as well as, against the O157 lipopolysaccharides have also been used to detect and support the diagnosis for EHEC infections. One such test platform, DIAPRO FAST-Q®, has provided results within 20 minutes for the direct detection of E. coli O157:H7 in stool samples from infected patients.[84] Polymerase chain reaction (PCR) has also become a part of routine testing and quantification of EHEC bacilli. A number of E. coli O157:H7 genes such as stx1 and stx2 (the genes for VT1 and VT2), eaeA, hlyA, fliC, and several genetic sequences from the O-antigen synthesis operon, have been selected for diagnostic amplification. Results from real-time PCR linked with a rapid cycling platform can be generated in ~30 minutes from the start of the thermal cycling.[85]

TREATMENT

Supportive therapy and the management of symptoms is presently the mainstay for the treatment of E. coli O157:H7 infections. As with all diarrheal diseases, fluid and electrolyte replacement is essential. Oral rehydration is the initial the course of action in the treatment of patients with mild or moderate dehydration. The World Health Organization (WHO) recommends an oral rehydration formula based on the physiological observation that the intestinal absorption of sodium is coupled with the absorption of glucose, even during a period of illness, when most substances are actively being excreted. Please examine Table 4 for the simple and inexpensive oral rehydration formula recommended by WHO, which has been credited with saving over a million lives around the world each year. When faced with a case of severe dehydration, clinicians are recommended to rehydrate patients intravenously with normal saline or Ringer's lactate.[4, 86]

Table 4: Oral rehydration formula recommended by WHO[4]

Ingredient	Amount (grams)
Table Salt (NaCl)	3.5
Sodium bicarbonate (NaHCO$_3$)	2.5
Potassium Chloride (KCl)	1.5
Glucose (C$_6$H$_{12}$O$_6$)	20

Body fluid management is essential, where water and electrolyte balance should be carefully monitored. During oliguric or anuric periods, clinicians should note that over hydration can easily cause the patients to develop fluid overload, hypertention and hyponatremia. During the course of the infection, hyperkalemia and hypokalemia may develop. Potassium supplements should be administered in cases of hypokalemia.[57] Antidiarrheal agents have been suggested to contribute in the retention of verocytotoxins in the colon enhancing the uptake of the toxins into the patients, therefore the administeration of antidiarrheal agents should be avoided.[87, 88]

Dialysis may be needed for patients with urine output less than 250mL/m^2 per day, or for patients who developed intractable fluid overload, hypertension, serum electrolyte disturbances and metabolic acidosis. Methods of dialysis for older children and adults are hemodialysis or peritoneal dialysis, while for younger children and infants, only peritoneal dialysis should be used.[56] Unfortunately, administering antibiotics does not demonstrate any effectiveness against the infection. In contrast, the administration of antibiotics during EHEC hemorrhagic colitis has actually resulted in a significantly higher risk in developing HUS.[89, 90] Studies have shown that E. coli O157:H7 is susceptible in vitro to various antibiotics such as ampicillin, carbenicilin, cephalothin, gentamicin, quinolones, trimetho-prim and trimethoprim-sulfamethoxazole, while in vivo administration of antibiotics did not reduce the duration of the illness in comparison to patients treated with antibiotics.[4, 51, 53, 91] Research has shown that exposure of patients to sub-lethal concentrations of ciprofloxin, trimethoprim-sulfamethoxazole, polymyxin B and tetracycline actually increased the release of verocytotoxin (VT1).[7, 92, 93] While administering inhibitory concentrations of roxithromycin, rokitamycin or clindamycin produced a decreased amount of verocytotoxins release, it showed no effect on the population of bacilli. In contrast, exposure to cefdinir, fosfomycin or levofloxacin decreased the number of bacilli but increased the amount of VT1 and VT2 released.[94] In addition, patients treated with trimethoprim-sulfametho-xazole had longer durations of diarrhea, bloody diarrhea and have a greater propensity of developing HUS.[95] In a study by Carter et al. (1987), antibiotic therapy administered after the onset of symptoms was actually associated with higher case fatality rate.[72]

Three mechanisms have been put forth in an attempt to explain why antibiotics are not effective against E. coli O157:H7 infections.

Table 5: Differential diagnosis of chronic EHEC with selected disease with similar symptoms. These diseases are pseudomembranous colitis (PC), ischemic colitis (IC), Salmonellosis (SAL), *Shigella*, *Campylobacter* (CAMP) and *Yersinia* enterocolitis (YE)

Symptoms	EHEC	PC	IC	SAL	Shigella	CAMP	YE
Fever	■		■	■			■
Chills	■		■	■			
Abdominal cramps	■	■	■		■		■
Headaches	■					■	
Nausea	■	■	■				■
Vomiting	■	■	■				■
Diarrhea (non-bloody or bloody)	■	■	■				■
Dehydration	■	■	■	■			
Colonic mucosal edema	■		■				
Colonic mucosal erosion	■		■				
Mucosal (colon) hemorrhage	■		■		■	■	
Pallor	■						
Somnolence	■						
Lethargy	■						
Microangiopathic hemo. anemia	■	■	■		■	■	
Thrombocytopenia	■	■	■			■	
Anuria	■				■	■	
Oliguria	■				■	■	
Renal failure	■				■	■	
Petechiae	■						
Hematuria or proteinuria	■			■			
Respiratory distress	■						
Liver dysfunctions	■					■	
Transient segmental narrow	■						
Bowel stenosis		■					
Rectal ulceration	■						
Friable mucosa	■						
Pseudomembranes	■						
Diffused colitis	■			■			
Seizures	■			■		■	■
Chronic seizures	■			■	■	■	■
Coma	■			■	■	■	
Cortical blindness	■						
Hemiparesis	■						
Rectal prolapse	■	■	■	■	■		
Toxic megacolon	■	■	■	■		■	
Ascites	■	■	■	■		■	

The first hypothesis is that antobiotics eliminate competing bowel flora of beneficial bacteria and allow an overgrowth of *E. coli* O157:H7, especially when the bacilli are resistant to the antibiotic administered. Secondly, the antibiotic may cause sublethal damage or lysis of the bacilli causing an increase in the release of Shiga-like toxin into the lumen of the intestinal tract. Finally, the administration of antibiotics may actually induce the transduction of Shiga-like toxin genes by bacteriophages.[50, 96, 97]

In light of the dangers associated with antibacterial therapy, it is suggested that antibiotics should be avoided in treating patients with hemorrhagic colitis or HUS. Nonetheless, antibacterial treatments after the onset of HUS have not shown to have any negative influences.[98]

DIFFERENTIAL DIAGNOSIS

Specific and accurate diagnosis of *E. coli* OH157:H7 (EHEC) requires clear documentation of patient history and laboratory analysis. The differential diagnosis for EHEC should also include *C. difficile*-related pseudomembranous colitis (PC), as well as, ischemic colitis (IC) caused by other medical conditions such as vasculitis, diabetes, colon cancer, etc. from which EHEC may be indistinguishable histologically. In addition, other symptomatic similar diseases such as Salmonellosis (SAL: genus *Salmonella*), *Shigella* (caused by genus bacteria in the genus *Shigella*

dysenteriae, *Campylobacter* (CAMP: caused by bacteria in the genus *Campylobacter*) and *Yersinia* enterocolitis (YE: caused by *Yersinia enterocolitica*) should also be considered in properly diagnosing EHEC (Table 5).

References:

1. Dembek Z. F., Anderson E.L. Food, Waterborne, and Agricultural Diseases. Medical Aspects of Biological Warfare. Chapter 2. Washington D.C.: The Surgeon General United States Army Medical Department Medical Center and School Borden Institute. 2007. pp. 21-38

2. Murray P.R., Rosenthal K.S., Kobayashi G.S., Pfaller M.A. Medical Microbiology. Fourth Edition. St. Louis: Mosby College Publishing, 2002. pp. 266-273

3. Tortora, Gerard J., Funke, Berdell R., Case, Christine L. Microbiology: An Introduction. Eighth edition. San Francisco: Pearson Education, 2004. pp. 314

4. Guerrant R.L., Walker D.H., Weller P.F. Tropical Infectious Diseases – Principles, Pathogens & Practice. Volume 1. Philadelphia: Churchill Livingstone Elsevier. 2006. pp. 201-219

5. Travelers' Health. Chapter 3, Infectious Disease Related to Travel. Center for Disease Control and Prevention (CDC). Revised August 1, 2014. Retrieved December 14, 2014. Website: http://wwwnc.cdc.gov/travel/yellowbook/ 2014/chapter-3-infectious-diseases-related-to-travel/esch erichia-coli

6. Salyers A., Whitt D.D. Bacterial Pathogenesis: A molecular Approach. Second Edition. Washington D.C.: American Society for Microbiology Press. 2002. pp. 9

7. Karmali M.A., Petric M., Lim C., Fleming P.C., Arbus G.S., Lior H. The Association between Idiopathic Hemolytic Uremic Syndrome and Infection by Verotoxin-producing *Escherichia coli*. The Journal of Infectious Diseases, 1985. 151: pp. 775-782

8. Rangel J.M., Sparling P.H., Crowe C., Griffin P.M., Swerdlow D.L. Epidemiology of *Escherichia Coli* O157:H7 Outbreaks, United States, 1982-2002. Emerging Infectious Diseases, 2005. 11: pp. 603-609

9. Disease Listing Enterohemorrhagic *Escherichia coli*. Centers for Disease Control and Prevention. October 6, 2005. Retrieved November 5, 2009. Website: http://cdc.gov/ncidod/dbmd/disease info/enterohemecoli_t.htm

10. Dewell G.A., Ransom J.R., Dewell R.D. McCurdy K., Gardner I.A., Hill A.E., Sofos J.N., Belk K.E., Smith G.C., Salman M.D. Prevalence of and Risk for *Escherichia coli* O157 in Market-ready Beef Cattle from 12 US Feedlots. Foodborne Pathogens and Disease,

2005. 2: pp. 70-76

11. US Department of Agriculture. Economic Opportunities for Dairy Cow Culling Management Options. Animal and Health Inspection Service. Revised: May 1996. Retrieved: November 6, 2009. Website: http://www.aphis.usda.gov/vs/ceah/ncahs/nahms/dairy/dai ry96/DR96fct3.pdf
12. Ferguson D.D., Scheftel J., Cronquist A., Smith K., Woo-Ming A., Anderson E., Knutsen J., De A.K., Gershman K. Temporally distinct *Escherichia coli* 0157 Outbreaks Associated with Alfalfa Sprouts Linked to a Common Seed Source – Colorado and Minnesota, 2003. Epidemiology and Infection, 2005. 133: pp. 439-447
13. Hilborn E.D., Mshar P.A., Fiorentino T.R., Dembek Z.F., Barrett T.J., Howard R.T., Carter M.L. An Outbreak of *Escherichia coli* 0157:H7 Infections and Haemolytic Uraemic Syndrome Associated with Consumption of Unpasteurized Apple Cider. Epidemiology and Infection, 2000. 124: pp. 31-36
14. Ackers M. L., Mahon B.E., Leahy E., Goode B., Damrow T., Hayes P.S., Bibb W.F., Rice D.H., Barrett T.J., Hutwagner L., Griffin P.M., Slutsker L. An Outbreak of *Escherichia coli* O157:H7 Infections Associated with Leaf Lettuce Consumption. The Journal of Infectious Diseases, 1998. 177: pp. 1588-1593
15. Naimi T.S., Wicklund J.H., Olsen S.J., Krause G., Wells J.G., Bartkus J.M., Boxrud D.J., Sullivan M., Kassenborg H., Besser J.M., Mintz E.D., Osterholm M.T., Hedberg C.W. Concurrent Outbreaks of *Sigella sonni* and Enterotoxigenic *Escherichia coli* Infections Associated with Parsley: Implications for Surveillance and Control of Foodborne Illness. Journal of Food Protection, 2003. 66: pp. 535-541
16. Keene W.E., Hedberg K., Herriott D.E., Hancock D.D., McKay R.W., Barrett T.J., Fleming D.W. A Prolonged Outbreak of *Escherichia coli* O157:H7 Infections Caused by Commercially Distributed Raw Milk. The Journal of Infectious Diseases, 1997. 176: pp. 815-818
17. Goh S., Newman C., Knowles M., Bolton F.J., Hollyoak V., Richards S., Daley P., Counter D., Smith H.R., Keppie N. *E. coli* O157 phage type 21/28 outbreak in North Cumbria Associated with Pasteurized Milk. Epidemiology and Infection, 2002. 129: pp. 451-457
18. MacDonald D.M., Fyfe M., Paccagnella A., Trinidad A., Louie K., Patrick D. *Escherichia coli* O157:H7 Outbreaks Linked to Salami, British Columbia, Canada, 1999. Epidemiology and Infection, 2004. 132: pp. 283-289
19. Honish L., Predy G., Hislop N., Chui L., Kowalewska-Grochowska K., Trottier L., Kreplin C., Zazulak I. An Outbreak of *E. coli* O157:H7 Hemorrhagic Colitis Associated with Unpasteurized Gouda Cheese. Canadian Journal of Public Health, 2005. 96: pp. 182-184
20. Michino H., Araki K., Minami S., Takaya S., Sakai N., Miyazaki M., Ono A., Yanagawa H. Massive Outbreak of *Escherichia coli* O157:H7 Infection in Schoolchildren in Sakai City, Japan, Associated with Consumption of White Radish Sprouts, American Journal of Epidemiology, 1999. 150: pp. 787-796
21. Swerdlow D.L., Woodruff B.A., Brady R.C., Griffin P.M., Tippen S., Donnell H.D. Jr, Geldreich E., Payne B.J., Meyer A. Jr, Wells J.G. A Water Borne Outbreak in Missouri of *Escherichia coli* O157:H7, Associated with Bloody Diarrhea and Death. Annals of Internal Medicine, 1992. 117: pp. 812-819
22. Bruneau A., Rodrigue H., Ismael J., Dion R., Allard R. Outbreak of E. coli O157:H7 Associated with Bathing at a Public Beach in the Montreal-Centre Region. Canada Communicable Disease Report, 2004. 30: pp. 133-136
23. Hanson, T. Inside Walkerton: Canada's Worst-Ever *E. coli* contamination. The Shock, The Investigation and The Aftermath. Revised May 17, 2010. Retrieved November 24, 2011. Website: http://www.cbc.ca/news/canada/story/ 2010/05/10/f-walkerton-water-ecoli.html
24. Knutton S., Baldwin T., Williams P.H., McNeish A.S. Actin Accumulation at Sites of Bacterial Adhesion to Tissue Culture Cells: Basis of a New Diagnostic Test for Enteropathogenic and Enterohemorrhagic *Escherichia coli*. Infection and Immunology, 1989. 57: pp. 1290–1298
25. Ritchie J.M., Waldor M.K. The Locus of Enterocyte Effacement-Encoded Effector Proteins All Promote Enterohemorrhagic *Escherichia coli* Pathogenicity in Infant Rabbits. Infection and Immunology, 2005. 73: pp. 1466-1474
26. Kresse A.U., Guzmann C.A., Ebel F. Modulation of Host Cell Signaling by Enteropathogenic and Shiga Toxin- Producing *Escherichia coli*. International Journal of Medical Microbiology, 2001. 291: pp. 277-285
27. Kresse A.U., Schulze K., Deibel C., Ebel F., Rohde M., Chakraborty T., Guzman C.A. Pas, a Novel Protein Required for Protein Secretion and Attaching and Effacing activities of Enterohemorrhagic *Escherichia coli*. The Journal of Bacteriology, 1998. 180: pp. 4370-4379
28. Hartland E.L., Leong J.M.Enteropathogenic and enterohemorrhagic *E. coli*: ecology, pathogenesis, and evolution. Frontiers in cellular and Infection Microbiology, 2013. 3: pp. 15
29. Perna N.T., Mayhew G.F., Pósfi G., Elliot S., Donnenberg M.S., Kaper J.B., Blattner F.R. Molecular Evolution of a Pathogenicity Island from Enterohemorrhagic *Escherichia coli* O157:H7. Infection and Immunity, 1998. pp. 3810-3817
30. Hueck C.J. Type III Protein Secretion System in Bacterial Pathogens of Animals and Plants. Microbiology and Molecular Biology Reviews, 1998. 62: pp. 379-433
31. Frankel G., Phillips A.D., Rosenshine I., Dougan G., Kaper J.B., Knutton S. Enteropathogenic and Enterohaemorrhagic *Escherichia coli*: More Subversive Elements. Molecular Microbiology, 1998. 30: pp. 911-921
32. Welinder-Olsson C., Kaijser B. Enterohemorrhagic *Escherichia coli*. Scandinavian Journal of Infectious Diseases, 2005. 37: pp. 405-416
33. Elliott S.J., Wainwright L.A., McDaniel T.K., Jarvis K.G., Deng Y.K., Lai L.C., McNamara B.P., Donnenberg M.S., Kaper J.B. The Complete Sequence of the Locus of Enterocyte Effacement (LEE) from Enteropathogenic *Escherichia coli* E2348/69. Molecular Microbiology, 1998. 28: pp. 1-4
34. Jerse A.E., Yu J., Tall B.D., Laper J.B. A Genetic Locus of Enteropathogenic *Escherichia coli* Necessay for the Production of Attaching and Effacing Lesions on Tissue Culture Cells. Proceeding of the National Academy of Science, 1990. 87: pp. 7839-7843
35. Kenny B., DeVinney B., Stein M., Reinscheid D.J., Frey E.A., Finlay B.B. Enteropathic *E. coli* (EPEC) transfers its Receptor for Intimate Adherence into Mammalian Cells. Cell, 1997. 91: 511-520
36. Campellone K.G., Rankin S., Pawson T., Kirschner M.W., Tipper D.J., Leong J.M. Clustering of Nck by a 12-Residue Tir Phosphopeptide is Sufficient to Trigger Localized Actin Assembly. The Journal of Cell Biology, 2004, 164: pp. 407-416
37. Campellone K.G., Robbins D., leong J.M. EspF (U) is a Translocated EHEC Effector that Interacts with Tir and N-WASP and Promotes Nck-independent Actin Assembly. Developmental Cell, 2004. 7: pp. 217-228
38. Tu X., Nisan I., Yona C., Hanski E., Rosenshine I. EspH, a New Cytoskeleton-modulating Effector of Enterohaemorrhagic and Enteropathogenic *Escherichia coli*. Molecular Microbiology, 2003. 47: pp. 595-606
39. Hamaguchi M., Kamikubo H., Suzuki K.N., Hagihara Y., Yanagihara I., Sakata I., Kataoka M., Hamada D. Structural Basis of a-Catenin Recognition by EspB from Enterohaemorrhagic E. coli Based on Hybrid Strategy Using Low-Resolution Structural and Protein Dissection. Public Library of Science (PLoS) One, 2013. 8: pp. e71618
40. Chiu H-J. , Syu W-J. Functional analysis of EspB from enterohaemorrhagic *Escherichia coli*. Microbiology, 2005. 151: pp. 3277-3286
41. Hamaguchi M., Hamada D. , Suzuki K.N., Sakata I., Yanagihara I. Molecular basis of actin reorganization promoted by binding of enterohaemorrhagic *Escherichia coli* EspB to α-catenin. Federation of European Microbiological Societies (FEMS) Journal, 2008. 275: pp. 6260–6267
42. Iizumi T., Sagara H., Kabe Y., Azuma M., Kume K., Ogawa M., Nagai T., Gillespie P.G., Sasakawa C., Handa H. The Enteropathogenic *E. coli* Effector EspB Facilitates Microvillus Effacing and Antiphagocytosis by Inhibiting Myosin Function. Cell Host and Microbe, 2007. 2: pp. 383–392
43. O'Brein A.D., LaVeck G.D. Purification and Characterization of a Shigella Dysenteriae 1-Like Toxin Produced by *Escherichia coli*. Infection and Immunity, 1983. 40: pp. 675-683
44. Paton J.C., Paton A.W. Pathogenesis and Diagnosis of Shiga Toxin-producing *Escherichia coli* Infections. Clinical Microbiology Reviews, 1998. 11: pp. 450-479
45. Schmidt H. Shiga-Toxin-Converting Bacteriophages. Research in Microbiology, 2001. 152: pp. 687-695
46. Salyers A.A., Whitt D.D. Bacterial Pathogenesis: A Molecular Approach. Second Edition. Washington D.C.: ASM Press, 2002. pp.416-420
47. Lingwood C.A. Role of Verotoxin Receptors in Pathogenesis. Trends in Microbiology, 1996. 4: pp. 147-153
48. Sandvig K. Shiga Toxin. Toxicon: Official Journal of the International Society of Toxinology, 2001. 39: pp. 1629-1635
49. Robinson C.M., Sinclair J.F., Smith M.J., O'Brien A.D. Siga Toxin of Enterohemorrhagic *Escherichia coli* Type 0157:H7 Promotes Intestinal Colonization. Proceedings of the National Academy of Science, 2006. 103: pp. 9667-9672
50. O'Brien A.D., Holmes R.K. Shiga and Shiga-like Toxins. Microbiological Reviews, 1987. 51: pp. 206-220
51. Su C., Brandt L.J. *Escherichia coli* O157:H7 Infection in Human. Annals of Internal Medicine, 1995. 123: pp. 698-707
52. Riley L.W. The Epidemiologic, Clinical, and microbiologic Features of Hemorrhagic Colitis. Annual Reviews of Microbiology, 1987. 41: pp. 383-407
53. Griffin P.M., Ostroff S.M., Tauxe R.V., Greene K.D., Wells J.G., Lewis J.H., Blake P.A. Illnesses Associated with *Escherichia coli* 0157:H7 Infections. A Broad Clinical Spectrum. Annals of Internal Medicine, 1988. 109: pp. 705-712
54. Slutsker L., Ries A.A., Greene K.D., Wells J.G., Hutwagner L., Griffin P.M. *Escherichia coli* O157:H7 Diarrhea in the United States: Clinical and Epidemiologic Features. Annals of Internal Medicine, 1997. 126: pp. 505-513
55. Neill M.A., Tarr P.I., Clausen C.R., Christie D.L., Hickman R.O. *Escherichia coli* O157:H7 as the Predominant Pathogen Associated with the Hemolytic Uremic Syndrome: A Prospective Study in the Pacific Northwest. Pediatrics, 1987. 80: pp. 37-40
56. Cleary T.G. Cytotoxin-producing *Escherichia coli* and the Hemolytic Uremic Syndrome. Pediatric Clinics of North America, 1988. 35: pp. 485-501
57. Japanese Pediatric Nephrology Association. Pediatrics International, 1999. 41: pp. 449-451
58. Fong J.S., de Chadarevian J.P., Kaplan B.S. Hemolytic-uremic Syndrome. Current Concepts and Management. Pediatric Clinics of North America, 1982. 29: pp. 835-856
59. Karmali M.A. Infection by Verocytotoxin-producing *Escherichia coli*. Clinical Microbiology Reviews, 1989. 2: pp. 15-38
60. Pickering L.K., Obrig T.G., Stapleton F.B. Hemolytic-uremic Syndrome and Enterohemorrhagic *Escherichia coli*. The Pediatric Infectious Disease Journal, 1994. 13: pp. 459-475
61. Martin D.L., MacDonald K.L., White K.E., Soler J.T., Osterholm M.T. The Epidemiology and Clinical Aspects of the Hemolytic-uremic Syndrome in Minnesota. The New England Journal of Medicine, 1990. 323: pp. 1161-1167
62. Peterson R.B., Meseroll W.P., Shrago G.G., Gooding C.A. Radiographic Features of Colitis Associated with the Hemolytic-uremic Syndrome. Radiology, 1976. 118: pp. 667-671
63. Whitington P.F., Friedman A.L., Chesney R.W. Gastrointestinal Disease in the Hemolytic-uremic Syndrome. Gastroenterology, 1979. 76: pp. 728-733
64. Bale J.F. Jr., Brasher C., Siegler R.I. CNS Manifestation of the Hemolytic-uremic Syndrome. Relationship to Metabolic Alterations and Prognosis. American Journal of Diseases of Children, 1980. 134: pp. 869-872
65. Cimolai N., Morrison B.J., Carter J.E. Risk Factors for the Central Nervous System Manifestations of Gastroenteritis-associated Hemolytic-uremic Syndrome. Pediatrics, 1992. 90: pp. 616-621
66. Schlieper A., Rowe P.C., Orrbine E., Zoubek M., Clark W., Wolfish N. McLaine P.N. Sequelae of Haemolytic Uraemic Syndrome, 1992. 67: pp. 930-934
67. Rooney J.C., Anderson R.M., Hopkins J.H. Clinical and Pathological Aspects of Central Nervous System Involvement in the Haemolytic Uraemic Syndrome. Australia Paediatric Journal, 1971. 7: pp. 28-33
68. Upadhyaya K., Barwick K., Fishaut M., Kashgarian M., Seigel N.J. The Importance of Nonrenal Involvement in Hemolytic-uremic Syndrome. Pediatrics, 1980. 65: pp. 115-120
69. Sheth K.J., Swick H.M., Haworth N. Neurologic Involvement in Hemolytic-uremic Syndrome. Annals of Neurology, 1986. 19: pp. 90-93
70. Argyle J.C., Hogg R.J., Pysher T.J., Silva F.G., Siegler R.L. A Clinicopathological Study of 24 Children with Hemolytic Uremic Syndrome. Pediatric Nephrology, 1990. 4: pp. 52-58
71. Karmali M.A., Petric M., Lim C., Fleming P.C., Arbus G.S., Lior H., The Association between idiopathic Hemolytic-uremic Syndrome and Infection by Verotoxin-producing *Escherichia coli*. The Journal of Infectious Diseases, 1985. 151: pp. 775-782
72. Carter A.O., Borczyk A.A., Carlsom J.A., Harvey B., Hockin J.C., Karmali M.A., Krishnan C., Korn D.A., Lior H. A Severe Outbreak of *Escherichia coli* O157:H7—Associated Hemorrhagic Colitis in a Nursing Home. The New England Journal of Medicine, 1987. 316: pp. 1496-1500
73. Reiss G., Kunz P., Koin D., Keefe E.B. *Escherichia coli* O157:H7 Infection in Nursing Homes: Review of Literature and Report of Recent Outbreak. Journal of the American Geriatrics Society, 2006. pp. 680-684
74. Farmer J.J. 3rd, Davis B.R. H7 antiserum-sorbitol Fermentation Medium: a Single Tube Screening Medium for Detecting *Escherichia coli* O157:H7 Associated with Hemorrhagic Colitis. Journal of Clinical Microbiology, 1985. 22: pp. 620-625
75. March S.B., Ratnam S. Sorbitol-MacConkey Medium for Detection of *Escherichia coli* O157:H7 Associated with Hemorrhagic Colitis. Journal of Clinical Microbiology, 1986. 23: pp. 869-872
76. Chapman P.A., Daly C.M. Comparison of Y1 Mouse Adrenal Cell and Coagglutination Assay for Detection of *Escherichia coli* heat labile enterotoxin. Journal of Clinical Pathology, 1989. 42: pp. 755-758
77. Tarr P.I., Neill M.A., Clausen C.R., Watkins S.L., Christie D.L., Hickman R.O. *Escherichia coli* O157:H7 and the Hemolytic-uremic Syndrome: Importance of Early Culture in Establishing the Etiology. The Journal of Infectious Diseases, 1990. 162: pp. 553-556
78. Scotland S.M., Rowe B., Smith H.R., Willshaw G.A., Gross R.J. Vero Cytotoxin-producing Strains of *Escherichia coli* from Children with Haemolytic-uremic Syndrome and Their Detection by Specific DNA Probes. Journal of Medical Microbiology, 1988. 25: pp. 237-243
79. Newland J.W., Neill R.J. DNA Probes for Shiga-like Toxin I and II and for Toxin-converting Bacteriophages. Journal of Clinical Microbiology, 1988. 26. pp. 1292-1297

80. Karch H. Meyer T. Evaluation of Oligonucleotide Probes for Identification of Shiga-like-toxin-producing *Escherichia coli*. Journal of Clinical Microbiology, 1989. 27. pp. 1180-1186

81. Kehl K.S., Havens P., Behnke C.E., Acheson D.W. Evaluation of the premier EHEC assay for detection of Shiga toxin-producing *Escherichia coli*. Journal of Clinical Microbiology, 1997. 35: pp. 2051-2054

82. Meridian Bioscience Receives FDA Clearance for New E. coli Test. Genetic Engineering & Biotechnology News. Revised: February 20, 2007. Retrieved: November 10, 2009. Website: www.genen gnews.com/news /bnitem_ print.aspx?name=13137091

83. Chui L., Lee M-C., Allen R., Bryks A., Haines L., Boras V. Comparison between ImmunoCard STAT!® and real-time PCR as screening tools for both O157:H7 and non-O157 Shiga toxin-producing *Escherichia coli* in Southern Alberta, Canada. Diagnostic Microbiology and Infectious Disease, 2013. 77: pp. 8-13

84. Ding S-F., Zhao Y-X., Liu L., Hatami S., Lea P. Rapid Test for Diagnosis of Enterohemorrhagic E.coli O157:H7 in Human Stool Samples. Journal of Rapid Methods & Automation in Microbiology, 2002. 10: pp. 255-261

85. Bono J.L., Keen J.E., Miller L.C., Fox J.M., Chitko-McKown C.G., Heaton M.P., Laegreid W.W. Evaluation of a Real-Time PCR Kit for Detecting *Escherichia coli* O157 in Bovine Fecal Samples. Applied and Environmental Microbiology, 2004. 70: pp. 1855-1857

86. Hirschhorn N., Greenough W.B. Progress in Oral Rehydration Therapy. Scientific American, 1991. 264: pp. 50-56

87. Tarr P.I., Gordon C.A., Chandler W.L. Shiga Toxin Producing *Escherichia coli* and Haemolytic Uraemic Syndrome. Lancet, 2005. 365: pp. 1073–1086

88. Siegler R., Oakes R. Hemolytic Uremic Syndrome, Pathogenesis, Treatment, and Outcome. Current Opinion in Pediatrics, 2005. 17: pp. 200–204

89. Slutsker L., Reis A.A., Maloney K., Wells J.G., Greene K.D., Griffin P.M. A Nation-wide Case-control Study of *Escherichia coli* O157:H7 Infection in the United States. The Journal of Infectious Diseases, 1998. 177: pp. 962-966

90. Zimmerhackl L.B., *E. coli*, Antibiotics, and the Hemolytic-uremic Syndrome. The New England Journal of Medicine, 2000. 342: pp. 1990-1991

91. Ostroff S.M., Kobayashi J.M., Lewis J.H. Infection with *Escherichia coli* O157:H7 in Washington State. The First Year of Statewide Disease Surveillance. The Journal of the American Medical Association, 1989. 262: p. 355-359

92. Walterspiel J.N., Ashkenazi S., Morrow A.L. Cleary T.G. Effect of Subinhibitory Concentration of Antibiotics on Extra-cellular Shiga-like Toxin I. Infection, 1992. 20: pp. 25-29

93. Karch H., Strockbine N.A., O'Brien A.D. Growth of *Escherichia coli* in the Presence of Trimethoprim-sulfamethoxazole Facilitates Detection of Shiga-like Toxin Producing Strains by Colony Blot Assay. Federation of European Microbiological Society Microbiology Letters, 1986. 35: pp. 141-145

94. Panos G.Z., Betsi G.I., Falagas M.E. Systemic Review: are Antibiotics Detrimental of Beneficial for the Treatment of Patients with *Escherichia coli* O157:H7 Infection? Alimentary Pharmacology & Therapeutics, 2006. 24: pp. 731-742

95. Pavia A.T., Nichols C.R., Green D.P., Tauxe R.V., Mottice S., Green K.D., Wells J.G., Siegler R.L., Brewer E.D., Hannon D. Hemolytic-Uremic Syndrome during an Outbreak of *Escherichia coli* O157:H7 Infections in Institutions for Mentally Retarded Persons: Clinical and Epidemiologic Observations. The Journal of pediatrics, 1990. 116: pp. 544-551

96. Sack R.B. Enetrohemorrhagic *Escherichia coli*. The New England Journal of Medicine, 1987. 317: pp. 1535-1537

97. Kimmitt P., Harwood C., Barer M. Toxin Gene Expression by Shiga Toxin-producing *Escherichia coli*: the Role of Antibiotics and the Bacterial SOS Response. Emerging Infectious Diseases, 2000. 6: pp. 458-465

98. Sheiring J., Andreoli S.P., Zimmerhackl L.B. Treatment and Outcome of Shiga-toxin-associated Hemolytic Uremic Syndrome (HUS). Pediatric Nephrology, 2008. 23: pp. 1749-1760

Photo Bibliography

Figure 2.7-1: Scanning electron micrograph (SEM) demonstrates numerous Gram-negative *Escherichia coli* bacteria of the strain O157:H7. This scanning electron micrograph was taken by Janice Haney Carr in 2006 and released by the CDC. Public domain photo

Figure 2.7-6: A 3D structure rendering of shiga toxin. The A subunit is shown in organge and B subunit is shown in blue. This graphic is produced by Fraser M.E., Fujinaga M., Cherney M.M., Melton-Celsa A.R., Twiddy E.M., O'Brien A.D., James M.N.G. and released via Structure of Shiga Toxin Type 2 (Stx2) from *Escherichia coli* O157:H7. The Journal of Biological Chemistry, 2004. 79: pp. 27511–27517. Public domain graphic

Francisella tularensis is an obligate anaerobic, non-motile, Gram negative coccobacillus, facultative intracellular parasite that is the causative agent of the zoonosis known as tularemia. *F. tularensis* was first identified in 1911 by G.W. McCoy as the cause of a plague-like disease among ground squirrels in Tulare County, California. Subsequently in 1921, Edward Francis described the transmission of the disease by deer flies via contaminated blood and coined the name tularemia.[1]

F. tularensis is an acute febrile and highly invasive infection that is characterized by its ability to rapidly multiply intracellularly to high bacterial densities, as well as, resulting in extensive tissue necrosis.[2] Due to its, highly infectious, debilitating, and at times, deadly characteristics, tularemia is classified as a Category A biological warfare agent by the Center for Disease Control (Figure 2.8-1).

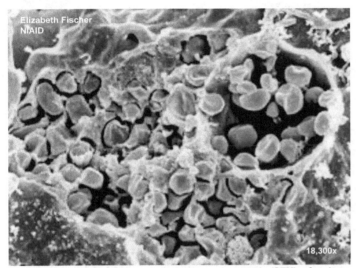

Figure 2.8-1: Colorized scanning electron micrograph (SEM) of a bone marrow-derived macrophage infected with *Francisella tularensis*

Presently, there are four subspecies of *F. tularensis* known and it is recognized that two out of the four subspecies are clinically significant in humans. These four subspecies are indistinguishable serologically and can only be identified through the analysis of their distinct 16S ribosomal RNA subunits.[3]

The first *F. tularensis* subspecie (subsp.) is *tularensis nearctica*, type A (or Biovar A). Subsp. *tularensis nearctica* is highly infectious to humans, as well as, a variety of rodents and is the most common isolate in the United States. Pulse field gel electrophoresis showed that subsp. *tularensis nearctica* can be further subdivided into three clades (sub-populations): A1a, A1b and A2, which differ with their clinical outcomes. Patients infected with A1b strain demonstrate higher mortality rates in comparison with individuals infected with A1a and A2 strains.[4] The second subspecies is *F. tularensis* subsp. *palaearctica holarctica*, type B (or Biovar B) which is more widely distributed around the world, but demonstrate less virulence in humans.[4, 5] The third subspecie is *F. tularensis* subsp. *mediaasiatica* was isolated in central Asia and appear to be closely related to *F. tularensis* subsp. *tularensis nearctica* based on the same hybridized sequence of 16S rRNA and its ability to ferment glycerol. Nonetheless, subsp. *mediaasiatica* exhibits only mild virulence in rabbits and humans. Lastly, *F. tularensis* subsp. *novicida* was first isolated from water samples in Utah and is

only mildly infectious in humans. *Novicida* is only capable of causing the disease in immunocompromised individuals.[6, 7, 8]

Genetic sequencing of *Francisella* has shown similarities among the four subspecies. The genome of each subspecie is ~1.8 Mb, however, *F. novicida* possesses the largest genome at 1.91 Mb. The G+C contents of all four subspecies are ~32% with 1,800-2,000 putative coding sequences, while between 70 to 90% of open reading frames have been predicted to encode functional proteins. Within the genome of all four serotypes of *Francisella*, a 30kb region with low G+C content has been identified as the pathogenic island which is required for the coccobacillus's survival within host cells. This pathogenic island demonstrated ~97-99% nucleotide similarities among the subspecies.[9, 10, 11]

It is interesting to note that the pathogenic *F. tularensis* subsp. *tularensis* and the slightly less pathogenic *F. tularensis* subsp. *holarctica* possesses 200 to 300 pseudogenes, while the least pathogenic *F. novicida* contains only 14 pseudogenes. It has been estimated that ~30% of annotated genes within all four subspecies of *F. tularensis* are described as proteins with unknown functions, therefore it is speculated that these isolates encode novel virulence determinants which remains to be elucidated.[9, 10, 11]

F. tularensis is an exceedingly effective biological warfare agent due to its unusually high infectivity after aerosolization. It has been reported that no more than 10 coccobacilli can cause an infection in humans if introduced subcutaneously, while 10 to 50 aerosolized virulent organisms can induce tularemia if introduced through the respiratory tract.[12, 13, 14] Nonetheless, there are no records indicating that the disease can spread through human-to-human contact. Understanding the effectiveness of this biological agent, the U.S. biological warfare production facility at Pine Bluff Arsenal, Arkansas, produced *F. tularensis* as one of its many biological warfare agents in 1954. Tularemia remained in the U.S. biological weapon arsenal until its termination in 1970 and the destruction of its entire stockpiles by 1973.[15, 16] The Soviet Union also experimented and produced large quantities of this agent as reported by Alibek (1999) in his autobiography Biohazard. As the First Deputy Director of the Soviet biological weapons agency, Biopreparat, he was responsible for all Soviet biological weapons facilities and had firsthand knowledge of this and many other agents.[17] According to his autobiography, Alibek stated that experimentation and testing of tularemia occurred in Omutninsk, Soviet Union. In 1983, Alibek, was accidentally infected with *F. tularensis* from a leaky fermentor at Building 107 located where the Biopreparat housed and experimented with some of the deadliest organisms on Earth. Classified as L2, *F. tularensis* was part of the Enzyme Project, launched by the Soviet Union in 1973 to explore the possibilities of genetically altering pathogens to become resistant to antibiotics and vaccines.[17]

In 1969, the World Healthy Organization estimated that an aerosolized dispersal of virulent *F. tularensis*, over a densely populated metropolitan area with approximately five million inhabitants, would result in 250,000 incapacitated and up to 19,000 fatalities. A 1997 study by the CDC reported that the estimated economic impact of a aerosolized virulent *F. tularensis* bioterrorist attack would result in 5.4 billion dollars for every 100,000 individuals infected.[18, 19]

Tularemia, also known as, Rabbit Fever or Deerfly Fever, occurs naturally in North America, parts of Europe (although rarely seen in the United Kingdom), the Middle East, Russia and Japan. In North America, there are more than 10 species of ticks (e.g. *Dermacentor spp.*) that serve as the principle reservoir of this coccobacillus. Additionally, *F. tularensis* has been isolated from 55 additional arthropod species, as well as, more than 100 non-arthropod organisms.[20] The natural transmission of this disease in North America is most often associated with rabbits, while in Russia, transmission is closely associated with water rats and other aquatic mammals (Figure 2.8-2).[1]

Tularemia is an acute febrile illness. The type and severity of this infection depends on the route by which the coccobacilli are introduced into the host, in addition to the biovar that is involved. *F. tularensis* can be introduced into the host via abrasions or cuts in the skin, or through the mucous membrane of the eyes.[1, 11, 20, 21] Moreover, the coccobacillus can also be transmitted through insect bites[11, 22, 23], inhalation of aerosolized microbes [11, 24, 25] or through ingestion (e.g. contaminated water supply).[11, 26, 27] The major target organs of the coccobacilli are the lymph nodes, lungs, pleura, spleen, liver and kidneys (Figure 2.8-3).[11, 21]

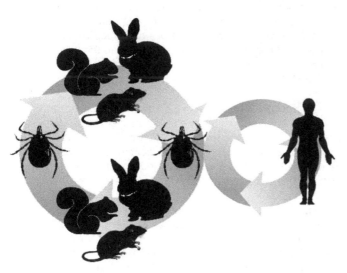

Figure 2.8-2: Sylvatic cycle of *F. tularensis*

It is not believed that *F. tularensis* produces any classical virulence factors, such as exotoxins. Nonetheless, a significant inflammatory response can be observed during the course of tularemia infections. Numerous studies have indicated that the lipopolysaccharide (LPS) of this microbe is not responsible for inducing the host inflammatory response. Therefore, it is theorized that the virulence of this coccobacillus may be attributed to its ability to proliferate within host macrophage, alveolar epithelial cells, hepato-cytes, neutrophils, and dendritic cells, thereby hindering normal functions, as well as, instigating a significant host inflammatory response. It is postulated that the host inflammatory response induced by the bacteria may contribute to the disease process. Unfortunately, the mechanisms that caused the inflammatory response are presently not understood.[28, 29, 30, 31, 32, 33, 34]

The host immune reaction against tularemia is primarily mediated by T-cell independent mechanisms, with secondary contributions by T-cell dependent mechanisms. It has been reported that both mechanisms begin within three days after the introduction of the microbe.[1] For example, in the T-cell independent mechanism, the cocco-bacillus is phagocytized by macrophages through a novel invasion strategy whereby the microbe induces the macrophage to produce asymmetric spacious pseudopod loops.[35] Once the

bacterium has been phagocytized, the macrophage begins to secrete tumor necrosis factor-alpha (TNF-α). It is known that TNF-α stimulates cytotoxic lymphocytes (natural killer - NK cells) to produce interferon-gamma (IFN-γ). The production of IFN-γ, in turn, feeds back to the macrophages and prompts the phagocytes to kill intracellular bacteria through the production of nitric oxide.[36, 37] However, the bacteria possesses a counter strategy for its intracellular survival. Once gaining intracellular access to the macrophage, the bacterium arrests the maturation of the phagosome at a late endosomal-like stage. For example, between 15 to 30 minutes after phagocytosis, the bacterium will limit the acidification of the phagosome and by 30 to 60 minutes, the phagosome's membrane is degraded, letting the bacterium escape and rapidly multiply within the cytoplasm of the macrophage.[28, 38]

- ▪ Mucous membrane
- ▪ Epidermal
- ▪ Respiratory
- ▪ Mastrointestinal

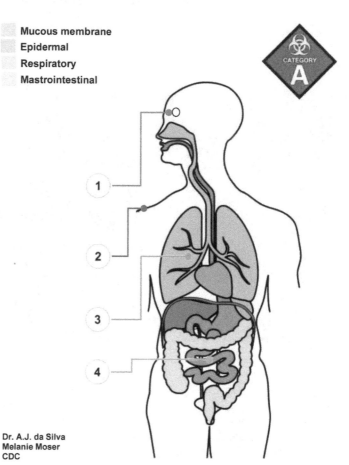

Dr. A.J. da Silva
Melanie Moser
CDC

Figure 2.8-3: *F. tularensis* infection diagram. ① *F. tularensis* spores could be introduced through mucous membrane of the eye. ② *F. tularensis* spores could be introduced through abrasion, cuts or insect bites via the epidermis. ③ *F. tularensis* spores could be introduced through respiratory tract. ④ *F. tularensis* spores could be introduced through gastrointestinal tract

The ability of *F. tularensis* to prompt the dissolution of the phagosome is apparently dependent on the expression of a pathogen-specific 23 kDA Ig1C intracellular growth locus protein, although the exact function of the protein is presently unknown. Nonetheless, studies have shown that the failure to express the Ig1C protein results in the complete loss of virulence.[38, 39] Ig1C is a component of the pathogenicity island that also comprises proteins such as Ig1A-D, pdpA and pdpD, which appear to be regulated by the macrophage growth locus genes Mg1A and Mg1B.[40, 41, 42] It has also been reported that the multiplied bacteria appear to have the capability to reenter the endocytic pathway by inducing an autophagy-mediated process and reside within large double membrane juxtanuclear LAMP-1 positive vacuoles. However, this observation requires further study.[43, 44]

Finally, bacteria are released from the infected cells, are believed to occur through bacterial induced apoptosis and/or through a process known as pyroptosis.[45, 46] Pyroptosis is an innate immune response that results from the detection of cytosolic bacteria and the subsequent activation of caspase-1 within a multi-molecular complex called inflammasome. The activation of the inflammasome results in the formation of discrete pores within the plasma membrane of the macrophage, leading to osmotic lysis. Pyroptosis results in apoptosis of the host cell and the release of pro-inflammatory cytokines as well as the enclosed bacteria.[47]

In the T-cell dependent mechanism, the macrophage will process the bacterial antigens with major histocompatibilty complex molecule II (MHC II) within its Golgi apparatus to form a MHC II and bacterial antigen complex, which begins rallying lymphocytes to recognize the complex. In particular, the MHC II and bacterial antigen complex will initiate the differentiation of CD4+ and CD8+ T Helper lymphocytes, which will respond by proliferating and secreting TNF-α, interleukin 2 (IL-2), interleukin 4 (IL-4) and IFN-γ.[48, 49] It has been reported that these responses can persist for up to 25 years after the initial infection. The secreted cytokines (TNF-α, interleukin 2 (IL-2) and IFN-γ) will in turn stimulate macrophages to kill intracellular bacteria while interleukin 4 (IL-4) will stimulate the antibody production of B-lymphocytes.[50, 51, 52]

SYMPTOMS

The clinical manifestations of tularemia are dependent on the biovar and the number of organisms that are introduced, as well as, the location of introduction. In general, tularemia can present as one of two general syndromes: ulceroglandular and typhoidal, although six different clinical syndromes can be described. These manifestations of disease suggest that the two general syndrome classifications are the result of differences in the immunoresponse of infected individuals.[1, 20, 21] In the ulceroglandular form of tularemia, which appears in 75% of patients, the pathogen is generally well contained by the host's immune system, pneumonia is rare and prognosis of a full recovery is high. Ulceroglandular form of tularemia is generally contracted from handling contaminated carcass or from an insect bite.[21] Patients suffering from the ulceroglandular tularemia will display lesions on their skin, mucous membrane (including conjunctiva) at the site of coccobacilli introduction, which is followed by painful swellings of the local lymph nodes (lymph nodes measuring <1 cm in diameter).[1, 11, 20, 21]

In the typhoidal form of tularemia which appears in 25% of patients, the immunoresponse seems deficient, demonstrating limited amounts of localized disease. For example, in patients suffering from the typhoidal tularemia, there will be no skin or mucous membrane lesions, and the lymph nodes will measure at >1 cm in diameter. In this form, pneumonia is common, the prognosis is poor and the mortality rates without treatment are much higher.[1, 20, 21]

The incubation period for both clinical forms of tularemia is generally 3 to 6 days.[1, 52, 53] The onset of disease for patients suffering from both the ulceroglandular and typhoidal forms of tularemia is generally abrupt with symptoms including fever (38-40° C or 100.4-104° F), headaches, chills, coryza (inflammation of the nasal mucous membrane), sore throat (pharyngitis), rigor and body aches, which often occurred as lower back pains. In 42% of the patients, pulse-temperature dissociation has been observed, in which the patient will display a pulse increase at less than 10 beats per minute for every 1° F increase in temperature above normal. In addition, a dry or slightly productive cough in association with substernal pain or tightness is also a common symptom. Furthermore, patients may also demonstrate vomiting, arthralgia, abdominal pain, diarrhea, dysuria, stiff neck, progressive weakness, malaise, and anorexia accompanied by weight loss as further signs of illness.[2, 20, 21]

In approximately 60% of patients suffering from ulceroglandular tularemia, cutaneous or mucosal, ulcers appear. Initially, localized cutaneous papules will appear at the site of the inoculation. Within a few days, the papules will be surrounded by a zone of inflammation and become pustular and ulcerated. These ulcers generally measure 0.4 to 3.0 cm in diameter, tender, possesses an indolent characteristic with heaped-up edges that may be covered by an eschar (Table 1).[1, 2, 21, 54]

Table 1: List of symptoms commonly appearing in both ulceroglandular and typhoidal forms of tularemia

Symptoms	+	++	+++
Fever			▪
Chills			▪
Malaise			▪
Progressive weakness			▪
Headache			▪
Coryza			▪
Pharyngitis			▪
Rigor			▪
Myalgia			▪
Arthralgia			▪
Stiff neck			▪
Abdominal pain			▪
Vomiting			▪
Diarrhea			▪
Dysuria			▪
Anorexia			▪
Weight loss			▪
Cutaneous papules			▪
Cutaneous ulcer			▪
Mucous mem. papules			▪
Mucous membrane ulcer			▪
Pneumonia			▪
Productive cough			▪
Nonproductive cough			▪
Pleuritic chest pain			▪
Dyspnea			▪
Headaches			▪
Profused sweating			▪
Drowsiness			▪
General weakness			▪
Shortness of breath			▪
Hemoptysis			▪
Hilar adenopathy	▪		
Pleural effusions	▪		
Cavitary lesions	▪		
Bronchopleural fistulae	▪		
Bronchopleural calci.	▪		
Appendicitis	▪		
Enteritis	▪		
Erythema nodosum	▪		
Meningitis	▪		
Pericarditis	▪		
Peritonitis	▪		

+ Rare ++ Common +++ Frequent

■ Both ulceroglandular and typhoidal tularemia
■ Ulceroglandular tularemia
■ Typhoidal tularemia

In the cases which involved the conjunctiva (e.g. oculoglandular tularemia), the ulcerations are generally accompanied by pronounced chemosis and vasculitis. These ulcerations are generally accompanied by regional lymphadenopathy in approximately 85% of cases. The swollen/ enlarged lymph nodes are generally measured at 0.5 to 10 cm in diameter and could appear as single, grouped or sporotrichoid distribution. These enlarged lymph nodes may become fluctuant, drain spontaneously and persist up to three years in this manner. It has been reported that affected lymph nodes may rupture, even with proper antibiotic treatment (Table 2).[1, 2, 21, 54]

there may be signs of erythema, exudate, petechiae, hemorrhage or ulcers. Affected individuals may commonly develop exudative pharyngitis or tonsillitis at times with ulcerations, while on occasion patients may also develop stomatitis. Rarely, patients suffering from pharyngitis may also develop retropharyngeal abscess or suppuration of regional lymph nodes (Table 3).[1, 21, 57, 58]

Table 2: List of symptoms commonly appearing in both ulceroglandular and oculoglandular forms of tularemia

Symptoms	+	++	+++
Fever			■
Chills			■
Malaise			■
Progressive weakness			■
Headache			■
Coryza			■
Pharyngitis			■
Rigor			■
Myalgia			■
Arthralgia			■
Stiff neck			■
Abdominal pain			■
Vomiting			■
Diarrhea			■
Dysuria			■
Anorexia			■
Weight loss			■
Mucosal papules			■
Mucosal ulcers			■
Chemosis			■
Vasculitis			■
Region lymphadenopathy			■
Pneumonia	■		
Productive cough	■		
Nonproductive cough	■		
Pleuritic chest pain	■		
Dyspnea	■		
Headaches	■		
Profused sweating	■		
Drowsiness	■		
General weakness	■		
Shortness of breath	■		
Hemoptysis	■		
Hilar adenopathy	■		
Pleural effusions	■		
Cavitary lesions	■		
Bronchopleural fistulae	■		
Bronchopleural calci.	■		
Appendicitis	■		
Enteritis	■		
Erythema nodosum	■		
Meningitis	■		
Pericarditis	■		
Peritonitis	■		

+ Rare ++ Common +++ Frequent

■ Both ulceroglandular and oculoglandular tularemia
■ Oculoglandular tularemia
■ Ulceroglandular tularemia with pharyngitis

Approximately 25% of patients suffering from the ulceroglandular tularemia will develop oropharyngeal tularemia. This form of tularemia is generally associated with drinking contaminated water and/or ingesting tainted food, but rarely from inhaling contaminated droplets of aerosolized coccobacilli.[54, 55, 56] In general, the posterior pharynx of patients may not be inflamed but

Table 3: List of symptoms commonly appearing in both ulceroglandular and oropharynxgeal tularemia forms

Symptoms	+	++	+++
Fever			■
Chills			■
Malaise			■
Progressive weakness			■
Headache			■
Coryza			■
Pharyngitis			■
Rigor			■
Myalgia			■
Arthralgia			■
Stiff neck			■
Abdominal pain			■
Vomiting			■
Diarrhea			■
Dysuria			■
Anorexia			■
Weight loss			■
Pharyngeal erythema		■	
Pharyngeal exudate		■	
Pharyngeal petechiae		■	
Pharyngeal hemorrhage		■	
Pharyngeal ulcers		■	
Exudative pharyngitis		■	
Tonsillitis		■	
Pneumonia		■	
Productive cough		■	
Nonproductive cough		■	
Pleuritic chest pain		■	
Dyspnea		■	
Profuse sweating		■	
Drowsiness		■	
General weakness		■	
Shortness of breath		■	
Hemoptysis		■	
Ulcer exudate pharyngitis	■		
Ulcerated tonsillitis	■		
Stomatitis	■		
Retropharyngeal abscess	■		
Supp. of lymph nodes	■		
Hilar adenopathy	■		
Pleural effusions	■		
Cavitary lesions	■		
Bronchopleural fistulae	■		
Bronchopleural calcifi.	■		
Appendicitis	■		
Enteritis	■		
Erythema nodosum	■		
Meningitis	■		
Pericarditis	■		
Peritonitis	■		

+ Rare ++ Common +++ Frequent

■ Both ulceroglandular & oropharynxgeal tularemia
■ Oropharynxgeal tularemia

In patients suffering from pharyngitis resulting from ulceroglandular tularemia, pneumonia may appear as an additional and more severe complication in approximately 30%

of patients. Out of these pneumonia cases, approximately 47 to 94% will demonstrate lower respiratory tract involvement. It is also estimated that 80% of patients with typhoidal tularemia also develop pneumonia. This higher incidence of pneumonia associated with typhoidal tularemia may account for the higher instances of mortality associated with the typhoidal form of infection.[1, 11, 18] In most cases of pneumonia, patients will commonly display symptoms such as productive or nonproductive cough, pleuritic chest pain, dyspnea, headaches, profused sweating, drowsiness, general weakness, shortness of breath or hemoptysis. It is estimated that ~1% or less of patients will develop hilar adenopathy without parenchymal involvement, while ~15% of patients have also been observed to develop pleural effusions. In addition, interstitial patterns such as cavitary lesions, bronchopleural fistulae and calcifications have also been observed in patients with tularemia pneumonia.[1, 20, 59] Other, less frequently observed clinical conditions induced by tularemia pneumonia may include appendicitis, enteritis, erythema nodosum, meningitis, pericarditis and peritonitis (Table 3).[1, 2, 20, 54, 60, 61, 62]

Table 4: List of symptoms commonly appearing in direct inhalation of *F. tularensis* subsp. *tularensis*

Symptoms	+	++	+++
Fever			■
Chills			■
Malaise			■
Progressive weakness			■
Headache			■
Pneumonia			■
Pharyngitis			■
Bronchiolitis			■
Pleura-pneumonitis			■
Hilar lymphadenitis			■
Coryza		■	
Rigor		■	
Myalgia		■	
Arthralgia		■	
Stiff neck		■	
Vomiting		■	
Diarrhea		■	
Anorexia		■	
Weight loss		■	
Peribronchial infiltration	■		
Bronchopneumonia	■		
Pleural effusions	■		
Hilar lymphadenopathy	■		
Respiratory failure	■		

+ Rare ++ Common +++ Frequent

Inhalation of *F. tularensis* subsp. *holarctica* results in a mild and generally non-life-threatening respiratory infection. However, direct inhalation of aerosolized *F. tularensis* subsp. *tularensis* can also result in tularemia pneumonia with possible symptoms of pharyngitis, bronchiolitis, pleura-pneumonitis and hilar lymphadenitis, along with various symptoms of systemic illness. This form of infection has been reported to cause initial clinical signs of systemic illness, without the prominent symptoms of respiratory infection.[25, 55] Initial pulmonary radiographic image of inhalational tularemia in 25 to 50% of infected individuals indicates peribronchial infiltration which generally advanced to bronchopneumonia in one or more lobes of the lung(s). This bronchopneumonia infection is often accompanied by pleural effusions and hilar lymphadenopathy. Nonetheless, some patients may display minimal or no symptoms, while others may display only one or several small pulmonary infiltrations or scattered granulomatous lesions of the parenchyma of the lungs

or pleura (Table 4).[21]

Untreated tularemia may progress into tularemia sepsis. Tularemia sepsis is a rare form of the disease and can be potentially severe and fatal. Symptoms of tularemia sepsis include fever, chills, headaches, abdominal pain, diarrhea and vomiting. Patients suffering from this condition appear toxic and may exhibits sign of confusion or laps into a coma. Unless treatment is immediately administered, septic shock and other systemic inflammatory response syndromes such as disseminated intravascular coagulation (DIC) and bleeding, acute respiratory distress syndrome and organ failure may ensue (Table 5).[21, 51]

Without antibiotic treatments, mortality rates associated with Biovar A are ~5 to 15%. Again, without the benefits of antibiotics, the mortality rate increased substantially to ~30 to 60% as patients deteriorated into pneumonia and other more severe form of the disease. Presently, the mortality rate associated with Biovar A tularemia with proper treatment is less than 2%, while Biovar B rarely causes fatalities in patients, although the protracted course of disease and frequent reoccurrence of complications may pose concerns.[2, 11, 20, 21]

Table 5: List of symptoms commonly appearing in tularemia sepsis

Symptoms	+	++	+++
Fever			■
Chills			■
Abdominal pain			■
Headache			■
Pneumonia			■
Vomiting			■
Diarrhea			■
Confusion			■
Coma			■
Septic shock			■
DIC			■
Bleeding			■
Acute respiratory distress			■
Organ failure			■

+ Rare ++ Common +++ Frequent

DETECTION

In contrast with other bacterial infections, tularemia is generally not associated with any dramatic changes in the patient's blood chemistry. For example, the leukocyte count may be normal or slightly elevated (a relative increase of mononuclear cells) during infection. Liver enzyme values may demonstrate a slight increase, mean C-reactive protein values have been found to peak at 53 mg/L. Nonetheless, the erythrocyte sedimentation rate remains increased at 30 to 50 mm/h for the first month, after the onset of the illness.[2, 20, 63]

F. tularensis is faintly stained by conventional reagents and is not easily recognizable through Gram staining. Therefore, one method of rapid and presumptive identification of *F. tularensis* can be made by examining secretions, exudates or biopsy specimens from infected individuals through the utilization of immunohistochemical (immunofluorescent) techniques. Numerous immunohistochemical assays have been privately developed by using fluoresce-inated monoclonal or polyclonal antibodies targeting the anti-*F. tularensis* lipopolysaccharide antigen or other coccobacilli surface antigens.[21, 64, 65, 66, 67] Commercially developed antibodies specifically targeting lipopolysaccharide and vegetative cells are available from HyTest

Table 6: Medication dosage, side effects of various treatment for tularemia in adults

Medication	Mechanism of Action	Side Effects	Recommended Dosage
Doxycycline	Inhibits protein synthesis	Nausea, diarrhea, bloody stools, severe stomach cramps, indigestion, heartburn, vomiting, photosensitivity, anorexia, dysphagia, headaches, blurred vision, rash, arthralgia, fever, feeling tired	200 mg daily for 14 days or 100 mg daily for 3 weeks
Streptomycin	Inhibits protein synthesis	Fever, headache, rash, hives, difficulty breathing, tightness in the chest, swellings (mouth, face, lips, or tongue), decreased urination, dizziness, hearing loss, light-headedness, loss of balance, muscle weakness, nausea, numbness, tingling, tinnitus, vaginal irritation, vaginal discharge and vomiting	1g intramuscular twice daily
Tetracycline	Inhibits protein synthesis	Hairy tongue, blurred vision, diarrhea, difficulty swallowing and breathing, fever, chills, headache, hives, hoarseness, indigestion, inflammation of tongue, swellings (mouth, face, lips, or tongue), arthalgia, anorexia, sores in the mouth, nausea, vomiting, rash, sensitivity to sunlight, sore throat, stomach pain, swelling and itching of the rectum, rash, itching, tightness in the chest, vaginal irritation or discharge	100 mg intravenously or orally twice daily for 14 days
Ciprofloxacin (Cipro)	Inhibits the function of DNA gyrase	Nausea, diarrhea, liver function tests abnormal, vomiting, and rash, headache, abdominal pain/discomfort, foot pain, pain in extremities, injection site reaction	750 mg twice daily
Gentamicin	Inhibits protein synthesis	Shortness of breath, increased thirst, loss of appetite, hives, swellings (lips, face, or tongue), rash, fainting, lack of urine, decreased hearing, tinnitus, dizziness, clumsiness, unsteadiness, numbness, skin tingling, muscle twitching, seizures, diarrhea, abdominal cramps, nausea, vomiting, rash	5 mg/kg intramuscularly or intra-venously once daily
Norfloxacin (Noroxin)	Inhibits the function of DNA gyrase	Nausea, headache, stomach upset, weakness, abdominal pains, cramping, dizziness, diarrhea or drowsiness, tremor, hypersensitivity to sunlight, seizures, mental/mood changes, persistent sore throat/fever, vision changes, hearing loss, rash, itching, swelling severe dizziness, fainting, trouble breathing change in amount or appearance of urine, yellowing of the eyes/skin, fast/slow/irregular heartbeat, easy bruising/bleeding, numbness/tingling of arms/legs	400 mg twice daily

Ltd.® and Tetracore Inc®.[68] Both immunofluorescent and immune-histochemical identification techniques can produce results within several hours and have been found useful in the absence of a recoverable culture or other specimen suitable for polymerase chain reaction (PCR).[51, 69, 70]

Definitive identification of F. tularensis can be made through cultures, although this organism is difficult to culture on standard media. In addition, culturing these coccobacilli may take days before positive identification can be made.[1, 13, 14, 25] Organisms may be isolated and grown from pharyngeal washing, sputum specimens, ulcers, blood samples, conjunctival exudates and from gastric aspirates from patients suffering from inhalational tularemia.[21, 24] It has been reported that these coccobacilli can be grown on cysteine enriched broth, thioglycollate broth, cysteine heart blood agar, buffered charcoal-yeast agar and chocolate agar. Media should be incubated at 37° C (98.6° F) and growth may be seen as early as 24 to 48 hours. On cysteine-enriched agar, F. tularensis colonies are typically 1.0 mm in diameter, small smooth, opaque colonies after 24 to 48 hours of incubation and 3.0 to 5.0 mm in diameter after 96 hours of incubation under ideal conditions. In comparison, F. tularensis grown on cysteine-enriched heart blood agar, with a similar incubation period, as indicated previously, appear opalescent and do not discolor the medium.[1, 2, 21, 68] Identification of colonies is generally tested through slide agglutination (~5 minutes) or direct fluorescent antibody staining (~30 minutes). In addition, DNA analysis targeting the fopA or tul4 genes of F. tularensis can be performed using PCR (~30 minutes to 4 hours).[2, 68, 71, 72, 73]

Often, identification of F. tularensis is made through serological methods, such as bacterial agglutination or enzyme-linked immunosorbent assay (ELISA). Nonetheless, adequate amounts of antibodies that agglutinate F. tularensis only appear within a week after infection, and measurable amounts for serological diagnosis (titer >1:160) do not appear until approximately 2 weeks after the onset of the infection.[19, 74, 75, 76] With this limitation, serology is only minimally applicable in managing an outbreak, but could be of value for epidemiological or forensic cases.[21] Traditionally, the serological tests most widely used were the whole-cell agglutination test (Widal's reaction) and passive hemagglutination.[77, 78]

Modification to the agglutination tests, though the introduction of the micro-agglutination assays, resulted in superior performance. Both whole-cell agglutination tests and microagglutination assays, are designed to detect combined IgM and IgG antibodies. Presently, agglutination assays are still widely used and are commercially available (e.g. Tube Agglutination Tests by Becton Dickinson, Franklin Lakes, NJ, USA).[18, 68, 76, 79, 80] It has been reported that ELISA, are superior to agglutination assays. This superiority is mainly due to the fact that ELISAs have the advantage that different antibody classes (e.g. IgM, IgG and IgA) can be determined separately.[68, 81, 82] ELISA assays detect antibodies against the lipopolysaccharides (LPS) from *F. tularensis*. An elevated ELISA titer can be important diagnostically at the end of the first week of illness where a significant increase of titer in consecutive serum samples indicates tularemia.[83]

TREATMENT

Ever since its introduction in the 1940's, streptomycin has remained the antibiotic of choice for tularemia. This medication has reduced the mortality rate of the most severe form of tularemia from more than 30% to 3%, with a clinical cure rate of 97%.[81] Nonetheless, due to the vestibular toxicity and the risk of hypersensitivity reaction for personnel handling the medication, streptomycin is now rarely available and is infrequently used in the treatment of tularemia.[2] An acceptable alternative is gentamicin, which is more widely available and may be administered intravenously. Gentamicin is administered at a dose of 5mg/kg, divided in two doses daily and the treatment should be continued for 10 days to achieve a 88% cure rate.[20, 84, 85]

During the 1950's and 1960's chloramphenicol was used as an alternative with a cure rate of 77%.[85] However, due to its rare but severe hematological side effects and the high rate of relapse, chloramphenicol is no longer used in routine treatments. Tetracycline has also been used at times and the chance treatment has been reported to have a cure rate of 86%. Nonetheless, treatment failure and relapse make this compound less desirable. It is suggested that tetracycline be administered for at least 14 days to reduce the possibilities of treatment failure and relapse.[2, 23, 86] Presently, tetracycline has been replaced by doxycycline. In the treatment of tularemia, a dose of 200 mg of doxycycline once daily for 14 days or 100 mg daily for three weeks is recommended to prevent relapse. Quinolones are now suggested as an effective alternative to conventional treatments with gentamicin and doxycycline. Quinolones are particularly attractive since they are well tolerated by patients, reach adequate blood levels after oral administration and have excellent intracellular penetration. Nonetheless, quinolones such as ciprofloxacin, norfloxacin and levofloxacin have only been used in trial bases for the treatment of tularemia.[2, 86, 87] Please examine Table 6 for more information with regards to the antibiotics used in the treatment of adults suffering from tularemia.

In children suffering from tularemia, the antibiotic of choice is gentamicin. Doxycycline is an acceptable alternative, however, it is not recommended for children under the age of eight due to its adverse side effects on developing teeth. Please examine Table 7 for more information in regards to the antibiotics used in the treatment of children suffering from tularemia. In treating pregnant women suffering from tularemia, the key medication for treating the illness is gentamicin administered at 5mg/kg intramuscularly or intravenously, two times daily.

An acceptable alternative is doxycycline, which is suggested to be administered at 100 mg intravenously twice daily (Table 6).[2, 21]

Ever since the 1930's, vaccines have been developed to combat tularemia. These vaccines include those made from killed *F. tularensis*, whole cell and live attenuated strains. In the 1930's, a whole-cell phenol-killed or acetone extract vaccine was developed by Foshay et al. (1989), but was shown to be limited in its effectiveness. It is believed that the failure of the killed vaccines to induce solid protection is due to their inability to elicit a robust cellular immune response.[1, 88, 89] In the 1940's and 1950's, live attenuated vaccines were developed in the Soviet Union, which lead to the vaccination of approximately sixty million of the population with great success. Samples of the Soviet vaccine were gifted to the United States as a part of a formal scientific exchange program. In 1961, at U.S. Army Medical Research Institute of Infectious Disease located at Fort Detrick, this Soviet produced vaccine was further purified and a derivative known as live vaccine strain (LVS) was developed. Under Operation Whitecoat, the vaccine was tested on human volunteers and has shown to provide 90 to 100% protection against subcutaneous challenges with *F. tularensis* and ~83% protection in aerosol challenges. Presently, LVS is approved by the FDA as investigational new drug.[1, 89, 90, 91]

DIFFERENTIAL DIAGNOSIS

Like most biological warfare agents, a high level of suspicion is required to diagnose tularemia due to the lack of available rapid and specific confirmatory tests. Additionally, it is known that the various forms of tularemia can have a nonspecific appearance and may resemble a wide range of much more

Table 7: Medication dosage, side effects of various treatment for tularemia in children

Medication	Mechanism of Action	Side Effects	Recommended Dosage
Levofloxacin	Inhibits the function of DNA gyrase	Nausea, stomach upset, loss of appetite, diarrhea, abdominal pains, cramping, drowsiness, dizziness, headache, or insomnia, joint/muscle/ tendon pain or swelling (tendonitis, tendon rupture), hypersensitivity to sunlight, rash itching, swelling, chest pain, change in the amount of urine, dark urine, easy bruising/ bleeding, dizziness, fainting, fast/irregular heart-beat, difficult breathing, mental/mood changes, severe depression, persistent nausea, vomiting, persistent sore throat, fever, seizures, fatigue, yellowing eyes and skin	500 mg twice daily
Gentamicin	Inhibits protein synthesis	Shortness of breath, increased thirst, anorexia, hives, swellings (lips, face, or tongue), rash, fainting, lack of urine, decreased hearing, ringing in the ears, dizziness, clumsiness, unsteadiness, numbness, skin tingling, muscle twitching, seizures, diarrhea, abdominal cramps, nausea, vomiting, rash	2.5 mg/kg intramuscularly or intravenously 3 times daily
Doxycycline	Inhibits protein synthesis	Nausea, diarrhea, bloody stools, severe stomach cramps, indigestion, heartburn, vomiting, photosensitivity, loss of appetite, dysphagia, headaches, blurred vision, rash, joint pain, fever, feeling tired	≥ 45 kg, 100 mg intravenously 2 times daily. ≤ 45 kg, 2.2 mg/kg intravenously 2 times daily. This medication is not recommended for children under the age of 8

Table 8: Differential diagnosis of tularemia with selected disease with similar symptoms. These diseases are brucellosis, plague, legionellosis (Legion), Q fever, sporotrichosis (Sporo) and typhus

Symptoms	Tularemia	Brucellosis	Plague	Legion	Q fever	Sporo	Typhus
Fever & chills	■	■	■	■	■		■
Headache	■	■	■	■	■		■
Malaise	■	■	■	■	■		■
Coryza	■						
Pharyngitis	■				■		
Rigor	■						
Myalgia	■	■	■	■	■		■
Arthralgia	■	■	■		■	■	
Stiff neck	■						
Non-productive cough	■	■	■	■	■		■
Productive cough	■	■	■	■	■	■	■
Substernal pain	■		■	■			
Pleuritic chest pain	■	■	■				
Shortness of breath	■					■	
Vomiting	■		■		■		■
Diarrhea	■		■	■			
Dysuria	■						
Anorexia	■	■		■	■		
Weight loss	■	■		■	■		
General weakness	■		■		■		
Drowsiness	■						
Abdominal pain	■		■		■		■
Skin lesions	■	■				■	■
Mucous membrane lesions	■					■	
Conjunctival lesions	■					■	
Conjunctival ulceration	■					■	
Mucous membrane ulcer	■					■	
Cutaneous ulcer	■	■				■	■
Lymphoadenopathy	■	■	■		■		■
Pneumonia	■		■	■	■	■	■
Pleuritic chest pain	■						
Dyspnea	■					■	
Hemoptysis	■						
Dyspnea	■		■				
Profused sweating	■	■			■		
Hemoptysis	■					■	
Bronchiolitis	■						
Pleuropneumonitis	■						
Hilar lymphadenitis	■						
Chemosis	■						
Vasculitis	■						
Pharyngeal involvement	■						
Retropharyngeal abcess	■						
Suppuration of lymph nodes	■						
Tonsillitis with ulcers	■						
Stomatitis	■					■	
Cavitary lesions	■						
Bronchopleural fistulae	■						
Bronchopleural calcification	■						
Pleural effusions	■						■
Hilar adenopathy	■						
Appendicitis	■						
Enteritis	■						
Erythema nodosum	■				■		
Meningitis	■		■	■		■	
Pericarditis	■						
Peritonitis	■						
Confusion	■		■	■	■		
Coma	■						

common illnesses. For example, differential diagnosis should include brucellosis, plague, legionellosis (Legion), Q fever, Lyme disease, sporotrichosis (Sporo) and typhus. Other differential diagnosis should include cat scratch disease, ehrlichiosis, pasteurella infections, psittacosis, pyoderma, Rocky Mountain spotted fever, staphylococcal or streptococcal infections (Table 8).[1, 92]

References

1.   Evans M.E., Friedlander A.M. Tularemia. Medical Aspects of Chemical and Biological

Warfare. Chapter 24. Washington D.D.: Office of the Surgeon General Department of the Army, United States of America. 1997. pp. 503-512
2. Tärnvik A., Chu M.C. New Approaches to Diagnosis and Therapy of Tularemia. Annals of the New York Academy of Science, 2007. 1105: pp. 378-404
3. Forsman M., Sandström G., Jaurin B. Identification of Francisella Species and Discrimination of Type A and Type B Strains of F. tularensis by 16S rRNA Analysis. Applied and Environmental Microbiology, 1990. 56: pp. 949-955
4. Kugeler K.J., Mead P.S., Janusz A.M., Staples J.E., Kubota K.A., Chalcraft L. G., Petersen J.M. Molecular epidemiology of Francisella tularensis in the United States. Clinical Infectious Diseases, 2009. 48: pp. 863–870
5. de la Puente-Redondo V.A., García del Blanco N., Gutiérrez-Martín C.B., García-Peña F.J., Rodríguez Ferri E.F. Comparison of Different PCR Approaches for Typing of Francisella tularensis Strains. Journal of Clinical Microbiology, 2000. 38: pp. 1016-1022
6. Sandström G., Sjöstedt A., Forsman M., Pavlovich N.V., Mishankin B.N. Characterization and Classification of Strains of Francisella tularensis isolated in Central Asian Focus of the Soviet Union and in Japan. Journal of Clinical Microbiology, 1992. 30: pp. 172-175
7. Jungblut P.R., Hecker M. Proteomics of Microbial Pathogens. Weinheim: Wiley-VCH. 2007. pp. 250-251
8. Larsson P.,Elfsmark D.,Svensson K.,Wikström P.,Forsman M.,Brettin T., Keim P., Johansson A. (2009). Molecular evolutionary consequences of niche restriction in Francisella tularensis, a facultative intracellular pathogen. Public Library of Science (PLoS) Pathogens, 2009. 5: pp. e1000472
9. Titball R. W., J. F. Petrosino. 2007. Francisella tularensis genomics and proteomics. Annals of the New York Academy of Sciences, 2007. 1105: pp. 98–121
10. Pechous R.D., McCarthy T.R., Zahrt T.C. Working toward the Future: Insights into Francisella tularensis Pathogenesis and Vaccine Development. Microbiology and Molecular Biology Reviews, 2009. 73: pp. 684-711
11. Kingry L.C., Petersen J.M. Comparative review of Francisella tularensis and Francisella novicida. Frontiers in Cellular and Infection Microbiology, 2014. 4:pp. 35
12. Bell J.F., Owen C.R., Larson C.L. Virulence of Bacterium tularense. I. A study of the virulence of Bacterium tularense in mice, guinea pigs, and rabbits. The Journal of Infectious Diseases, 1955. 97: pp. 162-166
13. Saslaw S., Eigelsbach H.T., Wilson H.E., Prior J.A., Carhart S. Tularemia Vaccine Study, I: Intracutaneous Challenge. Archives of Internal Medicine, 1961. 107: pp. 121-133
14. Saslaw S., Eigelsbach H.T., Wilson H.E., Prior J.A., Carhart S. Tularemia Vaccine Study, II: Respiratory Challenge. Archives of Internal Medicine, 1961. 107: pp. 134-146
15. Franz D.R., Parrott C.D., Takafuji E.T. The U.S. Biological Warfare and Biological Defense Programs. Medical Aspects of Chemical and Biological Warfare. Chapter 19. Washington D.D.: Office of the Surgeon General Department of the Army, United States of America. 1997. pp. 425-436
16. Chistopher G.W., Cieslak T.J., Pavlin J.A., Eitzen E.M. Biological Warfare: a Historical Perspective, The Journal of American Medical Association, 1997. 278: pp. 412-417
17. Alibek K. Biohazard. New York: Dell Publishing. 1999. pp. 29-38, 41-42, 63-79
18. Health Aspects of Chemical and Biological Weapons. Geneva: World Health Organization. 1970. pp. 105-107
19. Kaufmann A.F., Meltzer M.I., Schmid G.P. The Economic Impact of a Bioterrorist Attack: are Prevention and Post-attack Intervention Programs Justifiable? Emerging Infectious Diseases, 1997. 2: pp. 83-94
20. Evans M.E., Gregory D.W., Schaffner W., McGee Z.A. Tularemia: A 30-year Experience with 88 Cases. Medicine, 1985. 64: pp. 251-269
21. Dennis D.T., Inglesby T.V., Henderson D.A., Bartlett J.G., Ascher M.S., Eitzen E., Fine A.D., Friedlander A.M., Hauer J., Layton M., Lillibridge S.R., McDade J.E., Osterholm M.T., O'Toole T., Parker G., Perl T.M., Russell P.K., Tonat K. Tularemia as a Biological Weapon: Medical and Public Health Management. The Journal of American Medical Association, 2001. 285: pp. 2763-2773
22. Klock L.E., Olsen P.F., Fukushima T. Tularemia Epidemic Associated with Deerfly. The Journal of American Medical Association, 1973. 226: pp. 149-152
23. Markowitz L.E., Hynes N.A., de la Cruz P., Campos E., Barbaree J.M., Plikaytis B.D., Mosier D., Kaufmann A.F. Tick-borne Tularemia. An Outbreak of Lymphadenopathy in Children. The Journal of American Medical Association, 1985. 254: pp. 2922-2925
24. Overholt E.L., Tigertt W.D., Kadull P.J. Ward M.K., Charkes N.D., Rene R.M., Salzman T.E., Stephens M. An Analysis of Forty-Two Cases of Laboratory-Acquired Tularemia. American Journal of Medicine, 1961. 30: pp. 785-806
25. Syrjälä H., Kujala P., Myllylä V., Salminen A., Airborne Transmission of Tularemia in Farmers. Scandinavian Journal of Infectious Diseases, 1985. 17: pp. 371-375
26. Jellison W.L., Epler D.C., Kuhns E., Kohls G.M. Tularemia in Man from a Domestic Rural Water Supply. Public Health Report, 1950. 65: pp. 1219-1226
27. Mignani E., Palmieri F. Fontana M., Marigo S. Italian Epidemic of Waterborne Tularemia. Lancet, 1988. 2: pp. 1423
28. Oyston P.C.F. Francisella tularensis: Unravelling the Secrets of an Intracellular Pathogen. Journal of Medical Microbiology, 2008. 57: pp. 921-930
29. Ancuta P., Pedron T., Girard R., Sandstrom G., Chaby R. Inability of the Francisella tularensis Lipopolysaccharide to Mimic or to Antagonize the Induction of the cell Activation by Endotoxins. Infections and Immunity, 1996. 64: pp. 2041-2046
30. Sandstrom G., Sjostedt A., Johansson T., Kuoppa K. Williams J.C. Immunogenicity and Toxicity of Lipopolysaccharide from Francisella tularensis LVS. Federation of European Microbiological Societies Microbiology Reviews, 1992. 5: pp. 201-210
31. McCaffrey R.L., Allen L.A. Francisella tularensis LVS Evades Killing by Human Neutrophils via Inhibition of the Respiratory Burst and Phagosome Escape. Journal of Leukocyte Biology, 2006. 3: pp. 1224-1230
32. Sjöstedt A. Intracellular Survival Mechainiam of Francisella tularensis, a Stealth Pathogen. Microbes and Infection, 2006. 8: pp. 561-567
33. Clemens D.L., Horwitz M.A. Uptake and Intracellular Fate of Francisella tularensis in Human Macrophages. Annals of the New York Academy of Science, 2007. 1105: pp. 160-186
34. Rasmussen J.W., Cello J., Gil H., Forestal C.A., Furie M.B., Thanassi D.G., Benach J.L.. Mac-1+ Cells Are the Predominant Subset in the Early Hepatic Lesions of Mice Infected with Francisella tularensis. Infection and Immunity, 2006. 74: pp. 6590-6598
35. Clemens D.L., Lee B.Y., Horwitz M.A. Francisella tularensis enters Macrophages via a Novel Process Involving Pseudopod Loops. Infection and Immunity, 2005. 73: pp. 5892-5902
36. Anthony L.S.D., Ghadirian E., Nestel F.P., Kongshavn P.A.L. The Requirement for Gamma Interferon in Resistance of Mice to Experimental Tularemia. Microbial Pathogenesis, 1989. 7: pp. 421-428
37. Fortier A.H., Polsinelli T., Green S.J., Nacy C.A. Activation of Macrophages for Destruction of Francisella tularensis: Identification of Cytokines, Effector Cells, and Effector Molecules. Infection and Immunity, 1992. 60: pp. 817-825
38. Clemens D.L., Lee B.Y., Horwitz M.A. Virulent and Avirulent Strains of Francisella Tularensis Prevent Acidification and Maturation of Their Phagosomes and Escape into the Cytoplasm in Human Macrophages. Infection and Immunity, 2004. 72: pp. 3204-3217
39. Lindgren H., Golovliov I., Baranov V., Ernst R.K., Telepnev M., Sjöstedt A. Factors Affecting the escape of Francisella Tularensis from the Phagolysosome. Journal of Medical Microbiology, 2004. 53: pp. 1-6
40. Lauriano C.M., Barker J.R., Yoon S.S. Mg1A Regulates Transcription of Virulence Factors Necessary for Francisella tularensis Intraamoebae and Intramacrophage Survival. The Proceedings of the National Academy of Sciences United States of America, 2004. 101: pp. 4246-4249
41. Nano F.E., Zhang N., Cowley S.C., Klose K.E., Cheung K.K., Robert M.J., Ludu J.S., Letendre G.W., Meierovics A.I., Stephens G., Elkins K.L. A Francisella tularensis Pathogenicity Island Required for Intramacrophage Growth. The Journal of Bacteriology, 2004. 186: pp. 6430-6436
42. Santic M., Molmeret M., Klose K.E., Jones S., Kwaik Y.A. The Francisella tularensis Pathogenicity Island Protein ig1C and its Regulator mg1A are Essential for Modulating Phagosome Biogenesis and Subsequent Bacterial Escape into the Cytoplasm. Cellular Microbiology, 2005. 7: pp. 969-979
43. Santic M., Molmeret M., Barker J.R., Klose K.E., Dekanic A., Doric M., Abu Kwaik Y. A Francisella tularensis Pathogenicity Island Protien Essential for Bacterial Proliferation within the Host Cell Cytosol. Cellular Microbiology, 2007. 9: pp. 2391-2403
44. Checroun C., Wehrly T.D., Fischer E.R., Hayes S.F., Celli J. Autophagy-Mediated Reentry of Francisella tularensis into the Endocytic Compartment after Cytoplasmic Replication. The Proceedings of the National Academy of Sciences United States of America, 2006. 103: pp. 14578-14583
45. Lai X. H., Golovliov I., Sjostedt A. Francisella tularensis Induces Cytopathogenicity and Apoptosis in Murine Macrophages via a Mechanism that Requires Intracellular Bacterial Multiplication. Infection and Immunity, 2001. 69: pp. 4691-4694
46. Mariathasan S., Weiss D.S., Dixit V.M., Monack D.M. Innate Immunity Against Francisella tularensis is Dependent on the ASC/caspase-1 Axis. Journal of Experimental Medicine, 2005. 202: pp. 1043-1049
47. Henry T., Monack D.M. Activation of the Inflammasome upon Francisella tularensis Infection: Interplay of Innate Immune Pathways and Virulence Factors. Cellular Microbiology, 2007. 9: pp. 2543-2551
48. Surcel H., Ilonen J., Poikonen K., Herva E. Francisella tularensis-specific T-cell Clones are Human Leukocyte Antigen Classw II Restricted, Secrete Interleukin-2 and Gamma Interferon, and Induce Immunoglobulin Production. Infection and Immunity, 1989. 57: pp. 2906-2908
49. Surcel H., Syrjälä H., Karttunen R., Tapaninaho S., Herva E. Development of Francisella tularensis Antigen Responses Measured as T-lyphocyte Proliferation and Cytokine Production (Tumor Necrosis Factor Alpha, Gamma Interferon, and Interleukin-2 and -4) during Human Tularemia. Infection and Immunity, 1991. 59: pp. 1948-1953
50. Ericsson M., Sandström G., Sjöstedt A., Tärnvik A. Persistance of Cell-mediated Immunity and Decline of Humoral Immunity to the Intracellular Bacterium Francisella tularensis 25 Years after Natural Infection. Journal of Infectious Diseases, 1994. 170: pp. 110-117
51. Center for Biosecurity. University of Pittsburgh Medical Center Fact Sheet. Francisella tularensis (Tularemia). Updated November 19, 2007. Retrieved December 2, 2009. Website: http://www.upmc-biosecurity.org/website/focus/agents_diseases/fact_sheets/tularemia.html
52. Giddens W.R., Wilson J.W.J., Dienst F.T., Hargrove M.D. Tularemia, an Analysis of One-hundred Forty-seven Cases. Journal of the Louisiana Sate Medical Society, 1957. 109: pp. 93-98
53. Young L.S., Bicknell D.S., Archer B.G. Tularemia Epidemic: Vermont, 1968: Forty-seven Cases Linked Linked to contact with Muskrats. The New England Journal of Medicine, 1969. 280: pp. 1253-1260
54. Foshay L. Tularemia: a Summary of Certain Aspects of the Disease Including Methods for Early Diagnosis and the Results of Serum Treatment in 600 Patients. Medicine, 1940. 19: pp. 1-83
55. Dahlstrand S., Ringertz O., Zetterberg B. Airborne Tularemia in Sweden. Scandinavian Journal of Infectious Diseases, 1971. 3: pp. 7-16
56. Mignani E., Palmieri F., Fontana M., Marigo S. Italian Epidemic of Waterborne Tularemia. Lancet, 1988. 2: pp. 1423
57. Tärnvik A., Sandström G., Sjöstedt A. Epidemiological Analysis of Tularemia in Sweden 1931-1993. Federation of European Microbiological Societies Immunology and Medical Microbiology, 1996. 13: pp. 201-204
58. Hughes W.T., Etteldorf J.N. Oropharyngeal Tularemia. Journal of Pediatrics, 1957. 51: pp. 363-372
59. Everett D.E., Templer J.W. Oropharyngeal Tularemia. Archives of Otolaryngology, 1980. 106: pp. 237-238
60. Rubin S.A. Radiographic Spectrum of Pleuropulmonary Tularemia. American Journal of Roentgenology, 1978. 131: pp. 277-281
61. Lovell V.M., Cho C.T., Londsey N.J., Nelson P.L. Francisella tularensis Meningitis: A Rare Clinical Entity. Journal of Infectious Diseases, 1986. 154: pp. 916-918
62. Adams C.W. Tularemic Pericarditis. Diseases of the Chest, 1958. 34: pp. 1-8
63. Syrjälä H. Peripheral Blood Leukocyte Counts, Erythrocyte Sedimentation Rate and C-reactive Protein in Tularemia Caused by the Type B Strain of Francisella tularensis. Infection, 1986. 14: pp. 51-54
64. Zeidner N.S., Carter L.G., Monteneiri J.A., Peterson J.M., Schriefer M., Gage K.L., Hall G., Chu M.C. An Outbreak of Francisella tularensis in Captive Prairie Dogs: an Immunohostochemical Analysis. The Journal of Veterinary Diagnostic Investigation, 2004. 16: pp. 150-152
65. Greiser-Wilke I., Soine C., Moenning V. Monoclonal Antibodies Reacting Specifically with Francisella sp. Journal of Veterinary Medicine. Series B, 1989. 36: pp. 593-600
66. Lilliehook B., Sandström G. Production of Murine Monoclonal Antibodies Against Francisella tularensis Antigens and Characterization of Antibody-reactive Epitopes. International Archives of Allergy and Applied Immunology, 1989. 90: pp. 71-77
67. Fulop M., Webber T., Manchee R.J., Kelly D.C. Production and Characterization of Monoclonal Antibodies Directed Against the Lipopolysaccharide of Francisella tularensis. Journal of Clinical Microbiology, 1991. 29: pp. 1407-1412
68. Splettstoesser W.D., Tomaso H., Dahouk S. Al., Neubauer H., Schuff-Werner P. Diagnostic Procedures in Tularemia with Special Focus on Molecular and Immunological Techniques. Journal of Veterinary Medicine. Series B, 2005. 52: pp. 249-261
69. White J.D. McGavran M.H. Identification of Pasteurella tularensis by Immunofluorescence. The Journal of the American Medical Association, 1965. 194: pp. 180-182
70. Guarner J., Greer P.W., Bartlett J., Chu M.C., Shieh W.J., Zaki S.R. Immunohistochemical Detection of Francisella tularensis in Formalin-fixed Paraffin-embedded Tissue. Applied immunohistochemistry and Molecular Morphology, 1999. 7: pp. 122-126
71. Fulop M., Leslie D., Titball R. A Rapid, Highly Sensitive Method for the Detection of Francisella tularensis in Clinical Samples Using the Polymerase Chain Reaction. American Journal of Tropical Medicine and Hygiene, 1996. 54: pp. 364-366
72. Sjöstedt A., Eriksson U., Berglund L., Tärnvik A. Detection of *Francisella tularensis* in Ulcers of Patients with Tularemia by PCR. Journal of Clinical Microbiology, 1997. 35: pp. 1045-1048

73. Johansson A., Berglund L., Eriksson U., Göransson I, Wollin R, Forsman M, Tärnvik A, Sjöstedt A. Compative Analysis of PCR versus Culture for Diagnosis of Ulceroglandular Tularemia. Journal of Clinical Microbiology, 2000. 38: pp. 22-26

74. Syrjälä H., Herva E., Honen J., Saukkonen K., Salminen A. A Whole-blood Lymphocyte Stimulation Test for the Diagnosis of Human Tularemia. The Journal of Infectious Diseases, 1984. 150: pp. 912-915

75. Syrjälä H., Koskela P., Ripatti T., Salminen A., Herva E. Agglutination and ELISA Methods in the Diagnosis of Tularemia in Different Clinical Forms and Severities of the Disease. The Journal of Infectious Diseases, 1986. 153: pp. 142-145

76. Sato T., Fujita H., Ohara Y., Homma M. Microagglutination Test for Early and Specific Serodiagnosis of Tularemia. Journal of Clinical Microbiology, 1990. 28: pp. 2372-2374

77. Voller A., Bidwell D.E., Bartlett A. 1976. Enzyme Immunoassays in Diagnostic Medicine. Bulletin of the World Health Organization, 1976.53: pp. 55-65

78. Carlsson H. E., Lindberg A.A. 1978. Application of Enzyme Immunoassay for Diagnosis of Bacterial and Mycotic Infections. Scandinavian Journal of Immunology, 1978. 8: pp. 97-110

79. Levesque B., de Serres G., Higgins R., D'Halewyn M.A., Artsob H., Grondin J., Major M., Garvie M., Duval B. Seroepidemiologic Study of Three Zoonoses (Leptospirosis, Q Fever and Tularemia) among Trappers in Quebec, Canada. Clinical and Diagnostic Laboratory Immunology, 1989. 90: pp. 71-77

80. Gutierrez M.P., Bratos M.A., Garrote J.I., Duenas A., Almaraz A., Alamo R., Rodriguez Marcos H., Rodriguez Recio M.J., Munoz M.F., Orduna A., Rodriguez-Torres A. Serologic Evidence of Human Infection by Francisella tularensis in the Population of Castilla y Leon (Spain) prior to 1997. Federation of European Microbiological Societies Microbiology Reviews, 2003. 35: pp. 165-169

81. Koskela P., Salminen A. Humoral Immunity against Francisella tularensis after Natural Infection. Journal of Clinical Microbiology, 1985. 22: pp. 973-979

82. Bevanger L., Maeland J.A., Naess A.I. Cometitive Enzyme Immunoassay for Antibodies to a 43000-Molecular-Weight Francisella tularensis Outer Membrane Protein for the Diagnosis of Tularemia. Journal of Clinical Microbiology, 1989. 27: pp. 922-926

83. Carlsson H.E., Lindberg A.A., Lindberg G., Hederstedt B., Karlsson K-A., Agell B.O. Enzyme-Linked Immunosorbent Assay for Immunological Diagnosis of Human Tularemia. Journal of Clinical Microbiology, 1979. 10: pp. 615-621

84. Enderlin G., Morales L., Jacobs R.F., Cross T.J., Streptomycin and Alternative Agents for the Treatment of Tularemia: Review of the Literature. Clinical Infectious Diseases, 1994. 19: pp. 42-47

85. Mason W.L., Eigelsbach H.T., Little S.F., Bates J.H. Treatment of Tularemia, Including Pulmonary Tularemia, with Gentamicin. American Review of Respiratory Diseases, 1980. 121: pp. 39-45

86. Limaye A.P., Hooper C.J. Treatment of Tularemia with Fluoroquinolones: Two Cases and Review. Clinical Infectious Disease, 1999. 29: pp. 922-924

87. Aranda W.A. Treatment of Tularemia with Levofloxacin. European Society of Clinical Microbiology and Infectious Diseases, 2001. 7: pp. 167-169

88. Tärnvik A. Nature of Protective Immunity to Francisella tularensis. Reviews of Infectious Diseases, 1989. 11: pp. 440-451

89. Conlan J.W., Oyston P.C.F. Vaccines Against Francisella tularensis. Annals of the New York Academy of Sciences, 2007. 1105: pp. 325-350

90. Sjöstedt A., Tärnvik A., Sandström G. Francisella tularensis: Host-parasite Interaction. Federation of European Microbiological Societies Medical Microbiology, 1996. 13: pp. 181-184

91. Hornick R.B., Eigelsbach H.T. Aerogenic Immunization of Man with Live Tularemia Vaccine. Bacteriological Reviews, 1966. 30: pp. 532-538

92. Tularemia. Louisiana Office of Public Health – Infectious Disease Epidemiology Section. Revised July 17, 2011. Retrieved December 14, 2011. Website: http://www.dhh.state.la.us/ offices/miscdocs/ docs-249/Manual/TularemiaManual.pdf

Photo Bibliography

Figure 2.8-1: Colorized scanning electron micrograph (SEM) of a bone marrow-derived macrophage infected with Francisella tularensis strain LVS. This electron photomicrograph was taken by Elizabeth Fischer and released by the National Institute of Allergy and Infectious Diseases (NIAID). Public domain photo

Figure 2.8-3: F. tularensis infection diagram The human anatomical illustration was created by Dr. Alexander J. da Silva and Melanie Moser in 2003. The illustration is released by CDC. Public domain graphics

Shigellosis, also known as bacillary dysentery, is a disease most commonly associated with crowded, poverty stricken, unhygienic conditions. Typically found in developing or third world nations, bacillary dysentery is caused by organisms belonging to the genus *Shigella*. *Shigella* spp. are non-lactose fermenting, oxidase-negative, non-sporeforming, facultative anaerobic, Gram-negative bacilli. With the exception of *Shigella dysenteriae*, the remaining organisms of the genus *Shigella* are capable of fermenting mannitol.[1, 2] From the start of their discovery, *Shigella* spp. have been listed as non-motile and nonflagellated. However, in a 1995 study, *Shigella* spp. were shown to be capable of producing a single flagellum, 10 microns long, 12 to 14 nm in diameter, and typically arising from one pole of the bacterium. It is reported that the expression of the flagellum and motility of the microbe is strictly regulated by unidentified genetic and environmental factors.[3]

The genus *Shigella* consists of four species: *S. dysenteriae* (subgroup A), *S. flexneri* (subgroup B), *S. boydii* (subgroup C) and *S. sonnei* (subgroup D). Presently, within the four species, approximately 44 different O-antigen components of the lipopolysaccaride based serotypes have been described (Table 1).[1, 2]

The first description of *Shigella* was completed by Kiyoshi Shiga in 1898, from which the organism obtained its name. *Shigella* belongs to the family Enterobacteriaceae that naturally infects humans and other primates. These organisms cannot be distinguished from *Escherichia coli* through contemporary criteria of DNA relatedness, and if these organisms were discovered today they would be classified within the genus *Escherichia*. Nonetheless, *Shigella* has remained a separate genus due to its historical separation, as well as, its unique clinical symptoms (Figure 2.9-1).[1, 6]

Table 1: Shigella serotypes[4, 5]

Subgroups	Species	# Serotypes
A	S. dysenteriae	15
B	S. flexneri	8
C	S. boydii	20
D	S. sonnei	1

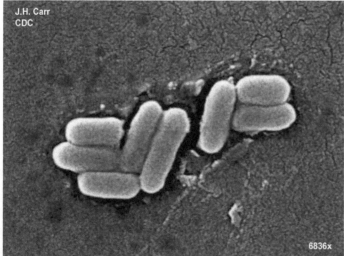

J.H. Carr
CDC

6836x

Figure 2.9-1: *Shigella* spp. belong to the family Enterobacteriaceae and cannot be distinguished from *Escherichia coli* through the contemporary criteria of DNA relatedness

Shigellosis is an important contributor to malnutrition in children in third world countries. It is responsible for infecting an average of 164.7 million people (~163.2 million infected in developing countries), with a global mortality rate of ~1.1 million, with 99% of deaths occurring in developing countries annually.[1, 2] It has been reported that 69% of all cases, as well as, 61% of all fatalities resulting from shigellosis are children under the age of five. The *Shigella* species responsible for the reported cases are *S. flexneri* (60%), *S. sonnei* (15%), *S. boydii* (6%), and *S. dysenteriae* (6%). Out of 6% of the total cases caused by *S. dysenteriae*, 30% were caused by *S. dysenteriae* serotype 1.[1, 2, 7, 8]

Of all the species belonging to the genus *Shigella*, *S. dysenteriae* serotype 1, also known as Shiga's bacillus, is the most virulent. *S. dysenteriae* serotype 1 is highly resistant to stomach acidity and requires a low infectious dose. It has been estimated that 10-100 *S. dysenteriae* serotype 1 bacilli can produce an active infection. Additionally, this bacillus possesses a high rate of mortality. *S. dysenteriae* is known to cause several systemic manifestations such as bacteremia, hemolytic uremic syndrome (HUS) and post-infectious arthritis (Reiter's syndrome).[1, 8, 9, 10, 11, 12, 13]

During World War II, the Japanese biological development center, Unit 731 headquartered near Pingfan (Harbin), China, experimented with *Shigella* as a potential biological warfare agent. During the war crimes prosecutions, members of Unit 731 admitted to intentionally contaminating water supplies, food items and/or spraying various bacteria, including *Shigella* spp. from aircrafts over 11 Chinese cities, infecting and causing the deaths of untold numbers of inhabitants.[14] In the past decade, *Shigella* has also been used as a biological terror weapon within the United States. In 1997, a laboratory worker intentionally contaminated muffins and donuts in the staff break room with *S. dysenteriae* serotype 2. This purposeful attack resulted in 12 of 45 laboratory staff developing severe acute diarrheal illness, with eight individuals having *S. dysenteriae* isolated from stool, while four were hospitalized. Luckily, no fatalities resulted from this attack. Due to the highly infectious nature, antibiotic resistance and absence of a vaccine, *S. dysenteriae* serotype 1 is an attractive biological weapon and is listed as a category B biological warfare agent by the Center for Disease Control and Prevention (CDC).[15]

S. dysenteriae serotype 1 does not have a natural reservoir in animals and can only be spread from human to human via fecal-oral transmission, generally in unsanitary conditions. Insects, such as flies may also serve as a mechanism of transferring the bacilli from person to person. The incidences of naturally occurring shigellosis are the highest among children under the age of five. At such a youthful age, good individual hygiene is more difficult to maintain. Additionally, children have yet to acquire the specific immunity to combat the disease (Figure 2.9-2 and 2.9-3).[1]

S. dysenteriae serotype 1, as with all other *Shigella* serotypes and related organisms such as *Escherichia coli*, are acid resistant and exit the human host via fecal matter. Similar to those acid resistant (AR) systems found in *E. coli*, *Shigella* spp. possess at least four AR systems which promote survival in the host digestive tract. Presently, three out of the four AR (AR1-AR3) are known to function within *Shigella* spp. AR1 is a stationary-phase, acid induced, glucose-repressed oxidative pathway, dependent on the alternative sigma factor δ^S, encoded by the general stress regulator sigma factor sigma-38 (σ38, or RpoS) gene and the global regulatory protein cAMP receptor protein (CRP). AR1 protects the bacilli in the absence of glutamate at pH 2.5; nonetheless, the exact manner by which AR1 protect the cells is presently unknown.[16, 17, 18] AR2 and AR3 are involved in the active removal of intracellular protons via decarboxy-lation of amino acids. These AR systems consist of pairs of amino acid decarboxylases and antiporters. The amino acid decarboxylases replace the alpha-carboxyl groups or their substrates with a proton that is acquired from the cytoplasm, which in turn, produces carbon dioxide and a byproduct that is actively transported by the antiporter. For example, the decarboxylation of glutamate and arginine is completed through the actions of AR2 and AR3 respectively. AR2 is a stationary-phase, glutamate-dependent acid resistance system (GDAR) pathway, which is regulated transcriptionally via the alternative sigma factor RpoS of bacterial RNA polymerase.[19, 20, 21] AR2 or GDAR pathway is a glutamate decarboxylase system, consisting of two homologous decarboxylase enzymes: GadA and GadB, as well as, an antiporter, GadC.[21] AR2 system acts on the acidic environment by mopping up protons leaking into the bacterial cytosol through the decarboxylation of glutamate into gamma aminobutyric acid (GABA). Subsequently, by exchanging GABA for external glutamate with the antiporter GadC, the bacterium is able to maintain the pH homeostasis within its cytoplasm. It has been reported that GadC is highly pH dependent, with no detectable activities at or above pH 6.5. AR3 is comprised of arginine decarboxylase (AdiA) which is responsible for decarboxylating arginine to create agmatine and the antiporter AdiC. [16, 17, 18, 21, 22]

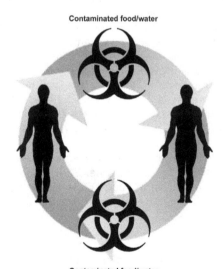

Contaminated food/water

Contaminated food/water

Figure 2.9-2: Transmission cycle of *S. dysenteriae*

The activation of acid resistance systems allows the organism to tolerate exposure to pH levels less than 2.5 (such as the environment within the stomach), for several hours. After the microbe passes through the stomach, it down regulates the acid-resistance genes and up regulates the invasion genes. Presently, there are two views with regards to the mechanism in which the bacilli invade the host's intestinal epithelial cells. [16, 17, 18, 21, 22]

The traditional view postulates that *Shigella* spp. invade the cells of the terminal ileum and colon through a complex mechanism mediated by both bacterial and host proteins.[1, 23, 24] For example, the use of a set of genes, known as the invasion plasmid antigen B (ipaB), ipaC, and ipaD; encoded on a large 180- to 220-kb plasmid induces bacterial uptake via a phagocytosis-like process on the apical surface of the intestinal mucosal cell. Following

phagocytosis, the microbes reach the cytoplasm of the host cell via membrane bounded endosome. The subsequent lysis of the endosome releases the bacteria into the cytoplasm where they multiply and eventually cause the death of the host epithelial cell. The manner by which the bacilli induce host epithelial cell death has not been adequately explained.[1, 25, 26, 27]

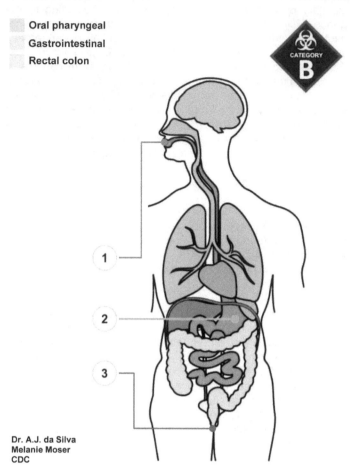

■ Oral pharyngeal
■ Gastrointestinal
■ Rectal colon

Dr. A.J. da Silva
Melanie Moser
CDC

Figure 2.9-3: *Shigella* spp. infection diagram. ①*Shigella* spp. enter the host through contaminated food and/or water. ②*Shigella* spp. cause systemic infection through the gastro-intestinal tract. ③*Shigella* spp. exit the host via fecal route

The alternative view, and now the more accepted view, postulates that the bacilli initially transverse the mucosa, not directly through the epithelial cells, but through the M (microfold) cells, which are found in the follicle-associated epithelium of the Peyer's Patches.[21, 28] After entry, *Shigella* spp. can be seen in an intercellular position where they are able to invade enterocytes baso-laterally.[29] Also during this same time, the bacilli are translocated to macrophages by the M cells, in association with the follicle structure of the Peyer's Patches and are phagocytized. Once phagocytized, the invasive *Shigella* triggers caspase 1 (activated by ipaB) and induces apoptosis in macrophages.[21, 30, 31] During the course of apoptosis, cellular fragments of the dying macrophages containing the bacilli are phagocytized by adjacent macrophages and remain inside these cells in large phago-lysosomes, from which live bacteria may escape.[21, 29, 32] In addition, to the disintegration of apoptotic macrophages, large stores of inflammatory cytokines such as interleukin-1β (IL-1β) and IL-18 are released, accounting for the early development of intense local inflammation.[21, 33, 34] For example, IL-1β triggers the strong intestinal inflammation characteristic with shigellosis, while IL-18 activates natural killers (NK) cells and promotes the production of gamma interferons (IFN-γ), thereby amplifying innate immune responses.[21, 35, 36]

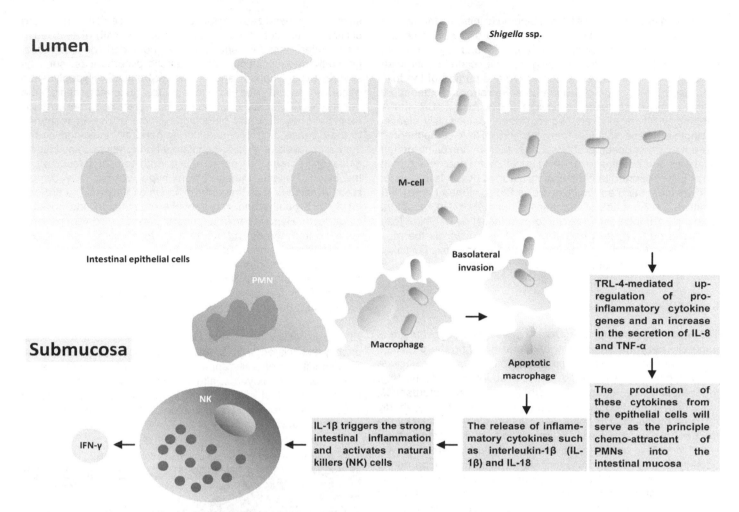

Lumen

Shigella ssp.

M-cell

Intestinal epithelial cells

Basolateral invasion

PMN

Macrophage

Submucosa

Apoptotic macrophage

NK

TRL-4-mediated up-regulation of pro-inflammatory cytokine genes and an increase in the secretion of IL-8 and TNF-α

IFN-γ

IL-1β triggers the strong intestinal inflammation and activates natural killers (NK) cells

The release of inflame-matory cytokines such as interleukin-1β (IL-1β) and IL-18

The production of these cytokines from the epithelial cells will serve as the principle chemo-attractant of PMNs into the intestinal mucosa

Figure 2.9-4: A diagrammtic display on the mechanism of invasion (alternative view on invasion) through the intestinal epithelium by *Shigella* spp.

Regardless of the traditional and alternative views, once the bacilli gain access to the cytoplasm (after lysing the phagocytic vacuole within the M cells), the microbe expresses a motility phenotype that allows for intracellular movement and cell to cell spread.[34, 37] The expression of the phenotype allows the bacilli to interact with the host cell cytoskeleton and reorganize the F-actin on the cell surfaces. The reorganization of the F-actin allows *Shigella* spp. to use it as a polarized motor that pushes the bacilli forward and permits the formation of long membrane bound protrusions, bringing it into the cytoplasmic compartment of the next cell.[38, 39, 40, 41] Through an E-cadherin (a calcium dependent cell adhesion molecule) mediated process, the protrusions formed by *Shigella* spp. are actively endocytized by adjacent epithelial cells through intercellular junctions. By using the above process, the bacilli can infect a large surface area of the intestinal epithelium, while being protected from the host immune system (Figure 2.9-4).[29, 42]

The invasion of the intestinal epithelium by *Shigella* spp. will result in toll-like receptor (TRL)-4-mediated up-regulation of pro-inflammatory cytokine genes and an increase in the secretion of IL-8 and tumor necrosis factor-α (TNF-α) by the epithelial cells.[43, 44] The production of pro-inflammatory cytokines will serve as the principle chemoattractant for polymorphonuclear leuko-cytes (PMNs) to the intestinal mucosa. This recruitment of PMNs will subsequently trigger an intense inflammatory response, that may lead to epithelial cell destruction and histopathological lesions of the terminal ileum and colon, indistinguishable from acute ulcerative colitis.[23, 25, 45]

S. dysenteriae serotype 1 produces a cytolethal verocytotoxin

called shiga toxin (Stx), which is identical to the toxin produced by *Escherichia coli* O157:H7.[46] Although, no other organisms belonging to the genus *Shigella* produce the exact same toxin, *S. flexneri* and *S sonnei* produce toxins that are biologically and antigenically similar, although they contain 10^4 to 10^5 fold less cytotoxic activity.[47, 48] The shiga toxin is composed of two moieties: single A subunit (~32 kDa) which is proteolytically cleaved to yield a 28 kDa peptide (A_1) and a 4 kDa peptide (A_2) which is non-covalently attached to a pentamere of five identical B subunits (Figure 2.9-5).[46, 49, 50]

M. E. Fraser *et al.*

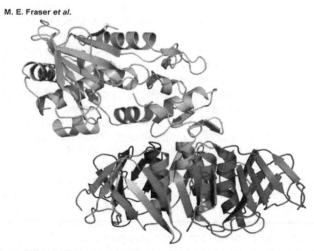

Figure 2.9-5: A 3D structure rendering of shiga toxin. The A subunit is shown top left and B subunit is shown bottom right

Once released by the bacilli, toxin binding is initiated through the B subunits which are known to connect to glycolipid receptors known as globotriaosylceramide (Gb$_3$), found commonly on human endothelial cells leading to the clathrin-dependent endocytosis.[51] Subsequently, the enzymatic portion of the toxin is transported to the Golgi apparatus via retrograde transports to the rough endoplasmic reticulum (rER). At the rER, the A$_1$ subunit, which is also an N-glycosidase, catalytically cleaves a single adenine residue from the 28S rRNA component of the eukaryotic ribosome 60S subunit, thereby inhibiting protein synthesis and eventually resulting in cell death and detachment. It has been reported that the toxicity induced by Stx is influenced by cytokines, such as tumor necrosis factor alpha (TNF-α). For example, TNF-α is able to increase the numbers of Gb$_3$ receptors, which in turn, increases toxicity to endothelial cells. Shiga toxin produced by *S. dysenteriae* serotype 1, is known as the most virulent agent of bacterial dysentery and is epidemically linked to the development of hemolytic uremic syndrome (HUS).[1, 2, 52, 53, 54, 55, 56 , 57]

SYMPTOMS

The incubation time for shigellosis caused by *S. dysenteriae* is generally between 24 to 72 hours after ingesting the organism via contaminated food and/or water. Initial symptoms include at least one of the following malaise: abdominal cramps (e.g. tenderness in the left lower quadrant), acid base disturbances, signs of systemic toxicity and fever (~38.5° C or 101.3° F), shortly followed by diarrhea or bacillary dysentery, characterized by the frequent passage of small volume, bloody and mucoid stools.[1, 2, 58, 59, 60, 61] The symptoms of bacillary dysentery are generally accompanied by tenesmus, defined as painful straining during defecation. Bacillary dysentery is the result of the inflammation and ulceration of colonic mucosa and an intense proctitis, which may result in rectal prolapsed, especially in young children.[1, 2]

Vomiting and sever dehydration are not prominent symptoms although some mild to moderate dehydration does occur due to water loss from diarrhea, dysentery, fever, reduced food and fluid intake.[1, 2] It has been estimated that the fluid loss during the dysentery phase of the disease is less than 30mL/kg/day. Due to the reduction in food and fluid intake, *Shigella* spp. dysentery is associated with anorexia, although the stomach and small intestines are not involved in the infection. Generally, the illness is self limiting and lasts only 4 to 7 days, after the initial onset of symptoms.[58, 62, 63, 64]

Shigella spp. infections generally do not progress beyond the lamina propria, however, in rare cases it can spread transmurally and lead to colonic and distal ileal perforation.[65, 66] Unfortunately, perforations are generally diagnosed postmortem during autopsies of fatal cases of shigellosis involving neonates and severely malnourished children. Death is generally the result of the persistent leakage of intestinal flora into the peritoneum, causing complications such as intravascular volume, shock caused by endotoxemia, sepsis, pooling of fluids in the peritoneum and bowl lumen, decrease venous return and respiratory complications involving diminished tidal volume.[67] Other prominent, but rare manifestations, are functional intestinal obstruction and toxic megacolon, stemming from severe inflammation which eventually results in necrosis of intestinal cells. In these conditions, the colon is grossly dilated, with its wall edematous and inflamed.[68] Bacteriemia is also a rare occurrence associated with this disease, but it exists in severely malnourished or immunocompromised patients. [69, 70, 71]

Shigellosis is associated with number of systemic manifestations, such as generalized motor seizures, especially in young children with high fever.[72] Some patients with the disease may suffer seizures and become obtunded or comatose, generally in association with metabolic disturbances, such as severe hypoglycemia and/or hyponatremia.[73] Hypoglycemia generally occurs due to inadequate gluconeogenesis (the generation of glucose from non-carbohydrate substances such as lactate, glycerol and glucogenic amino acids), in response to the disease, and this condition is generally indicated by the increased levels of glucose regulatory hormones such as insulin, glucagon, adrenaline, noradrenalin and cortisol circulating in the blood. Patients suffering from hypoglycemia may display blood glucose of less than 1mmol/L, which may lead to protein-losing enteropathy and may provoke malnutrition and possibly even death. Hyponatremia is generally associated with patients suffering from the dysenteric form of shigellosis. This condition is postulated to be caused by the inadequate secretion of vasopressin (anti-diuretic hormone). In general, the serum sodium concentrations for patients suffering from this condition are less than 125 mmol/L, which can result in cerebral edema and possibly death (Table 2).[1, 64]

Due to its ability to secrete Stx, the development of HUS is directly associated with *S. dysenteriae* serotype 1 infections. This condition generally appears in children between the ages of six months to six years, although in rare cases it does occur in adults. The first symptoms of HUS emerges approximately 7 days after the onset of dysentery, often with the intestinal conditions subsiding.[1, 74, 75]

Table 2: An overview of the clinical symptoms of shigellosis

Symptoms	+	++	+++
Malaise			■
Abdominal cramps			■
Acid base disturbances			■
Systemic toxicity signs			■
Fever			■
Diarrhea			■
Bloody diarrhea			■
Bacillary dysentery			■
Tenesmus			■
Reduced food intake			■
Reduced fluid intake			■
Nausea		■	
Vomiting		■	
Dehydration		■	
Intravascular volume	■		
Endotoxis shock	■		
Sepsis	■		
Pooling in peritoneum	■		
Pooling in bowl lumen	■		
Decrease venous return	■		
Diminished tidal volume	■		
Intestinal obstruction	■		
Toxic megacolon	■		
Rectal prolaps	■		
Bacteriemia	■		
Motor seizures (children)	■		
High fever (children)	■		
Seizure	■		
Obtunded	■		
Coma	■		
Hypoglycemia	■		
Hyponatremia	■		

+ Rare ++ Common +++ Frequent

HUS is diagnosed by the simultaneous appearance of

microangiopathic hemolytic anemia (anemia with the presence of fragmented erythrocytes and a hemoglobin concentration of less than 10 g/dL), thrombocytopenia (less than 100 thousand platelets/mm[3]) and acute renal failure (anuria, oliguria or elevated serum creatinine levels ~1.5 time higher than normal values in age matched controls).[76, 77] It is common to observe symptoms such as severe renal failure and hemolytic anemia, while thrombocytopenia is usually less dramatic, with platelet counts in the range of 25,000 to 100,000/mm[3] in patients suffering from *S. dysenteriae* type 1 induced HUS. It has been reported that the HUS manifestations caused by *S. dysenteriae* serotype 1 are incomplete, where any of the three manifestations may occur in isolation.[78, 79]

During the acute phase of illness, signs of central nervous system dysfunction maybe observed. These dysfunctions include lethargy, seizures or coma, and are observed more frequently in children. Post mortem examination shows evidence of raised intracranial pressure. Survivors of acute episodes of HUS may experience chronic seizures, cortical blindness, hemiparesis, and in children, developmental delays.[7, 80, 81, 82, 83, 84]

DETECTION

Presently specific diagnosis of *Shigella* infection requires the isolation of the bacilli from microbial cultures, generally from stool or rectal swabs. The organism can be cultured in selective medium for Gram-negative organisms such as MacConkey, deoxycholate citrate, xylose-lysine-deoxycholate, Hektoen enteric or *Salmonella-Shigella* agar.[1] Due to *Shigella*'s inability to ferment lactose, the color of the pH indicator does not change. This allows clear indication of lactose-negative colonies, which may warrant further examination by the investigators. Additional examinations may include subculture the colony on triple sugar iron, Kligler iron agar or use serological methods to separate it from other non-lactose fermenting bacteria such as *Salmonella*.[1] Subsequently, the colonies are identified via biochemical tests and agglutination assays. For example, in the methodology devised by Frankel *et al.* (1989), three pairs of synthetic oligonucleotide primers were prepared and shown to hybridize specifically to the genes encoding the heat-stable (ST) and the heat-labile (LT) enterotoxins located on the invasion-associated loci (ial) of the large *Shigella* virulence plasmid. When the three primer pairs were used in the polymerase chain reaction (PCR), the three corresponding genetic loci could be simultaneously amplified using DNA extracted directly from stool samples, and the amplified products could be readily detected by ST-, LT- and ial-specific, alkaline phosphatase-labelled oligonucleotide probes.[85] Nonetheless, cultivation of bacteria followed by biochemical and agglutination assays is time consuming (48 to 72 hours), and in many developing nations, the equipment necessary to perform these microbiological tests are not readily available. Therefore a more economical and rapid diagnostic method is necessary, such as immunofluorescent antibodies that have been developed specifically for *S. dysenteriae* type 1. This immunohistochemical methodology has demonstrated high sensitivity (92%) and high specificity (93%) towards identifying *Shigella* spp. infection.[86] Other methodologies have also been developed to rapidly identify these bacilli. For example, immunomagnetic isolation (IMS) and polymerase chain reaction (PCR) assays were developed to isolate *Shigella spp.* directly from fecal samples within three to four hours. DNA from the bacteria is captured by boiling the bacilli in water, and the IMS-PCR assay is sensitive in that it can detect 10 *Shigella* per gram of fecal matter.[87] Furthermore, another rapid detection method-ology using IMS assay, followed by the detection of the bacilli using monoclonal antibodies has been devised. The particles were coated with monoclonal antibodies

specific for the O-antigens of *Shigella dysenteriae* serotype 1 and these captured bacteria were detected by an enzyme-linked immunoassay with O-antigen specific rabbit antiserum. This assay takes approximately two to three hours to complete and the sensitivity limit was 10[3] cfu/ml, as determined by viable cell counting.[88]

Unfortunately, none of the above described diagnostic tests are available commercially. Presently, the only commercially available tests are monoclonal and polyclonal antibody enzyme-linked immuno-sorbent assays (ELISA), developed against Stx produced by *Shigella* spp. or EHEC. For example, a particular ELISA known as, Premier EHEC assay, developed by Meridian Diagnostics®, has been reported to be timely and cost effective and should be used as a routine screen for enteric pathogens in high-risk individuals, especially children.[89] Additionally, an assay called ImmunoCard STAT!® also developed by Meridian Bioscience®, is used to rapidly test for the presence of Stx. This detection kit has been reported to be an acceptable alternative to Premier EHEC assay.[90]

In 2013, Ojha *et al.* reported a pentaplex PCR assay to detect specific *Shigella* spp. For example, invC is used to identify shigella genus, rfc for *S. flexneri*, wbgZ for *S. sonnei*, and rfpB for *S. dysenteriae*, as well as, one internal control ompA gene. Validation of the procedure was completed with 120 *Shigella* strains and 37 non-Shigella strains; the result was reported to yield 100% specificity.[91]

TREATMENT

Although antimicrobial therapy is presently the cornerstone of treatment for shigellosis, the number of antibiotic resistant *Shigella* spp. that have appeared in recent years has placed drastic limitations on the medications useful for treatment. *Shigella* spp. have been progressively acquiring resistance to many of the antibiotics used in its treatment, mainly due to its ability to gain resistance genes from plasmids and transposons (Table 3).[92]

It has been reported that the spread of antibiotic resistance determinants by integrons triggers the rapid evolution of multi-drug resistance pheno-types in *Shigella* spp. Integrons are defined as genetic elements that acquire and exchange exogenous DNA, also known as gene cassettes, though a site-specific recombination mechanism. [111, 114] Within the various integrons that have been identified, integron classes 1 and 2 are the most common.[115] In various studies on *S. sonnei*, the class 1 integron was discovered to carry two gene cassettes: esterase/lipase (estX) and aminoglycoside adenyltransferase (aadA1), which are responsible for resistance to streptomycin and spectinomycin respectively.[111, 116] In the study by Ahmed *et al.* (2006), the class 2 integron was discovered to be associated with transponson Yn7, and carry 3 classic gene cassettes: dihydrofolate reductase (dfrA1), streptothricin acetyltransferase (sat1) and aadA1. Gene cassette dfrA1 is responsible for resistance to trimethoprim, sat1 is responsible for resistance to streptothricin and aadA1 responsible for resistance to both streptomycin and spectinomycin.[101, 110, 114]

Resistance to ampicillin is primarily mediated by beta-lactamases which hydrolyzes the beta-lactam ring, inactivating the antibiotic. Studies have shown that *oxa* genes (oxa-1-type beta-lactamase) predominates in ampicillin, cephalothin, oxacillin and cloxacillin resistant isolates.[101, 111] It has also been reported that the isolates possess the ability to produce the enzyme chloramphenicol acetyltransferase that breaks down this antimicrobial agent,

Table 3: Selected chronological list of antimicrobial resistance for *Shigella* spp.

Location	Years	Information Regarding Antimicrobial Resistance
England and Wales	1979-1983	*Shigella* subgroups A, B and C were found to be antibacterial resistant sulphonamides, streptomycin, tetracycline, ampicillin, trimethoprim-sulfamethoxazole (TMP-SMZ), furazolidone, nalidixic acid and chloramphenicol. [93]
India	1984	*S. dysenteriae* type 1 was discovered to be resistant to streptomyocin, tetracycline and chloramphenicol although it was highly sensitive to nalidixic acid, gentamicin, furazolidone and moderately sensitive to ampicillin and co-trimoxazole. [94]
India	1988	Nalidixic acid resistant stain of *S. dysenteriae* type 1 was identified. [95]
Israel	1990-1996	*Shigella* subgroups B, C and D were resistant to nalidixic acid, TMP-SMZ, amoxicillin and ampicillin. [96, 97]
India	1992	A new strain of *S. dysenteriae* type 1 was isolated form 24% of total bloody diarrhea case patients in India that demonstratrated resistance to nalidixic acid, furazolidone, ampicillin and co-trimoxazole. Luckily, this new strain was sensitive to fluoroquinolone derivatives such as norfloxacin and ciprofloxacin. [98]
Thailand	1992	A nalidixic acid resistant Shigella dysenteriae type 1 strain was discovered in Thailand. [99]
United States	1995-1998	Some *S. flexneri* and *S. sonnei* isolates were found in Oregon to be resistant to TMP-SMZ, ampicillin, tetracycline, nalidixic acid and cefixime. [100]
Spain	1995-2000	Isolates of *S. flexneri* and *S. sonnei* were found in Barcelona that has high levels of resistance to ampicillin, trimethoprim, tetracycline, chloramphenicol and nalidixic acid. [101]
Chile	1997-2001	Shigella subgroup B was resistant to tetracycline, ampicillin, co-trimoxazole, chloramphenicol, and amoxicillin. Shigella subgroup D was resistant to ampicillin, co-trimoxazole, tetracycline, chloramphenicol, and amoxicillin. [102]
Tanzania	1999	*Shigella dysenteriae* and *Shigella sonnei* discovered in Ifakara, Tanzania showed a high level of resistance to ampicillin, chloramphenicol, tetracycline, and co-trimoxazole. [103]
Indonesia	1998-1999	Various stains of Shigella from subgroups A, B, and D isolated were found to be resistant to ampicillin, TMP-SMZ, chloramphenicol and tetracycline. [104]
Indonesia	2000	Three strains of *S. dysenteriae* type 2 were discovered that are resistant to nalidixic acid, tetracycline, co-trimoxazole, ampicillin and chloramphenicol. [105]
Iran	1999-2001	Various strains from all four Shigella subgroups were found to have resistance towards nalidixic acid, co-trimoxazole, tetracycline, ampicillin and fourazolodon. [106]
Palestine	1999-2006	Most of the *Shigella* isolates (e.g. subgroup B) discovered in Gaza Palestine was resistant to trimethoprim-sulfamethoxazole, ampicillin and chloramphenicol. [107]
Brazil	2000-2002	All four subgroups of *Shigella* were isolated and tested for antimicrobial resistance in Brazil. The result of this experimentation was that these organisms showed resistance to TMP-SMZ, ampicillin, penicillin, co-trimoxazol, nalidixic acid, ciprofloxacin and norfloxacin. [108]
India	2002	Numerous strains of *S. dysenteriae* type 1 were discovered in Kolkata that is resistant to chloramphenicol, ampicillin, tetracycline, co-trimoxazole, furazolidone, nalidixic acid, ciprofloxacin, norfloxacin and amoxicillin. [109]
India	2003	Fluoroquinolones resistant *S. dysenteriae* type 1 in northeastern Bangladesh. [110]
Japan	2002-2004	Isolates of *S. flexneri* and *S. sonnei* were discovered in Hiroshima prefecture to be resistant to ampicillin, streptomycin, TMP, tetracycline, nalidixic acid and ciprofloxacin [111]
India	2002-2007	Various stains of *Shigella* from all subgroups (A, B, C and D) were discovered in Bangalore India to be resistant to chloramphenicol, ampicillin, co-trimoxazole, nalidixic acid and ciprofloxacin. [112]
China	1997-2009	Shigella spp. subgroups A, B and D and 13 distinct serotypes were discovered in China to be antimicrobial resistant. Subgroup B serotypes f2a and f4a were found to be Ciprofloxacin-resistant. Out of all the isolates, resistance to tetracycline was the most common (96.7%), followed by nalidixic acid (94.0%), ampicillin (85.7%), trimethoprim/sulfamethoxazole (79.4%) and chloramphenicol (76.7%). [113]

therefore are resistance to chloramphenicol. Nalidixic acid-resistant *Shigella* isolates possess a single point mutation in either codon 83 or 87 of *gyrA* gene.[101, 117] However, nalidixic acid resistance is not only due to mutations in the quinolone resistance determining regions, but also to an active efflux pump that appears likely to be sufficient to confer the 20- to 80-fold resistance to quinolones.[118] Please see Table 4 for more information on antimicrobial resistance of different *Shigella* spp.

With the large amount of information gathered that indicates *Shigella* spp. are antimicrobial resistant, the current options for antimicrobial treatment for shigellosis should be selected based upon the pattern of resistance in the community (geographical area), in order to devise the first line and second line of drugs for treatment. Since the resistance shown in various *Shigella* spp. in certain geographical areas may not appear in others, it is still possible to use certain antimicrobial agents that are resistant by certain subgroups and serotypes else where, to treat the disease. For example, in the United States it is still possible to use nalidixic acid to treat shigellosis caused by *Shigella* subgroups A and C, although both subgroups B and D are now resistant (Table 4). It is important that the physician utilizes empiric antimicrobial treatment in combating shigellosis. If a patient does not improve within 48 hours of treatment with a particular antimicrobial agent, then it can be assumed that the strain of *Shigella* is resistant to the antibiotic(s) (or infection with another organism

should be suspected) and a change to an appropriate agent is recommended. Presently the suggested drugs of choice effective towards all *Shigella* subgroups are listed in Table 5a and 5b.[1]

Severe dehydration in patients suffering from shigellosis is rare, therefore, general rehydration therapy is not usually necessary. An oral rehydration therapy is usually sufficient to reverse mild to moderate dehydration. The World Health Organization (WHO) recommends an oral rehydration formula based on the physiological observation that the intestinal absorption of sodium is coupled with the absorption of glucose, even during a period of illness when most substances are actively being excreted. Please examine Table 6 for the simple and inexpensive oral rehydration formula recommended by WHO. When faced with a case of severe dehydration, it is recommended that patients are rehydrated intravenously with normal saline or Ringer's lactate.[119, 120]

In the cases of hyponatremia, patients can be treated with saline solution or 3% NaCl solution intravenously (12 mL/kg should raise the sodium concentration by 10 mmol/L). If physicians choose the NaCl therapy for hyponatremia, close monitoring of the patient is necessary, since a rapid increase in sodium concentration may lead to CNS complications. It is important to note that *Shigella* spp. cause an inadequate secretion of vasopressin (anti-diuretic hormone), therefore the water intake of the patients needs to be closely monitored.[1, 121]

Table 4: Antibiotic resistance of *Shigella* spp.

Antibiotics	A	B	C	D
Amoxicillin	+	+	-	+
Ampicillin	+	+	+	+
Azithromycin	-	-	-	-
Cefixime	-	+	-	+
Ceftriaxone	-	-	-	-
Chloramphenicol	+	+	+	+
Ciprofloxacin	+	+	+	+
Co-trimoxazole	+	+	+	+
Furazolidone	+	+	+	+
Gentamicin	-	-	-	-
Nalidixic acid	+	+	+	+
Norfloxacin	+	+	+	+
Penicillin	+	+	+	+
Pivamdinocillin	-	-	-	-
Streptomycin	+	+	+	+
Sulphonamides	+	+	+	-
Tetracycline	+	+	+	+
TMP-SMZ	+	+	+	+
Trimethoprim	-	+	-	+

+ Resistant
- Non-resistant

Table 5a: Type of medications for the treatment of *Shigella* spp. and dosage required. Agent 1 is pivamdinocillin, Agent 2 is Ceftriaxone, Agent 3 is Enoxacin and Agent 4 is Azithromycin

Agent	Dosage	
	Adult	Pediatic
1	400 mg	25 mg/kg
2	1 g	50-75 mg/kg
3	200 mg	10 mg/kg
4	500 mg d1; 250 mg d2+	10 mg/kg d 1; 5 mg/kg d2+

Table 5b: The frequency and duration of the medication used for the treatment of *Shigella* spp. Agent 1 is pivamdinocillin, Agent 2 is Ceftriaxone, Agent 3 is Enoxacin and Agent 4 is Azithromycin

	Amount Administered	
	Frequency	Duration
1	4 times daily	5 days
2	1 time daily	5 days
3	2 times daily	3 days
4	1 time daily	5 days

Table 6: Oral rehydration formula recommended by WHO

Ingredient	Amount (Grams)
Table Salt (NaCl)	3.50
Sodium bicarbonate (NaHCO$_3$)	2.50
Potassium Chloride (KCl)	1.50
Glucose (C$_6$H$_{12}$O$_6$)	20.0

Since *Shigella* spp. cause an invasive disease of the human colonic mucosa, this infection generally places a heavy nutritional burden on patients, especially in the young, often resulting in hypoglycemia, anorexia, increased catabolism malabsorption and malnutrition. In cases of hypoglycemia, physicians should encourage the feeding of young children with breast milk and adults with a high calorie, protein-rich diet of solid food to prevent malnutrition.[1] Kabir *et al.* (1994), reported that patients responded well to a high protein diet as they demonstrated improved absorption rates of serum proteins, retinal binding protein, as well as other non-protein compounds such as vitamin A.[122, 123] In addition, zinc supplements have been shown to promote faster recovery from diarrhea and significantly higher weight gain.[124]

Unlike the ineffectiveness of antibiotics against EHEC infections,

early administration of antibiotics in *S. dysenteriae* infections greatly reduces the chances of individuals developing HUS. In a report by Bennish *et al.,* (2006) early administration of effective antibiotics showed a marked decrease in Stx concentrations in stool samples examined.[125] Nonetheless, patients suffering from HUS may require a heavy regiment of antibiotics, transfusions and peritoneal dialysis. Even with intervention, the fatality rate resulting from this condition is extremely high even when aggressively treated.[1, 126]

Toxic megacolon has a mortality rate of approximately 50%. Patients suffering from toxic megacolon should be placed on complete bowl rest and should receive adequate intravenous supplementation of fluids and electrolytes. It is suggested that all narcotic, antidarrheal and anticholinergic agents be avoided.[127] One possible treatment for this condition is colectomy, which may become necessary due to ulcerative colitis. Other treatments include, but are not limited to nasogastric or long tube suctions being used in colonic decompression, where the tubes must be placed into the ileum with fluoroscopic guidance.[128] Rectal prolapse generally will resolve on its own as the infection runs its course, although it is suggested that in the interim the prolapse tissue should be kept moist and be protected from damage. If bacteremia or sepsis develops, aggressive treatment of broad spectrum antibiotics should be administered (Table 4).[1]

Presently, there are no commercially available vaccines against *Shigella* spp. Nonetheless, many investigational vaccines are in clinical trials. There are two approaches to *Shigella* spp. vaccines. One is the utilization of live attenuated strategy and the other is utilizing the bacilli lipopolysaccharide (LPS)-conjugate strategy.[129, 130, 131]

In regards to the live attenuated vaccines, a *S. flexneri* 2a vaccine, known as SC602, was constructed at the Pasteur Institute and manufactured at Walter Reed Army Institute of Research. This live microbe is fully able to invade cultured cells, but with its *icsA* and *iuc* genes (invasion plasmid) deleted, the organism cannot spread intercellularlly. It has been reported that a single inoculation with SC602 protected 58 North American volunteers against the debilitating symptoms of shigellosis.[131] A second live attenuated vaccine against *S. dysenteriae* type 1, known as SC599, which was constructed at the Pasteur Institute in Paris, France, by creating deletions in several genes including *icsA*, *ent*, *fep* and *stxA*. Clinical trials of this experimental vaccine also showed promise, however, more examination is required.[132]

Another vaccine SSRW1 (*S. sonnei* vaccine: constructed and trials performed in Israel) was made using the deletion of *icsA*. CVD 1203, a vaccine against *S. flexneri* 2a, has deletions in *aroA* and *icsA*, also has shown against promised in protecting against shigellosis.[129, 133, 134] With regards to the bacilli lipopolysaccharide (LPS)-conjugate as a potential vaccine strategy, a Ty21a-based Shigella vaccine was developed which uses live, attenuated *Salmonella typhi* vaccine strain Ty21a, as a carrier for *Shigella* LPS antigens. Preliminary animal studies demonstrate protection in challenges, but further examination and experimentation is required.[135] Several other *Shigella* vaccines have been developed and have shown promise in clinical trials. The most promising is the O-specific polysaccharideprotein conjugate, which has demonstrated protective efficacy in human trials. There are also several other approaches in the development of a vaccine such as ribosomal vaccines and inactivated whole-cell vaccines.[129]

DIFFERENTIAL DIAGNOSIS

The differential diagnosis of shigellosis should include

Table 7: Differential diagnosis of chronic EHEC with selected disease with similar symptoms. Please note that YE abbreviates for _Yersinia enterocolitica_ and CDC abbreviates for _Clostridium difficile_ colitis

Symptoms	Shigellosis	O157:H7	Salmonella	YE	Amebiasis	Cholera	CDC
Malaise	■	■	■			■	■
Abdominal cramps	■	■	■	■		■	■
Acid base disturbances	■					■	
Signs of systemic toxicity	■	■	■			■	
Fever	■	■	■	■		■	■
Diarrhea	■	■	■	■		■	■
Bloody diarrhea	■	■	■				
Bacillary dysentery	■	■	■				
Tenesmus			■	■	■		
Reduced food intake							
Reduced fluid intake							
Nausea	■	■	■		■	■	
Vomiting		■	■			■	
Dehydration	■	■	■			■	■
Intravascular volume	■						
Endotoxis shock	■					■	
Sepsis	■						
Rectal prolaps	■	■					
Pooling in peritoneum	■						
Pooling in bowl lumen	■						
Decrease venous return	■						
Diminished tidal volume	■						
Intestinal obstruction	■						
Toxic megacolon	■	■			■		
Bacteriemia		■					
Motor seizures (children)	■	■					
High fever (children)	■	■					
Seizure	■						
Obtunded	■						
Coma	■	■					
Hypoglycemia	■						
Hyponatremia	■						

Escherichia coli O157:H7 infection, _Salmonella enteritidis_, _Yersinia enterocolitica_ (YE), amebiasis caused by _Entamoeba histolytica_, cholera, _Clostridium difficile_ colitis (CDC), and inflammatory bowel disease (IBD). For example, blood is a common symptom in both shigellosis and amebiasis but symptomatic display of blood in shigellosis is generally bright red rather than dark brown as presented by amebiasis. In addition, during microscopic examination of stool smears from patients, individual suffering from shigellosis will possess numerous PMNs while patients suffering from amebiasis will reveal erythrophagocytic trophozoites.[1, 136] Please examine Table 7 for more information.

References

1. Guerrant R.L., Walker D.H., Weller P.F. Tropical Infectious Diseases – Principles, Pathogens & Practice. Volume 1. Philadelphia: Churchill Livingstone Elsevier. 2006. pp. 255-264
2. Murray P.R., Rosenthal K.S., Kobayashi G.S., Pfaller M.A. Medical Microbiology. Fourth Edition. St. Louis: Mosby College Publishing, 2002. pp. 275-276
3. Girón J.A. Expression of Flagella and Motility by Shigella. Molecular Microbiology, 1995. 18: pp. 63-75
4. Shigella Annual Summary 2004. Department of Health and Human Services. Center for Disease Control and Prevention. Revised November 2005. Retrieved December 6, 2009. Website: http://www.cdc.gov/ncidod/DBMD/phlisdata/shigtab/2004/ShigellaIntroduction2004.pdf
5. Kaisar A.T., Islam Z., Islam M.A., Dutta D.K., Safa A., Ansaruzzaman M., Faruque A.S.G., Shahed S.N., Nair G.B., Sack S.A. Phenotypic and Genotypic Characterization of Provisional Serotype Shigella flexneri 1c and Clonal Relationships with 1a and 1b Strains Isolated in Bangladesh. Journal of Clinical Microbiology, 2003. 41: pp. 110-117
6. Lan R., Reeves P.R. Escherichia coli in Disguise: Molecular Origins of Shigella. Microbes and Infection, 2002. 4: pp. 1125-1132
7. Kotloff K.L., Winickoff J.P., Ivanoff B., Clemens J.D., Swerdlow D.L., Sansonetti P.J., Adak G.K., Levine M.M. Global Burden of Shigella Infections: Implications for Vaccine Development and Implementation of Control Strategies. Bulletin of the World Health Organization, 1999. 77: pp. 651-666
8. Pal P., Pal A., Niyogi S.K., Ramamurthy T., Bhadra R.K. Comparative analysis of the genomes of Shigella dysenteriae type 2 & type 7 isolates. The Indian Journal of Medical Research, 2013. 137: pp 169-177
9. Levine M.M., Dupont H.L., Formal S.B., Hornick R.B., Takeuchi A., Snyder M.J., Libonati J.P. Pathogenesis of Shigella dysenteriae 1 (Shiga) dysentery. The Journal of Infectious Diseases, 1973. 127: pp. 261-270
10. Levine M.M., Kaper J.B., Black R.E., Clements M.L. New Knowledge on Pathogenesis of Bacterial Enteric Infections as Applied to Vaccine Development. Microbiological Reviews, 1983. 47: pp. 510-550
11. DuPont H.L., Levine M.M., Hornick R.B., Formal S.B. Inoculum Size in Shigellosis and Implications for Expected Mode of Transmission. The Journal of Infectious Diseases, 1989. 159: pp. 1126-1128
12. Pavliak V., Nashed E.M., Pozsgay V., Kováč P., Karpas A., Chu C., Schneerson R., Robbins J.B., Glaudemans C.P.J. Binding of the O-antigen of Shigella dysenteriae Type 1 and 26 Related Synthetic Fragments to a Monoclonal IgM Antibody. The Journal of Biological Chemistry, 1993. 268: pp. 25797-25802
13. Tortora G.J., Funke B.R., Case C.L. Microbiology an Introduction. San Francisco: Benjamin Cummings. 2010. pp. 309-310
14. McIssac J.H. Hospital Preparation for Bioterror. A Medical and Biomedical System Approach. Burlington: Academic Press. 2006. pp. 21-22
15. Kolavic S.A., Kimura A., Simons S.L., Slutsker L., Barth S., Haley C.E. An Outbreak of Shigella dysenteriae Type 2 among Laboratory Workers due to Intentional Food Contamination. Journal of the American Medical Association, 1997. 278: pp. 396-398
16. Lin J., Soo Lee I., Frey J., Slonczewski J. L., Foster J. Comparative Analysis of Extreme Acid Survival in Salmonella typhimurium, Shigella flexneri and Escherichia coli. The Journal of Bacteriology, 1995. 177: pp. 4097–4104
17. Castani-cornet M-P., Penfound T.A., Smith D., Elliot J.F., Foster J.W. Control of Acid Resistance in Escherichia coli. Journal of Bacteriology, 1999. 181: pp. 3525-3535
18. Oglesby A.G., Murphy E.R., Iyer V.R., Payne S.M. Fur Regulates Acid Resistance in Shigella flexneri via RyhB and ydeP. Molecular Microbiology, 2005. 58: pp. 1354-1367
19. Small P., Blankenhorn D., Welty D. Zinser E., Slonczewski J.L. Acid and Base Resistance in Escherichia coli and Shigella flexneri:Role of rpoS and Growth pH. The Journal of Bacteriology, 1994. 176: pp. 1729-1737
20. Bhagwat A.A., Bhagwat M. Comparative Analysis of Transcriptional Regulatory Elements of Glutamate-dependent Acid-resistance System of Shigella flexneri and Escherichia coli O157:H7. Federation of European Microbiological Society Microbiology Letters, 2004. 234: pp. 139-147
21. Tang Y-W., Sussman M., Liu D., Poxton I., Schwartzman J. Molecular Medical Microbiology. London: Academic Press. 2014. pp. 1155-1158
22. Jennison A.V., Verma N.K. The Acid-resistance Pathway of Shigella flexneri 2457T. Microbiology, 2007. 153: pp. 2593-2602
23. Fleckenstein J.M., Kopecko D.J. Breaching the Mucosal Barrier by Stealth: an Emerging Pathogenic Mechanism for Enteroadherent Bacterial Pathogens. The Journal of Clinical Investigation, 2001. 107: pp/ 27-30
24. Sansonetti P.J., Tan Van Nhieu G., Egile C. Rupture of the Intestinal Epithelial Barrier and Mucosal Invasion by Shigella flexneri. Clinical Infectious Disease, 1999. 28: pp. 466-475
25. Maurelli A.T. Shigella Inside and Out: Lifestyle of the Invasive and Dysenteric. American Society for Microbiology News, 1992. 58: pp. 603-608
26. Vaudry B., Maurelli A.T., Clere P., Sadoff J.C., Sansonetti P.J. Localization of Plasmid Loci Necessary for the Entry of Shigella flexneri into HeLa Cells and Characterization of One locus Encoding Four Immunogenic Polypeptides. Journal of General Microbiology, 1987. 133: pp. 3403-3413

27. Watarai M., Tobe T., Yoshikawa M., Sasakawa C. Contact of Shigella with Host Cells Triggers Release of Ipa Invasins and is an Essential Function of Invasiveness. The European Molecular Biology Organization (EMBO) Journal, 1995. 14: pp. 2461-2470
28. Sansonetti P.J., Arondel J., Fontaine A., d'Hauteville H., Bernardini M.L. OmpB (Osmo-Regulation) and icsA (Cell to Cell Spread) Mutants of *Shigella flexneri*: Vaccine Candidates and Probes to Study the Pathogenesis of Shigellosis. Vaccine, 1991. 9: 416-422
29. Perdomo O.J.J., Cavaillon J.M., Huerre M., Ohayon H., Gounon P., Sansonetti P.J. Acute Inflammation Cause Epithelial Invasion and Mucosal Destruction in Experimental Shigellosis. The Journal of Experimental Medicine, 1994. 180: pp. 1307-1319
30. Zychlinsky A., Prevost M.C., Sansonetti P.J. *Shigella flexneri* Induces Apoptosis in Infected Macrophages. Nature, 1992. 358: pp. 167-169
31. Zychlinsky A., Kenny B., Ménard R., Prévost M.C., Holland I.B., Sansonetti P.J. IpaB Mediates Macrophage Apoptosis induced by *Shigella flexneri*. Molecular Microbiology, 1994. 358: pp. 619-627
32. Senerovic L., Tsunoda S.P., Goosmann C., Brinkmann V., Zychlinsky A., Meissner F., Kolbe M. Spontaneous formation of IpaB ion channels in host cell membranes reveals how Shigella induces pyroptosis in macrophages. Cell Death and Disease, 2012. 3: pp. e384
33. Zychlinsky A., Fitting C., Cavaillon J.M., Sansonetti P.J. Interleukin 1 is Released by Murine Macrophages during Apoptosis Induced by *Shigella flexneri*. The Journal of Clinical Investigation, 1994. 94: pp. 1328-1332
34. Sansonetti P.J., Ryter A., Clerc P., Maurelli A.T., Mounier J. Multiplication of *Shigella flexneri* within HeLa Cells: Lysis of the Phagocytic Vacuole and Plasmid Mediated Contact Hemolysis. Infection and Immunity, 1986. 51: pp. 461-469
35. Le-Barillec K., Magalhaes J.G., Corcuff E., Thuizat A., Sansonetti P.J., Phalipon A., Di Santo J.P. Role for T and NK Cells in the Innate Immune Response to *Shigella flexneri*. The Journal of Immunology, 2005. 175: pp. 1735-1740
36. Way S.S., Borczuk A.C., Dominitz R., Goldberg M.B. An Essential Role for Gamma Interferon in Innate Resistance to *Shigella flexneri* Infection. Infection and Immunity, 1998. 66: pp. 1342-1348
37. Makino S., Sasakawa C., Kamata K., Kurata T., Yoshikawa M. A Genetic Determinant Required for Continuous Reinfection of Adjacent Cells in Large Plasmid in *Shigella flexneri* 2a. Cell, 1986. 46: pp. 551-555
38. Bernardini M.L., Mounier J., d'Hauteville H., Coquis-Rondon M., Sansonetti P.J. Identification of icsA, a Plasmid Locus of *Shigella flexneri* that Governs Intra- and Intercellular Spread through Interaction with F-actin. The Proceedings of the National Academy of Sciences United States of America, 1989. 86: 3867-3871
39. Goldberg M.B., Bârzu O., Parsot C., Sansonetti P.J. Unipolar Localization and ATPase Activity of IcsA, a *Shigella Flexneri* Protein Involved in Intracellular Movement. The Journal of Bacteriology, 1993. 175: pp. 2189-2196
40. Kadurugamuwa J.L., Rhode M., Wehland J., Timmis K.N. Intercellular Spread of Shigella flexneri through a Monolayer Mediated by Membranous Protrusions and Associated with Reorganization of the Cytoskeletal Protein Vinculin. Infection and Immunity, 1991. 59: pp. 3463-3471
41. Nhieu G.T.V., Liu B.K., Zhang J., Pierre F., Prigent S., Sansonetti P., Erneux C., Kim J.K., Suh P-G., Dupont G., Combettes L., Actin-based confinement of calcium responses during Shigella invasion. Nature Communications, 2013. 4: pp. 1567
42. Sansonetti P.J., Mounier J., Prévost M.C., Mège R.G. Cadherin Expression is required for the spread of *Shigella flexneri* between epithelial cells. Cell, 1994. 76: pp. 829-839
43. Struelens M.J., Pate D., Kabir I., Salam A., Nath S.K., Butlerb T. Shigella Septicemia: Prevalence, Presentation, Risk Factors, and Outcome. The Journal of Infectious Diseases, 1985. 152: pp. 784-790
44. Jung H.C., Eckmann L., Yang S.K., Panja A., Fierer J., Morzycka-Wroblewska E., Kagnoff M.F. A Distinct Array of Proinflammatory Cytokines is Expressed in Human Colon Epithelial Cells in Response to Bacterial Invasion. The Journal of Clinical Investigation, 1995. 95: pp. 55-65
45. Sansonetti P.J., Arondel J., Huerre M., Harada A., Matsushima K. Interleukin-8 Controls Bacterial Transepithelial Translocation at the Cost of Epithelial Destruction in Experimental Shigellosis. Infection and Immunity, 1999. 67: pp. 1471-1480
46. Taylor M. Enterohaemorrhagic Escherichia coli and *Shigella dysenteriae* Type 1-Induced Haemolytic Uraemic Syndrome. Pediatric nephrology, 2008. 23: pp. 1425-1431
47. Keusch G.T., Jacewicz. The Pathogenesis of Shigella Diarrhea. VI. Toxin and Antitoxin in *Shigella flexneri* and *Shigella sonnei* Infections in Humans. The Journal of Infectious Diseases, 1977. 135: pp. 552-556
48. O'Brien A.D., Thompson M.R., Gemski P., Doctor B.P., Formal S.B. Biological Properties of Shigella flexneri 2A Toxin and its Serological Relationship to *Shigella dysenteriae* 1 Toxin. Infection and Immunity, 1977. 15: pp. 796-798
49. Lauvrak S.U., Wälchli S., Iversen T-G., Slagsvold H.H., Torgersen M.L.m Spilsberg B., Sandvig K. Shiga Toxin Regulates its Entry in a Syk-dependent Manner. Molecular Biology of the Cell, 2006. 17: pp. 1096-1109
50. Schiering J., Andreoli S.P., Zimmerhackl L.B. Treatment and Outcome of Shiga-toxin-associated Hemolytic Uremic Syndrome (HUS). Pediatric Nephrology, 2008. 23: pp. 1749-1760
51. Acheson D.W., Kane A.V., Keusch G.T. Shiga Toxin. Methods in Molecular Biology, 2000. 145: pp. 41-63
52. Lingwood C.A. Role of Verotoxin Receptors in Pathogenesis. Trends in Microbiology, 1996. 4: pp. 147-153
53. Sandvig K. Shiga Toxin. Toxicon: Official Journal of the International Society of Toxinology, 2001. 39: pp. 1629-1635
54. Sandvig K., Grimmer S., Lauvrak S.U., Torgersen M.L., Skretting G., van Deurs B., Iversen T.G. Pathways Followed by Ricin and Shiga Toxin into Cells. Histochemistry and Cell Biology, 2002. 117: pp. 131-141
55. Sandvig K., van Deurs B. Membrane Traffic Exploited by Protein Toxin. Annual Review of Cell and Development Biology, 2002. 18: pp. 1-24
56. Sandvig K.,, Olsnes S., Brown J.E., Petersen O.W., van Deurs B. Endocytosis from Coated Pits of Shiga Toxin: A Glycolipid-binding Protein from Shigella dysenteriae 1. The journal of Cell Biology, 1989. 108: pp. 1331-1343
57. Nestoridi E., Kushak R.I., Tsukurov O., Grabowski E.F., Ingelfinger J.R. Role of Renin Angiotensen System in TNF-alpha and Shiga-toxin-induced Tissue Factor Expression. Pediatric Nephrology, 2008. 23: pp. 221-231
58. Lending R.E., Buchsbaum H.W., Hyland R.N. Shigellosis Complicated by Acute Appendicitis. Southern Medical Journal, 1986. 79: pp. 1046-1047
59. Nussinovitch M., Shapiro R.P., Cohen A.H., Varsano I. Shigellosis Complicated by Perforated Appendix. The Pediatric Infectious Disease Journal, 1993. 12: pp. 352-353
60. Wang X-Y., Tao F., Xiao D., Lee H., Deen J., Gong J., Zhao Y., Zhou W., Li W., Shen B., Song Y., Ma J.,j Li Z-M., Wang Z., Su P-Y., Chang N., Xu J-H., Ouyang P-Y, von Seidlein L., Xu Z-Y., Clemens J.D. Trend and Disease Burden of Bacillary Dysentery in China (1991-2000). Bulletin of the World Health Organization, 2006. 84: pp. 561-569
61. Guerin P.J., Brasher C., Baron E., Mic D., Grimont F., Ryan M., Aavitsland P., Legros D. *Shigella dysenteriae* serotype 1 in west Africa: Intervention Strategy for an Outbreak in Sierra Leone. The Lancet, 2003. 362: pp. 705-706
62. Rahman M.M., Kabir I., Mahalanabis D., Malek M.A. Decreased Food Intake in Children with Severe Dysentery due to *Shigella dysenteriae* 1 Infection. European Journal of Clinical Nutrition, 1992. 46: pp. 833-838
63. Arazona Department of Health Services. Shigellosis Bioterrorism Agent Profiles for Health Care Workers. Revised August 2004. Retrieved December 11, 2009. Website: http://www.azdhs.gov /phs/edc/edrp/es/pdf/shi gellosisset.pdf
64. McMillan J.A., Feigin R.D., DeAngelis C., Jones M.D. Oski's Pediatrics: Principles & Practice. Fourth Edition. Philadelphia: Lippincott Williams & Wilkins. 2006. pp. 1116-1121
65. Starke J.R., Baker C.J. Neonatal Shigellosis with bowel perforation. The Pediatric Infectious Disease Journal, 1985. 4: pp. 405-407
66. Grant H.W., Hadley G.P., Wiersma R., Rollins N. Surgical Lessons Learned from the *Shigella dysenteriae* Type I Epidemic. Journal of the Royal College of Surgeons of Edinburgh, 1998. 43: pp. 160-162
67. Bennish M.L. Potentially Lethal Complications of Shigellosis. Reviews of Infectious Diseases, 1991. 13: pp. S319-S324
68. Wilson A.P.R., Ridgway G.L., Sarner M., Boulos P.B., Brook M.G., Cook G.C. Toxic Dilatation of the Colon in Shigellosis. British Medical Journal, 1990. 301: pp. 1325-1326
69. Christianson K.A. Toxic Megacolon Complicating Shigellosis. Journal of the Royal College of Surgeons of Edinburgh, 1992. 46: pp. 109-110
70. Harnadani J.D., Azad M.T., Chowdhury J.J., Kabir I. Intestinal Perforation in a Child with *Shigella dysenteriae* Type 1 Infection: A Rare Complication. Journal of Diarrhoeal Diseases Research, 1994 12: pp. 225-226
71. Struelens M.J., Patte D., Kabir I., Salam A., Samir K., Nath S.K., Butler T. Shigella Septicemia: Prevalence, Presentation, Risk Factors, and Outcome. The Journal of Infectious Diseases, 1985. 152: pp. 784-790
72. Khan W.A., Dhar U., Salam M.A., Griffiths J.K., Rand W., Bennish M.L. Central Nervous System Manifestations of Childhood Shigellosis: Prevalence, Risk Factors and Outcome. Pediatrics, 1999. 103: pp. E18
73. Bennish M.L. Potentially Lethal Complications of Shigellosis. Reviews of Infectious Diseases, 1991. 13: pp. S319-S324
74. Bhimma R., Rollins N.C., Coovadia H.M., Adhikari M. Post-dysenteric Hemolytic Uremic Syndrome in Children during an Epidemic of Shigella Dysentery in Kwazulu/Natal. Pediatric nephrology, 1997. 5: pp. 560-564
75. Fong J.S., de Chadarevian J.P., Kaplan B.S. Hemolytic-uremic Syndrome. Current Concepts and Management. Pediatric Clinics of North America, 1982. 29: pp. 835-856
76. Johnson S., Taylor M.C. What's New in Haemolytic Uraemic Syndrome? European Journal of Pediatrics, 2008. 167: pp. 965-971
77. Japanese Pediatric Nephrology Association. Pediatrics International, 1999. 41: pp. 449-451
78. Koster F., Levin J., Walker L., Tung K.S., Gilman R.H., Rahaman M.M., Majid M.A., Islam S., Williams R.C. Hemolytic-uremic Syndrome after Shigellosis: Relation to Endotoxemia and Circulating Immune Complexes. The New England Journal of Medicine, 1978. 298: pp. 927-933
79. Lopez E.L., Contrini M.M., Devoto S., DeRosa M., Graña M., Aversa L., Gomez H., Genero M., CVleary T. Incomplete Hemolytic-uremic Syndrome in Argentinean Children with Bloody Diarrhea. The Journal of Pediatrics, 1995. 127: pp. 364-367
80. Rooney J.C., Anderson R.M., Hopkins J.H. Clinical and Pathological Aspects of Central Nervous System Involvement in the Haemolytic Uraemic Syndrome. Australia Paediatric Journal, 1971. 7: pp. 28-33
81. Bale J.F. Jr., Brasher C., Siegler R.I. CNS Manifestation of the Hemolytic-uremic Syndrome. Relationship to Metabolic Alterations and Prognosis. American Journal of Diseases of Children, 1980. 134: pp. 869-872
82. Rowe P.C., Orrbine E., Wells G., McLaine P.N. The Epidemiology of Childhood Hemolytic Uremic Syndrome in Canada, 1986-1988. Journal of Pediatrics, 1991. 119: pp. 218-224
83. Sheth K.J., Swick H.M., Haworth N. Neurologic Involvement in Hemolytic-uremic Syndrome. Annals of Neurology, 1986. 19: pp. 90-93
84. Argyle J.C., Hogg R.J., Pysher T.J., Silva F.G., Siegler R.L. A Clinicopathological Study of 24 Children with Hemolytic Uremic Syndrome. Pediatric Nephrology, 1990. 4: pp. 52-58
85. Frankel G., Girón J.A., Valmassoi J., Schoolnik G.K. Multi-gene Amplification: Simultaneous Detection of Three Virulence Genes in Diarrheal Stool. Molecular Microbiology, 1989. 3: pp. 1729-1734
86. Albert M.J., Ansaruzzaman M., Alim A.R. Mitra A. K. Fluorescent Antibody Staining Test for Rapid Diagnosis of *Shigella dysenteriae* 1 Infection. Diagnostic Microbiology and Infectious Disease, 1992. 15: pp. 359-361
87. Islam D., Lindberg A.A. Detection of *Shigella dysenteriae* Type 1 and *Shigella flexneri* in Feces by Immunomagnetic Isolation and Polymerase Chain Reaction. Journal of Clinical Microbiology, 1992. 30: 2801-2806
88. Islam D., Tzipori S., Islam M., Lindberg A.A. Rapid Detection of *Shigella dysenteriae* and *Shigella flexneri* in faeces by Immunomagnetic Assay with Monoclonal Antibodies. European Journal of Clinical Microbiology and Infectious Diseases, 1993. 12: pp. 25-32
89. Kehl K.S., Havens P., Behnke C.E., Acheson D.W. Evaluation of the premier EHEC Assay for Detection of Shiga Toxin-Producing *Escherichia coli*. Journal of Clinical Microbiology, 1997. 35: pp. 2051-2054
90. Meridian Bioscience Receives FDA Clearance for New E. coli Test. Genetic Engineering & Biotechnology News. Revised: February 20, 2007. Retrieved: November 10, 2009. Website: www.genengnews .com/news/bnitemprint .aspx?name=13137091
91. Ojha S.C., Yean C.Y., Ismail A., Singh K-K. B. A Pentaplex PCR Assay for the Detection and Differentiation of Shigella Species. BioMed Research International, 2013. 2013: pp. 1-9
92. Sack B.R., Rahman M., Yunus M., Khan E.H. Antimicrobial Resistance in Organisms Causing Fiarrheal Disease. Clinical Infectious Diseases, 1997. 24: pp. S102-S105
93. Gross R.J., Threlfall E.J., Ward L.R., Rowe B. Drug Resistance in *Shigella dysenteriae*, *S. flexneri* and *S. boydii* in England and Wales: Increasing Incidence of Resistance to trimethoprim. British Medical Journal, 1984. 288: pp. 784-786
94. Pal S.C., Sengupa P.G., Sen D., Bhattacharya S.K., Deb B.C. Epidemic Shigellosis due to *Shigella dysentariae* Type 1 in South Asia. Indian Journal of Medical Research, 10989. 89: pp. 57-64
95. Sen D., Dutta P., Deb B.C., Pal S.C. Nalidixic Acid Resistant *Shigella dysenteriae* Type 1 in Eastern India. Lancet, 1988. 2: pp. 911
96. Mates A., Eyny D., Philo S., Antimicrobial Resistance Trends in Shigella Serogroups Isolated in Israel, 1990-1995. European Journal of Clinical Microbiology and Infectious Diseases, 2000. 19: 108-111
97. Dagan D., Orr N., Yavzori M., Yuhas Y., Meron D., Ashkenazi S., Cohen D. Retrospective Analysis of the First Clonal Outbreak of Nalidixic Acid-Resistant *Shigella sonnei* Shigellosis in Israel. European Journal of Clinical Microbiology & Infectious Diseases, 2002. 21: pp. 887-889
98. Bhattacharya M.K., Bhattacharya S.K., Pail M., Dutta D., Dutta P., Kole H., De D., Ghosh A.R., Das P., Nair G. Shigellosis in Calcutta during 1990-1992: Antibiotic Susceptibility Pattern and Clinical Features. Journal of Diarrhoeal Diseases Research, 1994. 12: pp. 121-124

99. Hoge C.W., Bodhidatta L., Tungtaem C., Echeverria P. Emergence of Nalidixic Acid Resistant *Shigella dysenteriae* Type 1 in Thailand: An Outbreak Associated with Consumption of a Coconut Milk Dessert. International Journal of Epidemiology, 1995. 24: pp. 1228-1232

100. Replogle M.L., Fleming D.W., Cieslak P.R. Emergence of Antimicrobial-Resistant Shigellosis in Oregon. Clinical Infectious Diseases, 1000. 30: pp. 515-519

101. Navia M.M., Gascón J., Vila J. Analysis of the Mechanism of Resistance to Several Antimicrobial Agents in *Shigella* spp. Causing Travellers' Diarrhoea. European Society of Clinical Microbiology and Infectious Diseases, 2005. 11: pp. 1035-1047

102. Fullá N., Prado V., Durán C., Lagos R., Levine M.M. Surveillance for Antimicrobial Resiatnce Profile Among *Shigella* Species Isolated from a Semirural Community in the Northern Administrative Area of Santiago, Chile. American Journal of Tropical Medicine and Hygiene, 2005. 72: pp. 851–854

103. Navia M.M., Capitano L., Ruiz J., Vargas M., Urassa H., Shellemberg D., Gascón J.M. Vila J. Typing and Characterization of Mechanisms of Resistance of *Shigella* spp. Isolated from Feces of Children Under 5 Years of Age from Ifakara, Tanzania. Journal of Clinical Microbiology, 1999. 37: pp. 3113-3117

104. Subekti D., Oyofo B.A., Tjaniadi P., Corwin A.L., Larasati W., Putri M., Simanjuntak C.H., Punjabi N.H., Taslim J., Setiawan B., Djelantik A.A.G.S., Sriwati L., Sumardiati A., Putra E., Campbell J.R., Lesmana M. *Shigella* spp. Surveillance in Indonesia: the Emergence of Reemergence of *S. dysenteriae*. Emerging Infectious Diseases, 2001. 7: pp. 137-140

105. Dutta S., Dutta D., Dutta P., Matsushita S., Bhattacharya S.K., Yoshida S. *Shigella dysenteriae* Serotype 1, Kolkata, India. Emerging Infectious Diseases, 2003. 9: pp. 1471-1474

106. Hosseini M.J., Ranjbar R., Ghasemi H., Jalalian H.R. The Prevalence and Antibiotic Resistance of *Shigella* spp. Recovered from Patients Admitted to Bouali Hospital, Tehran, Iran During 1999-2001. Pakistan Journal of Biological Sciences, 2007. 10: pp. 2778-2780

107. Farid H Abu Elamreen F.H.A., Sharif F.A., Deeb J.E. Elamreen A., Isolation and Antibiotic Susceptibility of Salmonella and Shigella Strains Isolated from Children in Gaza, Palestine from 1999 to 2006. Journal of Gastroenterology and Hepatology, 2008. 23: pp. e330-e333

108. Silva T., Nogueira P.A., Magalhães G.F., Grava A.F., da Silva L.H.P., Orlandi P.P. Characterization of *Shigella* spp. by Antimicrobial Resistance and PCR Detection of ipa Genes in an Infantile Population from Porto Velho (Western Amazon Region), Brazil. Memórias do Instituto Oswaldo Cruz, 2008. 103: pp./ 731-733

109. Dutta S., Ghosh A., Ghosh K., Dutta D., Bhattacharya S.K., Nair G.B., Yoshida S. Newly Emerged Multiple-Antibiotic-Resistant *Shigella dysenteriae* Type 1 Strains in and around Kolkata, India, are Clonal. Journal of Clinical Microbiology, 2003. 41: pp. 5833-5834

110. Naheed A., Kalluri P., Talukder K.A., Faruque A.S.G., Khatun F., Nair G.B., Mintz E.D., Breiman R.F. Fluoroquinolone-resistant *Shigella dysenteriae* type 1 in northeastern Bangladesh. The Lancet Infectious Diseases, 2004. 4: pp. 607 - 608

111. Ahmed A.M., Furuta K., Simomura K., Kasama Y., Shimamoto T. Genetic Characterization of Multidrug Resistnace in *Shigella* spp. from Japan. Journal of Medical Microbiology, 2006. 55: pp. 1685-1691

112. Srinivasa H., Baijayanti M., Raksha. Magnitude of Drug Resistant Shigellosis: a Report from Bangalore. Indian Journal of Medical Microbiology, 2009. 27: pp. 358-360

113. Zhang W., Luo Y., Li J., Lin L., Ma Y., Hu C., Jin S., Ran L., Cui S. Wide dissemination of multidrug-resistant Shigella isolates in China. The Journal of Antimicrobial Chemotherapy, 2011. 66: pp. 2527–2535

114. Stokes H.W., Hall R.M. A Novel Family of Potentially Mobile DNA Elements Encoding Site-specific Gene-integration Functions: Integrons. Molecular Microbiology, 1989. 3: pp. 1669-1683

115. Hansson K., Sundström L., Pelletier A., Roy P.H. Intl2 Integron Integrase in Tn7. The Journal of Bacteriology, 2002. 184: pp. 1712-1721

116. DeLappe N., O'Halloran F., Fanning S., Corbett-Feeney G., Cheasty T., Cormican M., Antimicrobial Resistance and Genetic Diversity of *Shigella sonnei* Isolates from Western Ireland, an Area of Low Incidence of Infection. Journal of Clinical Microbiology, 2003. 41: pp. 1919-1924

117. Hirose K., Terajima J., Izumiya H., Tamura K., Arakawa E., Takai N., Watanabe H. Antimicrobial Susceptibility of *Shigella sonnei* Isolates in Japan and Molecular Analysis of S. sonnei Isolates with Reduced Susceptibility to Fluoroquinolones. Antimicrobial Agents and Chemotherapy, 2005. 49: pp. 1203–1205

118. Ahamed J., Gangopadhyay J., Hundu M., Sinha A.K. Mechanisms of Quinolone Resistnace in Clinical Isolates of *Shigella dysenteriae*. Antimicrobial Agents and Chemotherapy, 1999. 43: pp. 2333-2334

119. Hirschhorn N., Greenough W.B. Progress in Oral Rehydration Therapy. Scientific American, 1991. 264: pp. 50-56

120. Khan A.M., Rabbani G.H., Faruque A.S.G., Fuchs G.J. WHO-ORS in Treatment of Shigellosis. Journal of Diarrhoeal Diseases Research, 1999. 17: pp. 88-89

121. Gorbach S.L., Bartlett J.G., Blacklow N.R. Infectious Diseases. Third Edition. Philidelphia: Lippincott, Williams and Wilkins. 2004. pp. 603-606

122. Kabir I., Butler T., Underwood L.E., Rahman M.M. Effects of a Protein-rich Diet During Convalescence from Shigellosis on Catch-up Growth, Serum Proteins, and Insulin-like Growth Factor-I. Pediatric Research, 1992. 32: pp. 689-692

123. Kabir I., Malek M.A., Mahalanabis D., Rahman M.M., Khatun M., Wahed M.A., Majid N. Absorption of Macrobutrients from High-Protein Diet in Children During Convalescence from Shigellosis. Journal of Pediatric Gastroenterology and Nutrition, 1994. 8: pp. 63-67

124. Roy S.K., Raqib R., Khatun W., Azim T., Chowdhury A., Fuch G.J., Sack D.A. Zinc Supplementation in the Management of Shigellosis in Malnourished Children in Bangladesh. European Journal of Clinical Nutrition, 2008. 62: pp. 849-855

125. Bennish M.L., Khan W.A., Begum M., Bridges E.A., Ahmed S., Saha D., Salam M.A., Acheson D., Ryan E.T. Low Risk of Hemolytic Uremic Syndrome after Early Effective Antimicrobial Therapy for *Shigella dysenteriae* Type 1 Infection in Bangladesh. Clinical Infectious Diseases, 2006. 42: pp. 356–362

126. Taneja N., Lyngdoh V.W., Sharma M. Haemolytic Uraemic Syndrome due to Ciprofloxacin-resistant *Shigella dysenteriae* Serotype 1. Journal of Medical Microbiology, 2005. 54: pp. 997-998

127. Gan S.I., Beck P.L. A New Look at Toxic Megacolon: an Update and Review of Incidence, Etiology, Pathogenesis, and Management. The American Journal of Gastoenterology, 2003. 98: pp. 2363-2371

128. Neschis M., Siegelman S.S., Parker J.G. The Megavolon of Ulcerative Colitis. Gastroenterology, 1968. 55: pp. 251-259

129. Future Needs and Directions for Shigella Vaccines. Weekly Epidemiological Records, 2006. 10: pp. 51-58

130. Fält I.C., Schweda E.K.H., Klee S., Singh M., Floderus E., Timmis K.N., Lindberg A.A. Expression of *Shigella dysenteriae* Serotype 1 O-antigenic Polysaccharide by Shigella flexneri aroD Vaccine Canditates and Different *S. flexneri* Serotypes. Journal of Bacteriology, 1995. 177: pp. 5310-5315

131. Ashkenazi S., Cohen D. An update on vaccines against Shigella. Therapeutic Advances in Vaccines, 2013. 1: pp. 113-123

132. Coster T.S., Hoge C.W., VanDeVerg L.L., Hartman A.B., Oaks E.V., Venkatesan M.M.,

Cohen D., Robin G., Fontaine-Thompson A., Sansonetti P.J., Hale T.L. Vaccination against Shigellosis with Attenuated *Shigella flexneri* 2a Strain SC602. Infection and Immunity, 1999. 67: pp. 3437–3443

133. Launay O., Sadorge C., Jolly N., Poirier B., Béchet S., van der Vliet D., Seffer V., Fenner N., Dowling K., Giemza R., Johnson J., Ndiaye A., Vray M., Sansonetti P., Morand P., Poyart C., Lewis D., Gougeon M.L. Safety and Immunogenicity of SC599, an Oral Live Attenuated *Shigella dysenteriae* type-1 Vaccine in Healthy Volunteers: Results of a Phase 2, Randomized, Double-blind Placebo-controlled Trial. Vaccine, 2009. 18: pp. 1184-1191

134. Hartman A.B., Venkatesan M.M. Construction of a Stable Attenuated *Shigella sonnei* ΔvirG Vaccine Strain, WRSS1, and Protective Efficacy and Immunogenicity in the Guinea Pig Keratoconjunctivitis Model. Infection and Immunity, 1998. 66: pp. 4572-4576

135. Kotloff K.L., Noriega F., Losonsky G.A., Sztein M.B., Wasserman S.S., Nataro J.P., Levine M.M. Safety, Immunogenicity, and Transmissibility in Humans of CVD 1203, A Live Oral *Shigella flexneri* 2a Vaccine Candidate Attenuated by Deletions in aroA and virG. Infection and Immunity, 1996. 64: pp. 4542–4548

136. Dearlove C.E., Forrest B.D., van den Bosch L., La Brooy J.T. The Antibody Response to an Oral Ty21a-Based Typhoid-Cholera Hybrid Is Unaffected by Prior Oral Vaccination with Ty21a. The Journal of Infectious Diseases, 1992. 165: pp. 182-183

137. Siegenthaler W. Differential Diagnosis in Internal Medicine. Stuttagrt: Thieme. 2007. pp. 148

Photo Bibliography

Figure 2.9-1: *Shigella* spp. belongs to the family Enterobacteriaceae and cannot be distinguished from *Escherichia coli* through the contemporary criteria of DNA relatedness. This scanning electron micrograph (SEM) was taken by Janice Haney Carr in 2006 and released by the CDC. Public domain photo

Figure 2.9-3: *Shigella* spp. infection diagram. The human anatomical illustration was created by Dr. Alexander J. da Silva and Melanie Moser in 2003. The illustration is released by the CDC. Public domain graphics

Figure 2.9-5: A 3D structure rendering of shiga toxin. The A subunit is shown in organge and B subunit is shown in blue. This graphic is produced by Fraser M.E., Fujinaga M., Cherney M.M., Melton-Celsa A.R., Twiddy E.M., O'Brien A.D., James M.N.G. and released via Structure of Shiga Toxin Type 2 (Stx2) from *Escherichia coli* O157:H7. The Journal of Biological Chemistry, 2004. 79: pp. 27511–27517. Public domain graphic

Yersinia pestis, is a non-fastidious and highly infective microbe, responsible for three deadly pandemics in recorded history. The first pandemic, known as the Justinian Plague, lasted from 542 to 767 AD. Historical records indicate that the disease swept through Asia Minor, Africa and Europe and then arrived in Constantinople, the capital of the Eastern Roman Empire (Byzantine Empire). It has been estimated that approximately 300,000 people died in the city of Constantinople alone, with the total deaths estimated at forty to one hundred million.[1, 2, 3] The second pandemic is known infamously as the Black Death (also known as the Bubonic Plague), which reached the height of its infection between 1347 to 1351. It is believed that the plague spread from central Asia, where it was responsible for an estimated 25 million deaths, before extending to Asia Minor, Asia and eventually to Europe where an additional 25 million people succumbed to the disease (Figure 2.10-1).[2]

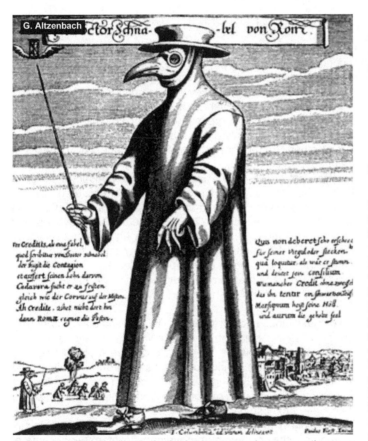

Figure 2.10-1: Believing that toxic air, also known as miasmas, was the cause of the plague, the doctors and the wealthy, wore costumes, for protection. The costume shown above is quite common in Venice and Florence. Note that the "beak" of the mask is generally filled with perfumed herbs and flowers in an attempt to counter the miasmas

The third pandemic began in the 1850s and lasted until 1959. Historical documentation indicates that this plague began in Yünnan Province then spread throughout China, reaching the port cities of Canton (Guangzhou) and Hong Kong by 1894. From these ports, the disease spread to India, Indochina, Egypt, Madagascar and Tunisia, and by 1899, the plague had extended its reach to the United States (e.g. Hawaii, San Francisco, New Orleans, New York etc.), as well as, South America.[2, 3, 4] It is estimated that during the first 30 years of the third pandemic, approximately 30 million people were affected, resulting in more than 12 million deaths.[1]

In nature, *Y. pestis* is a zoonotic infection of rodents and their fleas. The flea acquires *Y. pestis* from their host, an infected rodent, after a blood meal. Initially, the microbe multiplies in the flea's mid-gut, before extending into the oesophaghus and proventriculus. Eventually, the flea will reach a 'block stage', where it cannot feed without first regurgitating the newly divided bacteria onto the new host. Naturally occurring infection in humans are generally the result of incidental infections through flea bites and from handling or ingesting contaminated animal tissue (Figure 2.10-2).[1]

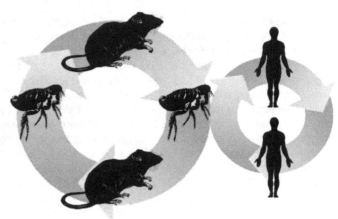

Figure 2.10-2: Sylvatic cycle of *Y. Pestis*

Being such an infamous and highly infectious agent, it is not surprising that military leaders throughout history have attempted to use this pathogen as a biological weapon. For example, in 1346, during the battle of Caffa, present day Feodossia, the bodies of Tartar soldiers, having succumbed to the plague, were catapulted over the city walls, spreading the disease to the city's Christian population. It is postulated by numerous historians that this action resulted in the spread of the bubonic plague throughout Europe, when infected Genoese merchants escaped the besieged city and became unwitting carriers of the disease.[5, 6] This same tactic was used again in 1422 during the battle of Carolstein, located in modern day Czech Republic. After an unsuccessful siege, Lithuanian soldiers catapulted the plague infected bodies, plus an additional 2000 cartloads of excrement, into the enemy ranks resulting in a great number of fatalities.[7] In 1936, Britain established a committee to examine issues regarding offensive and defensive biological warfare. By 1940, a biological warfare laboratory was established at Porton Down where numerous offensive biowarfare weapons, including the plague were examined. Similarly, the British Common Wealth Nation of Canada also initiated biological warfare research in 1939. Under the leadership of Sir Frederick Banting, Cannaught Laboratories was established at Ile Grosse and Suffield, Quebec where numerous offensive biological agents were developed, including the plague.[8, 9]

In 1933, the Japanese biological warfare research Unit 731, in Manchuria was experimenting and conducting live trials with the *Y. pestis*, as well as, many other biological agents. The Japanese used the human flea, *Pulex irritans*, as a stratagem to simultaneously protect the bacteria, while effectively spreading the microbe among the population. The fleas were capable of regurgitating ~24,000 organisms in a single feeding thereby making it an effective delivery system. Additionally, the fleas are extremely resilient and can withstand air drag; they naturally target humans and can also infect rat populations within the targeted area for an extended epidemic. Between the years of 1940 to 1941, porcelain bombs filled with plague infected fleas were developed and used on the Chinese populations with mixed results. It has been estimated that these biological attacks resulted in approximately 10,000 civilian casualties, as well as, 1700 deaths among Japanese occupation forces.[3, 10, 11] During this time, Japan's Axis ally, Germany, concentrated their efforts in developing an impressive chemical warfare program, but much less attention was placed on biological warfare. Nonetheless, most biological warfare efforts in Germany were aimed at weaponizing numerous deadly agents, including the plague (Figure 2.10-3).[8, 9]

In response to the apparent biological attacks on China by the Japanese forces, the United States began aggressively exploring the potential use of biological agents. Initially the U.S. biological warfare program was located at Edgewood Arsenal, Aberdeen, Maryland but by April 1943, a new facility was established at Camp Detrick (later renamed Fort Detrick), Maryland. The U.S. efforts in biological agents continued after World War II and by 1964, the American biological warfare program had researched and produced numerous offensive biological weapons, including the plague.[9, 12] However, the U.S. effort in developing a plague weapon was met with difficulties. The American bioweaponeers found that Y. pestis lost virulence too rapidly (sometimes within 30 minutes) and eventually lost interest in developing it as a biological weapon. The Soviets, however, were not so quick to dismiss the plague, and continued their research until they eventually solved the problem. The Soviet military labelled the plague as L1 and maintained 20 tons of this agent within their military arsenal until the collapse of the communist state in December, 1991.[10]

Y. pestis is a non-motile, non-sporulating, non-lactose fermenting, bipolar, microaerophilic, oxidase-negative, urease-negative, Gram-negative, facultative anaerobic and facultative intracellular coccobacillus. This bacterium measures 0.5 to 0.8 x 1.5 to 2.0 μm and is biochemically unreactive. These organisms belong to the family Enterobacteriaceae (genus XI) and are the causative agent of bubonic, pneumonic and septicemic plague (Figure 2.10-3).[1, 3, 4] Due to the potential of widespread person to person transmission, illness and death, the Center for Disease Control and Prevention (CDC) has classified Y. pestis as a biosafety level 4 and Category A biological warefare agent.

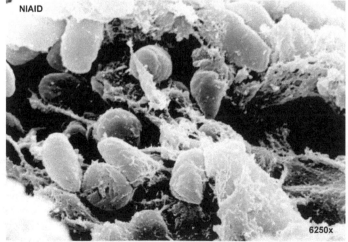

NIAID

6250x

Figure 2.10-3: Scanning electron micrograph (SEM) demonstraing a mass of *Yersinia pestis* bacteria in the foregut of the flea

Y. pestis possesses a typical cell wall, with a whole-cell lipid composition and an entero-bacterial antigen, similar to that of other enteric bacteria. Its lipopolysaccharides lacks extended O-group side chains, although it is characterized as rough, because it processes a core component. Y. pestis does not possess a true capsule, but when cultured above 33° C, this organism develops a carbohydrate-protein envelope, called capsular antigen or fraction 1 (F1).[13, 14] There are three biovars of Y. pestis, defined by their conversion of nitrate to nitrite and fermentation of glycerol. Biovar antiqua is positive for both characteristics; biovar orientalis forms only nitrite and is negative for fermentation of glycerol, while biovar mediaevalis ferments glycerol but does not form nitrite. All three biovars display no difference in virulence or pathology in humans or in animals.[13, 14]

Y. pestis expresses several virulence factors, enabling them to survive in rodents, fleas and humans. These virulence factors are encoded on the bacterial chromosome, as well as, located on three plasmids: pPCP1 (9.5 kb), pCD1 (70-75 kb) and pMT1, also known as pFra plasmid (100-110 kb).

CHROMOSOME ENCODED FACTORS

Y. pestis chromosomally encoded virulence factors include lipopolysaccharide endotoxin (LPS), AraC-type regulator YbtA, hemin storage locus products and the pH 6 antigen (also known as Psa). LPS is the major cell wall component of Y. pestis. The lipid A moiety of LPS, which is responsible for host immune system activation, is composed of a glucosamine-disaccharide back-bone carrying acyl chains and phosphate groups. Unlike many other Gram-negative bacteria, the lipid A of Y. pestis is heterogeneous (e.g. hexa-acylated to triacylated types) when the bacteria are grown at 27°C but shifts to the hypoacylated types (e.g. tetra- and triacylated types) when they are cultured at 37°C. Heterogeneous lipid A (Hexa-acylated type) is able to effectively activate Toll-like receptor 4 (TLR4), while the hypoacylated lipid A (tetra-acylated type) is a poor activator and serves instead as an antagonist in human hosts. The ability for Y. pestis to shift between heterogeneous and hypoacylated types enables the bacteria to evade the human innate immune response, thereby avoid elimination.[15, 16]

Like most other microorganisms, Y. pestis requires iron (Fe) as an essential element in a variety of informational cellular and metabolic pathways. Y. pestis produces a product termed yersiniabactin (Ybt), a siderophore-based iron acquisition and transport system. The genetic information required for the synthesis and utilization of Ybt are found within the region of the bacterial chromosome called psn loci located within the 35-45 kb Yersinia high-pathogenicity island (HPI) of the pgm locus. The pgm locus encodes numerous genetic information, some of which include irp1-irp2-ybtU-ybtT-ybtE, the ybtP-ybtQ-ybtX-ybtS, and of course, the psn loci that encode the yersiniabactin (Ybt). Additionally, within the pgm locus a gene called ybtA encodes a product called AraC-type regulator YbtA which is responsible for upregulating the expression of the yersiniabactin biosynthesis operon irp21 ybtUTE, the ybtPQXS operon and the psn gene. In contrast, the Ferric Uptake Regulator gene (Fur), which codes for Fur regulator, is responsible for the down-regulation of Ybt receptor and biosynthetic genes. Furthermore, the pgm locus also includes the haemin storage operon (hmsHFRS), which produces products that are essential for the production of a biofilm in the flea gut which induces the 'block stage'.[1, 17, 18, 19]

Reports have indicated that irp1 and irp2 loci encode two iron repressible high-molecular mass proteins designated HMWP1 (348 kDa) and HMWP2 (228 kDa). YbtU is believed to code for a product (YbtU) that has similar functions as NADPH-dependent reductase while *YbtT* is presumably coding a thioesterase-like enzyme (YbtT). *YbtS* transcribes a product (YbtS) that is presumably involved in the catalytic conversion of chorismate into salicylic acid and the product of *YbtE* is a salicylate-activating enzyme (YbtE). It is postulated that the HMWP 1 and 2, in conjunction with YbtU, YbtE, YbtS and possibly YbtT are required to synthesize the Ybt siderophore. The product of *ybtX* is a hydrophobic cytoplasmic membrane protein that does not appear to contribute any vital function to Ybt biosynthesis, while the products of *ybtP* and *ybtQ* are believed to be structurally unique subfamily of traffic ATPase/ABC transporter. Experiments have shown that cells with mutations in *ybtP* or *ybtQ* are still able to produce Ybt but were impaired in their ability to grow at 37ºC under iron-deficient conditions.[17, 20, 21]

The *psa* operon of *Y. pestis* encodes an adhesin containing surface fimbriae called pH 6 antigens. Previously thought to play a role in cell-to-cell transmission of the microbe within mammalian host, the pH 6 antigen is now believed to function as attachment sites for plasma apolipoprotein B (apoB)-containing lipoproteins (LDL). The attachment of apoB-LDL virtually eliminated any interactions between pH 6 antigens with macrophages. It is postulated that this interaction with apoB-LDL camouflages the bacteria and prevents recognition of the pathogen by host defense systems.[22, 23, 24]

pPCP1 PLASMID

pPCP1 plasmid encodes three protein products: plasminogen activator (Pla), bacteriocin pesticin (Pst) and pesticin immunity protein (Pim). The products of the pPCP1 plasmid are associated with the invasive characteristics of the plague (Figure 2.10-4).[4, 14, 25]

The structure of the Pla is comprised of a β-barrel fold with 10 membrane-spanning β strands, five surface loops and a barrel surface that binds to LPS. The biological activity of the Pla is influenced by the surface loops around the active site groove and by temperature-dependent shifts between heterogeneous to the hypoacylated LPS modifications.[1, 26, 27, 28, 29]

Pla is a bacterial surface protease that is capable of cleaving the C3 protein of the compliment system, thereby interfering with the activation of the compliment system and reducing chemo-attractants at the site of infection. Additionally, Pla possesses a temperature-dependent (regulated) coagulase and fibrinolytic activities. Coagulase activity is most evident at temperatures below 30ºC, but fibrinolytic activity increases with higher temperatures (< 30ºC). Coagulase facilitates the formation of a

bolus of blood, which permits for the bacteria to aggregate in the flea midgut. This bolus/aggregate of bacteria blocks the flea's proventriculus (a valve-like structure that connects the fleas' midgut to the esophagus) and leads to the regurgitation of up to 24,000 organisms while the flea is feeding. The fibrinolytic activity of the Pla is believed to enhance the invasiveness of *Y. pestis* by causing damage to host tissue barriers.[1, 23, 26, 27, 28, 29, 30, 31, 32] For example, Pla activity results in the proteolytic activation of plasminogen into plasmin resulting in fibrinolysis of fibrin clots as well as cleaving non-collagenous proteins of the mammalian basement membrane and extra-cellular matrix (e.g. laminin and fibronectin), thereby enhancing bacterial adherence. Additionally, plasmin also activates latent pro-collagenases, which may cause damage to the host tissue barrier, enhancing the invasiveness of the coccobacilli. These temperature-regulated coagulase and fibrinolytic activities may be a response to the nature of the vector, which is ectothermic versus the hosts which are endothermic.[23, 29 31, 32] Pla also inactivates alpha-2-antiplasmin, plasminogen activator inhibitor 1 (PAI-1) and inhibits the actions of thrombin-activatable fibrinolysis inhibitor (TAFI). These inhibitory actions of the Pla enhance uncontrollable fibrinolysis, which is believed to improve *Y. pestis* dissemination and survival within the mammalian host. However, Pla is also known to deactivate tissue factor (TF) pathway inhibitor, a counterintuitive action which causes an increase in fibrin formation and clotting. Therefore, the complex interactions between *Y. pestis* and the hemostatic system of the host require further elucidation.[29]

The pPCP1 plasmid is also responsible for encoding Pst, which is designed to defend their niche against other closely related species, such as *Y. pseudotuberculosis* 01, *Y. enterocolitica* biotype 1B, and various strains of *E. coli*.[33, 34, 35] Pst uses the FyuA receptor (responsible for the transport of the yersiniae iron chelator yersiniabactin) on targeted cells, thereby allowing for its transport through the bacterial outer membrane.[35, 36, 37] Once it gains access to the target cell, the Pst is believed to have two possible modes of action. First, it has been reported that Pst exhibits *N*-acetylglucos-aminidase activity and is believed to use murein-lipoprotein as a substrate where it catalyzes the hydrolysis of β-1, bond between *N*-acetylglucosamine and *N*-acetyl-muramic acid in the glycan backbone.[4, 35, 38] Second, Pst degrades murein after glycan cleavage at the C_1 position of the *N*-acetyl-murmuramic acid, producing muraminitol. Through either method described, the result is the conversion of sensitive cells into spheroplasts, where the cell wall of the targeted cell is almost completely removed, an action similar to that of antibacterial agents, such as penicillin.[37] While eliminating the competition though the synthesis and secretion of Pst, *Y. pestis* is protected from the agent via the immunity factor Pim. Pim is found in the periplasmic space anchored to the cytoplasmic

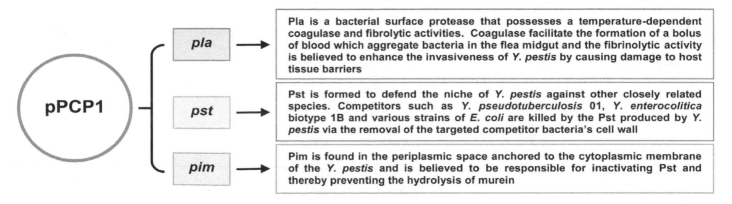

Figure 2.10-4: pPCP1 plasmid and its coded protein products and their functions

membrane of the *Y. pestis* by its N-terminal hydrophobic end and may be responsible for inactivating Pst, thereby preventing the hydrolysis of murein (Figure 2.10-5).[35, 39]

pCD1 PLASMID

The low-calcium response stimulon (*lcr*) plasmid, also known as pCD1, encodes a complex virulence property which includes regulatory genes that control the expression of secreted virulence surface proteins and a dedicated multiprotein secretory system, known as Type III secretion system (TTSS). It has been stated that *lcr* is necessary for virulence in all three biovars of *Y. pestis* and contains a set of regulatory genes and 12 identified coordinately regulated virulence genes. [4, 40, 41, 42]

The loci for which its functions have been classified include *lcrE*, which encodes a product called LcrE or YopN. LcrE functions in the down-regulation by calcium ions (Ca^{2+}), while *lcrF* is responsible for encoding a trans-actin factor (LcrF) that mediates the response to temperature (coordination of thermal induction of virulence determinants).[43, 44] *lcrG* is the first gene in the operon, encoding a protein called LcrG, which has been reported to suppress the secretion of YopN before host cell contact.[42, 45] The virulence gene *lcrV*, produces products that include a secreted protein called the V-antigen and 11 surface proteins called *Yersinia* outer proteins (Yops), which plays an important role in the virulence of the microbe. For example, some Yops function as effector proteins that directly attack the host cell, while others perform regulatory functions. [40, 41, 42, 47, 48] *lcrH* encodes LcrH, a protein that is used during the down-regulation of transcription in response to both calcium ions and nucleotides at 37° C. This loci has been found to negatively regulate V antigen and the operon encoding Yops.[46] *lcrK* encodes a protein called LcrK and is directly involved in the export process of Yops, and lcrR (protein product LcrR) has similar functions to LcrE, which is down-regulated by

calcium (Ca^{2+}) ions (Figure 2.10-5).[49, 50]

The V-antigen is a protective antigen that has been historically associated with resistance to phagocytosis and is believed to be essential for the survival of *Y. pestis* intracellularly within macrophages. V-antigen inhibits cytokine production through the Toll-like receptor 2 (TLR2) pathway, stimulating the production of interleukin-10 (IL-10) by macrophages. Being a potent anti-inflammatory cytokine, IL-10 acts to reduce the production of interferon-gamma (IFN-γ) and tumor necrosis factor-alpha (TNF-α). [49, 50, 51, 52, 53] Also involved in immunosuppression, Yop J has been shown to disrupt host cell signaling pathways involved in the production of proinflammatory cytokines, as well as, inducing macrophage apoptosis.[54]

Other products of the *lcrV* include various proteins that are involved in TTSS, a complex protein export pathway used to secrete effector proteins (e.g. V antigen) to counteract the immunodefenses after the pathogen has penetrated host tissues.[55, 56] Two proteins: YopB and YopD, are involved in the formation of a channel that is inserted through the eukaryotic plasma membrane. It has been reported that YopB and YopD have hydrophobic domains where they may act as transmembrane channel proteins, forming a small pore (diameter 6 to 23 Å), rather than causing membrane lysis. This channel is believed to be in continuous connection with an injectisome that exists within the bacteria. In this manner, effector Yops efficiently target the host cytosol without spilling into the extracellular environment.[55, 56, 57, 58, 59, 60] Additionally, it is believed that YopN (a product of *lcrE*) is responsible for sensing the interaction between the pathogen and the host eukaryotic cell and is the triggering mechanism that mediates the opening of the secretion channel.[61, 62]

It has been reported that the intimate contact between *Y. pestis* and the host result in increased expression of Yop proteins,

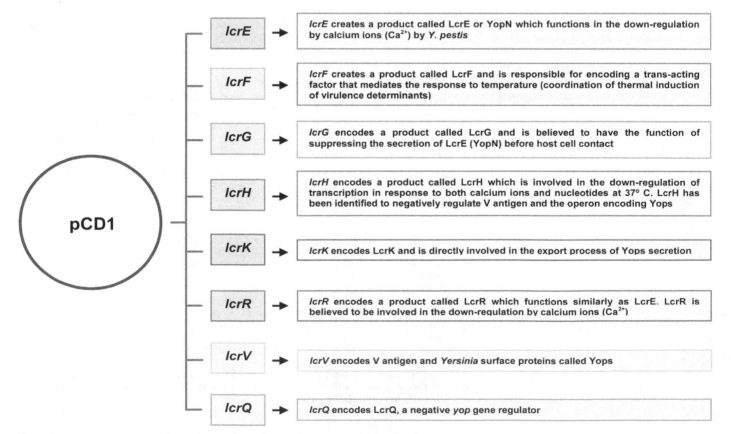

Figure 2.10-5: pCD1 plasmid and its products and their functions

suggesting intercellular communication, thereby linking Yop secretion and regulation. A hypothesis has been put forth that this contact-dependent regulation of Yop involves the concentration of LcrQ (product of *lcrQ*), a negative *Yop* gene regulator. In the model proposed, once the transmembrane channel is opened (via YopN), LcrQ is rapidly secreted from the pathogen and into the cytosol of the host. The reduction of the concentration of LcrQ within the bacterium also reduces the level of repression on the *Yop* genes resulting in increased Yop expression.[62, 63]

YopH is one of the many effector proteins secreted into the host cell and is a highly active tyrosine phosphatase (PTP). It has been reported that this effector protein's catalytic activities antagonizes several signaling pathways associated with phagocytosis. For example, the binding of integrin to the extracellular matrix proteins (i.e. invasin protein of *Y. pestis*) induces the focal adhesion structures where cellular actin cytoskeletons are connected to integrin via a protein complex containing a variety of molecules, including focal adhesion kinase (FAK), Src, Crk-associated substrate (p130Cas), α-actinin, vinculin, paxillin, and talin. YopH dephos-phorylates p130Cas, paxillin and FAK, thereby disrupting the focal adhesion structure and prohibiting phagocytosis, as well as, other associated activities such as oxidative bursts in macrophages and neutrophils.[56, 62, 64] Moreover, YopH also dephosphorolates other protein complexes associated with phagocytosis, such as the scaffolding protein SKAP-HOM, Fyb, Fyn-binding protein and Fak-homolog Pyk.[65, 66, 67]

YopE, YopT and YopO are effector proteins that target Rho (s) GTPases. It is known that Rho GTPases (e.g. RhoA, Rec-1 and Cdc42 etc.), which are small GTP-binding proteins, regulate a variety of cellular functions, such as the dynamic regulation of the actin cytoskeleton, as well as, gene expression.[68] When

bounded to GTP, Rho-GTPases adopt a conformation that allows interactions with 'down-stream' effectors and activation of their biological functions. However, if the GTP is hydrolyzed, presenting GDP bounded Rho-GTPases, the complex is rendered inactive (Figure 2.10-6).

YopE exhibits GTPase-activating/accelerating protein (GAP) activity toward RhoA, Rac-1 and Cdc42 by inserting an argenine-containing sequence into the GTPase catalytic site, by promoting GTP hydrolysis and the deactivation of Rho-GTPase. This activity reduces binding to the "down-stream" components of the signaling cascade and causes a disruption on the actin cytoskeleton where it counteracts phagocytosis and may eventually cause rounding and detachment of cells in culture, a phenomenon known as cytotoxicity.[56, 68] In addition to the anti-phagocytic activity, YopE also functions to counteract against proinflammatory cytokine production. For example, YopE was found to inhibit caspace-1 mediated maturation of prointerleukin-1β in macrophages through the deactivation of Rac-1, a Rho-GTPase.[56, 69]

The effector protein YopT has similar function as YopE, as it disrupts cytoskeletal structures, causing cell rounding and inhibition of phagocytosis. YopT acts as a cysteine protease to remove the lipid modification from RhoA, Rac or Cdc42. This cleavage releases the GTPase from the membrane and thereby inactivates this structure.[55, 70] YopO (also known as YpkA), on the other hand, is an effector protein with multiple functional domains. At the N-terminal portion of YopO, a serine/threonine kinase catalytic domain exists, activated by actin and acts as a cofactor. Once activated, this kinase undergoes autophosphorylation, and it phosphorylates actin and other artificial basic substrates. In addition, the N-terminal portion also allows YopO to interact with

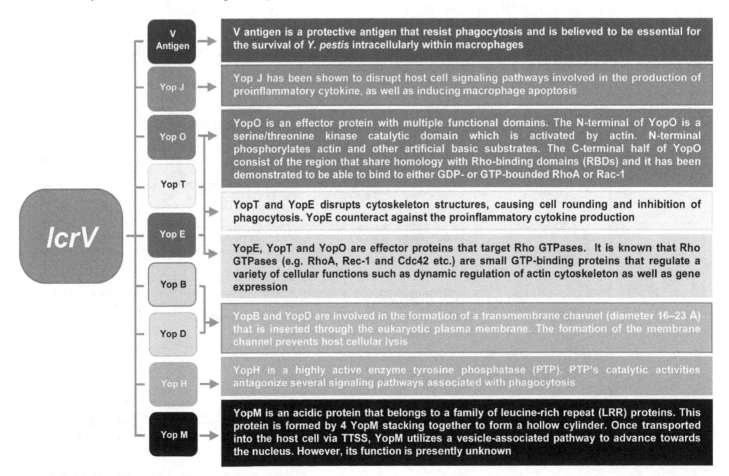

Figure 2.10-6: *IcrV* and its protein products and their function

eukaryotic cellular membranes. The C-terminal portion of YopO consists of the region with a share homology to Rho-binding domains (RBDs) and it has been demonstrated to be able to bind to either GDP- or GTP-bounded RhoA or Rac-1. YopO has the capability to disrupt actin cytoskeletons and cause cellular retraction and rounding in cultured cells.[56, 62, 71]

YopJ is a cysteine protease that functions to block the activation of mitogen-activated protein kinase (MAPK), a type of serine/threonine-specific protein kinase that responds to mitogens (extracellular stimuli) and regulates activities such as gene expression, mitosis, differentiation, proliferation, as well as, cell survival/apoptosis. In addition, YopJ is also responsible for blocking the actions of IκB Kinase (IKK), an enzyme complex that is part of the upstream NF-κB signal transduction cascade. It is believed that these inhibitory actions result in the suppression of cytokine production and trigger apoptosis of macrophage, although the exact manner by which YopJ causes apoptosis is presently unknown.[56, 72, 73, 74]

Out of all the effectors secreted by Y. pestis, YopM is the only one that is not an enzyme. YopM is an acidic protein that is 409 amino acids long, containing 15 leucine-rich repeats and belonging to a family of leucine-rich repeat (LRR) proteins. This protein has a horseshoe-like shape, formed by 4 YopMs stacking together to form a hollow cylinder with an inner diameter of 35Å. Once transported into the host cell via TTSS, YopM utilizes a vesicle-associated pathway to advance towards the nucleus, however the exact function of YopM in the eukaryotic nucleus is unknown.[75, 76] One study has shown that YopM regulates genes involved in the cell cycle and cell growth in macrophages, while another study provides contradictory evidence.[77, 78] An additional study has shown that YopM functions as an adaptor protein by forming a complex with ribosomal protein S6 kinase 1 (RSK1) and protein kinase C-like 2 (PRK2), which activates both enzymes. However, the exact cellular function that this complex performs remains to be elucidated.[79] Kerchen et al. (2004), demonstrated that YopM was required to induce a systemic depletion of natural killer (NK) cells. The depletion of NK cells causes a decrease of proinflammatory cytokines such as IL-12, IL-18 and IFN-γ. Nonetheless, the exact mechanism by which YopM causes the depletion of NK cells, and subsequently the reduction of

cytokines, is presently unknown.[80] In a 2006 study, Heusipp et al., demonstrated that α 1-antitrypsin (AAT), a glycoprotein that inhibits neutrophil elastase, interacts with at least eight LRR on YopM. However, with or without interacting with YopM, ATT efficiently inhibits elastase. Again, the exact function of YopM interacting with ATT remains to be elucidated (Figure 2.10-6).[81]

pMT1 PLASMID

pMT1 (also known as pFra, a 100 to 110 kb plasmid) encodes a 17 kDa polypeptide capsular antigen, fraction 1 (F1), and a multifunctional murine exotoxin (Ymt).[41] The F1 antigen is encoded by capsular antigen fraction 1 (caf1) genes produced by Y. pestis growing at 30° C or greater (~37° C). Synthesized as a monomer, the F1 antigen forms a large homopolymer (>200 kDa) on the cell surface of the bacteria in a stacked ring structure composed of hepamers.[23, 82] The F1 antigens have been shown to be homologous to interleukin-1β (IL-1β) and it has been suggested to interact with IL-1 receptors.[83] This capsular F1 antigen forms a large gel-like envelope, which is readily soluble and dissociates from the bacterium during in vitro cultivation and is involved in resisting phagocytosis in the absence of opsonizing antibodies, as well as, preventing adhesion to the epithelial cells thereby avoiding internalization.[1, 84, 85, 86, 87, 88, 89] The F1 antigen is highly immunogenic and has been shown to indirectly elicit a protective immunoresponse in humans.[90] In addition to caf1, the associated genes caf1M, caf1A and caf1R have also been cloned and sequenced. caf1M protein product has been found to share homology with PapD, a chaperone protein that is required for pilus assembly in Escherichia coli. It has been proposed that caf1M acts as a chaperone for F1, with a role in post-translational folding and secretion of the antigen.[91] The caf1A protein product is an outer membrane protein that has been reported to share homology with PapC, involved in the assembly and anchoring of the E.coli pilus and is believed to have similar function in Y. pestis.[92] caf1R protein products are positive activators that share homology with the AraC family of bacterial protein activators.[93]

Ymt, also known as phospholipase D (PLD), is a member of a newly described family of PLD enzymes found in all domains of life. Ymt is a β-adrenergic receptor antagonist and is responsible for blocking adrenaline-induced mobilization of glucose and fatty

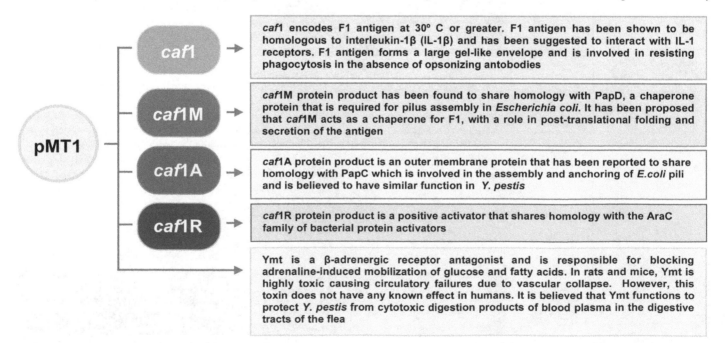

Figure 2.10-7: Protein products and function of pMT1 plasmid

acids. In rats and mice, Ymt is highly toxic causing circulatory failures, due to vascular collapse. However, this toxin does not appear to have any known effect in humans.[94, 95] It is believed that Ymt functions to protect the coccobacilli from the cytotoxic digestion products of blood plasma in the digestive tracts of the flea (Figure 2.10-7).[96]

SYMPTOMS

Y. pestis infection results in three main clinical manifestations: bubonic, pneumonic and septicemic plague. Additionally, two rare and unusual manifestations, meningeal and pharyngeal plague, may also occur. Bubonic plague generally affects individuals who have been bitten by a rodent flea that is carrying the plague bacterium or by handling infected animals. Pneumonic plague is generally a manifestation of the advanced bubonic form. However, once infected, this individual could perpetuate human-to-human spread of the disease through their respiratiry droplets without the involvement of insect or animal vectors. Septicemic plague is the manifested form of bubonic or pneumonic plague. This deadly condition occurs when the bacteria multiply in the blood, causing bacteremia and severe sepsis. Meningeal plague, is rare, and is the result of late complications from bubonic plague, while pharyngeal plague is a rare condition that is generally contracted via exposure to respiratory droplets or from ingestion of contaminated meats (Figure 2.10-8).[1]

Bubonic Plague

The typical incubation period for the bubonic plague is two to eight days and the disease generally begins with the sudden onset of headaches (~20 to 85% of cases), fever (38 to 40° C or 100.4 to 104° F), severe malaise (~75% of cases), chills (~40% of cases), altered mentations (~26 to 38% of cases), cough (~25% of cases), abdominal pains (18% of cases), chest pains (~13% of cases), myalgias, arthralgias and/or a general feeling of weakness. In addition, signs of prostrations, nausea and vomiting (~25 to 49% of cases) may follow within hours of the initial symptoms. Within 24 hours after the initial display of symptoms, the patients will observe tenderness and pain in one or more of the lymph nodes proximal to the site of the initial inoculation (flea bites or open wounds etc.), which will indicate the development of the bubo (es).[1, 3, 4, 97, 98] The development of bubo(es), which occurs in ~90% of cases, often appears at the femoral and inguinal lymph nodes (Figure 2.10-9), followed by axillary (Figures 2.10-10) and the cervical lymph nodes (Figure 2.10-11).[99, 100]

Within 24 hours, the enlarging bubo(es) will become progressively more swollen, tender and extremely painful. It has been reported that the pain is so intense that nearly comatose patients will attempt to shield themselves from trauma by abducting their extremities to decrease pressure.[1, 3, 4, 98] The tissue surrounding the bubo(es) will generally become edematous, while the overlaying skin may become warm, tense, and erythematous, as well as, desquamate. At this time, the patient will display signs of toxemia with the usual absence of cellulitis or of obvious ascending lymphangitis. Without effective anti-biotic treatment, bubonic plague may progress to an increasingly toxic state of fever, bladder distention, lethargy, tachycardia and hypotension.[100]

Leukocytosis often, occurs with a leukocyte count between 12 and 25 thousand/μL (could reach as high as 50 thousand/μL) with a predominance of immature polymorphonuclear leukocytes. Subsequently, patients will display signs of apathy, agitation,

confusion, fright, oliguria, anuria and eventually progress into convulsion and delirium.[1, 3, 4] Secondary septicemia will develop within 2 to 6 days after the onset of the previous symptoms. In a study by Butler *et al.*, (1976) the blood culture of *Y. pestis* colony count ranged from <10 to 4×10^7/ml (Figure 2.10-12).[100]

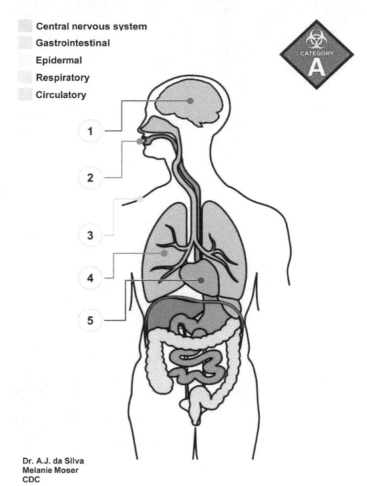

- ▨ Central nervous system
- ▨ Gastrointestinal
- ▨ Epidermal
- ▨ Respiratory
- ▨ Circulatory

Dr. A.J. da Silva
Melanie Moser
CDC

Figure 2.10-8: *Y. pestis* infection diagram. ① Complications from bubonic form that spread into the meninges causes the meningeal plague. ② Pharyngeal plague is spread via ingesting respiratory droplets or tainted food. ③ Bubonic plague is spread via an infected flea bite or handling contaminated animal. ④ Pneumonic plague is spread via infected droplets through the respiratory tract. ⑤ Septicemic plague is a manifestation from either bubonic or pneumonic form. *Y. pestis that* multiplied in the blood steams causing sepsis

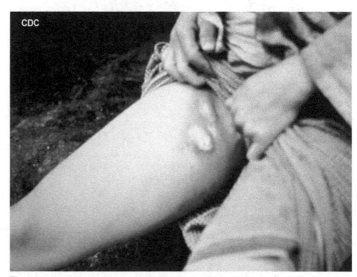

Figure 2.10-9: Photograph of a plague patient displaying inguinal buboes

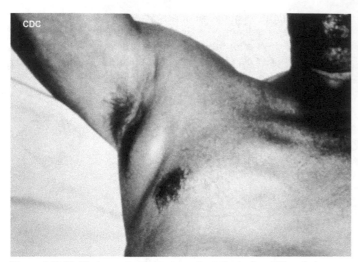

Figure 2.10-10: Photograph of a plague patient displaying axillary buboes

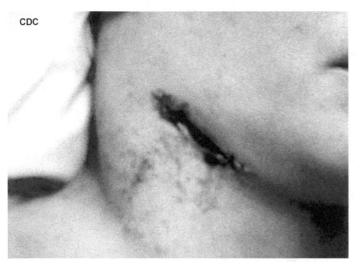

Figure 2.10-11: Photograph of a plague patient displaying cervical buboes

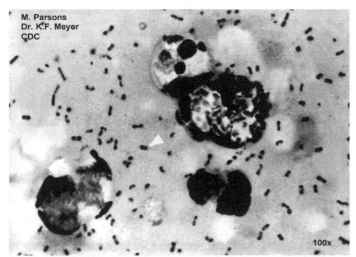

Figure 2.10-12: Bipolar staining of a plague smear prepared from lymph aspirated from a bubo of plague patient shown numerous *Y. pestis* bacteria (arrow) surrounding immature polymorphonuclear leukocytes

Approximately 5 to 15% of patients suffering from bubonic plague will develop secondary pneumonic plague, creating the potential for airborne transmission of the disease.[1, 3, 4, 89] Additional late stage pathology may include disseminated intravascular coagulopathy, as well as, multi-organ failure. Case fatalities for untreated bubonic plague are estimated at ~40 to 60% and generally result from septic shock (Table 1).[4, 101, 102]

Table 1: An overview of the clinical symptoms of bubonic plague. Note: Disseminated intravascular coagulopathy (DIC)

Symptoms	+	++	+++
Headaches			▪
Fever			▪
Prostrations			▪
Severe malaise			▪
Chills			▪
Nausea			▪
Vomiting			▪
Tender lymph nodes			▪
Painful lymph nodes			▪
Bubo (es) development			▪
Toxemia			▪
Bladder distention			▪
Lethargy			▪
Tachycardia			▪
Hypotension			▪
Leukocytosis			▪
Apathy			▪
Agitation			▪
Confusion			▪
Fright			▪
Oliguria			▪
Anuria			▪
Convulsion			▪
Delirium			▪
DIC			▪
Multi-organ failure			▪
Septic shock			▪
Altered mentations		▪	
Cough		▪	
Abdominal pains		▪	
Chest pains		▪	
Myalgias		▪	
Arthralgias		▪	
General weakness		▪	

+ Rare ++ Common +++ Frequent

Pneumonic Plague

Primary pneumonic plague is mainly the result of inhalation of aerosolized *Y. pestis*. The incubation of primary pneumonic plague is one to seven days, with the onset of symptoms being generally abrupt and may initially appear as a febrile flu-like illness. Initial symptoms include fever, chills, rigor, severe headaches, body pains, malaise, weakness, nausea, dizziness, discomfort in the chest and dyspnoea accompanied by increased respiratory and heart rates. These initial symptoms (~20 to 24 hours after the initial onset) are quickly followed by cough, which is dry at first, but becomes increasingly productive. Sputum may at first appear to be watery or mucoid and contain very little trace of *Y. pestis* coccobacilli. If left untreated, in a short period of time the sputum will become blood tinged or bloody, containing copious amounts of bacteria. During this time, patients will experience increasing chest pains with respiratory distress, prostration, tachypnea and dyspnea. These conditions are often accompanied by hemoptysis, cardio-pulmonary insufficiency, cyanosis and circulatory collapse (Table 2).[1, 3, 4, 103, 104, 105]

Radiographs of patients may initially indicate localized pulmonary involvement, with rapidly developing segmental consolidation before bronchoipneumonia finally spreads to other pulmonary segments and lobes of the same or opposite lung (Figure 2.10-13). Signs of liquification necrosis and cavitation may develop at the site of consolidation, which could result in significant residual scarring.[1, 3, 4, 106] Secondary pneumonic plague initially manifests as interstitial pneumonitis. During the progression of this condition sputum production is scant, and what little is produced is likely to be inspissated and tenacious in character when compared with sputum observed in primary pneumonic plague.[1, 3, 4] If left untreated pneumonic plague results in an almost 100% fatality.[1, 3, 4] Fatalities generally result from respiratory failure or sequelae of severe sepsis, including circulatory collapse, coagulopathy and hemorrhage (Table 2).[107]

Table 2: An overview of the clinical symptoms of pneumonic plague

Symptoms	+	++	+++
Fever			▪
Chills			▪
Rigor			▪
Severe headaches			▪
Body pains			▪
Malaise			▪
Weakness			▪
Nausea			▪
Dizziness			▪
Chest discomfort/pain			▪
Dyspnoea			▪
Increased respiration			▪
Increases heart rate			▪
Cough			▪
Respiratory distress			▪
Prostration			▪
Tachypnea			▪
Hemoptysis			▪
Cardiac insufficiency			▪
Pulmonary insufficiency			▪
Cyanosis			▪
Bronchoipneumonia			▪
Liquified necrosis (lungs)			▪
Cavitation of lung			▪
Interstitial pneumonitis			▪
Respiratory failure			▪
Severe sepsis			▪
Circulatory collapse			▪
Coagulopathy			▪
Hemorrhage			▪

+ Rare ++ Common +++ Frequent

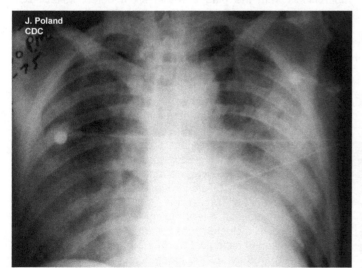

Figure 2.10-13: An anteroposterior x-ray reveals a bilaterally progressive pneumonic plague infection involving both lung fields

Septicemic Plague

Overwhelming endotoxemia, absence of local and apparent lymphadenitis, as well as, progressive dissemination of *Y. pestis* infection are the characteristics of primary septicemic plague. Initial symptoms of sepsis are fever, chills, nausea, vomiting, abdominal pains and initial constipation followed by diarrhea.[1, 3, 4, 100, 108, 109, 110] Systemic inflammatory response syndrome (SIRS), a condition related to sepsis, defined as an inflammatory state affecting the entire body, may progress rapidly. Petechiae and ecchymoses are manifestations of disseminated intravascular coagulation (DIC) (also known as consumptive coagulopathy), which is the pathological activation of clotting mechanisms causing small dispersed clots to form. This condition will progress to thrombi in microvasculatures of the acral parts of the body, such as tips of ears and phalanges, resulting in gangrene of infected tissues (Figure 2.10-14). Furthermore, refractory hypotension, acute renal failure, obtundation, shock and acute respiratory distress syndrome (ARDS) will also occur and are generally associated with pre-terminal events (Table 3).[1, 3]

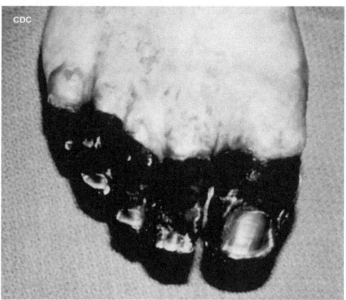

Figure 2.10-14: A photograph of a patient suffering from seticemic plague demonstrating gangrene of the right foot causing necrosis of the digits

Table 3: An overview of the clinical symptoms of septicemic plague

Symptoms	+	++	+++
Fever			▪
Chills			▪
Nausea			▪
Vomiting			▪
Abdominal pains			▪
Constipation			▪
Diarrhea			▪
SIRS			▪
Petechiae			▪
Ecchymoses			▪
DIC			▪
Gangrene of the ears			▪
Gangrene of phalanges			▪
Refractory hypotension			▪
Acute renal failure			▪
Obtundation			▪
Shock			▪
ARDS			▪

+ Rare ++ Common +++ Frequent

Meningeal Plague

Meningeal plague is a rare and unusual form of *Y. pestis* infection, and in most cases is the result of late complications from bubonic plague. Meningeal plague generally appears ~9 to

14 days after the onset of the initial infection. It is speculated that axillary or cervical bubo(es) may predispose the patient to meningitis since there are direct lymphatic connections to the meninges.[100] This form of the plague presents itself as a typical bacterial meningitis, although its onset may be delayed as the result of insufficient antibiotic treatment.[3, 111] Typical symptoms are high fever, malaise, stiff neck, headaches, diaphoresis, altered mental state, meningismus and polymorphonuclear leukocyte pleocytosis. Other symptoms that appear during the course of this infection are nausea, vomiting, abdominal pains, photophobia, confusion, and sleepiness.[1, 111, 112]

Pharyngeal Plague

Pharyngeal plague is also a rare condition, generally contracted through respiratory droplet exposure or from the ingestion of contaminated meats. In its early stages this infection may be clinically indistinguishable from other forms of pharyngitis, resembling tonsillitis. Initial symptoms include fever, sore throat and cervical lymphadenitis.[99] Cervical or submandibular bubo(es) will appear after the initial symptoms. Pharyngeal plague may develop into secondary pneumonic plague.[1, 3, 113]

DETECTION

Primary confirmation of the plague requires laboratory analysis, with *Y. pestis* being isolated from body fluids and/or tissue samples (e.g. blood, bubo aspirate, sputum, cerebral spinal fluid in patients suffering from meningeal plague and scrapings from skin lesions).[4] In patients with lymphadenopathy (buboes), aspirates should be taken by inserting a 20-guage needle attached to a 10 mL syringe containing 1mL of sterile saline. The clinician should inject the sterile saline into the bubo and withdraw the plunger several times until the solution withdrawn is tinged with blood. Bubo aspiration may also be done to decompress buboes, thereby relieving pain and discomfort. Once the aspirate is retrieved, several drops should be place on a slide, allowed to air-dry and then be stained. Various stains such as Gram stains, Wright-Giemsa stain, Wayson's stain and direct anti-F1 *Y. pestis* capsular antigen antibodies, with subsequent immunofluorescent stains, may be use for positive identification of the coccobacilli. Subsequent microscopic examination of the coccobacilli will show the characteristic "safety pin" (bipolar) appearance of the bacteria.[3, 4, 113, 114, 115]

Recently, a rapid, highly sensitive and effective test for the rapid identification of *Y. pestis* was developed by the Pasteur Institute in Madagascar. The F1-dipstick employs mono-clonal capture antibodies against F1 antigen from human or rodent samples; however, it cannot be used to identify *Y. pestis* in environmental or flea materials because the F1 capsule was produced at 37°C. F1-dipstick holds several advantages over the traditional microscopic identification method. First, this test does not require a skilled technologist or a microscope in a BSL-4 laboratory condition. Additionally, this test will provide accurate results rapidly (within 15 minutes) and not depend upon the judgment of an individual, no matter how skilled they may be.[116] A second, more sensitive method has been developed to rapidly and accurately identify *Y. pestis* under field conditions. Reported by Simon *et al.* (2013), this new test utilizes the monoclonal antibodies developed against plasminogen activator (PLA), a key virulence factor encoded by a *Y. pestis*-specific pPla plasmid. Unlike the F1-dipstick, this new one-step PLA-enzyme immunoassay (PLA-EIA) is capable of detecting *Y. pestis* in both human and rodent samples, as well as, environmental and flea materials under field conditions since the PLA-specific monoclonal antibodies was synthesized at both 20°C and 37°C.

This PLA-EIA (also known as the PLA-dipstick), coupled with the F1-dipstick will provide accurate results to confirm human plague diagnosis.[117]

Blood, bubo aspirate, sputum and cerebral spinal fluid (in patients suffering from meningeal plague) can be cultured on most routine laboratory media (e.g. blood agar, McConkey agar, trypticase soy broth or standard supplemented peptone broth) for the identification of the coccobacilli. Within 48 hours, small 1 to 3mm "hammered-metal" colonies will grow. Under the microscope, these colonies appear opaque and smooth with irregular edges.[3, 110, 113, 118]

Enzyme-linked immunosorbent assay (ELISA) is also available for detecting and measuring F1 antigens, antibodies (IgM and IgG) to the F1 capsule in the serum. This assay has been reported to detect F1 antigen levels as low as 0.4 ng/mL in sera samples.[1, 3, 118, 119] Polymerase chain reaction (PCR) tests using primers for the plasminogen activator (*pla* region of the pesticin plasmid) are available and can detect as few as 10 *Y. pestis* organisms. This test is presently used for the identification of *Y. pestis* in fleas, but has the potential to be adapted to aid in the diagnosis of human plague infection.[3, 120] Serological diagnoses are often used retro-spectively to confirm cases of the plague. Passive hemagglutination assays can be used to measure antibodies to the F1 capsule. Paired serum samples from either acute and/or convalescent phases or convalescent and post-convalescent samples can be used to provide presumptive evidence of plague infection. The fourfold rise or fall in titer of paired serum samples is considered a positive test for *Y. pestis*. Single serum sample can also be used to make a presumptive confirmation. For example, single serum sample with titer greater than 10 in a person not previously infected or vaccinated against the plague demonstrates a presumptive positive.[4, 121]

Two novel experimental detection methodologies have been developed to detect *Y. pestis*. The first is the matrix-assisted laser desorption /ionization time-of-flight mass spectrometry (MALDI-TOF), developed to accurately identify discriminate harmless environmental *Yersinia* species from the food-borne pathogens, such as *Yersinia enterocolitica* and *Yersinia pseudo-tuberculosis* from the plague within six minutes. MALDI-TOF was designed to identify and differentiate 39 different *Yersinia* strains representing 12 different *Yersinia* species, including 13 *Y. pestis* isolates representative of the Antiqua, Medievalis and Orientalis biotypes. Ayyadurai *et al.* (2010) reported that this new detection method circumvents the limitations of current phenotypic and PCR-based identification methods by eliminating errors associated with subjective assessments, saving valuable time needed for treatment and the need for expensive laboratory, equipment and materials.[122] The second novel technique is the PCR/electrospray ionization-mass spectrometry (PCR/ESI-MS) used to reveal the DNA signatures characteristic of *Y. pestis*, as well as other biological warfare agents. In this technique, the bacterial and viral agents are grouped along with their closely related near-neighbor organisms that may be completely harmless into biological threat clusters or biocluster for short. Detection of each bioclusters was validated by analysis of a wide-ranging collection of biological warfare organisms and their near neighbors prepared by spiking together biological threat nucleic acids into nucleic acids extracted from filtered environmental air. Sampath *et al.* (2012) reported that this biological threat assay was able to detect all the target organism clusters and did not misidentify any of the near-neighbor organisms as threats.[123]

A planar array immunosensor with a charge-coupled device (CCD) as a detector has been reported to be effective in simultaneously detecting 3 toxic analytes: ricin, staphylococcal enterotoxin B (SEB) and *Yersinia pestis*. Antibodies against these analytes are attached to the bottoms of the circular wells to form the sensing surface, while rectangular wells containing chicken immunoglobulin were used as alignment markers and to generate control signals. Once the optical adhesive is removed, the slides were mounted over a CCD operating at ambient temperature and a two-dimensional graded index of refraction lens array was used to focus the sensing surface onto the CCD. Once the solutions of toxins were placed on the slide, Cy5-labeled antibodies were introduced. Subsequently, by using quantitative image analysis, the identity and amount of toxin bound at each location on the slide were determined. It has been reported that amounts as low as 25 ng/mL of ricin, 15 ng/mL of *pestis* F1 antigen, and 5 ng/mL of SEB could be detected.[124]

TREATMENT

Within the last 50 years, the fatality rate in United States has been ~15% for plague sufferers. These fatalities are generally due to delays in seeking therapy, misdiagnosis and/or incorrect treatment. It is essential to rapidly diagnose the disease and to administer immediate treatment with antibiotics. If left untreated, bubonic plague has a 50% fatality rate, while both pneumonic and septicemic plagues are fatal in nearly all cases. [125]

Streptomycin has been the antibiotic of choice for the treatment of the plague since 1948. However, due to the vestibular toxicity and the risk of hypersensitivity reaction from personnel handling the medication, streptomycin is now rarely available and is infrequently used. In the United States, antibiotics such as gentamicin have since replaced streptomycin for the treatment. Nonetheless, in certain areas of the world streptomycin is still used regularly. Tetracycline and doxycycline (a member of the tetracycline family), as well as, chloramphenicol are considered to be effective alternatives.[111] Doxycycline is favored over tetracycline by clinicians due to its ease of administration, rapid absorption rate and its superior ability to achieve and maintain high concentrations after oral administration. Chloramphenicol is generally used when tissue penetration is essential. Such

Table 4a – Medication dosage, side effects for various treatment for the plague

Medication	Mechanism of Action	Side Effects	Dosage
Streptomycin	Inhibits protein synthesis	Fever, swelling, rash, hives, difficulty breathing, tightness in the chest, swellings (mouth, face, lips, or tongue), decreased urination, dizziness, headache, hearing loss, hives, lightheadedness, loss of balance, muscle weakness, nausea, numbness, tingling, tinnitus, skin rash, vaginal irritation, vaginal discharge and vomiting	Adult: 2g per day intramuscularly divided into 2 doses of 1 g per day for ~10 days Child: 30 mg/kg of body weight intramuscularly in 2 divided dose per day for ~10 days
Gentamicin	Inhibits protein synthesis	Shortness of breath, increased thirst, loss of appetite, closing of the throat, hives, swellings (lips, face, or tongue), rash, fainting, lack of urine, decreased hearing, ringing in the ears, dizziness, clumsiness, unsteadiness, numbness, skin tingling, muscle twitching, seizures, diarrhea, abdominal cramps, nausea, vomiting, rash	Adult: 3-5 mg/kg of body weight divided into 3 doses/day either intramuscularly or intravenously for ~10 days Child: 6-7.5 mg/kg of body weight divided into 3 times daily either intramuscularly or intravenously for ~10 days
Tetracycline	Inhibits protein synthesis	Lingua villosa, inflammation of tongue, swellings (mouth, face, lips, or tongue), difficulty swallowing, difficulty breathing, blurred vision, diarrhea, fever, headache, hives, hoarseness, indigestion, joint pain, loss of appetite, sores in the mouth, nausea, rash, sensitivity to sunlight, sore throat, stomach pain, swelling and itching of the rectum, rash, hives, itching, tightness in the chest, fever, chills, itching, nausea, vaginal irritation or discharge, vomiting	Adult: 2-4 g per day divided in 4 doses orally for ~10 days Child: 25-50 mg/kg of body weight per day divided into 4 doses orally for ~10 days
Doxycycline	Inhibits protein synthesis	Nausea, diarrhea, bloody stools, severe stomach cramps, indigestion, heartburn, vomiting, photosensitivity, loss of appetite, dysphagia, headaches, blurred vision, rash, joint pain, fever, feeling tired	Adult: Oral administration of 100-200 mg 2-4 times daily for ~10 days Child: 1 mg/kg of body weight on day 1 divided in two does per day. The remaining days of treatment use 0.5 mg/kg of body weight divided in two doses for ~10 days
Chloramphenicol	Inhibits protein synthesis	Diarrhea, headache, nausea, vomiting, fever, fatigue, sore throat, unusual bleeding or bruising, abdominal pain, bloating, vision changes, eye pain, rash, itching, swelling, dizziness, trouble breathing and tingling of the hands or feet	Intravenous administration of initial loading dose of 25 mg/kg of body weight followed by 4 g per day in 4 1g doses for ~10 days
Trimethoprim / sulfamethoxazole	Inhibit successive steps in the folate synthesis pathway in bacteria	Appetite loss, nausea, vomiting, rash, hives, itching, difficulty breathing, shortness of breath, severe or persistent cough, swellings (mouth, face, lips, or tongue), skin irritation (blistering, peeling, red, or swollen skin), bloody stools, severe diarrhea, nausea, vomiting, chest pain, chills, fever, sore throat, decreased urination, depression, hallucinations, joint or muscle pain, seizures, headache, vaginal irritation or discharge	4 mg/kg of body weight orally or intravenously every 12 hours
Ciprofloxacin (Cipro)	Inhibits the function of DNA gyrase	Nausea, diarrhea, liver function tests abnormal, vomiting, and rash, headache, abdominal pain/discomfort, foot pain, pain in extremities, injection site reaction	Oral administration of 40 mg/kg of body weight twice daily

conditions include, but not limited to, meningeal plague, pleuritis, endophthalmitis and myo-carditis. Chloramphenicol can be used independently or in conjunction with amino-glycosides such as gentamicin.[1, 126] Laboratory animal studies with ciprofloxin have shown promise, but no testing of its effectiveness in humans has been performed. Trimethoprim-sulfamethoxazole (TMP-SMZ) has been shown to be effective to treat bubonic plague but is not considered to be a first choice medication. Penicillins, cephalosporins and macrolides have had poor efficacy and should not be used to treat any form of the plague.[1, 127, 128]

Antibody treatment should be continued for at least 3 days after the patient has become afebrile and/or made a clinical recovery.[1] Please examine Tables 4a and 4b for more information regarding antimicrobial treatment for the plague.

The first plague vaccine, a heat-killed whole cell vaccine, was developed in 1897 and has been shown to protect against the bubonic form of the disease, although experimental evidence of this vaccine against other forms of the plague is limited and highly reactogenic.[129, 130, 131] A live attenuated vaccine, EV76 has also

Table 5: Differential diagnosis of Bubonic Plague (BP – in black), as well as, its secondary manifestations, meningeal (in purple) and pharyngeal plague (in yellow), with selected disease with similar symptoms. These diseases are streptococcal or staphylococcal adenitis (adenitis), Tularemia, Mycobacterial infection (Myco), Syphilis, *L. venereum* (LV) and Q fever

Symptoms	BP	Adenitis	Tularemia	Myco	LV	Q-fever	Syphilis
Fever	■		■		■		■
Chills	■		■		■		
Rigor	■		■				
Severe headaches	■		■	■		■	■
Lymphoadenopathy	■	■	■	■	■	■	■
Buboes	■				■		
Body pains	■		■	■		■	■
Malaise	■	■	■	■		■	■
Weakness	■		■			■	■
Nausea	■	■	■	■	■	■	
Dizziness	■						
Chest discomfort/pain	■	■		■		■	
Increased respiration	■		■				
Increases heart rate	■						
Cough	■		■	■		■	
Respiratory distress	■	■					
Pulmonary insufficiency	■	■	■				
Respiratory failure	■						
Cyanosis	■						
Bronchoipneumonia	■	■					
Liquified necrosis (lungs)	■						
Cavitation of lung	■	■					
Interstitial pneumonitis	■						
Prostration	■						
Tachypnea	■						
Dyspnea	■		■	■			
Hemoptysis	■		■	■			
Cardiac insufficiency	■						
Severe sepsis	■						
Circulatory collapse	■						
Coagulopathy	■						
Hemorrhage	■						
High fever	■	■	■	■	■	■	■
Malaise	■	■	■	■	■	■	■
Stiff neck	■						■
Headaches	■		■	■		■	■
Diaphoresis	■					■	
Nausea	■	■	■	■			
Vomiting	■	■	■	■			
Abdominal pains	■				■		
Altered mental state	■						■
Meningismus	■		■			■	
Leukocyte pleocytosis	■						
Photophobia	■						
Confusion	■					■	■
Sleepiness	■		■				
Fever	■	■	■	■	■		
Pharyngitis	■	■				■	■
Sore throat	■	■				■	■
Cervical lymphadenitis	■	■	■	■	■		

■ Bubonic Plague
■ Meningeal Plague
■ Pharyngeal plague

been developed and tested, but human trials have demonstrated severe reactions to the vaccines. It has been reported that live attenuated vaccines (1 mL) injected subcutaneously in human trials demonstrated marked systemic reactions including fever, malaise, aching and anorexia, while the vaccination sensitized less than 50% of the trial group towards the plague. Due to the severe side effects and lack of effectiveness, the trial was discontinued. During an outbreak of the plague in Dakar, Senegal, an intensive study of a live attenuated vaccine (EV strain from Madagascar) was undertaken by the French health authorities. Approximately 200,000 people were vaccinated but the results were less than desirable. Among the vaccinated, severe systemic and localizing reactions occurred; however, the fatality rate in these individuals was approximately 66%, compared to the 85% fatality rate of unvaccinated individuals.[129] The only plague vaccine available (previously licensed between 1946 to 1998), is USP, which is made from a formalin-killed Y. pestis (Indian isolate 195/P) and was developed by the United States military in the 1940's.[129, 132, 133] Primary side effects of this vaccine occuring in approximately 10% of the recipients include malaise, headache, fever, mild lymphadenopathy and erythema and induration at the site of injection. It is recommended that only individuals at high risk for plague should be immunized, such as military personnel and other field personnel working in plague endemic areas. The scheduled dose for adults is 1.0 ml initially with 0.2 mL between 1 to 3 months followed by a booster dose (0.2 mL) 5-6 months later. Additional booster doses should be given every six months for 1.5 years and subsequent inoculations should be given one to two years afterwards.[3, 130, 134]

Evidence that this plague vaccine is effective came indirectly, based on the number of confirmed plague cases in the United States military personnel during World War II (WWII) and Vietnam. In all of the vaccinated individuals there were no cases reported for WWII and only three observed cases in Vietnam.[129, 134] Nonetheless, the plague vaccine is ineffective toward aerosolized Y. pestis in animal studies.[10, 133]

There is no licensed vaccine available for the plague, however research and trials are ongoing. One of the current vaccines under study is a recombinant subunit vaccine for F1 and V antigens. It has been reported that individually the F1 and V antigens are immunogenic and protect against live organism challenges in animal trials.[50, 135] For example, vaccination with recombinant F1 protected mice against aerosolized Y. pestis, while similar protection can be obtained by transferring F1-specific monoclonal antibody. However, virulent F1-negative Y. pestis strains exists, therefore a vaccine based solely on the F1 antigen may fail to protect against all forms of plague (e.g. weaponized pneumonic plague).[136, 137, 138]

Similarly, a vaccine based solely on the V antigen protected mice from subcutaneous Y. pestis challenges, as well as, the transfer of anti-V- antigen specific antibodies. In addition, this type of vaccination protected mice against aerosolized Y. pestis challenges with both F1-positive and F1-negative strains. Nonetheless, a vaccine based solely on the V-antigen may fail to protect against weaponized pneumonic plague, since pathogenic Yersinia species may express V-antigen variants that do not fall under the protective immunity.[139, 140, 141] In combination, the two virulence factors have been reported to provide a high level of protection with virulent plague in animal models.[131, 135, 142, 143, 144]

DIFFERENTIAL DIAGNOSIS

Differential diagnosis of the plague should include *streptococcal* or *staphylococcal adenitis* (*Staphylococcal aureus*, *Staphylococcal pyogenes*), Tularemia, cat scratch disease (*Bartonella*

Table 6: Differential diagnosis of Pneumonic Plague with selected disease with similar symptoms. These diseases are *streptococcal* or *staphylococcal adenitis* (adenitis), Tularemia, Mycobacterial infection (Myco), Syphilis, *Lymphogranuloma venereum* (LV) and Q fever

Symptoms	BP	Adenitis	Tularemia	Myco	LV	Q-fever	Syphilis
Fever & chills	■	■	■				■
Rigor	■		■				
Severe headaches	■		■	■		■	■
Body pains	■		■	■	■	■	■
Malaise	■	■	■	■		■	
Weakness	■		■	■		■	
Nausea	■	■	■	■	■	■	
Dizziness	■						
Chest discomfort/pain	■		■	■		■	
Dyspnoea	■		■	■			
Increased respiration & heart rate	■						
Cough	■		■	■		■	
Respiratory distress	■						
Prostration	■						
Tachypnea	■						
Dyspnea	■		■	■			
Hemoptysis	■		■	■			
Cardiac insufficiency	■		■				
Pulmonary insufficiency	■						
Cyanosis	■						
Bronchoipneumonia	■		■				
Liquified necrosis (lungs)	■						
Cavitation of lung	■	■					
Interstitial pneumonitis	■						
Respiratory failure	■						
Severe sepsis	■						
Circulatory collapse	■						
Coagulopathy	■						
Hemorrhage	■						

Table 7: Differential diagnosis of Septicemic Plague with selected disease with similar symptoms. These diseases are streptococcal or staphylococcal adenitis (adenitis), Tularemia, Mycobacterial infection (Myco), Syphilis, *Lymphogranuloma venereum* (LV) and Q fever

Symptoms	BP	Adenitis	Tularemia	Myco	LV	Q-fever	Syphilis
Fever	■	■	■	■	■	■	■
Chills	■		■		■	■	
Nausea	■	■	■	■	■	■	
Vomiting	■	■	■	■	■	■	
Abdominal pains	■	■		■	■		
Constipation	■						
Diarrhea	■	■	■	■			
SIRS	■						
Petechiae	■						
Ecchymoses	■						
DIC	■						
Gangrene of the ears	■						
Gangrene of the phalanges	■						
Refractory hypotension	■						
Acute renal failure	■						
Obtundation	■						
Shock	■						
ARDS	■						

henselae), Mycobacterial infection (Myco: including scrofula, *Mycobacterium tuberculosis*), primary genital herpes, primary or secondary syphilis, *Lymphogranuloma venereum* (LV) and Q fever.[1, 145] Please examine Tables 5, 6 and 7 for more information.

References

1. Guerrant R.L., Walker D.H., Weller P.F. Tropical Infectious Diseases – Principles, Pathogens & Practice. Volume 1. Philadelphia: Churchill Livingstone Elsevier. 2006. pp. 471-481
2. Kohn G.C. Encyclopedia of Plague and Pestilence. New York: Facts on File Inc. 1995. pp. 25-27; 255-256; 260-261
3. McGovern T.W., Friedlander A.M. Plague. Medical Aspects of Biological Warfare. Chapter 23. Washington D.C.: The Surgeon General United States Army Medical Department Medical Center and School Borden Institute. 2007. pp. 479-502
4. Perry R.D., Fetherston J.D. *Yersinia pestis* – Etiologic Agent of Plague. Clinical Microbiology Reviews, 1997. 10: pp. 35-66
5. Ziegler P. The Black Death. New York: The John Day Company, 1969. pp 15
6. Derbes V.J., De Mussis and the Great Plague of 1348: a Forgotten Episode of Bacteriological War. Journal of the American Medical Association, 1996. 196: pp. 59-62
7. Derbes V.J. De Mussis and the Great Plague of 1348. The Journal of the American Medical Association, 1966. 196: pp. 59-62
8. Robertson A.G., Robertson L.J. From Asps to Allegations: Biological Warfare in History. Military Medicine, 1995. 160: pp. 369-372
9. Smart J.K. History of Chemical and Biological Warfare: An American Perspective. Medical Aspects of Biological Warfare. Chapter 2. Washington D.C.: The Surgeon General United States Army Medical Department Medical Center and School Borden Institute. 2007. pp. 9-86
10. Alibek K. Biohazard. New York: Dell Publishing. 1999. pp. 36-37; 166-167; 286
11. Eitzen E.M., Takafuji E.T. Historical Overview of Biological Warfare. Medical Aspects of Biological Warfare. Chapter 18. Washington D.C.: The Surgeon General United States Army Medical Department Medical Center and School Borden Institute. 2007. pp. 415-423
12. Franz D.R., Parrott C.D., Takafuji E.T. The U.S. Biological Warfare and Biological Defense Programs. Medical Aspects of Chemical and Biological Warfare. Chapter 19. Washington D.D.: Office of the Surgeon General Department of the Army, United States of America. 1997. pp. 425-436
13. Brubaker R.R. The Genus *Yersinia*: Biochemistry and Genetics of Virulence. Current Topics in Microbiology and Immunology, 1977. 57: pp. 111-158
14. Sodeinde O.A., Goguen J.D. Genetic Analysis of the 9.5-kilobase Virulence Plasmid of *Yersinia pestis*. Infection and Immunity, 1988. 56: 2743-2748
15. Matsuura M., Takahashi H., Watanabe H., Saito S., Kawahara K. Immunomodulatory Effects of *Yersinia pestis* Lipopolysaccharides on Human Macrophages. Clinical and Vaccine Immunology, 2010. 17: pp. 49-50
16. Matsuura M. Structural modifications of bacterial lipopolysaccharide that facilitate Gram-negative bacteria evasion of host innate immunity. Frontiers in Immunology, 2013. 4: pp. 109
17. Fetherston J.D.,Bertolino V.J., Perry R.D.YbtP and YbtQ: two ABC transporters required for iron uptake in Yersinia pestis. Molecular Microbiology, 1999. 32: pp. 289-299
18. Miethke M., Marahiel M.A. Siderophore-Based Iron Acquisition and Pathogen Control. Microbiology and Molecular Biology Reviews, 2007. 71: pp. 413-451
19. Bach S., de Almeida A., Carniel E. The Yersinia high-pathogenicity island is present in different members of the family Enterobacteriaceae. Federation of European Microbiological Societies (FEMS) Microbiology Letters, 2000. 183: pp. 289-294
20. Miller D.A., Luo L., Hillson N., Keating T.A., Walsh C.T. Yersiniabactin Synthetase: A Four-Protein Assembly Line Producing the Nonribosomal Peptide/Polyketide Hybrid Siderophore of *Yersinia pestis*. Chemistry and Biology, 2002. 9: pp. 333-344
21. Sebbane F., Jarrett C., Gardner D., Long D., Hinnebusch B.J. Role of the Yersinia pestis Yersiniabactin Iron Acquisition System in the Incidence of Flea-Borne Plague. Public Library of Science (PLoS) One, 2010. 5: pp. e14379
22. Huang X-Z., Lindler L.E. The pH 6 Antigen Is an Antiphagocytic Factor Produced by *Yersinia pestis* Independent of *Yersinia* Outer Proteins and Capsule Antigen. Infection and Immunity, 2004. 72: pp. 7212–7219
23. Williamson E.D., Oyston P.C.F. Protecting against plague: towards a next-generation vaccine. Clinical and Experimental Immunology, 2013. 172: pp. 1-8
24. Bao R., Nair M.K., Tang W.K., Esser L., Sadhukhan A., Holland R.L., Xia D., Schifferli

D.M. Structural basis for the specific recognition of dual receptors by the homopolymeric pH 6 antigen (Psa) fimbriae of Yersinia pestis. Proceedings of the National Academy of Sciences of the United States of America, 2013. 110: pp. 1065-1070
25. Straley S.C., Brubaker R.R. Lacalization in *Yersinia pestis* of Peptides Associated with Virulence. Infection and Immunity, 1982. 57: pp. 1517-1523
26. Perry R.D., Fetherston J.D. *Yersinia pestis* – Etiologic Agent of Plague. Clinical Microbiology Reviews, 1997. 10: pp. 35-66
27. Sodeinde O.A., Goguen J.D. Genetic Analysis of the 9.5-kilobase Virulence Plasmid of *Yersinia pestis*. Infection and Immunity, 1988. 56: pp. 2743-2748
28. Filippov A.A., Solodovnikov N.S., Kookleva I.M., Protsenko O.A. Plasmid Content in *Yersinia pestis* Strains of Different Origins. Federation of European Microbiological Societies (FEMS) Microbiology Letters, 1990. 67: pp. 45-48
29. Korhonen T.K., Haiko J., Laakkonen L., Järvinen H.M., Westerlund-Wikström B.Fibrinolytic and coagulative activities of *Yersinia pestis*. Frontiers in Cellular and Infection Microbiology, 2013. 3: pp. 35
30. McDonough K.A., Falkow S. A *Yersinia pestis*-specific DNA Fragment Encodes Temperature-dependent Coagulase and Fibrinolysin-associated Phenotype. Molecular Microbiology, 1989. 3: pp. 767-775
31. Lähteenmäki K., Virkola R., Sarém A., Emödy L., Korhonen T.K. Expression of Plasminogen Activator Pla of *Yersinia pestis* Enhances Bacterial Attachment to the Mammalian Extracellular Matrix. Infection and Immunity, 1998. 66: pp. 5755-5762
32. Sodeinde O.A., Subrahmanyam Y.B.V., Stark K., Quan T., Bao Y., Goguen J.D. A Surface Protease and the Invasive Character of Plague. Science, 1992. 258: pp. 1004-1007
33. Hu P.C., Yang G.C.H., Brubaker R.R. Specificity Induction, and Absorption of Pesticin. The Journal of Bacteriology, 1972. 112: pp. 212-219
34. Hu P.C., Brubaker R.R. Characterization of Pesticin: Separation of Antibacterial Activities. The Journal of Biological Chemistry, 1974. 249: pp. 4749-4753
35. Rakin A., Boolgakowa E., Hessemann J. Structural and Functional Organization of the *Yersinia pestis* Bacteriocin Pesticin Gene Cluster. Microbiology, 1996. 142: pp. 3415-3424
36. Ferber D.M., Fowler J.M., Brubaker R.R. Mutations to Tolerance and Resistance to Pesticin and Colicins in *Escherichia coli pbi*. The Journal of Bacteriology, 1981. 146: pp. 506-511
37. Vollmer W., Pilsl H., Hantke K., Höltje J-V., Braun V. Pesticin Displays Muramidase Activity. Journal of Bacteriology, 1997. 179: pp. 1580-1583
38. Ferber D.A., Brubaker R.R. Mode of Action of Pesticin: *N*-Acetylglucosaminidase Activity. Journal of Bacteriology, 1979. 139: pp. 495-501
39. Pilsl H., Hantke K., Braun V. Periplasmic Location of the Pesticin Immunity Protein Suggests Inactivation of Pesticin in the Periplasm. Journal of Bacteriology, 1996. 178: pp. 2431-2435
40. Smirnov G.B. Molecular Biology or the Factors Responsible for *Yersinia* Virulence. Biomedical Science, 1990. 1: pp. 223-232
41. Brubaker R.R. Factors Promoting Acute and Chronic Disease Caused by *Yersiniae*. Clinical Microbiology Reviews, 1991. 4: pp. 309-324
42. Price S.B., Cowan C., Perry R.D., Straley S.C. The *Yersinia pestis* V Antigen is a Regulatory Protein Necessary for Ca2+-dependent Growth and Maximal Expression of low-Ca2+ Response Virulence Genes. Journal of Bacteriology, 1991. 173: pp. 2649-2657
43. Yother J., Goguen J.D. Isolation and Characterization of Ca2+-blind Mutants of *Yersinia pestis*. Journal of Bacteriology, 1985. 164: pp. 704-711
44. Yother J., Chamness T.W., Goguen J.D. Temperature-controlled Plasmid Regulon Associated with Low-calcium Response in *Yersinia pestis*. Journal of Bacteriology, 1986. 165: pp. 443-447
45. Day J.B., Ferracci F., Plano G.V. Translocation of TopE and RopN into Eukaryotic Cells by *Yersinia pestis* YopN, tyeA, sycN, yscB and IcrG Deletion Mutants Measured Using a Phosphorylatable Peptide Tag and Phosphospecific Antibodies. Molecular Microbiology, 2003. 47L pp. 807-823
46. Price S.B., Straley S.C. LcrH, a Gene Necessary for Virulence of *Yersinia pestis* and for the Normal Response of *Y. pestis* to ATP and Calcium. Infection and Immunity, 1989. 57: pp. 1491-1498
47. Une T., Brubaker R.R. Roles of V Antigen in Promoting Virulence and Immunity in *Yersiniae*. The Journal of Immunology, 1984. 133: pp. 2226-2230
48. Motin V.L., Nakajima R., Smirov G.B., Brubaker R.R. Passive Immunity to Yersiniae Mediated by Anti-recombinant V Antigen and Protein A-V Antigen Fusion Peptide. Infection and Immunity, 1994. 4192-4201
49. Rosqvist R., Forsberg A., Rimpilainen M., Bergman T., Wolf-Watz H. The Cytotoxic TopE of *Yersinia* Obstructs the Primary Host Defense. Molecular Microbiology, 1990. 4: pp. 657-667
50. Barve S.S., Straley S.C. LcrR, a low-Ca2+-response Locus with Dual Ca2+-dependent Functions in *Yersinia pestis*. Journal of Bacteriology, 1990. 172: pp. 6441-4671

51. Leary S.E.C., Williamson E.D., Griffin K.F., Russell P., Eley S.M., Titball R.W. Active Immunization with Recombinant V Antigen from *Yersinia pestis Protects* Mice Against Plague. Infection and Immunity, 1995. 63: pp. 2854-2858
52. Nakajima R., Brubaker R.R. Association Between Virulence of *Yersinia pestis* and Suppression of Gamma Interferon and Tumor Necrosis Factor Alpha. Infection and Immunity, 1993. 61: pp. 23-31
53. Brubaker R.R. Interleukin-10 and Inhibition of Innate Immunity to *Yersiniae*: Role of Yops and LcrV (V Antigen). Infection and Immunity, 2003. 71: pp. 3673-3681
54. Lemaître N., Sebbane F., Long D., Hinnebusch B.J. *Yersinia pestis* YopJ Suppresses Tumor Necrosis Factor Alpha Induction and Contributes to Apoptosis of Immune Cells in the Lymph Node but is Not Required for Virulence in a Rat Model of Bubonic Plague. Infection and Immunity, 2006. 74: pp. 5126-5131
55. Cornelis G.R. *Yersinia* Type III Secretion: Send in the Effectors. The Journal of Cell Biology, 2002. 158: pp. 401-408
56. Viboud G.I., Bliska J.B. Yersinia Outer Proteins: Role in Modulation of Host Cell Signaling Responses and Pathogenesis. Annual Review of Microbiology, 2005. 59: pp. 69-89
57. Neyt C., Cornelis G.R. Insertion of a Yop Translocation Pore into the Macrophage Plasma Membrane by *Yersinia enterocolitica*: Requirement for Translocators YopB and YopD, but not LcrG. Molecular Microbiology, 1999. 33: pp. 971–981
58. Rosqvist R., Magnusson K.E., Wolf-Watz H. Target Cell Contact Triggers Expression and Polarized Transfer of *Yersinia* YopE Cytotoxin into Mammalian Cells. European Molecular Biology Organization (EMBO) Journal, 1994. 13: pp. 964–972
59. Sory M.P., Cornelis G.R. 1994. Translocation of a Hybrid YopE-adenylate cyclase from *Yersinia enterocolitica* into HeLa Cells. Molecular Microbiology, 1994. 14: pp. 583–594
60. Boland A., Sory M.P., Iriarte M., Kerbourch C., Wattiau P., Cornelis G.R. Status of YopM and YopN in the *Yersinia* Yop Virulon: YopM of *Y. enterocolitica* is Internalized Inside the Cytosol of PU5-1.8 Macrophages by the YopB, D, N Delivery Apparatus. European Molecular Biology Organization (EMBO) Journal, 1996. 15: pp. 5191–5201
61. Persson C., Nordfelth A., Holmström A., Håkansson S., Rosqvist R., Eolf-Watz H. Cell-surface-bound *Yersinia* Translocate the Protein Tyrosine Phosphatase YopH by a Polarized Mechanism into the Target Cell. Molecular Microbiology, 1995. 18: pp. 135-150
62. Fällman M., Persson C., Wolf-Watz H. Prospective Series: Host/Pathogen Interactions. *Yersinia* Protein that Target Host Cell Signaling Pathways. The Journal of Clinical Investigation, 1997. 99: pp. 1153-1157
63. Petersson J., Nordfelth R., Dubinina E., Bergman T., Gustafsson M., Magnusson K-E., Wolf-Watz H. Modulation of Virulence Factor Expre4ssion by Pathogen Target Cell Contact. Science, 1996. 273: pp. 1231-1233
64. Gustavsson A., Armulik A., Brakebusch C., Fässler R., Johansson S. Fällman M. Role of the β1-integrin Cytoplasmic Tail in Mediating Invasin-promoted Internalization of *Yersinia*. Journal of Cell Sciences, 2002. 115: pp. 2669-2678
65. Hamid N. Gustavsson A., Andersson K., McGee K., Persson C., Rudd C.E., Fallman M. YopH Dephosphorylates Cas and Fyn-binding Protein in Macrophages. Microbial Pathogenesis, 1999. 27: pp. 231–242
66. Black D.S., Marie-Cardine A., Schraven B., Bliska J.B. The *Yersinia* Tyrosine Phosphatase YopH Targets a Novel Adhesion-regulated Signalling Complex in Macrophages. Cellular Microbiology, *2000.* 2: pp. 401–414
67. Yuan M., Deleuil F., Fällman M. Interaction between the *Yersinia* Tyrosine Phosphatase YopH and Its Macrophage Substrate, Fyn-Binding Protein, Fyb. Journal of Molecular Microbiology and Biotechnology, 2005. 9: pp. 214-223
68. Barbieri J.T., Riese M.J., Aktories K. Bacterial Toxins that Modify the Actin Cytoskeleton. Annual Review of cell and Developmental Biology, 2002. 18: pp. 315-344
69. Schotte P., Denecker G., Van Den Broeke A., Bandenabeele P., Cornelis G.R., Beyaert R. Targeting Rac1 by the *Yersinia* Effector Protein YopE Inhibits Caspase-1-mediated Maturation and Release of Interleukin-1beta. The Journal of Biochemistry, 2004. 279: pp. 25134-25142
70. Shao F., Vacratsis P.O., Bao Z., Bowers K.E., Fierke C.A., Dixon J.E. Biochemical Characterization of the *Yersinia* YopT protease: Cleavage Site and Recongnition Elements in Rho GTPases. Proceedings of the National Academy of Sciences United States of America, 2003. 100: pp. 904-909
71. Juris S.J., Shao F., Dixon J.E. *Yersinia* Effctors Targets Mammalian Signalling Pathways. Cellular Microbiology, 2002. 4: pp. 201-211
72. Ruckdeschel K. Immunomodulation of Macrophages by Pathogenic *Yersinia* Species. Archivum Immunologiae et Therapiae Experimentalis, 2002. 50: pp. 131-137
73. Aepfelbacher M. Modulation of Rho GTPases by Type III Secretion System Translocated Effectors of *Yersinia*. Reviews of Physiology, Biochemistry and Pharmacology, 2004. 152: pp. 65-77
74. Zhang Y., Bliska J.B. Role of Macrophage Apoptosis in the Pathogenesis of *Yersinia*. Current Topics in Microbiology and Immunology, 2005. 289: pp. 151-174
75. Evdokimov A.G., Anderson D.E., Routzahn K.M., Waugh D.S. Unusual Molecular Architecture of the Yersinia pestis Cytotoxin TopM: a Leucine-rich Repeat Protein with the Shortest Repeating Unit. Journal of Molecular Biology, 2001. 312: pp. 807-821
76. Skrzpek E., Myers-Morales T., Whiteheart S.W., Straley S.C. Application of a Saccharomyces cerevisiae Model to Study Requirements for Trafficking of *Yersinia pestis* YopM in Eukaryotic Cells. Infection and Immunity, 2003. 71: pp. 937-947
77. Sauvonnet N., Pradet-Balade B., Garcia-Sanz J.A., Cornelis G.R. Regulation of mRNA Expression in Macrophages after *Yersinia enterocolitica* Infection. Role of Different Yop Effectors. The Journal of Biochemistry, 2002. 277: pp. 25133-25142
78. Hoffmann R., vanErp K., Trulzsch K., Heesemann J. Transcriptional Responses of Murine Macrophage to Infection with *Yersinia enterocolitica.* Cellular Microbiology, 2004. 6: pp. 377-390
79. McDonald C., Vacratsis P.O., Bliska J.B., Dixon J.E. The *Yersinia* Virulence Factor YopM forms a Novel Protein Complex with Two Cellular Kinases. The Hournal of Biochemistry, 2003. 278: pp. 18514-18523
80. Kerschen E.J., Cohen D.A., Kaplan A.M., Straley S.C. The Plague Virulence Protein YopM Targets the Innate Immune Response by Causing a Global Depletion of NK cells. Infections and Immunity, 2004. 72: pp. 4589-4602
81. Heusipp G., Spekker K., Brast S., Fälker S., Schmidt A. YopM of *Yersinia enterocolitica* Specifically Interacts with α1-Antitrypsin without Affecting the Anti-Protease Activity. Microbiology, 2006. 152: pp. 1327-1335
82. Tito M.A., Miller J., Griffin K.F., Williamson E.D., Titball R.W., Robinson C.V. Macromolecular organization of the *Yersinia pestis* capsular F1-antigen: insights from ToF mass spectrometry. Protein Science, 2001. 10: pp. 2408–241
83. Abramov V. M., Vasiliev A.M., Vasilenko R.N., Kulikova N.L., Kosarev I.V., Khlebnikov V.S., Ishchenko A.T., MacIntyre S., Gillespie J.R., Khurana R., Korpela T., Fink A.L., Uversky V.N.. 2001. Structural and Functional Similarity between *Yersinia pestis* Capsular Protein Caf1 and Human Interleukin-1β. Biochemistry, 2001. 40: pp. 6076–608
84. Galyov E.E., Smirnov O.Y., Karlishev A.V., Volkovoy K.I., Denesyuk A.L., Nazimov I.V., Rubtsov K.S., Abramov V.M., Dalvadyanz S.M., Zav'yalov V.P. Nucleotide Sequence of the *Yersinia pestis* Gene Encoding F1 Antigen and the Primary Structure of the Protein. Federation of European Biochemical Societies (FEBS) Letters, 1990. 277: pp. 230–232
85. Vorontsov E.D., Dubichev A.G., Serdobinstev L.N., Naumov A.V. Association-dissociation Process and Spermolecular Organization of the Capsule Antigen (protein F1) of *Yersinia pestis*. Biomedical Science, 1990. 1: pp. 391-396
86. Du Y., Rosqvist R., Forsberg Å. Role of Fraction 1 Antigen of *Yersinia pestis* in Inhibition of Phagocytosis. Infection and Immunity, 2002. 70: pp/ 1453-1460
87. Williams R.C., Gewurz H., Quie P.G. Effects of Fraction I from *Yersinia pestis* on phagocytosis *in vitro*. The Journal of Infectious Diseases, 1972. 126: pp. 235-241
88. Salyers A., Whitt D.D. Bacterial Pathogenesis: A Molecular Approach. Second Edition. Washington D.C.: American Society for Microbiology Press. 2002. pp. 202-215
89. Weening E.H., Cathelyn J.S., Kaufman G., Lawrenz M.B., Price P., Goldman W.E., Miller V.L. The dependence of the *Yersinia pestis* capsule on pathogenesis is influenced by the mouse background. Infection and Immunity, 2011. 79: pp. 644–652
90. Meyers K.F., Hightower J.A., McCrumb F.R. Plague Immunization. VI. Vaccination with the Fraction 1 Antigen of *Yersinia pestis*. The Journal of Infectious Diseases, 1974. 129: pp. S41-S45\
91. Zav'yalov V. P., Zav'yalova G.A., Denesyuk A.I., Korpela T. Modelling of Steric Structure of a Periplasmic Molecular Chaperone Caf1M of *Yersinia pestis*, a Prototype Member of a Subfamily with Characteristic Structural and Functional Features. Federation of European Microbiological Society Immunology and Medical Microbiology, 1995. 11: pp. 19–24
92. Karlyshev A. V., Galyov E.E., Smirnov O.Y., Guzayev A.P., Abramov V.M., Zav'yalov V.P. A New Gene of the F1 Operon of *Y. pestis* Involved in the Capsule Biogenesis. Federation of European Biochemical Societies (FEBS) Letters, 1992. 297: pp. 77–80
93. Karlyshev A. V., Galyov E.E., Abramov V.M., Zav'yalov V.P. *caf1R* Gene and its Role in the Regulation of Capsule Formation of *Y. pestis*. Federation of European Biochemical Societies (FEBS) Letters, 1992. 305: pp. 37-40
94. Brown S.D., Montie T.C. Beta-adrenergic blocking Activity of *Yersinia pestis* Murine Toxin. Infection and Immunity, 1977. 18: pp. 85-93
95. Hinnebusch B.J. The Evolution of Flea-borne Transmission in *Yersina pestis*. Current Issues in Molecular Biology, 2005. 7: pp. 197-212
96. Hinnebusch B.J., Rudolph A.E., Cherepenov P., Dixon J.E., Schwan T.G., Forsberg A. Role of *Yersinia* Murine Toxin in Survival of *Yersinia pestis* in the Midgut of the Vector Flea. Science, 2002. 296: pp. 733-735
97. von Teyn C.F., Weber N.S., Tempest B., Barnes A.M., Poland J.D., Boyce J.M., Zalma V. Epidemiologic and Clinical Features of an Outbreak of Bubonic Plague in New Mexico. The Journal of Infectious Diseases, 1977. 136: pp. 489-494
98. Barry M., Blackburn B.G. Bubonic and Pneumonic Plague in Uganda. Travel Medicine Advisor, 2009. 19: pp. 57-59
99. Conrad F.G., LeCocq F.R., Krain R. A Recent Epidemic of Plague in Vietnam. Archives of Internal Medicine, 1968. 122: pp. 193-198
100. Butler T., Levin J., Linh N.N., Chau D.M., Adickman M., Arnold K. *Yersinia pestis* Infection in Vietnam. II. Quantitative Blood Cultures and Detection of Endotoxin in the Cerebral Spinal Fluid of Patients with Meningitis. The Journal of Infectious Diseases, 1976. 133: pp. 493-499
101. Butler T. The Black Death Past and Present. 1. Plague in the 1980s. Transactions of the Royal Society of Tropical Medicine and Hygiene, 1989. 83: pp. 458-460
102. Prentice M.B., Rahalison L. Plague. The Lancet, 2007. 369: pp. 1196-1207
103. Lal G.M., Anuradha S. Pneumonic Plague, Northern India, 2002. Emerging Infectious Diseases, 2007. 13: pp. 664-666\
104. Kool J.L. Risk of Person-to-Person Transmission of Pneumonic Plague. Healthcare Epidemiology, 2005. 40: pp. 1166-1172
105. Ratsitorahina M., Chanteau S., Rahalison L., Ratsifasoamanana L., Boisier P. Epidemiological and Diagnostic Aspects of the Outbreak of Pneumonic Plague in Madagascar. The Lancet, 2000. 355: pp. 111-113
106. Alsofrom D.J., Mettler F.A.J., Mann J.M. Radiographic Manifestations of Plague in New Mexico, 1975-1980: A Review of 42 Proved Cases. Radiology, 1981. 139: pp. 561-565
107. Smiley S.T. Immune Defense against pneumonic plague. Immunological Reviews, 2008. 225: pp. 256-271
108. Hull H.F., Montes J.M., Mann J.M. Plague Masquerading as Gastrointestinal Illness. The Western Journal of Medicine, 1986. 145: pp. 485-487
109. Hull H.F., Montes J.M., Mann J.M. Septicemic Plague in New Mexico. The Journal of Infectious Diseases, 1987. 155: pp. 113-118
110. Crook L.D., Tempest B. Plague – A Clinical Review of 27 Cases. Archives of Internal Medicine, 1992. 152: pp. 1253-1256
111. Becker T.M., Poland J.D., Quan T.J., White M.E., Mann J.M., Barnes A.M. Plague Meningitis – A Retrospective Analysis of Reported Cases in the United States, 1970-1979. The Western Journal of Medicine, 1987. 147: pp. 554-557
112. Christie A.B., Chen T.H., Elberg S.S. Plague in Camels and Goats: Their Role in Human Epidemics. The Journal of Infectious Diseases, 1980. 141: 724-726
113. Poland J.D., Barnes A.M. Plague. Bacterial, Rickettisial and Mycotic Diseases, Volume I. Boca Raton: Chemical and Rubber Company (CRC) Press, 1979. pp. 515-559
114. Sharp S.E., Saubolle M.A., Baselski V., Carey R.B., Gilligan P.H., Krisher K., Lovchik J., Gray L., Humes R., Mangal C.N., Shapiro D.S., Weissfeld A., Welch D., York M.K., Sentinel Laboratory Guidelines for Suspected Agents of Bioterrorism *Yersinia pestis*. American Society for Microbiology, 2005. pp. 1-19
115. Guarner J., Shieh W.J., Greer P.W., Gabastou J.M., Chu M., Hayes E., Nolte K.B., Zaki S.R. Immunohistochemical Detection of *Yersinia pestis* in Formalin-fixed, Paraffin-embedded Tissue. American Journal of Clinical Pathology, 2002. 117: pp. 205-209
116. Butler T. Plague Gives Surprises in the First Decade of the 21st Century in the United States and Worldwide. The American Journal of Tropical Medicine and Hygiene, 2013. 89: pp. 788-793
117. Simon S., Demeure C., Lamourette P., Filali S., Plaisance M., Créminon C., Volland H., Carniel E. Fast and Simple Detection of Yersinia pestis Applicable to Field Investigation of Plague Foci. Public Library of Science One, 2013. 8: pp. e54947
118. Cavanaugh D.C., Fortier M.K., Robinson D.M., Williams J.E., Rust Jr J.H. Application of the ELISA Technique to Problems in the Serologic Diagnosis of Plague. Bulletin of the Pan American Health Organization, 1979. 13: pp. 399-402
119. Williams J.E., Gentry M.K., Braden C.A., Leister F., Yolken R.H. Use of an Enzyme-Linked Immunosorbant Assay to Measure Antigenaemia During Acute Plague. Bulletin of the World Health Organization, 1984. 62: pp. 463-466
120. Hinnebusch J., Schwan T.G. New Method for Plague Surveillance using Polymerase Chain Reaction to Detect *Yersinia pestis* in Fleas. Journal of Clinical Microbiology, 1993. 31: pp. 1511-1514
121. Chen T.H., Meyer K.F. An Evaluation of *Pasteurella pestis* Fraction-1-specific Antibody for the Confirmation of Plague Infections. Bulletin of the World Health Organization, 1966. 34: pp. 911-918
122. Ayyadurai S., Flaudrops C., Raoult D., Drancourt M. Rapid identification and typing of *Yersinia pestis* and other *Yersinia* species by matrix-assisted laser desorption/ionization time-of-flight (MALDI-TOF) mass spectrometry. Biomed Central (BMC), 2010. 10: pp. 285
123. Sampath R., Mulholland N., Blyn L.B., Massire C., Whitehouse C.A., Waybright N., Harter C., Bogan J., Miranda M.S., Smith D., Baldwin C., Wolcott M., Norwood D., Kreft R.,

Frinder M., Lovari R., Yasuda I., Matthews H., Toleno D., Housley R., Duncan D., Li F., Warren R., Eshoo M.W., Hall T.A., Hofstadler S.A., Ecker D.J. Comprehensive Biothreat Cluster Identification by PCR/Electrospray-Ionization Mass Spectrometry. Public Library of Science (PLoS) One, 2012. 7: pp. e36528

124. Vo-Dinh T. Biomedical Photonics Handbook. Danvers: Chemical Rubber Company (CRC) Press. 2010. pp. 20-14-20-16

125. Center for Disease Control and Prevention. Fatal Human Plague – Arizona and Colorado, 1996. Morbidity and Mortality Weekly Report, 1997. 46: pp. 617-636

126. Boulanger L., Ettestad P., Fogarty J., Dennis DT, Romig D, Mertz G. Gentamicin and Tetracyclines for the Treatment of Human Plague: Review of 75 Cases in New Mexico, 1985-1999. Clinical Infectious Disease, 2004. 38: pp. 663-669

127. Frean J.A., Arntzen L., Capper T., Bryskier A., Klugman K.P. In Vitro Activities of 14 Antibiotics against 100 Human isolates of Yersinia pestis from a Southern African Plague Focus. Antimicrobial Agents and Chemotherapy, 1996. 40: pp. 2646-2647

128. Russell P., Eley S.M., Bell D.L., Manchee R.J., Titball R.W. Doxycycline or Ciprofloxacin prophylaxis and Therapy Against Experimental Yersinia pestis Infection in Mice. Journal of Antimicrobial Chemotherapy, 1996. 37: pp. 769-774

129. Meyer K.F. Effectiveness of Live of Killed Plague Vaccines in Man. Bulletin of the World Health Organization, 1970. 42: pp. 653-666

130. Center for Disease control and Prevention. Plague Vaccine. Morbidity and Mortality Weekly Report, 1982. 31: pp. 301-304

131. Williamson E.D., Eley S.M., Stagg A.J., Green M., Russell P., Titball R.W. A Subunit Vaccine Elicits IgG in Serum, Spleen Cell Cultures and Bronchial Washings and Protects Immunized Animals Against Pneumonic Plague. Vaccine, 1997. 15: pp. 1079-1084

132. Williams J.E., Altieri P.L., Berman S., Lowenthal J.P., Cavanaugh D.C. Potency of Killed Plague Vaccines Prepared from Avirulent Yersinia pestis. Bulletin of the World Health Organization, 1980. 58: pp. 753-756

133. Darling R.G., Woods, J.B. USAMRIID's Medical Management of Biological Casulties Handbook. Fifth Edition. Fort Detrick: US Army Medical Research Institute of Infectious Diseases, 2004. pp. 40-44

134. Meyer K.F., Cavanaugh D.C., Bartelloni P.J., Marshall Jr J.D. Plague Immunization, I: Past and Present Trends. The Journal of Infectious Diseases, 1974. 129: pp. S13-S18

135. Andrews G.P., Heath D.G., Anderson Jr G.W., Welkos S.L., Friedlander A.M. Fraction 1 Capsular Antigen (F1) Purification from Yersinia pestis CO92 and from an Escherichia coli Recombinant Strain and Efficacy against Lethal Plague Challenge. Infection and Immunity, 1996. 64: pp. 2180-2187

136. Friedlander A.M., Welkos S.L., Worsham P.L., Andrews G.P., Heath D.G., Anderson Jr G.W., Pitt M.L., Estep J., Davis K. Relationship between Virulence and Immunity as Revealed in Recent Studies of F1 Capsule of Yersinia pestis. Clinical Infectious Diseases, 1995. 21: pp. S178-S181

137. Welkos S.L., Davis K., Pitt M.L., Worsham P.L., Friedlander A.M. Studies on the Contribution of the F1 Capsule-associated Plasmid pFra to the Virulence of Yersinia pestis. Contribution to Microbiology and Immunology, 1995. 13: pp. 299-305

138. David K.J., Fritz D.L., Pitt M.L., Welkos S.L., Worsham P.L., Friedlander A.M. Pathology of Experimental Pneumonic Plague Produced by Fraction-1-oisitve and Fraction-1-negative Yersinia pestis in African Green Monkeys (Cercopithecus aethiops). Archives of Pathology and Laboratory Medicine, 1996. 120: pp. 156-163

139. Une T., Brubaker R.R. Role of V Antigen in Promoting Virulence and Immunity in Yersiniae. The Journal of Immunology, 1984. 133: pp. 2226-2230

140. Sato K., Nakajima R., Hara F., Une T., Osada Y. Preparation of Monoclonal Antibody to V Antigen from Yersinia pestis. Contribution to Microbiology and Immunology, 1991. 12: pp. 225-229

141. Roggenkamp A., Geiger A.M., Leitritz L., Kessler A., Heesemann J. Passive Immunity to Infection with Yersinia spp. Mediated by Anti-recombinant V Antigen is Dependent on Polymorphism of V Antigen. Infection and Immunity, 1997. 65: pp. 446-451

142. Hill J., Copse C., Leary S., Stagg A.J., Williamson E.D., Titball R.W. Synergistic Production of mice against Plague with Monoclonal Antibodies Specific for the F1 and V Antigens of Yersinia pestis. Infection and Immunity, 2003. 71: pp. 2234-2238

143. Williamson E.D. Plague Vaccine Research and Development. Journal of Applied Microbiology, 2001. 91: pp. 606-608

144. Williamson E.D., Eley S.M., Stagg A.J., Green M., Russell P., Titball R.W. A Single Dose Subunit Vaccine Protects Against Pneumonic Plague. Vaccine, 2001. 19: pp. 566-571

145. McIsaac J.H., Hospital Preparation for Bioterror. A Medical and Biomedical System Approach. Burlington: Academic Press. 2006. pp. 51

Photo Bibliography

Figure 2.10-1: Believing that toxic air, also known as miasmas, were the cause of the plague, the doctors and the wealthy, wore costumes, for protection. This engraving by Gerhart Altzenbach is from the 17th century. Public domain graphics

Figure 2.10-4: Scanning electron micrograph (SEM) showing a mass of Yersinia pestis bacteria in the foregut of the flea. The scanning electron photomicrograph was taken by and released by the National Institute of Allergy and Infectious Diseases (NIAID). Pubic domain photo

Figure 2.10-9: Y. pestis infection diagram. The human anatomical illustration is created by Dr. Alexander J. da Silva and Melanie Moser in 2003. The illustration is released by the CDC. Public domain graphics

Figure 2.10-10: A photograph of a plague patient displaying inguinal buboes. Photograph was taken and released in 1993 by the CDC. Public domain photo

Figure 2.10-11: A photograph of a plague patient displaying axillary buboes. Photograph was taken and released in 1993 by the CDC. Public domain photo

Figure 2.10-12: A photograph of a plague patient displaying cervical buboes. Photograph was taken and released in 1993 by the CDC. Public domain photo

Figure 2.10-13: Bipolar staining of a plague smear prepared from lymph aspirated from a bubo of plague patient showing numerous Y. pestis bacteria. Photomicrograph was taken by Margaret Parsons, Dr. Karl F. Meyer and released by the CDC. Public domain photo

Figure 2.10-14: An anteroposterior X-ray revealing a bilaterally progressive pneumonic plague infection involving both lung fields. This X-ray was taken by Dr. Jack Poland and released by the CDC. Public domain photo

Figure 2.10-15: A photograph of a patient suffering from septicemic plague demonstrating gangrene of the right foot causing necrosis of the toes. Photograph was taken by William Archibald in 1977 and released by the CDC. Public domain photo

Ricin is one of the most poisonous and easily produced protein toxins known to man. This toxin is found in all regions of the castor plant, *Ricinus communis,* but is particularly concentrated in the seeds, also known as castor beans (Figure 3.1-1).

Ricin is a lectin consisting of two polypeptide chains, an A-chain and a B-chain, linked by a disulfide bond. This compound belongs to the type II family of dichain ribosome-inactivating proteins (RIPs); their function is to depurinate a single adenosine in the ribosomal ribonucleic acid (rRNA), thereby inactivating the ribosome. The active chain, A-chain, has the ability to catalytically modify the 28S rRNA loop contained in the 60S subunit of the ribosome effectively blocking protein synthesis in eukaryotic cells. Purified ricin can be produced in a crystalline form as a dry lyophilized powder or it can be dissolved in a solvent (Figure 3.1-2).[1, 2, 3]

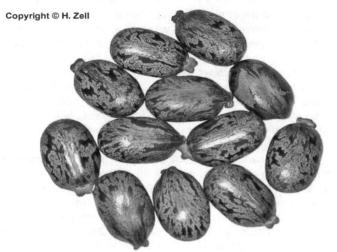

Figure 3.1-1: Castor beans from *Ricinus communis,* which possess a high concentration of ricin

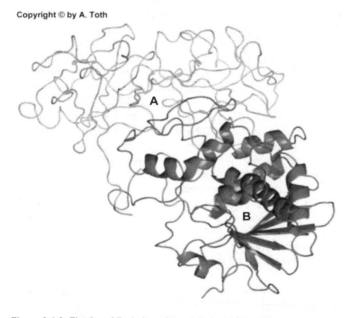

Figure 3.1-2: The A and B chains of the ricin toxin

The castor plant has been widely cultivated since ancient times for its oil. In ancient Egypt, the oil pressed from castor plant seeds were used as a lubricant and as a laxative. The purgative effects are the direct result of ricinoleic acid, which was freed from the castor oil through enzymatic hydrolysis, on the smooth musculature of the small intestines.[4] During World Wars I and II, the extract from castor plants was used to lubricate the rotary engines of aircrafts. Castor oil was continuously manufactured for that purpose until it was replaced by synthetic oils.[1]

The toxic effects of *R. communis* seeds in humans were recognized early in recorded history. Castor beans were commonly used in ancient Egyptian and Greek medicine, with therapies described in the *Susruta Ayurveda,* dating from the sixth century B.C.[5] In 1888, Peter Stillmark isolated a toxic protein from the seed of the castor plant, which he termed ricin. Stillmark discovered that ricin caused the agglutination of erythrocytes and precipitation of serum proteins.[6] In 1891, Paul Ehrlich was able to induce immunity in mice and rabbits by feeding them small numbers of castor beans on a regular basis. He was able to provide evidence to demonstrate the specific serum proteins produced are capable of precipitating and neutralizing the toxin. Interestingly, it was Ehrlich's work that provided the foundations for the discipline of immunology.[7]

In 1951, research into native ricin, which consists of only the A-chain, showed it to inhibit tumor growth. Developments in the last 3 decades have led to the creation of A-chain conjugated monoclonal antibodies, known as immunotoxins (chimeric toxins), which selectively target tumor cells for destruction. Additionally, toxin conjugated to growth factors (e.g. epidermal growth factors), transferrin, hormones and lectins that preferentially bind to certain cell types have also been developed as therapeutic remedies. Recently, genetic coupled conjugates of the immunotoxins have been developed which involves the preparation of hybrid genes to produce toxin fusion proteins in *Escherichia coli*. In recent years, a number of these chimeric toxins have gone through Phase I and/or II of clinical trials as anticancer agents.[8, 9, 10, 11, 12, 13]

While ricin is 1000 times less toxic than botulinum toxin (BoNT), its ease of production make it a capable candidate for an offensive biological weapon. In WWI, ricin was investigated as an offensive retaliatory weapon by the United States. Ricin laced shrapnel and bullets were developed. Additionally, a ricin dust cloud was created as a mass casualty weapon. Although these weapons were laboratory tested, they were never perfected before the end of the war.[14, 15] Nonetheless, research in the development of ricin as an offensive biological weapon continued into WWII. Code-named Compound W, ricin was weaponized by the United States and United Kingdom, and a W bomb was developed, but was never used in the conflict.[1, 5]

In 1978, Georgi Markov, a Bulgarian exile, was attacked in London, United Kingdom with a device disguised as an umbrella that fired a double drilled ricin coated pellet. The assassin discharged the pellet into the subcutaneous tissue of his leg, which resulted in his death several days later.[15, 16, 17] Another assassination attempt in Paris, France, on the life of another Bulgarian exile, Vladimir Kostov, a defector who worked for Radio Free Europe, also occurred in 1978. Kostov was also struck by a ricin coated pellet and only his heavy clothing prevented the pellet from penetrating any deeper than the epidermis of his back, sparing his life.[17] It is believed that similar pellet-firing weapons may have been responsible for at least six assassinations in the late 1970s and the early 1980s (Figure 3.1-3).[16, 19]

van Keuren R.T.
Borden Institute

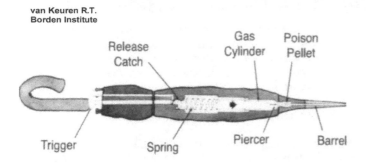

Figure 3.1-3: A diagram of the umbrella gun that was used to assassinate Bulgarian exile Georgi Markov in London in 1978. The weapon consisted of a spring-loaded piston, which would drive a carbon dioxide cartridge forward into a firing pin. The gas would then propel a poison projectile out of the hollow tip of the umbrella gun, through the clothing, and into the flesh of the intended victim

In 1994 and 1995, four men from the Minnesota Patriots Council, a tax-protest group, were convicted of possessing and conspiring to use ricin for the assassination of law enforcement officials. In 1995, a Kansas City oncologist Deborah Green was convicted of the attempted murder of her husband by contaminating his food with ricin. Again in 1995, Thomas Leahy, a Wisconsin resident, was arrested and charged with the possession of ricin. In October 2003, ricin was discovered in a South Carolina postal facility and on February 3, 2004, three US Senate office buildings were closed after ricin was found in a mailroom that served Senate Majority Leader Bill Frist's office, forcing the decontamination of 16 employees and the shutdown of several government buildings.[16, 20, 21, 22] On the fifth of January 2003, British authorities raided and arrested six suspected terrorists from Algeria and other northern African countries in their north London apartment. The British authorities believed that they were using their residence as a factory for producing ricin. It was reported that at least one of these six men had attended an Al-Qaida training camp in Afghanistan, while others received their training in Chechnya and the Pankisi Gorge region, State of Georgia.[23] More recently, on February 29, 2008, Reuters reported that ricin was found in a Las Vegas hotel room. Roger von Bergendorff was later charged with producing and possessing this biological weapon, although it is believed that he had no direct connection to any terrorist groups.[24]

STRUCTURE AND FUNCTION

Structurally, ricin is a 66 kd globular protein made up of two hemagglutinins and two distinct toxins. The toxins are heterodimmers, known as RCL III and RCL IV, and are made up of two polypeptide chains: a 32 kd A-chain and a 32 kd B-chain. The A-chain consists of 267 amino acid residues with 8 alpha helices and 8 beta sheets, while the B-chain consists of 262 amino acid residues arranged in a barbell-like tertiary protein structure with two homologous domains. The toxin is stored together with a 120 kd ricinus lectin in the matrix of the castor bean. The exact function of the lectin is presently unknown, but it is believed that this protein is involved in metabolic functions of the seed.[1, 3, 16, 25, 26, 27]

The A-chain is tucked between the roughly spherical domains of the B-chain where a lactose disaccharide moiety is bounded to each of the spherical domains of the B-chain. The 259th amino acid of the A-chain is linked by disulfide bond with the amino acid 4 of the B-chain. Both A- and B-chains are glycoproteins

containing mannose carbohydrate groups, essential for their toxicity (Figure 3.1-2).[1, 16, 28, 29]

Ricin does not require sophisticated or expensive equipment to be produced and can be lyophilized (freeze-dried) or crystallized to create a dry powder. The crystal structure is 2.5 Å and demonstrates a putative active cleft in the A-chain, believed to be the enzymatic active site of the toxin.[1, 16, 26]

It has been reported that the ricin B-chain binds to eukaryotic cell surface glycoproteins or glycolipids that are rich in galactose and N-acetylglucosamine, as well as, containing low amounts of sialic acid and N-actetylgalactosamine.[30] Presently, the specific host receptor(s) that ricin targets remain unknown and requires further elucidation. Nonetheless, the multiple manners by which ricin are internalized have been well documented. For example, Clathrin dependent endocytosis was first reported by van Deurs et al. (1985) where the toxin was internalized by Vero cells via receptor-mediated endocytosis via the coated pit-endosomal pathway.[31] However, ricin endocytosis can also occur by clathrin and caveolae independent mechanisms via uncoated pits[30, 32] Additionally, Rodal et al. (1999) reported that ricin could even be endocytosed when cholesterol was extracted from the cellular membrane of the targeted cell.[33] No matter the methodology of cellular entry, once ricin is internalized, it is initially delivered to early endosomes, from where the majority of the toxin recycles back to the cell surface, begins to be degraded and proceeds to late endosomes/lysosomes where further degradation is conducted.[34] Only a minor fraction (~5%) of ricin is transported from early endosomes to the trans-Golgi network through Rab-7, Rab-11 and clathrin independent manner.[13] Nonetheless, the toxin's transport to the trans-Golgi network is affected by changes in the cholesterol level. Grimmer et al. (2000) reported that depletion of cholesterol by treating cells with methyl-β-cyclodextrin (mβCD) inhibits the intracellular transport of ricin to the Golgi apparatus. Similarly, by increasing the level of cholesterol by treating cells with mβCD saturated with cholesterol (mβCD/chol) also reduced the intracellular transport of ricin to the Golgi apparatus.[35] Endosome to Golgi transport of ricin is also regulated by the presence of the Golgi-localized RII alpha isozyme, a regulatory subunit of cAMP-dependent protein kinase A (PKA). It has been shown that PKA type II alpha is involved in both endosome-to-Golgi and Golgi-to-ER transport of ricin.[36]

Once ricin is transported to the Golgi apparatus, it is retrogradely transported to the endoplasmic reticulum (ER) via coatomer protein I coated vesicles using calreticulin as a retrograde carrier.[37] The translocation of ricin A-chain from the ER to the cytosol occurs after reduction of internal disulfide bond connecting the ricin A-and B-chains. The breakage and isomerisation of disulfide bridges is catalyzed by the protein disulfide isomerase (PDI). Once the ricin A-chain is separated from the B-chain, it is transported to the cytosol via the Sec61p ER translocation channel and the ER-associated degradation pathway.[38, 39] Once the toxin appears in the cytoplasm, the A-chain enzymatically attacks the 28S loop of the 60S ribosomal subunit by cleaving one adenine residue (A^{4324}) near the 3' end of the molecule, causing elongation factor-2 to fail to bind, blocking and inhibiting protein synthesis, resulting in cell death.[40, 41, 42, 43, 44]

The toxicity of ricin varies with the route of entry. In experimental mice models, the approximate dose that is lethal to 50% of the exposed population (LD_{50}) is 3-5 µg/kg of body weight in 60 hours via inhalation, 5 µg/kg of body weight in 90 hours via intravenous inoculation, 22 µg/kg of body weight in 100 hours via intraperitoneal injection, 24 µg/kg of body weight in 100 hours via subcutaneous injection and 20 µg/kg of body weight in 85 hours via intravenous/intramuscular injection of the toxin. It is estimated that the lethal dose of ricin is ~1.0 µg/kg for all routes of introduction for humans.[1, 4, 45]

SYMPTOMS

Clinical symptoms and the pathological manifestation of ricin poisoning are dose and route of exposure dependent. This route specific pathology is likely the result of the properties of the B-chain, which binds readily to cell surface glycoproteins and glycolipids and triggers its uptake via endocytosis.[1, 46] No matter the route of entry into the human body, toxicity results from the inhibition of protein synthesis, as well as, mechanisms within the apoptosis pathways, direct cell membrane damage, alteration of membrane structure and function and the release of cytokine inflammatory mediators.[47, 48, 49, 50, 51, 52]

Ingestion

The introduction of ricin through the gastrointestinal tract is the least efficient manner by which the toxin enters the human body. It is believed that ricin is poorly absorbed, where some enzymatic digestion of the toxin may occur in the digestive tract thereby limiting their effectiveness. Fortunately, there is no data on the ingestion of purified ricin; most information is on the ingestion of castor beans. Nonetheless, it is estimated that the lethal dosage in humans is 1 to 20 mg of ricin per kilogram of body weight.[53] In 751 cases of castor bean ingestion and poisoning, there were 14 fatalities, constituting a death rate of 1.9%.[54] four to six hours (may be as late as 10 hours) after ingesting the toxin.[54, 55, 56, 57] These initial symptoms are followed by fever, headache, dilation of the pupils, diarrhea, rectal bleeding, anuria, cramps and thirst. Fluid loss may lead to electrolyte imbalance, hypotension, vascular collapse and shock. Death of the affected individual occurs on approximately the third day after the initial onset of symptoms.[54, 55, 56, 58]

Autopsy findings show multifocal ulcerations and severe hemorrhage of stomach and small intestinal mucosa. In addition, lymphoid necrosis is found in the mesenteric lymph nodes, gut-associated lymphoid tissue (GALT) and the spleen. Furthermore, necrosis of the Kupffer cells and hepatocytes, diffuse nephritis and diffused splenitis are also commonly seen (Table 1).[1, 2, 59]

Injection

The effects of intramuscular or subcutaneous injection of ricin have been obtained from the limited number of assassination attempts, which occurred during the Cold War. The best example is Georgi Markov, a Bulgarian exile who was injected with a lethal dose of ricin (~500µg) in 1978. Immediately after the injection, localized pain was felt by the individual and the onset of general weakness occurred within five hours. In 15 to 24 hours, symptoms including high fever, nausea and vomiting begin. It was not until 36 hours after the incident that Mr. Markov was admitted into the hospital with signs of tachycardia (with normal blood pressure), and sore and swollen lymph nodes in the region of the initial inoculation. Approximately 48 hours after the attack, the patient became hypotensive and tachycardic with a pulse rate of 160 beats per minute. Soon after, the patient displayed vascular collapse and shock. The white blood cell count at this time was measured at 26,300/mm³. Approximately 72 hours after the attack, the patient became anuric and began vomiting blood, while an electro-cardiogram demonstrated a complete atrio-ventricular (AV) conduction block. Mr. Markov passed away shortly after and at the time of death, his white blood cell count was 33,200/mm³ (Table 2).[1, 2, 59]

Table 1: An overview of the clinical symptoms after ricin ingestion

Symptoms	+	++	+++
Nausea			▪
Vomiting			▪
Oropharyngeal pain			▪
Heart burn			▪
Abdominal pain			▪
Fever			▪
Headache			▪
Dilation of the pupils			▪
Diarrhea			▪
Rectal bleeding			▪
Anuria			▪
Cramps			▪
Thirst			▪
Electrolyte imbalance			▪
Hypotension			▪
Vascular collapse			▪
Shock			▪

+ Rare ++ Common +++ Frequent

Table 2: An overview of the clinical symptoms after ricin inoculation

Symptoms	+	++	+++
General weakness			▪
High fever			▪
Nausea			▪
Vomiting			▪
Tachycardia (normal bp)			▪
Swollen lymph node			▪
Hypotension			▪
Vascular collapse			▪
Shock			▪
Anuric			▪
Vomiting blood			▪
AV conduction block			▪

+ Rare ++ Common +++ Frequent

Inhalation

There are no data available on the toxicity of aerosolized ricin in humans. The limited available data is based upon an allergic reaction by a worker who was exposed to the dust from castor beans and an accidental, sublethal aerosol exposure which occurred in 1940. The clinical symptoms are the sudden onset of congestion of the nose and throat, itchiness of the eyes, urticaria (e.g. hives) and tightness of the chest. In severe cases, wheezing and bronchial asthma have also been reported. In the accidental aerosol exposure of ricin fever, coughing, dyspnea, nausea and arthalgias will appear within four to eight hours. The onset of profuse sweating several hours later indicates the termination of most of the symptoms. There were no reported fatalities in the above stated cases and the patients responded to symptomatic therapy.[2, 16, 27, 59, 60, 61]

In animal models, rats exposed to lethal challenges of aerosolized ricin developed diffuse necrotizing pneumonia, coupled with interstitial and alveolar inflammation, as well as, edema. Aerosolized ricin binds to the ciliated cells of the bronchiolar lining, alveolar macrophages and epithelial cells lining the alveolar spaces. It has been reported that by 12 hours post inhalation, the inflammatory cell counts increased, as well as, the total protein concentration in the fluids obtained through bronchoalveolar lavage suggesting both the increased permeability of the air-blood barrier and cytotoxicity. At 18 hours and continuing up to 30 hours post inhalation, alveolar flooding is evident where extravascular lung water increased in volume. At 30 hours after inhalation, arterial hypoxemia and acidosis are present and significant alveolar flooding is observed through histological examinations. Death generally results from acute respiratory distress syndrome (ARDS).[1, 16, 27]

In a study by Wilhelmsen and Pitt (1996), five unimmunized adult rhesus monkeys were challenged with inhaled doses of 20.95-41.8 micrograms/kg of aerosolized ricin. Between 36 and 48 hours post-ricin inhalation, the monkeys either died or were euthanized at the onset of respiratory distress and were necropsied. The authors reported consistent gross and microscopic lesions were confined to the thoracic cavity, and multifocal to coalescing fibrinopurulent pneumonia was evident. In addition, diffuse necrosis, acute inflammation of airways, and diffuse alveolar flooding with peribronchovascular edema were also observed. Furthermore, purulent tracheitis, fibrinopurulent pleuritis, and purulent mediastinal lymphadenitis were also evident in the necropsid samples. Two monkeys had bilateral adrenocortical necrosis. The authors attributed the cause of death to asphyxiation following massive pulmonary alveolar flooding.[27, 62, 63]

DETECTION

There are numerous methods used to detect ricin. One of the earliest detection techniques is radioimmunoassay (RIA), which could be used to quantify amounts as low as 100 pg of ricin. Although, RIA has been proven effective in detecting ricin, its major shortcomings are lengthy incubation time, as well as, the dangers in handling and disposing of radioisotopes. Enzyme-linked immunosorbent assay (ELISA) involves shorter assay time and does not involve radioisotopes. The principle of ELISA is based upon antibody-antigen interaction and the test could be completed via a direct, competitive or sandwich format. For example, a sandwich ELISA using rabbit anti-ricin antibody could detect amounts as low as 40 ng/ml of ricin in body fluids through colorimetric measurement.[64, 65] A sandwich ELISA using affinity-purified goat polyclonal antibodies could detect amounts as low as 100 pg/ml of ricin in buffer, human urine and serum.[64, 66] In experimental challenges via laboratory animals, ELISA allowed the toxin to be identified after ~24 hours. In addition, due to the highly immunogenic nature of ricin, individuals who survive a ricin attack would have circulating antibodies within 2 weeks after exposure, therefore ELISA and chemilumine-scence (ECL) analysis can be used to identify the antibodies. Distinguishing ricin from other forms of poisoning can be difficult since ricin binds quickly and is metabolized before excretion. Nonetheless, ricin can be isolated from blood or other bodily fluids and examined via ELISA or through immunohistochemical analysis of tissues.[1, 2, 16] Fluorescence immunoassay have been developed to detect ricin at concentration of 10 fg/ml in assay buffer and 20 fg/ml in plasma and red blood cells,[67] while a sensitized latex agglutination test for ricin will provide a detection limit of 200 ng/ml.[68] The introduction of laser-induced fluorescence detection, also known as the fluorescence-based fiber optic immunoassay, reduced the assay time for toxin detection. This method is able to detect amounts as low as 100 pg/ml of ricin in buffer and 1 ng/ml of ricin in river water within 20 minutes.[69] Recently, a rapid and effective field detection system has been developed utilizing immunochromatography technique (ICT)-based assay. The ICT uses a capturing antibody (Mab 4C13) coated on a nitrocellulose membrane and the tracing antibody (MAb 3D74) labeled with colloidal gold in a convenient test strip format. Wu et al. (2011) reported that the assay time for the test strip was ~15 minutes and is able to detect amounts as low as 10 ng/ml of ricin in water and 25 ng/ml of ricin in human serum. However, when no ricin control samples were tested in parallel, soft drinks such as Sprite® and Coca Cola® showed false positive bands even

without toxin pollution.[70]

A planar array immunosensor with a charge-coupled device (CCD) as a detector has been reported to be effective in simultaneously detecting 3 toxic analytes: ricin, staphylococcal enterotoxin B (SEB) and Yersinia pestis. Antibodies against these analytes were attached to the bottoms of the circular wells to form the sensing surface, while rectangular wells containing chicken immunoglobulin were used as alignment markers and to generate control signals. Once the optical adhesive was removed, the slides were mounted over a CCD operating at ambient temperature and a two-dimensional graded index of refraction lens array was used to focus the sensing surface onto the CCD. Once the solutions of toxins were placed on the slide, Cy5-labeled antibodies were introduced. Subsequently, by using quantitative image analysis, the identity and amount of toxin bound at each location on the slide were determined. It has been reported that amounts as low as 25 ng/mL of ricin, 15 ng/mL of Y. pestis F1 antigen, and 5 ng/mL of SEB could be detected.[71]

An immunopolymerase chain reaction (IPCR) has been developed for the detection of ricin in buffer solution, as well as, in human serum samples. IPCR combines the specificity of immunological analysis with the exponential amplification of PCR (by 100 to 10,000 times). This technique is able to detect amounts as low as 10 fg/ml in human serum and is capable of detecting trace amounts of ricin 8 million times lower than that of conventional ELISA. Nonetheless, IPCR requires greater amount of time to perform the assay due to PCR and post-PCR analysis, as well as, the use of more expensive reagents.[64, 72, 73]

TREATMENT

Clinical management of ricin intoxicated patients will depend on the route of entry. The treatments that are presently available are supportive. For example, in inhalational cases, patients are provided with appropriate respiratory support such as oxygen, intubation, positive end-expiratory ventilation therapy, and hemodynamic monitoring. Anti-inflammatory agents and analgesics should be administered, since they would most likely benefit the patient. In addition, treatment for pulmonary edema should be appropriately performed as the patient's condition dictates. In gastrointestinal cases, the management should be through vigorous gastric lavage followed by the use of cathartics, such as magnesium citrate to remove the toxin from the digestive system. Fluid volume and electrolyte replacement, as well as, vasopressor therapy are very important to prevent the patient from experiencing vascular collapse and shock.[1, 2, 16]

There are no approved active prophylaxes via immunization at this time; however, research and testing are ongoing. Prophylactic immunization in animal models (e.g. mice, rats and non-human primates) with two to three doses of ricin toxoid (3 to 5 μg per dose) with or without adjuvant (e.g. aluminum hydroxide), have shown to be effective in protecting the animals following inhalational challenges with ricin. The toxoid could be made from a native toxin (e.g. formalin treated ricin toxin) or a preparation of the purified A-chain, which are capable of producing a measurable antibody response that correlates with protection from lethal exposure. It has been reported that the toxoid microencapsulated in Poly (lactide-co-glycolide) Microparticles have shown to be highly effective after only one immunization in mice.[74, 75]

In 2006, Dor BioPharma announced that it made progress with RiVax, a new drug that could be the world's first vaccine for the deadly ricin toxin. RiVax contains a recombinant subunit of the

Table 3: Differential diagnosis of ricin poisoning with selected disease with similar symptoms. These diseases are staphylococcal enterotoxin B (Staph-B), anthrax, Q-fever, pneumonic plague (PN), salmonella and shigella

Symptoms	Ricin	Staph-B	Anthrax	Q-fever	PN	Salmonella	Shigella
Fever	■	■	■	■	■	■	■
Nausea	■	■	■	■	■	■	■
Vomiting	■	■	■			■	■
Vomiting blood	■	■	■				
Headache	■	■	■	■		■	
Oropharyngeal pain	■						
Heart burn	■						
Abdominal pain	■	■				■	■
Diarrhea	■	■	■			■	■
Dilation of the pupils	■						
Anal hemorrhage	■						
Anuria	■						
Cramps	■	■					
Thirst	■	■					
Electrolyte imbalance	■						
Hypotension	■	■					
Vascular collapse	■						
General weakness	■	■		■	■		
Tachycardia (normal bp)	■		■				
Swollen lymph node	■		■	■			
Vascular collapse	■						
Shock	■		■				■
Anuric	■						
AV conduction block	■						

A-chain of the ricin toxin and has been shown to induce antibodies in humans that neutralised the ricin toxin during Phase I of clinical trials. RiVax has been reported to contain an adjuvant system, necessary to increase the level of ricin neutralizing antibodies and also to lengthen the period of immunity to ricin exposure.[76, 77]

DIFFERENTIAL DIAGNOSIS

The route of ricin exposure will determine the differential diagnosis of the toxic effect of the poison. For example, the differential diagnosis of inhalational ricin poisoning should include exposure to staphylococcal enterotoxin B (Staph-B), pyrolysis byproducts of organoflourines (e.g. Teflon or Kevlar), nitrogen oxides, and phosgene. In addition, diseases such as influenza, anthrax, Q-fever, and pneumonic plague (PN) should also be included into the diagnosis. The differential diagnosis of gastrointestinal ricin poisoning should include ingestion of caustics such as overdose iron or other metals, arsenic, colchicines. In addition, diseases such as anthrax, salmonella and shigella should also be considered (Table 3).[78, 79]

References

1. Franz D.R., Jaax N.K. Ricin Toxin. Medical Aspects of Chemical and Biological Warfare. Chapter 32. Washington D.C.: Office of the Surgeon General Department of the Army, United States of America. 1997. pp, 631-642
2. The Center for Food Security & Public Health. Iowa State University. Ricin. Revised January 2004. Retrieved December 24, 2009. Website: http://www.cfsph.iastate. edu/Factsheets/pdfs/ricin .pdf
3. Barbieri L., Baltelli M., Stirpe F. Ribosome-inactivating Proteins from Plants. Biochemica et Biophysica Acta, 1993. 1154: pp. 237-282
4. Alexander J., Benford D., Cockburn A., Cravedi J-P., Dogliotti E., Di Domenico A., Férnandez-Cruz M.L., Fürst P., Fink-Gremmels J., Galli C.L., Grandjean P., Gzyl J., Heinemeyer G., Johansson N., Mutti A., Schlatter J., van Leeuwen R., van Peteghem C., Verger P. Ricin (from Ricinus communis) as Undesirable Substances in Animal Feed. Scientific Opinion of the Panel on Contaminants in the Food Chain. European Food Safety Authority Journal, 2008. 726: pp. 1-38
5. Olsnes S. 2004. The History of Ricin, Abrin and Related Toxins. Toxicon, 2004. 44: pp. 361-370
6. Stillmark H. Über Ricin, Eines Gifiges Ferment aus den Samen von Ricinus communis L. und anderen Euphorbiacen. Inaugiral Dissertation, 1888. Eustonia: University of Dorpat
7. Ehrlich P. Experimentelle Untersuchungen über Immunität, I: Euber Ricin. Deutsch Med Wochenschr, 1891. 17: pp. 976–979
8. Olsnes S., Pihl A. Abrin, Ricin, and Their Associated Agglutinins. Receptors and Recognition: The Specificity and Action of Animal, Bacterial, and Plant Toxins. London: Chapman and Hall. 1976. pp. 129–173
9. Olsnes S., Pihl A. Construction and Properties of Chimeric Toxins Target Specific Cytotoxic Agents.Pharmacology of Bacterial Toxins. Oxford: Pergamon Press. 1986. pp. 709-739
10. Pharmacology of Bacterial Toxins. New York: Pergamon Press. 1986. pp. 709-739

11. Ucken F., Frankel A. The Current Status of Immunotoxins: An Overview of Experimental and Clinical Studies as Presented at the 3rd International Symposium on Immunotoxins. Leukemia, 1993. 7: pp. 341–348
12. Avila A.D., Calderón C.F., Perez R.M., Pons C., Pereda C.M., Ortiz A.R. Construction of an immunotoxin by linking a monoclonal antibody against the human epidermal growth factor receptor and a hemolytic toxin. Biological Research, 2007. 40: pp. 173-183
13. Słomińska-Wojewódzka M., Sandvig K. Ricin and Ricin-Containing Immunotoxins: Insights into Intracellular Transport and Mechanism of action in Vitro. Antibodies, 2013. 2: pp. 236-269
14. Giuseppe B., Giulio F., Rodolfo I., Gianfranco M., Anders R., Silvia S., Silvia U., Rossella T., Giuseppe T., Marco C. Reductive Activation of Ricin and Ricin A-chain Immunotoxins by Protein Disulfide Isomerase and Thioredoxin Reductase. Biochemical pharmacology, 2004. 67: pp. 1721-1731
15. Hunt R. Ricin. Washington, DC: American University Experiment Station. Chemical Warfare Monograph 37. 1918. pp. 107–117
16. Smart J.K. The U.S. Biological Warfare and Biological Defense Programs. Medical Aspects of Chemical and Biological Warfare. Chapter 2. Washington D.C.: Office of the Surgeon General Department of the Army, United States of America. 1997. pp. 9-86
17. Darling R.G., Woods, J.B. USAMRIID's Medical Management of Biological Casulties Handbook. Fifth Edition. Fort Detrick; US Army Medical Research Institute of Infectious Diseases, 2004. pp. 88-91
18. Crompton R., Gall D. Georgi Markov: Death in a Pellet. The Medico-legal Journal, 1980. 48: pp. 51-62
19. Harris R., Paxman J. A Higher Form of Killing: The Secret Story of Chemical and Biological Warfare. New York: Hill and Wang. 1982. pp. 217-218
20. Eitzen E.M., Takafuji E.T. Historical Overview of Biological Warfare. Medical Aspects of Biological Warfare. Chapter 18. Washington D.C.: The Surgeon General United States Army Medical Department Medical Center and School Borden Institute. 2007. pp. 415-423
21. Kifner J. Man is Arrested in a Case Involving Deadly Poison. New York Times. 23 December, 1995. pp. A-7
22. Goodman P.S. Seized Poison Set Off Few Alarms. Anchorage Daily News. 4 January, 1996. B-1
23. Weil M. Suspicious Powder Found in Frist Office: 6 of 8 Tests Positive for Lethal Toxin Ricin. The New York Times, Tuesday, February 3, 2004; Page A01
24. Bale J., Bhattacharjee A. Croddy E., Pilch R. Ricin Found in London: An al-Qa`ida Connection? Center for Nonproliferation Studies, Chemical and Biological Weapons Nonproliferation Program. Update February 29, 2008. Website: http://cns.miis.edu/pubs/reports/ricin.htm
25. Mylchreest I. Man Critical in Las Vegas After Poison Ricin Found. February 29, 2008, from Reuter. Web site: http://www.reuters.com/article/topNews/idUSN2915050420080229?feedType=RSS&feedName=topNews
26. Youle R., Huang A. Protein Bodies from the Endosperm of Castor Beans, Subfraction, Protein Components, Lectins, and Changes during Germination. Plant Physiology, 1976. 58: pp. 703-709
27. Rutenber E., Katzin B., Ernst S., Collins E.J., Mlsna D., Ready M.P., Robertus J.D. Crystallographic refinement of ricin to 2.5 Å. Proteins: Structure, Function, and Bioinformatics, 2004. 10: pp. 240-250
28. Hicks R.P., Hartell M.G., Nichols D.A., Bhattacharjee A.K., van Hamont J.E., Skillman D.R. The Medicinal Chemistry of Botulinum, Ricin and Anthrax Toxins. Current Medicinal Chemistry, 2005. 12: pp. 667-690
29. Olsnes S., Pihl A. Isolation and Properties of Abrin: a Toxic Protein Inhibiting Protein Synthesis. Evidence for Different Biological Functions of its Two Constituent-peptide Chains. European Journal of Biochemistry, 1973. 35: pp. 179–185
30. Olsnes S., Pihl A. Different Biological Properties of the Two Constituent Peptide Chains of Ricin, a Toxic Protein Inhibiting Protein Synthesis. Biochemistry, 1973. 12: pp. 3121–3126
31. van Deurs B., Pedersen L.R., Sundan A., Olsnes S., Sandvig K. Receptor-mediated endocytosis of a ricin-colloidal gold conjugate in vero cells. Intracellular routing to vacuolar and tubulo-vesicular portions of the endosomal system. Experimental Cell Research, 1985. 159: pp. 287-304

32. Sandvig K., Pust S., Skotland T., van Deurs B. Clathrin-independent endocytosis: mechanisms and function. Current Opinion in Cell Biology, 2011. 23: pp. 413-420

33. Rodal S.K., Skretting G., Garred O., Vilhardt F., van Deurs B., Sandvig K. Extraction of cholesterol with metyl-β-cyclodextrin perturbs formation of clathn-coated endocytic vesicles. Molecular Biology of the Cell, 1999. 10: pp. 961-974

34. Sandvig K., van Deurs B. Membrane traffic exploited by protein toxins. Annual Review of Cell and Developmental Biology, 2002. 18: pp. 1-14

35. Grimmer S., Iversen T.G., van Deurs B., Sandvig K. Endosome to Golgi transport of ricin is regulated by cholesterol. Molecular Biology of the Cell, 2000. 11: pp. 4205-4216

36. Birkeli K.A., Llorente A., Torgersen M.L., Keryer G., Taskén K., Sandvig K. Endosome-to-Golgi transport is regulated by protein kinase A type II alpha. The Journal of Biological Chemistry, 2003. 278: pp. 1991-1997

37. Day P.J., Owens S.R., Wesche J., Olsnes S., Roberts L.M., Lord J.M. An interaction between ricin and calreticulin that may have implications for toxin trafficking. The Journal of Biological Chemistry, 2001. 267: pp. 7202-7208

38. Wesche J., Rapak A., Olsnes S. Dependence of ricin toxicity on translocation of the toxin A chain from the endoplasmic reticulum to the cytosol. The Journal of Biological Chemistry, 1999,274: pp.34443-34449

39. Molinari M., Calanca V., Galli C., Lucca P., Paganetti P. Role of EDEM in the release of misfolded glycoproteins from the calnexin cycle. Science, 2003. 299: pp. 1397-1400

40. Larsson S.L.,Sloma M.S., Nygård O. Conformational changes in the structure of domains II and V of 28S rRNA in ribosomes treated with the translational inhibitors ricin or alpha-sarcin. Biochimica et Biophysica Acta, 2002. 1577: pp.53-62.

41. Sandvig K., Olsnes S., Pihl A. Kenetics of Binding of the Toxic Lectins Abrin and Ricin to Surface Receptors of Human Cells. The Journal of Biological Chemistry, 1976. 251: pp. 3977-3984

42. oule R., Neville D. Kinetics of Protein Synthesis Inactivation by Ricin-anti-thy.1.1 Monoclonal Antibody Hybrids: Role of the Ricin B subunit Demonstrated by Reconstitution. The Journal of Biological Chemistry, 1982. 267: pp. 1598–1601

43. Endo Y., Mitsui K., Motizuki M., Tsurugi K. The Mechanism of Action of Ricin and Related Toxic Lectins on Eukaryotic Ribosomes: The Site and the Characteristics of the Modification in 28S Ribosomal RNA caused by the Toxins. The Journal of Biological Chemistry, 1987. 262: pp. 5908–5912

44. Olsnes S. Closing in on Ricin Action. Nature, 1987. 328: pp. 474–475

45. Day P.J., Ernst S.R., Frankel A.E., Monzingo A.F., Pascal J.M., Molina-Svinth M.C., Robertus J.D. Structure and Activity of an Active Site Substitution of Ricin A Chain. Biochemistry, 1996. 35: pp. 11098-11103

46. Guerrant R.L., Walker D.H., Weller P.F. Tropical Infectious Diseases – Principles, Pathogens & Practice. Volume 1. Philadelphia: Churchill Livingstone Elsevier. 2006. pp.110-112

47. Olsnes S., Pihl A. Toxic Lectins and Related Proteins. Molecular Action of Toxins and Viruses. Amsterdam: Elsevier Biomedical Press. 1982. pp. 51–105

48. Day P.J., Pinheiro T.J., Roberts L.M., Lord J.M. Binding of Ricin A-chain to Negatively Charged Phospholipid Vesicles Leads to Protein Structural Changes and Destabilizes the Lipid Bilayer. Biochemistry, 2002. 41: pp. 2836-2843

49. Griffiths G.D., Leek M.D., Gee D.J. The Toxic Plant Proteins Ricin and Abrin Induce Apoptotic Changes in Mammalian Lymphoid Tissues and Intestine. The Journal of Pathology, 1987. 151: pp. 221-222

50. Hughes J.N., Lindsay C.D., Griffiths G.D.. Morphology of Ricin and Abrin Exposed Endothelial Cells is Consistent with Apoptotic Cell Death. Human & Experimental Toxicology, 1996. 15: pp. 443-451

51. Kumar O., Sugendran K., Vijayaraghavan R. Oxidative Stress Associated Hepatic and Renal Toxicity Induced by Ricin in Mice. Toxicon, 2003. 41: pp. 333-338

52. Lombard S., Helmy M.E., Pieroni G. Lipolytic Activity of Ricin from Ricinus sanguineus and Ricinus communis on Neutral Lipids. Biochemical Journal, 2001. 358: pp. 773-781

53. Morlon-Guyot J., Helmy M., Lombard-Frasca S., Pignol D., Piéroni G., Beaumelle B. Identification of the Ricin Lipase Site and Implication in Cytotoxicity. The Journal of Biological Chemistry, 2003. 278: pp. 17006-17011

54. Audi J., Belson M., Patel M., Schier J., Osterloh J. Ricin Poisoning a Comprehensive Review. Journal of American Medical Association, 2005. 294: pp. 2342-2351

55. Rauber A., Heard J. Castor Bean Toxicity Re-examined: A New Perspective. Veterinary and Human Toxicology, 1985. 27: pp. 498–502

56. Challoner K.R., McCarron M.M. Castor Bean Intoxication: Review of Reported Cases. Annals of Emergency Medicine, 1990. 19: pp. 1177-1183

57. Kopferschmitt J., Flesch F., Lugnier A., Sauder P., Jaeger A., Mantz J.M. Acute Voluntary Intoxication by Ricin. Human Toxicology, 1983. 2: pp. 239-242

58. Kinamore P.A., Jaeger R.W., de Castro F.J. Abrus and Ricinus Ingestion: Management of Three Cases. Clinical Toxicology, 1980. 17: pp. 401-405

59. Reed R.P. Castor Oil Seed Poisoning: a Concern for Children. The Medical Journal of Australia, 1998. 168: pp. 423-424

60. Shea D., Gottron F. Ricin: Technical Background and Potential Role in Terrorism. Congressional Research Service (CRS) Report for Congress. Revised February 4, 2004. Retrieved December 30, 2009. Website: http://www.fas.org/irp/crs/ RS21383.pdf

61. Brugsch H.G. Toxic Hazards: The Castor Bean. Massachusetts Medical Society, 1960. 262: pp. 1039–1040

62. Army Field Manual FM-8-284. Treatment of Biological Warfare Agent Casualties Headquarters, Department of the Army, the Navy, and the Air Force, and Commandant, Marine Corps. 2000. pp. 4-7-4-9

63. Wilhelmsen C., Pitt L. Lesions of Acute Inhaled Lethal Ricin Intoxication in Rhesus Monkeys. Veterinary Pathology, 1996. 33: pp. 296-302

64. Puri P., Kumar O. Integrating Immunobased Detection and Identification Methods for Ricin Analysis: An Overview. Bioterrorism and Biodefense, 2011. S2: pp. 003

65. Koja N., Shibata T., Mochida K. Enzyme-linked immunoassay of ricin. Toxicon, 1980. 18: pp. 611-618

66. Poli M.A., Rivera V.R., Hewetson J.F., Merill G.A. Detection of ricin by colorimetric and chemiluminescence ELISA. Toxicon, 1994. 32: pp. 1371–1377

67. Pradhan S., Kumar O., Jatav P.C., Singh S. (2009) Detection of ricin by comparative indirect ELISA using fluorscence probe in blood and red blood cells. Journal of Medical, Chemical, Biological, & Radiological Defense, 2009. 7

68. Kumar O., Rai G.P., Parida M., Vijayaraghavan R. (2004). Rapid detection of ricin by sensitizing carboxylated latex particles by ricin antibodies. Defense Science Journal, 2004. 54: pp. 57-63

69. Narang U., Anderson G.P., Lifler F.S., Burans J. (1997) Fiber optic based biosensor for ricin. Biosensors and Bioelectronics, 1997. 12: pp. 937-945

70. Wu J., Wang Y., jia P., Wang C., Zhao Y., Peng H., Wei W., Li H. Immunochromatography detection of ricin in environmental and biological samples. Nano Biomedicine and Engineering, 2011. 3: pp. 169-173

71. Vo-Dinh T. Biomedical Photonics Handbook. Danvers: Chemical Rubber Company (CRC) Press. 2010. pp. 20-14-20-16

72. Lubelli C., Chatgilialoglu A., Bolognesi A., Strocchi P., Colombatti M., Stirpe F. Detection of ricin and other ribosome-inactivating proteins by an immuno-polymerase chain reaction assay. Analytical Biochemistry, 2006. 355: pp. 102-109

73. He X., McMahon S., McKeon T.A., Brandon D.L. Development of a novel immuno-PCR assay for detection of ricin in ground beef, liquid chicken egg, and milk. The Journal of Food Protection, 2010. 73: pp. 695-700

74. Hewetson J., Rivera V., Lemley P., Pitt M., Creasia D., Thompson W. A Formalinized Toxoid for Protection of Mice from Inhaled Ricin. Vaccine Research, 1996. 4: pp. 179–187

75. Yan C., Resau J.H., Hewetson J., West M., Rill W., Kende M. Characterization and Morphological Analysis of Protein-loaded Poly(lactide-co-glycolide) Microparticles Prepared by Water-in-oil-in-water Emulsion Technique. Journal of Controlled Release, 1994. 32: pp. 231–241

76. Reymond E. Dor makes Ground with Ricin Vaccine. Pharmasutical Technology. Revised November 16, 2006. Retrieved December 30, 2009. Website: http://www.in-pharmatechnologist.com/Materials-Formulation/Dor-makes-ground-with-ricin-vaccine

77. Legler P.M., Brey R.N., Smallshaw J.E., Vitetta E.S., Millard C.B. Structure of RiVax: a recombinant ricin vaccine. Acta Crystallographica Section D: Biological Crystallography, 2011. 67: pp. 826-830

78. Schier J. Summary, Center for Disease Control and Prevention Clinician Outreach and Communication Activity Clinician Briefing Ricin as a Biologic Agent. Revised January, 27, 2004. Retrieved December 5, 2011. Website: http://www.aha.org/content/00-10/ricin.pdf

79. McIsaac J.H. Hospital Preparation for Bioterror. A Medical and Biomedical System Approach. Burlington: Academic Press. 2006. pp. 58

Photo Bibliography

Figure 3.1-1: Castor beans from Ricinus communis which possesses a high concentration of ricin. This copyrighted © photograph was taken and released in July, 2010 by H. Zell

Figure 3.1-2: The A- and B-chain of the ricin toxin. Note: A chain is in clue while B chain is in orange. This copyrighted © graphic was designed and released by A. Toth in Februrary, 2008

Figure 3.1-3: A diagram of the umbrella gun that was used to assassinate Bulgarian exile Georgi Markov in London in 1978. The weapon consisted of a spring-loaded piston, which would drive a carbon dioxide cartridge forward into a firing pin. The gas would then propel a poison projectile out of the hollow tip of the umbrella gun, through the clothing, and into the flesh of the intended victim. The diagram was reproduced from van Keuren RT. Chemical and Biological Warfare, An Investigative Guide. Washington, DC: Office of Enforcement, Strategic Investigations Division, US Customs Service; October 1990: 89. Public domain graphic

Staphylococcal enterotoxin (SE) consists of a family of highly hydrophilic molecules with molecular mass of 24-30 kDa produced by strains of *Staphylococcus aureus* (Figure 3.2-1). According to the surveillance report released by Centers for Disease Control and Prevention in 2011, staphylococcal food poisoning (SFP) is among the top five pathogens in the United States, affecting 241,148 persons annually.[1] Presently, 22 types of SE designated with letters A–V are currently known.[2] SEs that are most commonly implicated in staphylococcal food poisoning (SFP) are type A (SEA), B (SEB), C (SEC), D (SED), while another enterotoxin originally designated as type F (SEF), has been renamed toxic shock syndrome toxin 1 (TSST-1).[3, 4, 5, 6, 7, 8] SE molecules exhibit a low α-helix and a high β-pleated sheet content suggesting a flexible and highly accessible structure. SEs are commonly referred to as superantigens or pyrogenic toxins, because of their profound effect on the human immune system. For example, SEs have the capability to stimulate lymphocyte proliferation and lympho-kine production concentrations as low as 10^{-13} to 10^{-16} M, making them among the most potent activators of T lymphocytes known.[3, 4, 5, 6, 9]

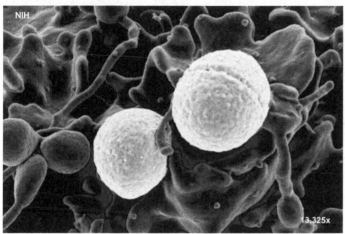

Figure 3.2-1: Colorized scanning electron photomicrograph (SEM) of *Staphylococcus aureus* bacteria, shown outside a white blood cell

During conventional antigen recognition, the CD4 co-receptor of a T-lymphocyte stabilizes the contacts between the T-cell antigen receptors and the major histocompatibility complex (MHC) class II molecules. This stabilizing function of CD4 is thought to be of primary importance for enhancing low-affinity interactions.[10, 11] The NH_2-terminal region of the SEs binds with the α-helical region of the major histocompatibility complex (MHC) class II molecules located on antigen presenting cells. It has been reported that unlike conventional antigens, SEs are neither processed, nor do they stimulate proteolysis of the peptide fragments that are generally required for protein antigens; rather they bind to MHC class II molecules outside of the peptide-binding groove and form a trimolecular complex with the T-lymphocyte antigen receptors (TcR). This complex formed between SEs and MHC class II molecules is required for binding to the Vβ region of the TcR, thereby supporting a mechanism for signal transduction that involves cross-linking of T-cells with MHC class II molecules.[4, 12, 13, 14, 15, 16] Alternatively, it has also been proposed that superantigens bind to T-cell receptors indirectly through another endogenous co-ligand. No matter the mechanism of action of these superantigens, it is believed that these molecules may directly replace CD4 binding and stimulate a large number of T-cells independently of conventional antigen

recognition.[17, 18, 19, 20]

The activation of T-helper cells causes the substantial release of cytokines, such as interferon gamma (IFN-γ), interleukin-1 (IL-1), IL-2, IL-6 and tumor necrosis factor alpha (TNFα) which is responsible for the systemic effects of the enterotoxin. In contrast, during a gastrointestinal illness, the superantigens stimulate a massive release of histamine and leukotriene from mast cells.[21, 22, 23]

Staphylococcal enterotoxin B, a 28 kDa exotoxin is the best understood of the enterotoxins. Like all other SEs, SEB is heat stable and is able to withstand boiling temperatures for several minutes. Additionally, SEB is able to withstand extremes of pH (pH 3-11) and protease digestion by gastric enzymes.[24] SEB, code-named PG, was examined by the Special Operations Division at Camp Detrick in 1964 and tested on animals at the Deseret Island in the Pacific Ocean and at Dugway Proving Ground in Utah.[25, 26] This toxin was especially attractive as an offensive biological agent, as much lower quantities were required to produce the desired effects than were needed with synthetic chemicals. It was calculated that the inhalation dose needed for incapacitating 50% of the average human population exposed (ED_{50}) is 0.0004 µg/ kg of the average individual body weight, while the lethal dose for 50% (LD_{50}) of the population exposed was calculated at 0.02 µg/kg of average body weight of the individual.[3, 4]

SYMPTOMS

SEB is highly incapacitating, but not very lethal. The incubation of SEB varies depending upon the route of entry. For example, the incubation period after ingestion of SEB is generally 4-10 hours, while the incubation period after inhalation of SEB is generally 3 to 12 hours.[4, 27]

Clinical symptoms caused by the ingestion of the enterotoxin include mild to severe headaches, myalgia, prostration, weakness, dizziness, nausea, abdominal cramps and explosive vomiting (at times bloody), which may last for several hours. It is known that SEB stimulates the vagus nerve endings in the stomach, which control the vomiting reflex. Additional symptoms includes leg cramps, thirst, anorexia and diarrhea (at times bloody).[4, 27, 28, 29, 30, 31] Fever, a prominent sign of aerosolized exposure, is generally not observed in gastrointestinal cases of SEB poisoning (Table 1).[3]

Clinical symptoms involved in the inhalation of the enterotoxin include fever (~41.1° C or 106° F), chills, mild to severe headaches, myalgia, prostration, nonproductive cough, chest pains, orthopnea and moist inspiratory and expiratory rales with dyspnea. In severe cases, pulmonary (alveolar) edema, interstitial edema and respiratory failure may result. In addition, SEB may also be associated with non-menstrual toxic shock syndrome, which generally consists of a cytokine storm followed by a rapid drop in blood pressure, elevated temperature, and multi-organ failure. This condition is due to the systemic spread of the SEB within a patent's body, without a staphlococcus infection. Gastrointestinal signs may also present themselves after an aerosolized exposure since enterotoxins may be swallowed during mucociliary clearance. These gastrointestinal symptoms include nausea, vomiting and diarrhea (Table 2).[3, 27, 29, 32, 33]

Table 1: An overview of the clinical symptoms after ingestion of SEB

Symptoms	+	++	+++
Headaches			■
Myalgia			■
Prostration			■
Weakness			■
Dizziness			■
Nausea			■
Abdominal cramps			■
Explosive vomiting			■
Bloody vomiting			■
Leg cramps			■
Thirst			■
Anorexia			■
Diarrhea			■
Bloody diarrhea		■	

+ Rare ++ Common +++ Frequent

Table 2: An overview of the clinical symptoms after inhalation of SEB

Symptoms	+	++	+++
Fever			■
Chills			■
Headaches			■
Myalgia			■
Prostration			■
Nonproductive cough			■
Chest pains			■
Orthopnea			■
Moist inspiratory rales			■
Moist expiratory rales			■
Dyspnea			■
Alveolar edema			■
Interstitial edema			■
Respiratory failure			■
Toxic shock syn.		■	
Cytokine storm		■	
Hypotension (rapid drop)		■	

+ Rare ++ Common +++ Frequent

DETECTION

Diagnosis of SEB intoxication is primarily based on clinical symptoms, nonetheless confirmation of such intoxication is through epidemiologic assays of tissue, body fluids or examination of environmental samples. SEB is a relatively stable molecule and may be found in blood serum, urine, stool, and gastric aspirate. Respiratory secretions (sputum) and nasal swabs collected within 24 hours of exposure can also be used to collect enterotoxin samples.[3, 27]

Numerous methods have been developed for SE detection. The most commonly used method, also known as the "double-antibody sandwich" protocol enzyme-linked imnmunosorbent assay (ELISA), recognizes SEB and other staphylo-coccal enterotoxins. In this double-sandwich format, the "bottom" monoclonal antibodies (MAbs) are used to capture the antigen (SEB) and the "top" MAbs are used to detect SEB. In order to prevent cross-reactivity, the MAbs used are generally developed from different animal species. The "bottom" detector MAbs can be directly labeled with a signal-generating molecule, or it can be detected with another antibody, labeled with an enzyme. For example, the labeled enzyme can catalyze a chemical reaction with the substrate that results in a colorimetric change. The intensity of this color can be measured by a spectrophotometer, which determines the optical density of the reaction, using a specific wavelength of light. This protocol for ELISA is highly sensitive and can detect SEB in body fluids at very low concentrations.[34, 35, 36]

Electrochemiluminescence (ECL), is in many ways similar to ELISA, except that the detector antibody is directly labeled with a chemiluminescent molecule.[37, 38] Examples of ECL are known as ORIGEN® (IGEN International), Elecsys® Immunoanalyzer (Roche Diagnostics), NucliSens® amplification technology (Organon Teknika), and the QPCR® System 5000 (PerkinElmer) which may be commercially purchased. All of these systems make use of antigen-capture assays, a ruthenium chemi-luminescent label and include magnetic beads to concentrate target agents. The magnetic beads are coated with capture antibody, and in the presence of a biological agent, immune complexes are formed between the agent and the labeled detector antibody. Subsequently, the samples are analyzed via an ECL analyzer which is composed of an electrochemical flow cell with a photon detector placed above the electrode. A magnet positioned below the electrode captures the magnetic bead-Ru-tagged immune complex allowing for rapid reaction kinetics and a short incubation time.[3, 27, 36, 39, 40]

Another method includes reversed passive latex agglutination (RPLA), available as a commercial test kit called SET-RPLA®, available from Denka Seiken Co., Ltd. Based on similar methodologies, a more sensitive and less time consuming RPLA using high density latex particles has been developed by Fujikawa and Igarashi (1988). This improved methodology takes only 3 hours of incubation time in comparison to the 16 hours required for SET-RPLA.[41] Detection of SEB may also be accomplished through biomolecular interaction analysis mass spectro-metry (BIA/MS). This experimental method utilizes a surface plasmon resonance (SPR) MS immunoassay that detects affinity-captured SEB both via SPR and by means of exact and direct mass measurement by matrix-assisted laser desorption/ionization time-of-flight (MALDI-TOF) mass spectrometry.[42] A newly proposed technique known as lateral flow assay (LFA), is based upon a double-antibody sandwich format on a porous nitrocellulose membrane. The LFA method has been reported as a rapid and sensitive technique and has been used successfully to detect SEB.[43]

A planar array immunosensor with a charge-coupled device (CCD) as a detector has been reported to be effective in simultaneously detecting three toxic analytes: ricin, staphylococcal enterotoxin B (SEB) and Yersinia pestis.[44]

Antibodies against these analytes are attached to the bottoms of the circular wells to form the sensing surface, while rectangular wells containing chicken immunoglobulin were used as alignment markers and to generate control signals. Once the optical adhesive is removed, the slides are mounted over a CCD operating at ambient temperature and a two-dimensional graded index of refraction lens array was used to focus the sensing surface onto the CCD. Once the solutions of toxins are placed on the slide, Cy5-labeled antibodies are then introduced. Subsequently, by using quantitative image analysis, the identity and amount of toxin bound at each location on the slide is determined. It has been reported that amounts as low as 25 ng/mL of ricin, 15 ng/mL of pestis F1 antigen, and 5 ng/mL of SEB could be detected.[44]

TREATMENT

Supportive management is generally adequate in the treatment of SEB intoxicated individuals. Using cold compresses, acetaminophen and/or aspirin are effective to relieve the symptoms of fever, muscle aches and arthralgias. Diphhydra-

Table 3: Differential diagnosis of staphylococcal enterotoxin with selected disease with similar symptoms. These diseases and toxins are staphylococcal enterotoxin (SE), ricin, Q-fever, tularemia, pneumonic plague (PN), anthrax, and shigella

Symptoms	SE	Ricin	Q-fever	Tularemia	PN	Anthrax	Shigella
Fever	■		■	■	■	■	
Chills	■		■	■	■	■	
Headaches	■	■	■	■	■	■	
Myalgia	■		■			■	
Prostration	■						
Weakness	■		■		■		
Dizziness	■				■		
Nonproductive cough	■		■	■		■	
Chest pains	■		■	■	■		
Orthopnea	■						
Nausea	■	■	■	■			■
Abdominal cramps	■	■					■
Explosive vomiting	■	■	■	■		■	
Bloody vomiting	■	■					
Thirst	■	■					
Anorexia	■		■			■	
Diarrhea	■	■	■	■		■	■
Diarrhea (bloody)	■						■
Moist inspiratory rales	■						
Moist expiratory rales	■						
Dyspnea	■						
Pulmonary (alveolar) edema	■						
Interstitial edema	■						
Respiratory failure	■				■		
Toxic shock syndrome	■					■	■
Cytokine storm	■						
Hypotension (rapid drop)	■	■					
Leg cramps	■						

mine and prochlorperazine have been successful in controlling nausea. Cough suppressants, containing dextromethorphan or codeine, could be used, while dihydrocodeinone may be employed during cases of prolong coughing. Fluid and electrolyte replacement may be needed to replace the losses experienced during episodes of vomiting and diarrhea in the course of gastrointestinal cases. Antidiarrheal medication may be use as the symptoms dictate.

Presently there are no approved immune-therapies or vaccines available for treating SEB intoxication.[3, 27]

DIFFERENTIAL DIAGNOSIS

The route of staphylococcal enterotoxin (SE) exposure will determine the differential diagnosis of the toxic effect of the poison. For example, the differential diagnosis of inhalational exposure to SE should include toxins such as ricin and phosgene. In addition, diseases such as Q-fever, tularemia, pneumonic plague (PN) and influenza should also be considered within the differential diagnosis. The differential diagnosis of gastrointestinal exposure to staphylococcal enterotoxin should include diseases such as anthrax, salmonella and shigella (Table 3).[4, 45]

References

1. Tallent S.M., Hait J., Bennett R.W. Staphylococcal Enterotoxin B-Specific Electrochemiluminescence and Lateral Flow Device Assays Cross-React with Staphylococcal Enterotoxin D. Journal of Association of Official Agricultural Chemists (AOAC) International, 2014. 97: pp. 862-867
2. Argudín, M. A., Mendoza, M. C., Rodicio M. R. Food poisoning and Staphylococcus aureus enterotoxins. Toxins, 2010. 2: pp. 1751–1773
3. Ulrich R.G., Sidell S., Taylor T.J., Wilhelmsen C.L., Franz D.R. Staphylococcal Enterotoxin B and Related Pyrogenic Toxins. Medical Aspects of Chemical and Biological Warfare. Chapter 32. Washington D.C.: Office of the Surgeon General Department of the Army, United States of America. 1997. pp. 621-630
4. Guerrant R.L., Walker D.H., Weller P.F. Tropical Infectious Diseases – Principles, Pathogens & Practice. Volume 2. Philadelphia: Churchill Livingstone Elsevier. 2006. pp. 1392-1396
5. Kamboj D.V., Nema V., Pandey A.K., Goel A.K., Singh L. Heterologous Expression of Staphylococcal Enterotoxin B (seb) gene for Antibody Production. Electronic Journal of Biotechnology, 2006. 9: pp. 551-558
6. Johnson H.M., Russell J.K., Pontzer C.H. Staphylococcal Enterotoxin Microbial Superantigens. The Federation of American Societies for Experimental Biology (FASEB) Journal, 1991. 5: pp. 2706-2712
7. Bergdoll M.S. The Staphylococcal Enterotoxins: an Update. The Staphylococci. New York: Gustav Fischer Verlag. 1985. pp. 247-254
8. Munson S.H., Tremaine M.T., Betley M.J., Welch R.A. Identification and Characterization of Staphylococcal Enterotoxin Type G and I from Staphylococcus aureus. Infection and Immunity, 1998. pp. 3337-3348
9. Carlsson R., Sjörgen H.O. Kinetics of IL-2 and Interferon-γ Production, Expression of IL-2 Receptors, and Cell Proliferation in Human Mononuclear Cells Exposed to Staphylococcal Enterotoxin A. Cellular Immunology, 1985. 96: pp. 175-183
10. Marrack P., Endres R., Shimonkevitz R., Zlotnick A., Dialynas D., Fitch F., Kappler J. 1993. The Major Histocompatibility Complex Restricted Antigen on T cells. II. Role of the L3T4 Product. The Journal of Experimental Medicine, 1993. 158: pp. 1077–1091
11. Greenstein J. L., Kappler, J., Marrack P., Burakoff S.J. The Role of the L3T4 in Recognition of Ia by a Cytotoxic H-2Dd-specific T cell Hybridoma. The Journal of Experimental Medicine, 1984.159: pp. 1213–1224
12. Dellabonna P., Peccoud J., Kappler J., Marrack P., Benoist C., Mathis D. Suprantigens Interact with MHC Class II Molecules Outside of the Antigen Groove. Cell, 1990. 62: pp. 1115-1121
13. Gascoigne N.R.J., Ames K.T. Direct Binding of Secreted T-cell Receptor Chain to Superantigen Associated with Class II Major Histocompatibility Complex Protein. Proceedings of the National Academy of Science United States of America, 1991. 88: pp. 613-616
14. Irwin M. J., Hudson K.R., Fraser J.D., Gascoigne N.R.J. 1992. Enterotoxin Residues Determining T-cell Receptor Vb Binding Specificity. Nature,1992. 359: pp. 841–843
15. Yagi J., Baron J., Buxser S., Janeway Jr C.A. 1990. Bacterial Proteins that Mediate the Association of a Defined Subset of T Cell Receptor: CD4 Complexes with Class II MHC. The Journal of Immunology, 1990. 144: pp. 892–901
16. Thomas R.J., Zhang L. Assessment of the Functional Regions of the Superantigen Staphylococcal Enterotoxin B. Toxins, 2013. 5: pp. 1859-1871
17. Yagi J., Uchiyama T., Janeway Jr C.A. 1994. Stimulator Cell Type Influences the Response of T Cells to Staphylococcal Enterotoxins. The Journal of Immunology, 1994. 152: pp. 1154–1162
18. Carlsson R., Fischer H., Sjögren H.O. Binding of Staphylococcal Enterotoxin A to Accessory Cells is a Requirement for its Ability to Activate Human T-cells. The Journal of Immunology, 1988. 140: pp. 2484-2488
19. Fleischer B., Schrezenmeier H. T-cell stimulation by Staphylococcal Enterotoxins. Clonally Variable Response and Requirement for Major Histochompatibility Complex II Molecules on Accessory or Target Cells. The Journal of Experimental Medicine, 1988. 167: pp. 1697-1708
20. Bavari S., Ulrich R.G. Staphylococcal Enterotoxin A and Toxic Shock Syndrome Toxin Compete with CD4 for Human Major Compatibility Complex Class II Binding. Infection and Immunity, 1995. 63: pp. 423-429
21. Stiles B.G., Bavari S., Krakauer T., Ulrich R.G. Toxicity of Staphylococcal Enterotoxins Potentiated by Lipopolysaccharide: Major Histocompatibility Complex Class II Molecule Dependency and Cytokine Release. Infection and Immunity, 1993. 61: pp. 5333-5338
22. Scheuber P. H., Denzlinger C., Wilker D., Beck G., Keppler D., Hammer D.K. 1987. Staphylococcal Enterotoxin B as a Nonimmunological Mast Cell Stimulus in Primates: the Role of Endogenous Cysteinyl Leukotrienes. International Archives of Allergy and Applied Immunology, 1987. 82: pp. 289-291
23. Marrack P., Kappler J. The Staphylococcal Enterotoxins and Their Relatives. Science,

1990. 248: pp. 705-717

24. Soriano J.M., Font G., Molto J.C., Mañes J. Enterotoxigenic Staphylococci and Their Toxins in Restaurant Foods. Trends in Food Scinece and Technology, 2002. 13: pp. 60-67

25. Franz D.R., Parrott C.D., Takafuji E.T. The U.S. Biological Warfare and Biological Defense Programs. Medical Aspects of Chemical and Biological Warfare. Chapter 32. Washington D.C.: Office of the Surgeon General Department of the Army, United States of America. 1997. 425-436

26. Alibek K. Biohazard. New York: Dell Publishing. 1999. pp. 233-234

27. The Center for Food Security & Public Health. Iowa State University. Staphylococcal Enterotoxin B. Revised January 2004. Retrieved December 24, 2009. Website: http://www.cfs ph.iastate.edu/Factsheets/pdfs/staphyloco ccal_enterotoxin_b.pdf

28. Do Carmo L.S., Cummings C., Linardi V.R., Dias R.S., dos Santos D.A., Shupp J.W., Peres Pereira R.K., Jett M. A Case Study of a Massive Staphylococcal Food Poisoning incident. Food Borne Pathogens and Disease, 2004. 1: pp. 241-246

29. Feig M. Staphylococcal Food Poisoning A Report of Two Related Outbreaks, and a Discussion of the Data Presented. American Journal of Public Health, 1950. 40: pp. 279-285

30. Do Carmo L.S., Dia R.S., Linardi V.R., de Sena M.J., dos Santos D.A. An Outbreak of Staphylococcal Food Poisoning in the Municipality of Passos, Mg, Brazil. Brazilian Archives of Biology and Technology, 2003. 46: pp. 581-586

31. Salyers A., Whitt D.D. Bacterial Pathogenesis: A Molecular Approach. Second Edition. Washington D.C.: American Society for Microbiology Press. 2002. pp. 216-231

32. Rajagopalan G., Sen M.M., Singh M., Murali N.S., Nath K.A., Iijima K., Kita H., Leontovich A.A., Gopinathan U., Patel R., David C.S. Intranasal Exposure to Staphylococcal Enterotoxin B Elicits an Acute Systemic Inflammatory Response. Shock, 2006. 25: pp. 647-656

33. Schlievert P.M. Staphylococcal Enterotoxin B and Toxic Shock Syndrome Toxic Shock Syndrome Toxin-1 are Significantly Associated with Non-menstrual TSS. Lancet, 1986. 1: pp. 1149-1150

34. Cook E., Wang X., Robiou N., Fries B.C. Measurement of Staphylococcal Enterotoxin B in Serum and Culture Supernatant with a Capture Enzyme-Linked Immunosorbent Assay. Clinical and Vaccine Immunology, 2007. 14: pp. 1094-1101

35. Bennett R.W. An Antibody Modified Automated Enzyme-linked Immunosorbant Assay-based Method for Detection of Staphylococcal Enterotoxin. Journal of Rapid Methods and Automation in Microbiology, 2008. 16: pp. 320-329

36. Andreotti P.E., Ludwig G.V., Peruski A.H., Tuite J.J., Morse S.S., Peruski L.F. Immunoassay of Infectious Agents. BioTechniques, 2003. 35: pp. 850-859

37. Henchal E.A., Teska J.D., Ludwig G.V., Shoemaker D.R., Ezzell J.W. 2001. Current Laboratory Methods for Biological Threat Agent Identification. Clinical Laboratory Medicine, 2001. 21: pp. 661-678

38. Peruski A.H., Peruski Jr L.F., 2003. Immunological Methods for Detection and Identification of Infectious Disease and Biological Warfare Agents. Clinical and Diagnostic Laboratory Immunology, 2003. 10: pp. 506-513

39. Bard A.J. Electrogenerated chemiluminescence. New York: Marcel Dekker Inc. 2004. pp. 381-396

40. Yang H., Leland J.K., Yost D., Massey R.J. Electrochemiluminescence: a New Diagnostic and Research Tool. ECL Detection Technology Promises Scientists New "Yardsticks" for Quantification. Biotechnology, 1994. 12: pp. 193-194

41. Fujikawa H., Igarashi H. Rapid Latex Agglutination Test for Detection of Staphylococcal Enterotoxins A to E That Uses High-Density Latex Particles. Applied and Environmental Microbiology, 1988. 54: pp. 2345-2348

42. Nedelkov D., Nelson R.W. Detection of Staphylococcal Enterotoxin B via Biomolecular Interaction Analysis Mass Spectrometry. Applied and Environmental Microbiology, 2003. 69: pp. 5212–5215

43. Shyu R-H., Tang S-S., Chiao D-J., Hung Y-W. Gold Nanoparticle-based Lateral Flow Assay for Detection of Staphylococcal Enterotoxin B. Food Chemistry, 2010. 118: pp. 462-466

44. Vo-Dinh T. Biomedical Photonics Handbook. Danvers: Chemical Rubber Company (CRC) Press. 2010. pp. 20-14-20-16

45. J.H. McIsaac. Hospital Preparation for Bioterror. A Medical and Biomedical System Approach. Burlington: Academic Press. 2006. pp. 58

Photo Bibliography

Figure 3.1-3: Colorized scanning electron photomicrograph of *Staphylococcus aureus* bacteria, shown outside a white blood cell. Electron photomicrograph was taken and released by the National Institute of Health, United States Department of Health and Human Services. Public domain photo

The trichothecene mycotoxin belongs to a diverse group of chemically related compounds made as secondary metabolites of fungi. Trichothecenes are mainly produced by species of organisms belonging to the genus *Fusarium*. Nonetheless, other fungal genera such as *Myrothecium, Spicellum, Verticimonosporium trichoderma, Stachybotrys* and *Cephalosporium* produce similar toxins. These trichothecene producing fungi are globally distributed and can be found in all environments (Figure 3.3-1).[1, 2]

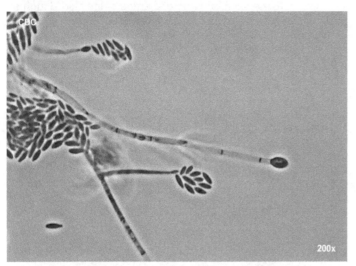

Figure 3.3-1: a photomicrograph of *Fusarium* spp. conidiophores

Trichothecene have a low molecular weight of 250 to 550 Da and are nonvolatile compounds. Trichothecene mycotoxins are a family of ~200 toxins that possess a common tricyclic 12,13-epoxytrichothec-9-ene (EPT) core structure.[3, 4, 5] Based on the substitution pattern of EPT, these toxins have been classified into four groups: types A, B, C and D. Types A, B and C, also known as simple trichothecenes can be differentiated based on the substitution at the C-8 position. For example, type A trichothecenes include toxins that has a hydroxyl group at C-8, an ester function at C-8 or no oxygen substitution at C-8. Type B trichothecenes generally possess a keto (carbonyl) function at C-8, although *Fusarium* type B trichothecenes typically have a hydroxyl group at the C-7 position. Type C trichothecenes have an epoxide located at the C-7/C-8 position, while type D trichothecenes, also known as macrocyclic trichothecenes, demonstrate an additional ring linking the C-4 and C-15 position. Although this classification system broadly differentiates the various forms of trichothecene mycotoxins, there are structural features that are not clearly defined with this arrangement. For example, all *Fusarium* trichothecenes possess either a hydroxyl or an acetyl group at the C-3 position, a characteristic not shared by toxins produced by organisms belonging to the genus *Trichoderma, Trichothecium, Myrothecium* or *Stachybotrys*.[5]

Mycotoxin T-2 is a highly toxic trichothecene produced by *Fusarium* species. This mycotoxin is believed to be the biological warfare agent used in numerous conflicts between the years of 1975 to 1984 (Figure 3.3-2). For example, during the years 1975 to 1981, it has been alleged that the Soviet Union supplied T-2 mycotoxin to the Lao People's Liberation Army and the North Vietnamese to be used against Hmong villagers and resistance forces.[6, 7, 8, 9, 10] Between 1979 to 1981, the Soviets were again accused of suppling mycotoxin to the North Vietnamese for

use against Khmer Rouge forces in Tuol Chrey, Kampuchea, Cambodia. Both alleged Laos and Kampuchea mycotoxin attacks have been described by eye witnesses as "yellow rain," which consisted of a shower of sticky yellow liquid and clouds of dust/powder or mists, which resonated like rain as it showered from the sky.[8, 9, 10, 11, 12] In Afghanistan (1979 to 1981), the Soviet Union and their Afghan allies were accused of using mycotoxin against the Mujahidin guerrillas.[8, 9, 13] These accusations and evidence of the use of a "yellow rain" by the Soviets were presented by Secretary of State Alexander M. Haig Jr. to United States Congress in 1982 in a report entitled Chemical Warfare in Southeast Asia and Afghanistan. Nonetheless, there are those in the scientific community who have challenged the accusations and stating that the "yellow rain" was nothing more than the fecal matter of honeybees dropped during their cleansing flights." [8, 14, 15] Unconfirmed reports implying that trichothecenes were used during the Egyptian attacks against Yemeni Royalists in Yemen, while Iraq has been accused of using the toxin during the 1983-1984 Iran-Iraq War.[8, 9, 16]

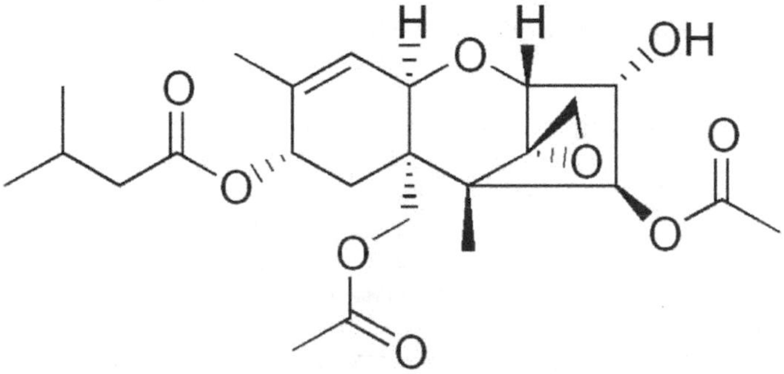

Figure 3.3-2: Molecular structre of T-2 mycotoxin. Note the olefinic bond ar C-9 and -10 and the epoxide group at C-12 and C-13

T-2 is considered to be primarily a blistering agent at lower exposure and concentrations, but can produce considerable incapacitation and death within minutes to hours at high concentrations. T-2 is easy to produce in mass quantities and can be delivered as dust, droplets or aerosolized form from aircrafts, rockets, artillery shells, mines or portable sprayers. At microgram (µg) amounts, T-2 can cause severe eye irritation, corneal damage and impaired vision.[1, 17, 18] At nanogram (ng) amounts, the T-2 can cause severe skin irritations, such as erythema, edema and necrosis, being about 400 times more potent than mustard agents.[1, 8, 19] It has been reported that the lethality of T-2 by aerosol exposure can be 10 to 50 times greater than introducing the toxin parenterally (e.g. through the skin or mucous membrane). It has been estimated that during an aerosolized attack, the LCt_{50} (the concentration and time that is lethal to 50% of the population exposed) is 200-5800 mg·min/m³. In addition, the lethality of T-2 via dermal route is estimated at LD_{50} (lethal dose to 50% of the population) 2 to 12 mg/kg.[19, 20, 21, 22]

Unlike other mycotoxins such as aflatoxin, T-2 does not require metabolic activation to exert its biological activities. Put simply, T-2 has the capability of direct interaction with eukaryotic cellular components. The lipophilic nature of T-2 allows it to be easily absorbed through the intestinal and pulmonary mucosa, where it rapidly enters systemic circulation and causes toxin-related toxicoses. Animal models have demonstrated that after exposure to high doses of aerosolized T-2, the creatures die without any apparent lung lesions or pulmonary edema.[20, 21, 22] By comparison to the absorption through the intestinal and pulmonary route, the absorption of T-2 via the integumentary system is relatively slow when it is in dust or powder form.[8, 23]

Once the toxin enters the individual, it immediately induces alterations in the membrane structure, which subsequently stimulates lipid peroxidation, causing excessive free radical damage in the liver, spleen, kidneys, thymus and bone marrow.[8, 24] Once T-2 crosses the plasma membrane of a cell, it immediately begins to interact with numerous targets including mitochondria and ribosomes.[5, 25, 26] Bin-Umer *et al.* (2011) reported that T-2 inhibited mitochondrial translation, as well as, a dose-dependent inhibition of mitochondrial membrane potential and reactive oxygen species. Additionally, T-2 prevents mitochondrial electron transport though the inhibition of succinate dehydrogenase (SDH) activity. SDH is a four subunit complex, also known as complex II. Complex II oxidizes succunate to form fumarate, while passing electrons to FAD, reducing it to $FDAH_2$.[8, 26, 27] At the ribosome, T-2 mycotoxin prevents the formation of peptide bonds at the peptidyl transferase center of the 60S ribosomal subunit. This inhibition manily affects polypeptide chain initiation and elongation, although some reports also suggest that T-2 mycotoxin also affects polypeptide chain termination. It has been calculated that inhibition of protein synthesis occurs approximately five minutes after exposure of Vero cells to T-2, with maximum response noted after 60 minutes. [5, 8, 25, 28, 29, 30, 31, 32, 33, 34]

Mycotoxins also possesses the ability to indirectly inhibit scheduled deoxyribonucleic acid (DNA) synthesis that occurs with rapidly proliferating tissues, such as the bone marrow, lymphoid tissues, skin, mucosal epithelia, and germ cells.[18] For example, in order to complete mitosis, cells require newly synthesized proteins, thereby allowing it to proceed from G_1 to S phase. By inhibiting protein synthesis, T-2 prevents the cell from completing replication.[34, 35, 36] It has also been reported that T-2 has a minor effect on ribonucleic acid (RNA) synthesis, which is believed to be a secondary effect of protein synthesis inhibition.[28]

SYMPTOMS

During T-2 mycotoxin exposure, the toxin can adhere to the skin, where it slowly penetrates. Clothing on an individual exposed to T-2 would be contaminated and serve as a reservoir for further toxin exposure. Additionally, T-2 could also be inhaled and enter through the respiratory tract and/or ingested and enter through the digestive tract.[8]

The degree of illness exhibited because of T-2 mycotoxin intoxication is affected by the route of exposure, as well as, the status of an individual's nutrition and health. For instance, previous liver damage, intestinal infections and stress could exacerbate the symptoms. Indications of T-2 intoxication can vary depending on acute or chronic exposure. The acute exposure occurs through a purposeful biological attack, where massive amounts of mycotoxin are delivered into a preselected area. Chronic exposure generally results from multiple exposures to subacute doses of mycotoxin. Chronic intoxications can occur naturally or when repeated subacute doses of mycotoxin are administered intravenously as chemotherapy to treat colon adenocarcinoma.[8]

Irrespective of the route of exposure to T-2 mycotoxin, certain symptoms remain consistent. For example, through all routes of exposure gastric and intestinal lesions will be present. In addition, exposed individuals will suffer from hematopoietic and immunosuppressive effects, similar to the symptoms experienced by individuals suffering from radiation poisoning. Toxic effects to the central nervous system will cause anorexia, lassitude, nausea, suppression of reproductive organ functions and acute vascular effects leading to hypotension and shock.[20, 21, 22, 38, 39, 40, 41]

Dermal exposure to the mycotoxin will result in local cutaneous necrosis and inflammation. Early symptoms on the areas of the skin that were exposed may begin within minutes. These symptoms include burning skin pain, redness, tenderness, swellings and severe itching of undamaged skin (pruritic). Subsequently, small to large vesicles and bullae (blisters) may form in combination with petechiae and ecchymoses of the exposed area. Soon after, black and leathery areas of necrosis may appear. It has been reported that after the individual has succumbed to the toxin, the necrotic areas of the skin slough off easily when the corpse is moved.[8, 42] Cutaneous contamination of the skin with T-2 mycotoxin may result in systemic infections (Table 1).

Table 1: An overview of the clinical symptoms of dermal exposure of mycotoxin

Symptoms	+	++	+++
Local skin necrosis			■
Local inflammation (skin)			■
Burning skin pain			■
Redness			■
Tenderness			■
Swellings			■
Pruritic			■
Bullae formation			■
Petechiae			■
Ecchymoses			■
Severe nausea			■
Vomiting			■
Lethargy			■
Weakness			■
Dizziness			■
Loss of coordination			■
Diarrhea (watery)			■
Diarrhea (bloody)			■
Dyspnea			■
Coughing			■
Sore mouth			■
Bleeding gums			■
Epistaxis			■
Hematemesis			■
Abdominal pain			■
Central chest pain			■
Anorexia			■
Dehydration			■
Hypothermic			■
Hypotensive			■
Tachycardia			■
Blood oozing from mouth			■
Oozing blood from nares			■
Tremors			■
Seizures			■
Coma			■

+ Rare ++ Common +++ Frequent

Subacute ingestion of trichothecene mycotoxin will result in systemic infections. Ingesting T-2 mycotoxin will result in a chronic condition known as atoxic alimentary aleukia, consisting of gastric and intestinal mucosa inflammation. This condition may progress into leucopenia, with progressive lymphocytosis and bleeding diathesis, depending on the quantity of toxins ingested.[43, 44]

In animal models (chickens), the ingestion of acute amounts

of T-2 mycotoxin will initially result in lesions to the upper gastrointestinal tract followed by asthenia, inappetence, diarrhea and panting. At higher doses of T-2 toxin, these animals will proceed into coma, while death occurs within 48 hours after exposure.[43, 44] In guinea pigs, an acute dose of T-2 resulted in lethargy and death within 48 hours. Postmortem examinations showed gastric and cecal hyperemia with watery-fluid distension of the cecum and edematous intestinal lymphoid tissue. Histological examination showed necrosis and ulceration of the gastrointestinal tract (Table 2).[45, 46]

Table 2: An overview of the clinical symptoms of subacute ingestion of mycotoxin

Symptoms	+	++	+++
Gastric inflammation			■
Intestinal inflammation			■
Leucopenia			■
Lymphocytosis			■
Bleeding diathesis			■
Severe nausea			■
Vomiting			■
Lethargy			■
Weakness			■
Dizziness			■
Loss of coordination			■
Diarrhea (watery)			■
Diarrhea (bloody)			■
Dyspnea			■
Coughing			■
Sore mouth			■
Bleeding gums			■
Epistaxis			■
Hematemesis			■
Abdominal pain			■
Central chest pain			■
Anorexia			■
Dehydration			■
Hypothermic			■
Hypotensive			■
Tachycardia			■
Blood oozing from mouth			■
Oozing blood from nares			■
Tremors			■
Seizures			■
Coma			■

+ Rare ++ Common +++ Frequent

Subacute doses of trichothecene induces chronic symptoms of upper respiratory tract, which includes nasal itching, burning, pain and bleeding, as well as, flu-like symptoms including non-productive coughing, sneezing, epistaxis and rhinorrhea. Other symptoms include sore throat, headache, general malaise dyspnea, wheezing, fatigue, dermatitis and intermittent focal alopecia.[47, 48] Acute aerosolized doses of T-2 (2.4 mg/L) in animal models result in signs of prostration, while fatalities occur within 18 hours. At lower acute aerosolized doses, 0.24 mg/L, the animals became lethargic, prostrate and died within 30 to 48 hours. However, postmortem examinations did not demonstrate any significant lesions in the respiratory tracts, although histological examinations showed microscopic lesions in the lymphoid system and intestinal tract (Table 3).[20, 21, 22]

Intoxication through the skin, gastrointestinal or respiratory tract may result in other early systemic symptoms. These symptoms include severe nausea, vomiting, lethargy, weakness, dizziness and loss of coordination. Depending on the individual, diarrhea may appear within minutes to hours. Diarrhea will at first appear watery brown then turn grossly bloody. Within 3 to 12 hours,

dyspnea, coughing, sore mouth, bleeding gums, epistaxis, hematemesis, abdominal pain and central chest pains may also occur. During the later course of intoxication, marked anorexia and dehydration are frequently observed. Dying patients will become hypothermic and hypotensive. Tachycardia is a common sign at this later stage of intoxication. In addition, bloody ooze from the nares and mouth, as well as, the passage of a maroon colored stool, marking the sign of hematochezia, will also appear. Death may occur in minutes, hours or days, and is commonly preceded by tremors, seizures and coma.[8, 49, 50, 51]

Table 3: An overview of the clinical symptoms of subacute inhalation of mycotoxin

Symptoms	Rare	Common	Frequent
Nasal itching			■
Nasal burning			■
Nasal pain			■
Non-productive cough			■
Sneezing			■
Epistaxis			■
Rhinorrhea			■
Sore throat			■
Headaches			■
Dyspnea			■
Wheezing			■
Fatigue			■
Dermatitis			■
Intermit. focal alopecia			■
General malaise			■
Severe nausea			■
Vomiting			■
Lethargy			■
Weakness			■
Dizziness			■
Loss of coordination			■
Diarrhea (watery)			■
Diarrhea (bloody)			■
Sore mouth			■
Bleeding gums			■
Hematemesis			■
Abdominal pain			■
Central chest pain			■
Anorexia			■
Dehydration			■
Hypothermic			■
Hypotensive			■
Tachycardia			■
Blood oozing from mouth			■
Oozing blood from nares			■
Tremors			■
Seizures			■
Coma			■
Tearing			■
Eye pain			■
Conjunctivitis			■
Photophobia			■
Decrease vision acuity			■

+ Rare ++ Common +++ Frequent

▨ Ocular exposure

Ocular exposure will result in tearing, eye pain, conjunctivitis and blurred vision. In rat models, the administration of low doses of T-2 toxin (1 μg) into the eyes, corneal irregularities developed within 12 to 24 hours, and it is thought that this condition may result in photophobia and decreased vision acuity. Histological examination of the rat cornea showed extreme thinning of the corneal epithelium which may be irreversible. At higher doses, rats displayed scleral, and conjunctival vasodilation and inflammation, which lasted up to 6 months. There are no reports of systemic toxicity via ocular exposure of T-2 toxin.[8, 45, 50]

DETECTION

Diagnosis of T-2 intoxication is primarily based on clinical observations; nonetheless, confirmation of such intoxication is through epidemiologic assays of tissue, body fluids or examination of environmental samples. Early symptoms of an aerosolized exposure to T-2 would greatly depend upon the particle size. For example, for large particles (>10 µm), similar to those of "yellow rain", early symptoms will include rhinorrhea, sore throat, dyspnea, blurred vision, vomiting, diarrhea and the burning and itching of skin. During a small particle (1 to 4 µm) attack, which would result in deep respiratory tract exposure, the early symptoms will likely include vomiting, diarrhea, skin irritation, and blurred vision. The later symptoms for both large-particle and deep respiratory tract aerosol exposure are similar. These symptoms include fever, chills, hypotension, nausea, vomiting, diarrhea, burning erythema, skin rash, blisters, confusion, ataxia and bleeding.[8, 45]

Analysis of blood and serum may aid in the diagnosis of T-2 intoxication. Although, there are no records of humans suffering from acute T-2 intoxication, experimental models involving lesser primates have demonstrated non-specific changes in serum chemistry and hematology. For example, intoxicated monkeys have presented elevated serum creatinine, serum enzymes (e.g. creatine kinase), serum amino acid levels and elevated electrolyte levels such as potassium and phosphorous. An initial increase in the number of neutrophils and lymphocytes may occur early in the intoxication followed by a decrease in lymphocytes within 48 hours. It has been reported that experimental animals that managed to survive beyond several days may demonstrate a decrease in all blood cellular elements.[19]

Specific and rapid diagnosis of T-2 mycotoxin is presently not available in the field. All testing (e.g. blood, serum and urine) needs to be performed in a laboratory for antigen detection. It has been reported that T-2 toxin is readily metabolized by microflora of the guts of mammals to several metabolites and that 50-75% of mycotoxins and its metabolites are eliminated in the urine and feces within 24 hours. Nonetheless, metabolites can still be detected as late as 28 days after exposure.[8, 45, 49, 52] Screens for T-2 mycotoxin include thin-layer chroma-tography (TLC) and cytotoxic assays.[53, 54] TLC is the most commonly used physicochemical test and is based on the separation of compounds by how far they migrate on a specific matrix with a specific solvent. The distance that a compound will travel is the unique identifier for that compound, whereby a retention factor (Rf) has been determined for most mycotoxins.[52]

Mycotoxin T-2 is not immunogenic and will not stimulate antibody production by the infected individual. Nonetheless, both

Table 4: Differential diagnosis of dermal exposure to T-2 mycotoxin. This differential diagnosis should include radiation poisoning, exposure to lewisite, mustard gas (MG), staphylococcal enterotoxin B (SEB) and ricin poisoning

Symptoms	T2	Radiation	Lewisite	MG	SEB	Ricin
Local skin necrosis	■	■	■	■		
Local inflammation (skin)	■	■	■	■		
Burning skin pain	■	■	■	■		
Redness	■	■	■	■		
Tenderness	■	■	■	■		
Swellings	■	■	■	■		
Pruritic	■	■	■	■		
Bullae formation	■	■	■	■		
Petechiae	■		■			
Ecchymoses	■		■			
Severe nausea	■	■		■	■	■
Vomiting	■	■		■	■	■
Lethargy	■	■				
Weakness	■	■			■	■
Dizziness	■	■			■	
Loss of coordination	■	■				
Diarrhea (watery)	■		■	■	■	■
Diarrhea (bloody)	■	■		■	■	
Dyspnea	■			■	■	
Coughing	■		■	■	■	
Sore mouth	■					
Bleeding gums	■	■				
Epistaxis	■		■	■		
Hematemesis	■				■	■
Abdominal pain	■				■	■
Central chest pain	■				■	
Anorexia	■					
Dehydration	■					
Hypothermic	■					
Hypotensive	■				■	■
Tachycardia	■					■
Blood oozing from mouth	■		■	■		
Oozing blood from nares	■		■	■		
Tremors	■	■				
Seizures	■	■				
Coma	■					

monoclonal and polyclonal antibodies have been created for T-2 to be used in ELISA radioimmunological assay and immuno-affinity chromatography (IAC).[52, 55, 56, 57] Pathology specimens, including blood, urine, lung, liver, and stomach contents, as well as, environmental samples can be tested using gas-liquid chromatography (GLC), high performance liquid chromatography (HPLC) and mass spectrometry (MS). GLC and HPLC are the most common methods used for identifying mycotoxins in both biomedical samples and agricultural products. Detection limits for trichothecene mycotoxins are 10 ppb; this is limited to a presumptive analysis of an unknown sample. MS is the physicochemical method of choice for definitive identification of trichothecene mycotoxins. Nonetheless, time consuming and extensive cleanup is needed for GLC, HPLC and MS methodologies after the tests are completed.[8, 45]

A combination of GLC and MS (MLC-MS) technique has been used to specifically identify mycotoxins. This methodology has been reported to be able to detect as little as 1 ppb of T-2 toxin without extensive cleanup. A combination of HPLC and MS (HPLC-MS) techniques have also been devised and proven to be a reliable and specific method for identifying T-2. This methodology has been reported to achieve a sensitivity of 0.1 ppb, without extensive cleanup.[52, 58, 59, 60]

Recently, an immunochip have been developed for quantifying the concentrations of T-2 mycotoxin, as well as, 5 other mycotoxins: aflatoxin B1, aflatoxin M1, deoxynivalenol, ochratoxin A and zearalenone. The complete antigens of mycotoxins were contact printed onto agarose-modified glass slides with 12 physically isolated subarrays, based on the reaction of both diffusion and covalent bond. Wang et al. (2012) reported that all six mycotoxin were successfully detected within four hours using only minimal samples. However, a commercial version of this immunochip is presently unavailable.[61]

TREATMENT

Presently there is no specific therapy, antidote and/or vaccine designed for T-2 mycotoxin intoxication; only supportive therapy and direct treatment of symptoms are available. Nonetheless, therapeutic approaches using animal models have demonstrated reduced mortality rates for T2 exposure.[8, 45]

Subsequent to an aerosolized exposure, mycotoxins may still be trapped within the nose, throat, upper respiratory tract and have the potential to be swallowed via cilliary action, potentially increasing the chances of systemic infection. Superactive charcoal absorbs swallowed T-2 and has been effective in treating mice within an hour of exposure.[62]

Irrigation of the eyes with large volumes of isotonic saline solution may aid in mechanically removing T-2 mycotoxin, but may not prevent ocular damage. Detailed ophthalmological evaluation for corneal lesions and appropriate treatment needs to be administered to prevent loss of vision, secondary infection and the development of posterior synechie. The skin of the individual will need to be decontaminated, generally done through washing with soap and water within 12 hours of exposure. Careful washing will reduce the blistering effects of the toxin but will not prevent mild dermal irritations. Calamine and other lotions and creams may help to alleviate the itching and burning symptoms of the exposed skin.[8, 45]

One of the main concerns of aerosolized dissemination of T-2 mycotoxin is respiratory irritations. These symptoms include

Table 5: Differential diagnosis of subacute ingestion of T-2 mycotoxin. This differential diagnosis should include radiation poisoning, exposure to lewisite, mustard gas (MG), staphylococcal enterotoxin B (SEB) and ricin poisoning

Symptoms	T2	Radiation	Lewisite	MG	SEB	Ricin
Gastric/intestinal inflammation	■					
Leucopenia	■					
Lymphocytosis	■					
Bleeding diathesis	■	■				
Severe nausea	■	■	■	■	■	■
Vomiting	■	■	■	■	■	■
Lethargy	■	■				
Weakness	■				■	■
Dizziness	■	■			■	
Loss of coordination	■	■				
Diarrhea (watery)	■	■	■	■	■	■
Diarrhea (bloody)	■	■		■	■	
Dyspnea	■			■	■	
Coughing	■		■	■	■	
Sore mouth	■					
Bleeding gums	■	■				
Epistaxis	■		■	■		
Hematemesis	■		■		■	■
Abdominal pain	■				■	■
Central chest pain	■				■	
Anorexia	■				■	
Dehydration	■					
Hypothermic	■					
Hypotensive	■		■		■	■
Tachycardia	■					■
Blood oozing from mouth	■		■			
Oozing blood from nares	■		■			
Tremors	■	■				
Seizures	■	■				
Coma	■					

Table 6: Differential diagnosis of subacute inhalation of T-2 mycotoxin. This differential diagnosis should include radiation poisoning, exposure to lewisite, mustard gas (MG), staphylococcal enterotoxin B (SEB) and ricin poisoning

Symptoms	T2	Radiation	Lewisite	MG	SEB	Ricin
Nasal itching	■		■	■		
Nasal burning	■		■	■		
Nasal pain	■		■	■		
Non-productive cough	■		■	■	■	
Sneezing	■					
Epistaxis	■	■	■			
Rhinorrhea	■		■	■		
Sore throat	■					
Headaches	■	■				■
Dyspnea	■			■	■	
Wheezing	■		■	■		
Fatigue	■	■				
Dermatitis	■					
Intermit. focal alopecia	■					
General malaise	■					
Severe nausea	■	■	■	■	■	■
Vomiting	■	■	■	■	■	■
Lethargy	■	■				
Weakness	■	■			■	■
Dizziness	■	■			■	
Loss of coordination	■					
Diarrhea (watery)	■	■	■	■	■	■
Diarrhea (bloody)	■	■		■		
Sore mouth	■					
Bleeding gums	■	■				
Hematemesis	■				■	■
Abdominal pain	■				■	■
Central chest pain	■				■	
Anorexia	■				■	
Dehydration	■					
Hypothermic	■					
Hypotensive	■		■		■	■
Tachycardia	■					■
Blood oozing from mouth	■		■	■		
Oozing blood from nares	■		■	■		
Tremors	■	■				
Seizures	■	■				
Coma	■					
Tearing	■		■	■		
Eye pain	■		■	■		
Conjunctivitis	■		■	■		
Photophobia	■		■	■		
Decrease vision acuity	■		■	■		

sore throat, hoarseness and a non-productive cough, which may be alleviated through steam inhalation, codeine, or cough suppressants, etc. Severe respiratory cases may require endotracheal intubation with positive pressure ventilation.[8, 45]

Bone marrow and rapidly diving cells are the first targets of mycotoxin. Theoretically, clinicians can administer granulocyte-stimulating factor to counteract the toxins effects. Again in animal models, the early use of high doses of systemic glucocorticosterioids has shown to increase the survival rate in trials. In addition, dosing animals before and after subcutaneous exposure to the toxin with diphenhydramine or naloxone has also shown to reduce the mortality rates. Finally, the treatment of experimental animals with methylthiazolidine-4-carboxylate has shown to have detoxification effects for the mycotoxin.[8, 45, 63, 64, 65]

DIFFERENTIAL DIAGNOSIS

Mycotoxin T-2 intoxication should be considered when multiple patients demonstrate similar clinical symptoms, especially when reports of "yellow rain" or if droplets of yellow fluid contaminate clothing or the environment. The differential Diagnosis of mycotoxin intoxification should include radiation poisoning, exposure to lewisite, mustard gas, staphylococcal enterotoxin B and ricin poisoning.[66, 67, 68, 69] Please examine Table 4 for the differential diagnosis of dermal exposure to T-2 mycotoxin, Table 5 for the differential diagnosis of subacute ingestion of T-2 mycotoxin and 6 for the differential diagnosis of subacute inhalation of T-2 mycotoxin.

References

1. Ueno T. Trichothecene Mycotoxins: Mycology, Cheistry, and Toxicology. Advanced Nutritional Research, 1989. 3: pp. 301-353
2. Desjardins A.E. Fusarium Mycotoxins Chemistry, Genetics and Biology. Eagan: American Phytopathological Society (APS) Press. 2006. pp. 1-260
3. Godtfredsen W.O., Grove J.F., Tamm C.H. Trichothecenes. Helvetica Chimica Acta, 1967. 50: pp. 1666-1668
4. Ciegler A. Trichothecenes: Occurrence and Toxicoses. Journal of Food Protection, 1978. 41: pp. 399-403
5. McCormick S.P., Stanley A.M., Stover N.A., Alexander N.J. Trichothecenes: From Simple to Complex Mycotoxins. Toxins, 2011. 3: pp. 802-814
6. Mirocha C.J. Hazards of Scientific Investigation: Analysis of Samples Implicated in Biological Warfare. Journal of Toxicology-Toxin Reviews. 1982. 1: pp. 199-203
7. Rosen R.T., Rosen J.D. Presence of Four Fusarium mycotoxin and Synthetic Material

in "Yellow Rain": Evidence for the Use of Chemical Weapons in Laos. Biomedical Mass Spectrometry, 1982. 9: pp. 443-450
8. Wannemacher R.W., Weiner S.L. Trichothecene Mycotoxins. Medical Aspects of Chemical and Biological Warfare. Chapter 34. Washington D.C.: Office of the Surgeon General Department of the Army, United States of America. 1997. pp. 655-676
9. Smart J.K. The U.S. Biological Warfare and Biological Defense Programs. Medical Aspects of Chemical and Biological Warfare. Chapter 2. Washington D.C.: Office of the Surgeon General Department of the Army, United States of America. 1997. pp. 9-86
10. Eitzen E.M., Takafuji E.T. Historical Overview of Biological Warfare. Medical Aspects of Biological Warfare. Chapter 18. Washington D.C.: The Surgeon General United States Army Medical Department Medical Center and School Borden Institute. 2007. pp. 415-423
11. Tucker J.B. The "Yellow Rain" Controversy: Lessens for Arms Control Compliance. The Nonproliferation Review, 2001. pp. 25-42
12. Ember L.R. Yellow Rain. Chemical and Engineering News, 1984. 62: pp. 8-34
13. Agarwal R., Shukla S.K., Dharmani S., Gandhi A. Biological Warfare – an Emerging Threat. Journal of Association of Physicians of India, 2004. 52: pp. 733-738
14. Haig Jr A.M. Chemical Warfare in Southeast Asia and Afghanistan. Report to the Congress from Secretary of State. Washington D.C.: United States Department of State, Bureau of Public Affairs, Office of Public Communication, Editorial Division. March 22, 1982. pp. 31
15. Robinson J., Guillemin J., Meselson M. Yellow Rain: The Story Collapses. Foreign Policy, 1987. 68: pp. 101–117
16. Ember L.R., Sorenson W.G., Lewis D.M. Charges of Toxic Arms Use by Iraq Escalate. Chemical and Engineering News, 1984. 62: pp. 16-18
17. Watson S.A., Mirocha C.J., Hayes A.W. Analysis for Trichothecenes in Samples from Southeast Asia Associated with "Yellow Rain." Fundamental and Applied Toxicology, 1984. 4: pp. 700-717
18. Stahl C.J., Green C.C., Farnum J.B. The Incident at Tuol Chrey: Pathological and Toxicological Examination of a Casualty after Chemical Attack. Journal of Forensic Science, 1985. 30: pp. 317-337
19. Wannemacher Jr R.W., Bunner D.L., Neufeld H.A. Toxicity of Trichothecenes and Other Related Mycotoxins in Laboratory Animals. Mycotoxins and Animal Foods. Boca Raton: Chemical and Rubber Company (CRC) Press. 1991. pp. 499-552
20. Creasia D.A., Thurman J.D., Wannemacher Jr R.W., Bunner D.L. Acute Inhalation Toxicity of T-2 Mycotoxin in the Rat and Guinea Pig. Fundamental and Applied Toxicology, 1990. 14: pp. 54–59
21. Marrs T.C., Edginton J.A., Price P.N., Upshall D.G. Acute Toxicity of T2 Mycotoxin to the Guinea-pig by Inhalation and Subcutaneous Routes. British Journal of Experimental Pathology, 1986. 67: pp. 259–268
22. Creasia DA, Thurman JD, Jones III LJ, Nealley M.L., York C.G., Wannemacher Jr R.W., Bunner D.L. Acute Inhalation Toxicity of T-2 Mycotoxin in Mice. Fundamental and Applied Toxicology, 1987. 8: pp. 230–235
23. Kemppainen B.W., Riley R.T. Penetration of [3H] T-2 Toxin through Excised Human and Guinea-pig Skin during Exposure to [3H] T-2 Toxin Adsorbed to Corn Dust. Food and Chemical Toxicology, 1984. 22: pp. 893–896
24. Suneja S.K., Wagle D.S., Ram G.C. Effect of Oral Administration of T-2 Toxin on Glutathione Shuttle Enzymes, Microsomal Reductase and Lipid Peroxidation in Rat Liver. Toxicon, 1989. 27: pp. 995–1001
25. McLaughlin C.S., Vaughan M.H., Campbell I.M., Wei C.M., Stafford M.E., Hansen B.S. Inhibition of Protein Synthesis by Trichothecenes. Mycotoxins in Human and Animal Health. Park Forest South: Pathotox Publishers. 1977. pp. 263–275
26. Pace J.G., Watts M.R., Canterbury W.J. T-2 Mycotoxin Inhibits Mitochondrial Protein Synthesis. Toxicon, 1988. 26: pp. 77–85
27. Bin-Umer M.A., McLaughlin J.E., Basu D., McCormick S., Tumer N.E. Trichothecene Mycotoxins Inhibit Mitochondrial Translation—Implication for the Mechanism of Toxicity. Toxins, 2011. 3: pp. 1484–1501
28. Cannon M., Smith K.E., Carter C.J. Prevention by Ribosome-bound Nascent Polyphenylalanine Chains of the Functional Interaction of T-2 toxin with its Receptor Site. Biochemical Journal, 1976. 156:289–294
29. Wei C.M., McLaughlin C.S. Structure-function Relationship in the 12,13-epoxytrichothecenes. Novel Inhibitors of Protein Synthesis. Biochemical and Biophysical Reseach Communications, 1974. 57: pp. 838–844
30. Tate W.P., Caskey C.T. Peptidyltransferase Inhibition by Trichodermin. Journal of Biological Chemistry, 1973. 248: pp. 7970–7972
31. Thompson W.L., Wannemacher Jr R.W. Detection and Quantitation of T-2 Mycotoxin with a Simplified Protein Synthesis Inhibition Assay. Applied and Environmental Microbiology, 1984. 48: pp. 1176–1180
32. Yoshizawa T., Morooka N. Trichothecenes from Mold Infested Cereals in Japan. Mycotoxins in Human and Animal Health. Park Forest South: Pathotox Publishers. 1977. pp. 309–321
33. Feinberg B., McLaughlin C.S. Biochemical Mechanism of Action of Trichothecene Mycotoxins. Trichothecene Mycotoxicoses: Pathophysiologic Effect. Volume I. Boca Raton: Chemical and Rubber Company (CRC) Press. 1991. pp. 27-35
34. Bennett J.W., Klich M., Mycotoxins. Clinical Microbiology Reviews, 2003. 16: pp. 497-516
35. Rosenstein Y., Lafarge-Frayssinet C. Inhibitory Effect of Fusarium T2-toxin on Lymphoid DNA and Protein Synthesis. Toxicology and Applied Pharmacology, 1983. 70: pp. 283–288
36. Suneja S.K., Ram G.C., Wagle D.S. Effects of Feeding T-2 toxin on RNA, DNA and Protein Contents of Liver and Intestinal Mucosa of Rats. Toxicology Letters, 1983. 18: pp. 73–76
37. Thompson W.L., Wannemacher Jr R.W. In vivo Effects of T-2 Mycotoxin on Synthesis of Proteins and DNA in Rat Tissues. Toxicology and Applied Pharmacology, 1990. 105: pp. 483–491
38. Sharma R.P., Kim Y-W. Trichothecenes. Mycotoxins and Phytoalexins. Boca Raton: Chemical and Rubber Company (CRC) Press. 1991. pp. 339–359
39. Pang V.F., Felsburg P.J., Beasley V.R., Buck W.B., Haschek W.M. Experimental T-2 Toxicosis in Swine following Topical Application: Effect on Hematology, Serum Biochemistry and Immune Response. Fundamental and Applied Toxicology, 1987. 9: pp. 50–59
40. Lundeen G.R., Poppenga R.H., Beasley V.R., Buck W.B., Tranquilli W.J., Lambert R.J. Systemic Distribution of Blood Flow during T-2 Toxin Induced Shock in Swine. Fundamental and Applied Toxicology, 1986. 7: pp. 309–323
41. Beasley V.R., Lundeen G.R., Poppenga R.H., Buck W.B. Distribution of Blood Flow to the Gastrointestinal Tract of Swine during T-2 toxin-induced Shock. Fundamental and Applied Toxicology, 1987. 9: pp. 588–594
42. Bamburg J.R., Strong F.M. 12,13-Epoxytrichothecenes. Microbial Toxins. Volume VII. New York: Academic Press. 1971. pp. 207–292
43. Chi M.S., Mirocha C.J., Kurtz H.J., Weaver G., Bates F., Shimoda W., Burmeister H.R. Acute Toxicity of T-2 Toxin in Broiler Chicks and Laying Hens. Poultry Science, 1977. 56: pp. 103–116
44. Hoerr F.J., Carlton EW.W., Tuite J., Vesonder R.F., Rohwedder W.K., Szigett G. Experimental Trichothecene Mycotoxicosis Produced in Boiler Chickens by Fusarium sporotrichiella var sporotrichioides. Avian Pathology, 1982. 11: pp. 385-405
45. Huebner K.D., Wannemacher R.W., Stiles B.G., Popoff M.R., Poli M.A. Additional Toxins of Clinical Concern. Medical Aspect of Biological Warfare. Chapter 17. Washington D.C.: Office of the Surgeon General Department of the Army, United States of America. 2007. pp. 355-389
46. DeNicola D.B., Rebar A.H., Cartlow W.W., Yagen B. T-2 Toxin Mycotoxicosis in the Guinea Pig. Food and Cosmetics Toxicology, 1978. 16: pp. 601–609
47. Hintikka E-L. Stachybotryotoxicosis as a Veterinary Problem. Mycotoxins in Human and Animal Health. Park Forest South: Pathotox Publishers Inc. 1977. pp. 277–284
48. Eppley R.M. Chemistry of Stachybotryotoxicosis. Mycotoxins in Human and Animal Health. Park Forest South: Pathotox Publishers Inc. 1977. pp. 285–293
49. Darling R.G., Woods, J.B. USAMRIID's Medical Management of Biological Casulties Handbook. Fifth Edition. Fort Detrick: US Army Medical Research Institute of Infectious Diseases, 2004. pp. 96-99
50. Freeman G.G. Further Biological Properties of Trichothecin, an Antifungal Substance from Tichothecium roseum Link, and its Derivatives. Journal of General Microbiology, 1955. 12: pp. 213–221
51. McIsaac J.H. Preparing Hospitals for Bioterror: a Medical and Biomedical Systems Approach. Burlington: Elsevier. 2006. pp. 59
52. Muro-Cacho C.A., Stedeford T., Banasik M., Suchecki T.T., Persad A.S. Mycotoxins: Mechanisms of toxicity and methods of detection for identifying exposed individuals. Journal of Land Use, 2004. 19: pp. 537-545
53. Robb J., Norval M. Comparison of Cytotoxicity and Thin-Layer Chromatography Methods for Detection of Mycotoxins. Applied and Environmental Microbiology, 1983. 46: pp. 948-950
54. Chu F.S. Detection and Determination of Mycotoxins. Mycotoxins and Phytoalexins. Boca Raton: Chemical and Rubber Company (CRC) Press, 1991. pp. 33–79
55. Fan T.S.L., Zhang G.S., Chu F.S. An Indirect Enzyme-linked Immunosorbent Assay for T-2 Toxin in Biological Fluids. Journal of Food Protection, 1984. 47: pp. 964–967
56. Rivers D.B., Coleman D.R. Development of a Direct ELISA for Anti-T-2 Toxin Immunoglobulin G. Biotechnology Techniques, 1987. 1: pp. 275-278
57. Candlish A.A.G., Smith J.E., Stimson W.H. Monoclonal Antibody Technology for Mycotoxin. Biotechnology Advances, 1989. 7: pp. 401-418
58. Mirocha C.J., Panthre S.V., Pawlosky R.J., Hewetson D.W. Mass Spectra of Selected Trichothecenes. Modern Methods in the Analysis and Structure Elucidation of Mycotoxins. New York: Academic Press. 1986. pp. 353–392
59. Vesonder R.F., Rohwedder W.K. Gas Chromatographic-mass Spectrometric Analysis of Mycotoxins. Modern Methods in the Analysis and Structure Elucidation of Mycotoxins. New York: Academic Press. 1986. pp. 335–352
60. Kostiainen R., Matsuura K., Nojima K. Identification of Trichothecenes by Frit-fast Atom Bombardment Liquid Chromatography High-resolution Mass spectrometry. Journal of Chromatography, 1991. 538: pp. 323–330
61. Wang Y., Liu N., Ning B., Liu M., Lv Z., Sun Z., Peng Y., Chen C., Li J., Gao Z. Simultaneous and rapid detection of six different mycotoxins using an immunochip. Biosensors and Bioelectronics, 2012. 34: pp. 44-50
62. Fricke R.F., Jorge J. Assessment of Efficacy of Activated Charcoal for Treatment of Acute T-2 Toxin Poisoning. Journal of Toxicology - Clinical Toxicology, 1990. 28: pp. 421–431
63. Shohami E., Wisotsky B., Kempski O., Feuerstein G. Therapeutic Effect of Dexamethasone in T-2 Toxicosis. Pharmacologic Researchm 1987. 4: pp. 527–530
64. Ryu J., Shiraki N., Ueno Y. Effects of Drugs and Metabolic Inhibitors on the Acute Toxicity of T-2 toxin in Mice. Toxicon, 1987. 25: pp. 743–750
65. Fricke R.F., Jorge J. Methylthiazolidine-4-carboxylate for Treatment of Acute T-2 Toxin Exposure. Journal of Applied Toxicology, 1991. 11: pp. 135–140
66. J.H. McIsaac. Hospital Preparation for Bioterror. A Medical and Biomedical System Approach. Burlington: Academic Press. 2006. pp. 59
67. Trichothecene Mycotoxin (T2) Information for Professionals. Texas Department of State Health Services. Retrieved December 14, 2011. Website: www.dshs.state.tx.us/preparedness/factsheet_T2_pro.pdf
68. T-2 Mycotoxicosis. Division of Environmental Health and Communicable Disease Prevention. Missouri Department of Health and Senior Serviecs Communicable Disease Investigation Reference Manual. Retrieved December 14, 2011. Website: http://health.mo.gov/living/healthcon diseases/communicable/communicabledisease/cdmanual/pdf/T2_sec.pdf
69. Hurst C.G., Petrali J.P., Barillo D.J., Graham J.S., Smith W.J., Urbanetti J.S., Sidell F.R. Vesicants Medical Aspects of Chemical Warfare. Chapter 8. Washington D.C.: The Surgeon General United States Army Medical Department Medical Center and School Borden Institute. 2007. pp. 259-309

Photo Bibliography

Figure 3.3-1: A photomicrograph of *Trichoderma* spp. conidiophores. The photograph was taken at 200x magnification and released by the CDC. Public domain photo

In the United States, agriculture contributes over one trillion dollars a year to the national gross domestic product (GDP), which is approximately one-sixth of the total GDP of the nation.[1] Therefore, it is not surprising that U.S. agriculture infrastructure is one of the main targets identified in the al Qaeda training manual captured by U.S. forces in Afghanistan.[2, 3] There are five potential targets for agricultural terrorism (agroterrorism): field crops, farm animals, food items during processing or distribution, wholesale or retail agricultural facilities (e.g. processing plants, storage facilities, food outlets etc.), infrastructure of agricultural transportation, as well as, research laboratories.[3, 4] Unfortunately, at the present time, gaining access to all of the potential terrorism targets is comparatively easy, since there are few if any security checks. Furthermore, most of the U.S. agricultural industry is restricted to monoculture of crops or livestock; moreover, the locations for food processing, as well as the distribution centers are highly clustered, making it relatively simple for terrorist to commit mass dissemination of a contagion. For example, a non-purposeful antimicrobial salmonellosis outbreak in the milk supply in Minnesota during 1985 affected more than 16,000 individuals. This outbreak demonstrated the potential for a successful large scale agro-terrorism attack.[5] Zemco Industries, a New York based company that supplies deli meats for Walmart, has recalled 380,000 pounds of its products fearing that they may be contaminated with *Listeria monocytogenes*.[6] More recently, The Happy Apples company has voluntary recalled their product, caramel apples, due to the potential contamination with *Listeria monocytogenes*. The Happy Apples Company is the supplier of Kroger Brand caramel apples.[7]

On December 3, 2004, the former Secretary of the Department of Health and Human Services, Tommy Thompson, warned of the potential for an agroterrorism attack. He stated "for the life of me, I cannot understand why the terrorists have not attacked our food supply, because it is so easy to do."[8] In spite of the importance of agriculture to the US economy, very little attention has been paid to protecting the nation from agricultural terrorism.[9, 10, 11]

Agroterrorism used against the infrastructure and economy of enemies has occurred throughout the history of warfare. For example, during 1915 to 1917 at the height of WWI, the Germans initiated a biological warfare attack using *Burkholderia mallei*, which causes the disease known as glanders, and *Bacillus anthracis* against horses and cattle used in the Allies' war effort.[12, 13] The Japanese during WWII were much more aggressive in maintaining and using biological warfare agents than other combatants. Unit 731, tested numerous anti-personnel biological weapons and also experimented with anti-livestock agents. For example, it has been alleged that the Japanese troops entered the Soviet Union to poison animals with anthrax and other undisclosed diseases.[13]

During WWII, the Germans experimented with foot-and-mouth disease virus (FMDV), a member of the genus *Aphthovirus* in the family *Picornaviridae*. Field trials were conducted and considerations were made in regard to aerial dissemination of the disease. Fortunately, the pathogen was never used during the war.[14] Also during this time, the British prepared and tested over five million anthrax laced cattle cakes that were intended to be air-dropped into German cattle fields.[15] Similarly during WWII, the United States Biological Weapons Program experimented with anti-crop biological agents. For example, the US possessed plans to use the spores of the brown spot rice fungus, and chemical agents to target Japanese and German crops.[13]

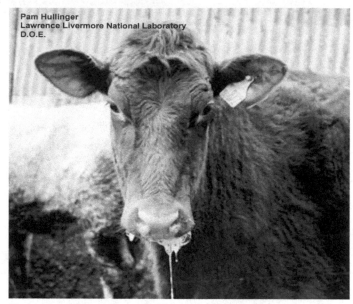

Pam Hullinger
Lawrence Livermore National Laboratory
D.O.E.

Figure 4.1-1: A cow stricken with foot and mouth disease (FMD)

Presently, it is believed that the US livestock population maybe more susceptible to agroterrorism, in comparison to crops. This susceptibility is partly due to the great success of the US disease eradication efforts with livestock herds. The success rate of disease eradication has formed complacency, where much of the nation's domestic animals are unvaccinated or unmonitored by farmers and veterinarians. It is believed that once purposely infected, livestock has the potential to become a vector or a reservoir of the pathogen.[9] This potential was demonstrated by the 2001 outbreak of foot and mouth disease (FMD) in the United Kingdom. It has been estimated that this outbreak cost the island nation over 4.6 billion dollars (Figure 4.1-1).[12]

Compared with a potential biological attack against humans, attacks on agriculture are less risky to terrorists. For example, most anti-agriculture pathogens are generally safer to work with and easier to develop than human pathogens. Furthermore, many of the potential biological agents used against agriculture are endemic, thereby posing difficulties in controlling the pathogen.[4]

The results of a successful agroterrorism would cause major economic/financial crises in the agricultural and food industries. In addition, such an attack would cause large scale economic losses to individuals, businesses and the government through costs to contain and eradicate the disease, as well as, to dispose of contaminated products. The supply chain of agricultural goods to the markets would also be disrupted. Moreover, the immediate aftermath of such an attack would most likely cause the population to lose confidence in local and federal governments, due to their inability to protect and defend against agroterrorism.[16]

References

1. General Accounting Office. U.S. Agriculture: Status of the Farm Sector, Fact Sheet for Congressional committees. GAO/RCED–95–104FS, 1995
2. Nganje W., Bier V., Han H., Zack L. Models of Interdependent Security Along the Milk Supply Chain. Effect of Biosecurity Risk and Food Scare Events on Food Prices. American Journal of Agricultural Economics, 2008. 90: pp. 1265-1271
3. Kosal M.E., Anderson D.E. An Underaddressed Issue of Agricultural Terrorism: A Case Study on Feed Security. Journal of Animal Science, 2004. 2: p. 3394-3400
4. Parker H.S. Agricultural Bioterrorism: A Federal Strategy to Meet the Threat. Institute for

National Strategic Studies. National Defense University. Washington D.C.: United States Government Printing Office. 2002. pp. 11-23

5. Ryan C.A., Nickels M.K., Hargrett-Brean N.T. Massive Outbreak of Antimicrobial-resistant Salmonellosis Traced to Pasteurized Milk. The Journal of the American Medical Association, 1987. 258: pp. 3269-3274

6. New York Firm Recalls Deli Meat Products for Possible Listeria Contamination. United States Department of Agriculture, Food Safety and Inspection Services. Revised December 10, 2010. Retrieved December 14, 2011. Website: http://www.fsis. usda.gov/ News_&_Events/Recall_049_2010_Release/index.asp

7. Happy Apple Company Expands Voluntary Recall of Caramel Apples To Include Kroger Brand Caramel Apples. Revised December 31, 2014. Food and Drugs Administration. Retrieved January 7, 2015. Website: http://www.fda.gov/Safety/Recalls /ucm428852.htm

8. Branigin W., Allen M., Mintz J. Tommy Thompson Resigns from the HHS. Washington Post. Revised: December 3, 2004. Retrieved: December 21, 2009. Website: http://www. washingtonpost.com/wp-dyn/articles /A31377-2004Dec3.html

9. Chalk P. The U.S. Agricultural System: a Target for Al-Qaeda? Terrorism Monitor. Revised: May 5, 2005. Retrieved: December 21, 2009. Website: http://www.jamestown. org/programs/gta/single/?_tx_ttne_ws%5Btt_news%5D=27669&tx_ttnews%5BbackPid%5 D=180&no_cache=1

10. Taylor D.L. Agroterrorism: A looming threat to food supply. Revised September 15, 2014. Retrieved January 7, 2015. The Californian. Website: http://www.thecalifornian.com/story/ news/local/2014/09/12/agroterrorism-looming-threat-food-supply/15541125/

11. Schneider R.G., Schneider K.R., Webb C.D., Hubbard M., Archer D.L. Agroterrorism in the U.S.: An Overview. University of Florida, The Institute of Food and agricultural Sciences (IFAS) Extension. Revised 2011. Retrieved January 7, 2015. Website: http://edis.ifas.ufl. edu/fs126

12. Dembek Z.F., Anderson E.L. Food, Waterborne and Agriculture Diseases. Medical Aspects of Chemical and Biological Warfare. Chapter 2. Washington D.C.: Office of the Surgeon General Department of the Army, United States of America. 1997. pp. 21-38

13. Smart J.K. The U.S. Biological Warfare and Biological Defense Programs. Medical Aspects of Chemical and Biological Warfare. Chapter 2. Washington D.C.: Office of the Surgeon General Department of the Army, United States of America. 1997. pp. 9-86

14. Hugh-Jones M. Wickham Steed and German Biological Warfare Research. Intelligence and National Security, 1992. 7: pp. 379-402

15. Rosie G. UK Planned to Wipe Out German with Anthrax. Sunday Herald. October 14, 2001. pp. A2

16. Monke J. Agroterrorism: Threats and Preparedness. CRS Report for Congress. Revised: August 13, 2004. Retrieved: December 23, 2009. Website: http://www.fas_.org/irp/crs/ RL32521.pdf

Photo Bibliography

Figure 4.1-1: Figure 4.1-1: A cow stricken with foot and mouth disease (FMD). The photograph was taken by Pam Hullinger of the Lawrence Livermore National Laboratory, Department of Energy. Public domain photo

African swine fever (ASF) is one of the most severe and potentially deadly diseases of domestic pigs (Family: *Suidae*). ASF occurs in two forms: an acute hemorrhagic infection which may produce mortality rates, as high as 100%, or a less virulent, chronic form of the disease.[1]

ASF is caused by the African swine fever virus (ASFV), the sole member of *Asfarvirdae*. ASFV is an enveloped icosahedral virus that possesses structure and genetic characteristics similar to both the *poxviridae* and the *iridoviridae*. *Asfavirdae* possess a linear, covalently close-ended, double-stranded DNA (170-192 kbp) genome (Figure 4.2-1).[2, 3]

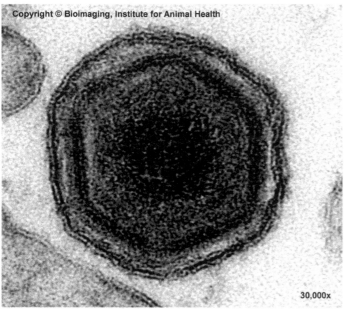

Copyright © Bioimaging, Institute for Animal Health

30,000x

Figure 4.2-1: A transmission electron photomicrograph (TEM) of African swine fever virus (ASFV)

Due to the seriousness of this disease, World Organization for Animal Health (OIE) has categorized ASF as a highly contagious disease that can spread rapidly and may cause serious socioeconomic effects on international trade of pig and pork products. Presently, there are no treatments or vaccines available for this disease and the only manner of controlling this infection is through sanitary measures.[2, 4, 5]

Recognizing ASF as a potential anti-livestock weapon, the Soviet Union established the Main Directorate for Scientific and Production Enterprises (Biokombinat) and the project named Ecology, to develop ASF as an agricultural biological weapon. According to Alibek (1999), ASF was engineered to be spread from Ilyushin bombers and flown over a target area in a line source pattern (e.g. straight line) for an extended coverage area. Even if only a few animals were infected, the contagious nature of the disease would ensure its spread and could potentially wipe out pork based agriculture activities in that region for an extended period of time.[6]

ASF was first described in East Africa in 1921 and is indigenous to the African continent including the island of Madagascar. Outbreaks of this disease have occurred elsewhere around the world, but have since been eradicated, with the exception of Sardinia, Italy, where the disease took root and became endemic.[1, 4]

ASF circulates in one of three distinct cycles. The first cycle is referred to as an ancient sylvatic cycle involving an eyeless *Ornithodoros moubata* (argasid ticks), *Phaecochoerus aethiopicus* (warthogs), *Hylochoerus* spp. (giant forest hogs), *Tayassu* spp. (peccaries) and *Potamochoerus porcus* (bushpigs). ASFV infections in warthogs, giant forest hogs and bushpigs are generally asymptomatic, therefore, it is believed that these species serve as reservoirs for the virus.[7, 8] The second cycle involves an infected tick (e.g. *Ornithodoros erraticus*) bite on domestic pigs. The third cycle occurs when the virus spreads among the domestic pig population through oronasal spread, formites and/or ingestion of contaminated meats.[1, 4, 7, 9, 10, 11]

ASFV is shed in all bodily excretions and is found in all tissues and bodily fluids, especially the blood of clinically ill domestic pigs. This virus is extremely resistant to harsh environmental conditions, which make introduction of ASFV into a domestic pig population a serious threat.[7, 12, 13] For example, it is known that this virus can survive for ~6 months in blood stored at 3.9° C (39° F), 150 days in boned meat stored at 3.9° C (39° F), 140 days in salted dry hams, several years in frozen carcasses, 11 days in feces at room temperature, and approximately a month in contaminated pens.[7] In the event of an ASF outbreak, culling the infected animals and animals that come in contact with them, as well as, restricting the movement (isolation) of healthy domestic herds are the only main control measures.[4] Rapid laboratory conformation of the virus is essential. Initial identification of ASFV of various distinct viral genetic genotypes (genotype I though XXII) is generally performed through polymerase chain reaction (PCR) amplification and the sequencing of the *p72* gene coding for the major capsid protein, although serological tests are available (ELISA etc.).[14, 15, 16, 17, 18] Of the 16 known genotypes of ASFV, genotype I, comprising viruses from Europe, South America, Caribbean and West Africa represents the most widespread and homogeneous genotype identified so far.[7, 17, 18]

ASFV replicates initially in porcine mononuclear phagocyte system cells (MPS) and subsequently in non-MPS cells.[19, 20, 21, 22, 23] The entry of the virus into the host cells involves receptor-mediated endocytosis. During an acute infection macrophages infected by this virus are concentrated in specific areas of lymphoid organs, while they are virtually absent in others. Additionally, only a limited percentage (6 to 30%) of monocytes are infected by ASFV.[24, 25, 26] These observations suggest that only a subpopulation of monocyte/macrophage are susceptible to ASFV. It has been suggested that the difference in permissiveness among cell subtypes may be explained either by the expression of virus specific membrane molecules, necessary for virus attachment and entry, or through intracellular factors, essential for viral replication.[27, 28, 29]

The bone marrow, as well as liver, spleen and lymph nodes are considered to be the secondary viral replication sites for ASFV.[30] In a report by Gómez-Villamandos *et al.* (1997), the effects of ASFV (intramuscularly inoculated) on swine bone marrow was examined chronologically. These researchers reported that from day five, post inoculated (PI), viral replication could be observed in promonocytes, monocytes/ macrophages, reticular cells and immature neutrophils. By day seven, viral replication could also be detected in megakaryocytes, endothelial cells and pericytes.[31]

After infection with ASFV, domesticated pigs may shed infective amounts of the virus for 24 to 48 hours before the first clinical signs of the disease occur. ASF can occur in four forms: chronic, peracute, acute or subacute. The incubation period of the virus during a chronic infection is approximately 5-19 days after direct contact with infected pigs or less than five days after exposure to ticks. The incubation period for peracute, acute and subacute forms of the disease is approximately 5-7 days.[7, 32]

Characteristically, peracute ASF displays the sudden death of infected animals with few lesions. Very few signs appear prior to death, although recumbency and high fever (42°C or 107.6° F) may be seen. On the other hand, the acute form of the disease displays a myriad of symptoms. These symptoms include high fever (42°C or 107.6° F), listless, weakness (e.g. ataxia of the hind-limb), anorexia, erythema lethargy, recumbency, dyspnea, vomiting, nasal and conjunctival discharges, that at times may be bloody, which may indicate lung edema, a major cause of death (Figure 4.2-3). Acute infections may also cause severe lymphopenia, neutrophilia with proliferation of immature forms of these blood cells. Neurological signs may also develop which include convulsions from viral encephalitis/ vasculitis. Additional symptoms include abdominal pains, constipation and diarrhea. Diarrhea will first appear mucoid and later turn bloody. Other signs include cyanotic skin blotching on the ears, tail, lower legs, thigh and rump, while generalized hemorrhages may occur on the skin or internal organs. Animals that are pregnant frequently abort. Animals suffering from the acute form of ASF may shed enormous amounts of virus through all secretions and excretions, while high levels of the virus are present in the tissues and blood. These animals often succumb to the disease within 7 to 10 days. Animals that survive the acute form of the disease will continue to shed viruses for approximately 30 days, although they may remain infected for months.[7, 31, 32]

The subacute form of ASF is a condition caused by less virulent strains of ASFV. This condition shares the same symptoms as the acute form, but is less severe. Fatalities from this form of ASF are generally lower in adults but are still high in young swine. Infected animals may die within three to four weeks or may recover to exhibit the chronic form of disease. Animals suffering from the chronic form of the disease generally display low fever, loss of appetite and may become emaciated. Animals suffering from the subacute form of the disease generally display moist coughing, a sign of respiratory distress (e.g. pneumonia). Other signs include coughing, diarrhea, vomiting and skin ulcers or necrotic skin foci which may also appear over body protrusions, as well as, areas of the swine that are subjected to trauma. Animals that survive the chronic form of ASF may survive for several months, but recovery is unlikely.[7, 32]

References

1. Penrith M.L., Thomson G.R., Bastos A.D.S. African Swine Fever. Infectious Diseases of Lifestock. New York: Oxford University Press. 2005. pp. 1087-1119
2. Arias M., Sánchez-Vizcaíno J.M. African Swine Fever. Trends in Emerging Viral Infections of Swine. Iowa City: Iowa State University Press. 2002. pp. 119-124
3. Dixon L.K., Costa J.V., Escribano J.M., Rock D.L., Viñuela E., Wilkinson P.J. Asfarviridae. Virus Taxonomy. Seventh Report of the International Committee on Taxonomy of Viruses. New York: Academic Press. 2000. pp. 159-165
4. Rowlands R.J., Michaud V., Heath L., Hutchings G., Oura C., Vosloss W., Dwarka R., Onashvilli T., Albina E., Dixon L.K. African Swine Fever Virus Isolate, Georgia, 2007. Emerging Infectious Diseases, 2008. 14: pp. 1870-1874
5. Gallardo C., Fernández-Pinero J., Pelayo V., Gazaev I., Markowska-Daniel I., Pridotkas G., Nieto R., Fernández-Pacheco P., Bokhan S., Nevolko O., Drozhzhe Z., Pérez C., Soler A., , Kolvasov D., Arias M. Genetic Variation among African Swine Fever Genotype II Viruses, Eastern and Central Europe. Emerging Infectious Diseases, 2014. 20: pp. 1544-1547
6. Alibek K. Biohazard. New York: Dell Publishing. 1999. pp. 37-38
7. The Center for Food Security & Public Health. Iowa State University. African Swine Fever. Revised December 19, 2006. Retrieved December 24, 2009. Website: www.cfsph.iastate. edu/factsheets/pdfs/classical_swine_fever.pdf
8. Oura C.A.L., Powell P.P., Abderson E., Parkhourse R.M.E. The Pathogenesis of African Swine Fever in the Resistant Bushpig. Journal of General Virology, 1998. 79: pp. 1439-1443
9. Lubisi B.A., Bastos A.D.S., Dwarka R.M., Vosloo W. Molecular Epidemiology of African Swine Fever in East Africa. Archives of Virology, 2005. 150: pp. 2439-2452
10. Groocock C.M., Hess W.R., Gladney W.J. Experimental Transmission of African Swine Fever Virus by *Ornithodoro coriaceus*, an Argasid Tick Indigenous to the United States. American Journal of Veterinary Research, 1980. 41: pp. 591-594
11. Oleaga-Pérez A., Pérez-Sanchez R., Encinas-Grandes A. Distribution and Biology of Ornithodoros erraticus in Parts of Spain Affected by African Swine Fever. Veterinary Record, 1990. 126: pp. 32-37
12. Plowright W., Parker J., Pierce M.A. The Stability of African Swine Fever Virus with Particular Reference to Heat and pH Inactivation. Archiv für die gesamte Virusforschung, 1967. 21: pp. 383-402
13. Donaldson A.I., Ferris N.P. The Survival of Some Airborne Animal Viruses in Relation to Relative Humidity. Veterinary Microbiology, 1976. 1: pp. 413-420
14. Bastos A.D.S., Penrith M-L, Crucière C., Edrich J.L., Hutchings G., Roger F., Couacy-Hymann E., Thomson G.R. Genotyping Field Dtrains of African Swine Fever Virus by Partial p72 Gene Characterization. Archives of Virology, 2003. 148: pp. 693-706
15. Bastos A.D.S., Penrith M-L, Macome F., Pinto F., Thomson G.R. Co-circulation of Two Genetically Distinct Viruses in an Outbreak of African Swine Fever in Mozambique: No Evidence for Individual Co-infection. Veterinary Microbiology, 2004. 103: pp. 169-182
16. Gonzague M., Roger F., Bastos A. Burger C., Randriamparany T., Smondack S., Cruciere C. Isolation of a Non-haemadsorbing, Non-cytopathic Strain of African Swine Fever Virus in Madagascar. Epidemiology and Infection, 2001. 41: pp. 591-594
17. Dixon L.K., Escribano J.M., Martins C., Rock D.L., Salas M.L., Wilkinson P.J., Asfarviridae. Virus Taxonomy. VIIIth Report of the International Committee on Taxonomy of Viruses. London: Academic Press. 2005. pp. 135-143
18. Boshoff C.I., Bastos A.D., Gerber L.J., Vosloo W. Genetic Characterization of African Swine Fever Viruses from Outbreaks in Southern Africa (1973-1999). Veterinary Microbiology, 2007. 121: pp. 45-55
19. Pan I.C. Spontaneously Susceptible Cells and Cell Culture Methodologies for African Swine Fever Virus. African Swine Fever. Boston: Matinus Nijhoff. 1987. pp. 81-126
20. Sierra M.A., Carrasco L., Gómez-Villamandos J.C., Martín de las Mulas J., Méndez A., Jover A. Pulmonary intravascular Macrophages in Pigs Inoculated with African Swine Fever Virus of Different Virulence. Journal of Comparative Pathology, 1990. 102: pp. 323-334
21. Sierra M.A., Gómez-Villamandos J.C., Carrasco L., Fernández A., Mozos E. In Vivo Study of the Haemadsorption Reaction in Afican Swine Fever Virus Infected Cells. Veterinary Pathology, 1991. 28: pp. 178-181
22. Gómez-Villamandos J.C., Hervás J., Méndez A., Carrasco L., Villeda C.J., Wilkinson P.J., Sierra M.A. Experimental ASF: Apoptosis of Lymphocytes and Virus Replication in Other cells. Journal of General Virology, 1995. 76: pp. 2399-2405
23. Gómez-Villamandos J.C., Hervás J., Méndez A., Carrasco L., Villeda C.J., Wilkinson P.J., Sierra M.A. Pathological Changes in the Renal Interstitial Capillaries of Pigs Inoculated with Two Different Strains of African Swiune Fever Virus. Journal of Comparative Pathology, 1995. 112: pp. 283-298
24. Minguez I., Rueda A., Dominguez J., Sánchez-Vizcaíno J.M. Double Labeling Immunohistological Study of African Swine Fever-infected Spleen and Lymph Nodes. Veterinary Pathology, 1988. 25: pp. 193-198
25. Gonzalez-Juarrero M., Lunney J.K., Sánchez-Vizcaíno J.M., Mebus C. Modulation of Splenic Macrophages, and Swine Leukocyte Antigen (SLA) and Viral Antigen Expression Following African Swine Fever Virus (ASFV) Inoculation. Archives of Virology, 1992. 123: pp. 145-156
26. Ramiro-Ibañez F., Escribano J.M., Alonso C. Application of a Monoclonal Antibody Recognizing Portein p30 to Detect African Swine Fever Virus-infected Cells in the Peripheral Blood. Journal of Virological Methods, 1995. 55: pp. 339-345
27. Sánchez-Torres C., Gómez-Puertas P., Gómez-del-Moral M., Alonso F., Escribano J.M., Ezquerra A., Domínguez J. Expression of Porcine CD163 on Monocyte/macrophages Correlates with Permissiveness to African Swine Fever Infection. Archives of Virology, 2003. 148: pp. 2307-2323
28. Cheng-Mayer C., Liu R., Landau N.R., Stamatatos L. Macrophage Tropism of Immunodeficiency Viirus Type I and Utilization of the CC-CKR5 Coreceptor. The Journal of Virology, 1997. 71: pp. 1657-1661
29. Carracosa A.L., Bustos M.J., Galindo I., Viñuela E. Virus-specific Cell Receptors are Necessary, but not Sufficient, to Confer Cell Susceptibility to African Swine Fever Virus. Archives of Virology, 1999. 144: pp. 1309-1321
30. Greig A. Pathogenesis of African Swine Fever in Pigs Natually Exposed to the Disease. Journal of Comparative Pathology, 1972. 82: pp. 73-79
31. Gómez-Villamandos J.C., Bautista M.J., Carrasco M.J., Caballero M.J., Hervás J., Villeda C.J., Wilkinson P.J., Sierra M.A. African Swine Fever Virus Infection of Bone Marrow: Lesion and Pathogenesis. Veterinary Pathology, 1997. 34: pp. 97-107
32. Penrith M-L., Guberti V., Depner K., Lubroth J. Preparation of African Swine Fever Contingency Plans. Rome: Food and Agriculture Organization of the United Nations. 2009. pp. 5-17

Photo Bibliography

Figure 4.2-1: A transmission electron photomicrograph (TEM) of African swine fever virus (ASFV). The electron photomicrograph was taken and released by Bioimaging, Institute for Animal Health. Copyrighted © work. CC BY-SA 3.0. Permission is granted to copy, distribute and/or modify this document under the terms of the GNU Free Documentation License

Avian influenza (AI) virus is a type A influenza that belongs to the *Influenzavirus A* genus of the *Orthomyxovirdae* virus. This virus is enveloped, pleiomorphic, appearing tubular or spherical, segmented, negative sense RNA genomes (890 to 2340 bases) with diameters ranging from 80 to 120 nm. It is believed that the segmented genome allows for these viruses to develop new strains through mutation and re-assortment of the gene fragments. The genetic instability of these viruses is responsible for the epidemics, which result from mutation, as well as, periodic pandemics, the result of genetic reassortment (Figure 4.3-1).[1, 2]

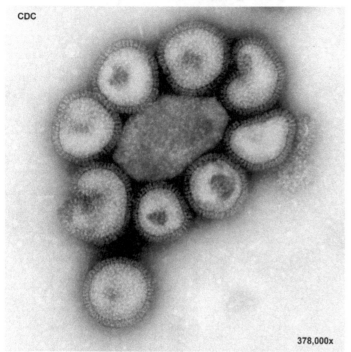

CDC

378,000x

Figure 4.3-1: A colorized negative stained transmission electron photomicrograph (TEM) of an avian influenza virus (H1N1)

Orthomyxovirdae are distributed into three genera classified as A, B, and C, based on the antigenicity of the nucleoproteins (NP) and matrix proteins. Influenza A subtypes are primarily viruses of aquatic birds, although they are known to infect swine, horses, humans, marine mammals and other animals. Influenza B mostly infects humans, although infection in seals, dogs, cats and swine have been reported. Influenza C is mostly known for its infections in humans. [1, 2, 3, 4, 5, 6]

Influenza A and B viruses contain eight helical nucleocapsid segments, while influenza C viruses contain seven helical nucleocapsid segments. Each of the nucleocapsid segments is associated with a negative-sense RNA (vial genome) linked with the trimeric viral RNA polymerase components PB1, PB2, and PA, and coated with multiple nucleoproteins (NPs) to form viral ribonucleoproteins (vRNPs). The outer layer of the influenza virus is surrounded by a lipid envelope spiked with multiple copies of glycoprotein hemaglutinin (HA), neuraminidase (NA), a small number of matrix protein 2 (M_2) and high quantities of matrix protein 1 (M_1). M_1 is responsible for keeping vRNPs attached to the inner layer, while associating with the M_1 protein and NS2 proteins (Figure 4.3-2).[1, 2, 3, 4, 5, 6] Type A influenza strains are further classified by the serological subtypes of the primary viral surface proteins (viral envelope): HA and NA. It is known that HA has 17 subtypes (H1–H17) and contains neutralizing epitopes

and 10 NA subtypes (N1-N10) which do not contain neutralizing epitopes. Among the HA subtypes, seven (H1, H2, H3, H5, H7, H9 and H10) have been identified in human isolates, whereas, among the NA subtypes six (N1, N2, N3, N7, N8 and N9) have been identified in human isolates. [1, 2, 7, 8, 9, 10, 11, 12, 13] One unique feature of the influenza virus is its ability to undergo antigenic variations via antigenic drift and antigenic shift.[14] Antigenic drift occurs continuously due to selection pressures from the host immune system and it comprises minor mutational alterations in the antigenicity of HA or NA. On the other hand, antigenic drift involves the genetic reassortment of the 8 gene segments of the type A influenza virus. This genetic reassortment can result in the creation of a novel HA and NA combination.[14, 15] For example, in 2012, Tong *et al.* reported that a unique H17N10 genome of type A influenza virus was found in bat populations of Guatemala.[16]

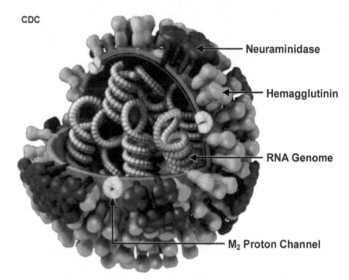

CDC

Neuraminidase

Hemagglutinin

RNA Genome

M_2 Proton Channel

Figure 4.3-2: A 3D graphical representation of an influenza virion's ultrastructure

Glycoprotein HA (a spike shaped trimer) are responsible for the attachment of the virus to the sialic acid-containing host cellular receptors, which induces internalization via endosomes, fusion of the viral and endosomal membrane and the subsequent release of the genome into the host cell cytoplasm.[1, 2, 17, 18] It has been reported that Amino acids found within the HA receptor binding domain, which is formed by the 190-helix, 220-loop and 130-loop, determine the receptor binding preference of the influenza viruses.[19, 20]   Human influenza A viruses preferentially bind to sialic acid with galactose α-2-6 linkages in the cells of the respiratory epithelium, while avian influenza A viruses preferentially bind to sialic acid with galactose α-2-3 linkages, found within the intestinal epithelial cells. Co-infections of both types of influenza A viruses may occur in the porcine tracheal epithelial cells and human respiratory epithelium since these cells include both sialic acid galactose α-2-6 and α-2-3 linkages. This co-infection allows for the mixing of the viruses and is the possible source of forming new virus types. In addition, HA also bind and aggregate erythrocytes from various species (e.g. chickens and humans etc.), and are responsible for the neutralization of host antibodies.[1, 2, 17, 18, 20]

NA (a glycoprotein tetramer) is responsible for cleaving terminal sialic acid residules from the glycolconjugates present on respiratory mucins, the host cells, as well as, progeny virions.

This enzymatic action destroys the sialic acid-containing host cellular receptor allowing the budding virus to be released by the infected cell to spread into the respiratory tract.[1, 2, 17, 20]

The matrix 1 and 2 (M_1 and M_2) proteins line the interior of the viral envelope. M_1 is one of the most abundant protein in the viral particle and is responsible for virion assembly while M_2 is responsible for forming a proton channel, as well as facilitating the dissociation of the viral RNA segments from the virion interior.[1, 2, 17, 21, 22] NS2 are found within the structural component of the viral particle and mediates the export of vRNPs from the nucleus to the cytoplasm through its interaction with exportin 1 (XPO1). Additionally, NS2 has been reported to interact with nucleoporins and serve as an adaptor between vRNPs and the nuclear pore complex.[23, 24, 25, 26] NS1 is one of the translated proteins of the influenza virus but is not incorporated in the viral particle. NS1 is a multifunctional protein and a virulence factor where it exerts a large spectrum of functions through interactions with a variety of cellular components residing either in the cytoplasm or in the nucleus. The NS1 protein plays a role in suppressing the production of host mRNAs by inhibiting the 3'-end processing of host pre-mRNAs. Additionally, NS1 also interferes with type I interferon system through direct interaction with PKR protein kinase and the ubiquitin ligase TRIM25, or through the sequestration of double-stranded RNA.[20, 27, 28, 29, 30]

Type A influenza infection begins with the binding of the viral HA to a specific sialic acid structure on the host cell surface glycoprotein. The virus is then internalized into a coated vesicle and transferred to an endosome. The acidification of the endosome causes the HA to bend-over, exposing its hydrophobic fusion-promoting regions, which allows for the fusion of the viral envelope with the endosome membrane. The M_2 protein then promotes the acidification of the envelope by allowing the flow of protons into the virus. This acidification breaks the interactions between M_1 protein and vRNP to allow the uncoating and delivery of the vRNP into the cytoplasm. Once the vRNP enters the cytoplasm of the host cell, it is transported to the nucleus by recognition of the nuclear localization sequences (NLSs) on nucleoproteins. Once the transport is complete, the M_1 protein dissociates.[1, 2, 31] Within the nucleus, the influenza polymerase components of the vRNP initiates viral positive sense RNA synthesis, as well as, the formation of complimentary RNA (cRNA). For example, the PB2 subunit binds with the 5' cap of the host's pre-mRNAs, while the endonuclease domain in PA subunit cleaves the pre-mRNA 10–13 nucleotides downstream from the cap via a process known as 'cap snaching'. Subsequently, the transcription of the positive sense viral RNA is initiated from the cleaved 3' end of the capped RNA segment. Once the transcription is completed, the positive sense viral RNA, also known as viral messenger RNA (VmRNA), is sent to the cytoplasm for translation. The translated M_2, HA and NA are sent to the endoplasmic reticulum (ER) for processing, glycosylated within the Golgi apparatus and then transported to the cell membrane.[32, 33, 34] The newly formed M_2 proteins insert themselves into the host cellular membrane and create proton channels. The proton channels prevent the acidification of the Golgi apparatus and other vesicles, thereby preventing acid-induced folding and inactivation of HA within the cell.[1, 2] The translated NS1 immdiately interacts with the cellular component and begins suppressing the production of host mRNA, as well as interfering with the host cell's type I interferon system.[27, 28, 29, 30] On the other hand, the cRNA (positive-sense viral RNA) will remain in the nucleus and serve as templates to synthesize negative-strands of the virions RNA genome before being transported into the cytoplasm. The transport of the negative-strands of the virions RNA genome is mediated by a M1–NS2 complex. Once the virions RNA genome reaches the cytoplasm it is grouped with polymerase components, as well as, NP proteins to form nucleocapsids before being transported to the cellular membrane. Once the nucleocapsids are completed, they will interact with the M_1 proteins lining the host cell membrane (also containing M_2 proteins, HAs and NAs). The formation of envelopes for the virus particles occurs in a random manner where 11 nucleocapsid segments are used per virion. Through this approach, a small number of virion will contain a complete genome while numerous defective particles are also created, these are antigenic and may cause interference. Consequently, the virus selectively buds out of the apical surface of the host cell through the enzymatic action of NA and allows for the preferential insertion of the HA within the envelope.[1, 2, 25, 34]

Type A influenza viruses occurs naturally in birds, especially in shorebirds and waterfowl where they serve as the virus's natural reservoir.[3, 5, 6, 17] The influenza A virus of all HA and NA subtypes can be found in these aquatic birds and do not usually cause overt disease among them. For example, in waterfowls, all nine NA subtypes and 14 HA (out of 15 HA) subtypes have been discovered, while in shorebirds eight NA and 10 HA subtypes have been found. The virus replicates mainly in the intestinal tract of these birds and is transmitted through the feces.[35] Avian influenza is transmitted by oral-fecal route from aquatic birds to domesticated poultry, and generally results in a mild unapparent disease, which is designated as low path avian influenza (LPAI) viruses. However, since commercial poultry farms raise thousands of animals in extremely close proximity, avian flu infection with time and opportunity will mutate and re-assort into a more virulent form. For example, highly pathogenic avian influenza (HPAI) can result from mutation and re-assortment producing a severe disease with high mortality.[36, 37, 38, 39, 40]

In domesticated birds, the clinical signs of influenza A infection vary according to the host species, age of the animal, the presence of other microorganisms and environmental factors. In susceptible avian species (e.g. chickens), uncomplicated infections can be divided into forms LPAI and HPAI. It is known that viral hemagglutinin subtypes H5 and H7 are associated with HPAI and high mortality rates (nearly 100% fatality rate) in chickens and turkeys.[19] Symptoms of HPAI infection include lack of energy and appetite, decreased egg production, laying soft-shelled or misshapen eggs, cyanosis of the head (including comb and wattle), edema of the head, ecchymoses of the shanks and feet, sinusitis, blood tinged oral and nasal discharge, coughing, sneezing, lacrimation, lack of coordination, green and white diarrhea and/or sudden death. In a report by Bouma et al. (2009), H5N1 viruses were used to infect chickens in a controlled environment. The infected birds showed signs of depression and labored breathing, sheding viruses from both the trachea and cloaca (e.g. saliva nasal secretions and fecal matter). These initially infected birds died within day two to three of exposure. All other birds that subsequently came into contact with these initially infected animals died on day four to five post contact.[37, 38, 40, 41, 42]

It is known that HPAI infections are generally self-limiting or can be rapidly controlled by culling.[17] All other influenza viruses cause a much milder form of the disease. Symptoms include signs of respiratory disease (e.g. coughing and sneezing), depression (e.g. low food consumption) and reduced production of eggs in laying birds. Asymptomatic infections may also occur where these less pathogenic viruses may simply replicate within the intestinal epithelial cells of these birds and shed in high concentrations in the fecal matter.[43, 44, 45]

General diagnosis is based upon clinical and epidemiological information. Laboratory diagnosis is needed to determine the exact subtype of the influenza virus. Viral isolation from respiratory specimens may be performed in several types of cell lines (e.g. PRMK, MDCK and LLC-MK2). The presence of the virus could be determined by hemadsorption with guinea pig erythrocytes before and after the cytopathic effect is visible. These viral isolates could be confirmed through hemagglutination inhibition or immunofluore-scence with viral type-specific antisera (Figure 4.3-3). Other techniques could also be used. For example, influenza antigens (M, NA or NP) could be detected through immunofluorescence or enzyme immunoassay. Commercially available kits can provide results within 15-30 minutes. Other commercially available kits use reverse transcription-polymerase chain reaction (RT-PCR) for the confirmation of specific genome of the virus.[1, 2]

Protective immunity is developed, where antibodies are produced against HA and NA. These two proteins are also the basis for conventional influenza vaccines.[17] The conventional vaccines available include inactivated homologous and inactivated heterologous vaccines which are produced from an inactivated whole avian influenza virus antigen (HA and NA) in oil based emulsion adjuvant. Recombinant vaccines are also available or presently under development. For example, several fowlpox virus vaccines that express H5 antigen have been developed. Other vaccines under development include subunit vaccines and DNA vaccines.[41, 46]

References

1. Guerrant R.L., Walker D.H., Weller P.F. Tropical Infectious Diseases – Principles, Pathogens & Practice. Volume 1. Philadelphia: Churchill Livingstone Elsevier. 2006. pp. 637-642
2. Murray P.R., Rosenthal K.S., Kobayashi G.S., Pfaller M.A. Medical Microbiology. Fourth Edition. St. Louis: Mosby College Publishing. 2002. pp. 535-542
3. Webster R.G., Bean W.J., Gorman O.T., Chambers T.M., Kawaoka Y. Evolution and Ecology of Influenza A Viruses. Microbiological Reviews, 1992. 56: pp. 152-179
4. Murphy B.R., Webster R.G. Orthomyxoviruses. Field Virology. Third Edition. Philadelphia: Lippincott-Raven. 1996. pp. 1397-1445
5. Osterhaus A.D.M.E., Rimmelzwaan G.F., Martina B.E., Bestebroer T.M., Fouchier R.A.M. Influenza B Virus in Seals. Science, 2000. 288: pp. 1051-1053
6. Guo Y.J., Jin F.G., Wang P., Wang M., Zhu J.M. Isololation of Influenza C Virus from Pigs and Experimental Infection of Pigs with Influenza C Virus. Journal of General Virology, 1983. 64: pp. 177-182
7. Fouchier R.A., Munster V., Wallenstan A., Bestebroer T.M., Herfst S., Smith D., Rimmelzwaan G.F., Olsen B., Osterhaus A.D. Characterization of a Novel Influenza A Virus Hemagglutinin Subtype (H16) Obtained from Vlack-Headed Gulls. The Journal of Virology, 2005. 79: pp. 2814-2822
8. Wong S.S., Tuen K. Avian Influenza Virus Infections in Human. Chest, 2006. 129: pp. 156-168
9. Ma W., Gramer M., Rossow K., Yoon K-J. Isolation and Genetic Characterization of New Reassortant H3N1 Swine Influenza Virus from Pigs in the Midwestern United States. Journal of Virology, 2006. 80: pp. 5092-5096
10. Puzelli S., Rossini G., Facchini M.,Vaccari G., Di Trani L.,Di Martino A., Gaibani P., Vocale C., Cattoli G., Bennett M., McCauley J.W., Rezza G., Moro M.L.,Rangoni R., Finarelli A.C., Landini M.P., Castrucci M.R., Donatelli I., Influenza Task Force. Human Infection with Highly Pathogenic A(H7N7) Avian Influenza Virus, Italy, 2013. Emerging Infectious Diseases, 2013. 20: pp. 1745-1749
11. Li Q., Zhou L., Zhou M., Chen Z., Li F., Wu H., Xiang N., Chen E., Tang F., Wang D., Meng L., Hong Z., Tu W., Cao Y., Li L., Ding F., Liu B., Wang M., Xie R., Gao R., Li X., Bai T., Zou S., He J., Hu J., Xu Y., Chai C., Wang S., Gao Y., Jin L., Zhang Y., Luo H., Yu H., He J., Li Q., Wang X., Gao L., Pang X., Liu G., Yan Y., Yuan H., Shu Y., Yang W., Wang Y., Wu F., Uyeki T.M., Feng Z. Epidemiology of Human Infections with Avian Influenza A(H7N9) Virus in China. The New England Journal of Medicine, 2014. 370: pp. 520-532
12. Zhang T., Bi Y., Tian H., Li X., Liu D., Wu Y., Jin T., Wang Y., Chen Q., Chen Z., Chang J., Gao G.F., Xu B. Human Infection with Influenza Virus A(H10N8) from Live Poultry Markets, China, 2014. Emerging Infectious Diseases, 2014. 20: pp. 2076-2079
13. Lopez-Martinez I., Balish A., Barrera-Badillo G., Jones J., Nuñez-García T.E., Jang Y., Aparicio-Antonio R., Azziz-Baumgartner E., Belser J.A., Ramirez-Gonzalez J.E., Pedersen J.C., Ortiz-Alcantara J., Gonzalez-Duran E., Shu B., Emery S.L., Poh M.K., Reyes-Teran G., Vazquez-Perez J.A., Avila-Rios S., Uyeki T., Lindstrom S., Villanueva J., Tokars J., Ruiz-Matus C., Gonzalez-Roldan J.F., Schmitt B., Klimov A., Cox N., Kuri-Morales P., Davis T.C., Diaz-Quiñonez J.A. Highly Pathogenic Avian Influenza A(H7N3) Virus in Poultry Workers, Mexico, 2012. Emerging Infectious Diseases, 2013. 19: pp. 1531-1534
14. Shoham D. The modes of evolutionary emergence of primal and late pandemic influenza virus strains from viral reservoir in animals: an interdisciplinary analysis. Influenza Research and Treatment, 2011. 2011: pp. 1-27
15. Taubenberger J.K., Morens D.M. Influenza: the once and future pandemic. Public Health Reports, 2010. 125: pp. 16–26
16. Tong S., Li Y., Rivailler P., Conrardy C., Castillo D.A., Chen L-M., Recuenco S., Ellison J.A., Davis C.T., York I.A., Turmelle A.S., Moran D., Rogers S., Shi M., Tao Y., Weil M.R., Tang K., Rowe L.A., Sammons S., Xu X., Frace M., Lindblade K.A., Cox N.J., Anderson L.J., Rupprecht C.E., Donis R.O. A distinct lineage of influenza A virus from bats. Proceedings of the National Academy of Sciences, United States of America, 2012. 109: pp. 4269–4274
17. Treanor J.J. Part III Infectious Diseases and Their Etiologic Agents, Influenza Virus. Principle and Practice of Infectious Disease. Sixth Edition. Philadelphia: Elsevier. 2005. pp. 2060-2065
18. Thomas J.K., Noppenberger J. Avian Influenza: A Review. American Journal of Health-system Pharmacy, 2007. 64: pp. 149-165
19. Xu R., McBride R., Paulson J.C., Basler C.F., Wilson I.A. Structure, receptor binding, and antigenicity of influenza virus hemagglutinins from the 1957 H2N2 pandemic. Journal of Virology, 2010. 84: pp. 1715–1721
20. Liu Q., Liu D-Y., Yang Z-Q. Characteristics of human infection with avian influenza viruses and development of new antiviral agents. Acta Pharmacologica Sinica, 2013. 34: pp. 1257–1269
21. Shtykova E.V., Baratova L.A., Fedorova N.V., Radyukhin V.A., Ksenofontov A.I., Volkov V.V., Shishkov A.V., Dolgov A.A., Shilova L.A., Batishchev O.V., Jeffries C.M., Svergun D.I. Structural Analysis of Influenza A Virus Matrix Protein M1 and Its Self-Assemblies at Low pH. Public Library of Science (PLoS) One, 2013. 8: pp. e82431
22. Cady S.D., Luo W., Hu F., Hong M. Structure and function of the influenza A M2 proton channel. Biochemistry,2009. 48: pp. 7356–7364
23. Yasuda J., Nakada S., Kato A., Toyoda T., Ishihama A. Molecular assembly of influenza virus: association of the NS2 protein with virion matrix. Virology, 1993. 196: pp. 249–255
24. O'Neill R.E., Talon J., Palese P. (1998) The influenza virus NEP (NS2 protein) mediates the nuclear export of viral ribonucleoproteins. European Molecular Biology Organization (EMBO) Journal, 1998. 17: pp. 288–296
25. Neumann G., Hughes M.T., Kawaoka Y. (2000) Influenza A virus NS2 protein mediates vRNP nuclear export through NES-independent interaction with hCRM1. European Molecular Biology Organization (EMBO) Journal, 2000. 19: pp. 6751–6758
26. de Chassey B., Aublin-Gex A., Ruggieri A., Meyniel-Schicklin L., Pradezynski F., Davoust N., Chantier T., Tafforeau L., Mangeot P-E., Ciancia C., Perrin-Cocon L., Bartenschlager R., André P., Lotteau V., Chanda S.K. The Interactomes of Influenza Virus NS1 and NS2 Proteins Identify New Host Factors and Provide Insights for ADAR1 Playing a Supportive Role in Virus Replication. Public Library of Science (PloS) Pathogens, 2013. 9: pp. e1003440.
27. Gack M.U., Albrecht R.A., Urano T., Inn K.S., Huang I.C., Carnero E., Farzan M., Inoue S., Jung J.U., García-Sastre A. (2009) Influenza A virus NS1 targets the ubiquitin ligase TRIM25 to evade recognition by the host viral RNA sensor RIG-I. Cell Host and Microbe, 2009. 5: pp. 439–449
28. Min J.Y., Li S., Sen G.C., Krug R.M. (2007) A site on the influenza A virus NS1 protein mediates both inhibition of PKR activation and temporal regulation of viral RNA synthesis. Virology, 2007. 363: pp. 236–243
29. Falcon A.M., Fortes P., Marion R.M., Beloso A., Ortin J. (1999) Interaction of influenza virus NS1 protein and the human homologue of Staufen in vivo and in vitro. Nucleic Acids Research, 1999. 27: pp. 2241–2247
30. Marion R.M., Fortes P., Beloso A., Dotti C., Ortin J. (1999) A human sequence homologue of Staufen is an RNA-binding protein that is associated with polysomes and localizes to the rough endoplasmic reticulum. Molecular and Cellular Biology, 1999. 19: pp. 2212–2219
31. Wu W.W., Pante N. The directionality of the nuclear transport of the influenza A genome is driven by selective exposure of nuclear localization sequences on nucleoprotein. Virology Journal, 2009. 6: pp. 68
32. Plotch S.J., Bouloy M., Ulmanen I., Krug R.M. A unique cap (m^7GpppXm)-dependent influenza virion endonucleaase cleaves capped RNAs to generate the primers that initiate viral RNA transcription. Cell, 1981. 23: pp. 847–858
33. Hagen M., Chung T.D.Y., Butcher A., Krystal M. Recombinant influenza virus polymerase: requirement of both 5' and 3' viral ends for endonuclease activity. The Journal of Virology, 1994. 68: pp. 1509–1515
34. Das K., Aramini J.M., Ma L-C., Krug R.M., Arnold E. Structure of influenze A proteins and insights into antiviral drug targets. Nature Structural and Molecular Biology, 2010. 17: pp. 530-538
35. Fouchier R.A.M., Osterhaus A.D.M.E., Brown I.H. Animal Influenza Virus Surveillance. Vaccine, 2003. 21: pp. 1754-1757
36. Friend, M., Franson J.C., Ciganovich E.A. Field Manual of Wildlife Diseases. General Field Procedures and Disease of Birds. Washington D.C.: United States Geological Survey. 1999. pp. 181-184
37. Center for Disease Control and Prevention. Avian Influenza (Bird Flu). Key Facts about Avian Influenza (Bird Flu) and Avian Influenza A (H5N1) Virus. Revised June 30, 2006. Retrieved December 25, 2009. Website: www.cdc.gov/flu/avian/gen-info/pdf/ avianflufacts.pdf
38. United States Geological Survey. The Avian Influenza H5N1 Threat. Revised August 2005. Retrieved December 25, 2009. Website: www.nwhc.usgs.gov/publications/fact_sheets/pdfs/... /HPAI082005.pdf
39. Berhane Y., Hisanaga T., Kehler H., Neufeld J., Manning L., Argue C., Handel K., Hooper-McGrevy K., Jonas M., Robinson J., Webster R.G., Pasick J. Highly Pathogenic Avian Influenza Virus A (H7N3) in Domestic Poultry, Saskatchewan, Canada, 2007. Emerging Infectious Diseases, 2009. 15: pp. 1492-1495
40. Bouma A.,. Classen I., Natih K., Klinkenberg D., Donnelly C.A., Koch G., van Boven M. Estimation of Transmission Parameters of H5N1 Avian Influenza Virus in Chickens. Public Library of Science (PLoS) Pathogens, 2009. 5: pp. 1-13
41. Saif M., Espinoza M. Avian Influenza: an Internal Report for the College of Food, Agricultural, and Environmental Sciences. The Ohio State University. Revised February 2006. Retrieved December 26, 2009. Website: http://ohioline.osu.edu/avi-fact/pdf/0001.pdf
42. The Center for Food Security & Public Health. Iowa State University. High Pathogenicity Avian Influenza. Revised January 8, 2009, Retrieved December 24, 2009. Website: http://www.cfsph.iastate.edu/FactSheets/pdfs/highly_pathogenic_avian_influenza.pdf
43. Slemons R.D., Easterday B.C. Virus Replication in the Digestive Tract of Ducks Exposed by Aerosol to Type-A Influenza. Avian Diseases, 1978. 22: pp. 367-377
44. Kida H., Yanagawa R., Matsuoka Y. Duck Influenza Lacking Evidence of Disease Signs and Immune Response. Infection and Immunity, 1980. 30: pp. 547-553
45. Kanegae Y., Sugita S., Shortridge K.F., Yoshioka Y., Nerome K. Origin and Evolutionary Pathways of the H1 Hemagglutinin Gene of Avian. Archives of Virology, 1994. 134: pp. 17-28
46. Rao S.S., Styles D., Kong W., Andrews C., Gorres J.P., Nabel G.J. A Gene-based Avian Influenza Vaccine in Poultry. Poultry Science, 2009. 88: pp. 860-866

Photo Bibliography

Figure 4.3-1: A colorized negative stained transmission electron photomicrograph (TEM) of an avian influenza virus (H1N1). This photomicrograph was taken by Dr. F. A. Murphyin 1976 and released by the CDC. Public domain photo

Figure 4.3-2: A 3D graphical representation of an influenza virion's ultrastructure. The graphics were developed by Douglas Jordan in 2009 and released by the CDC. Public domain graphic

Classical swine fever (CSF), also known as hog cholera or pig plague, is a highly contagious and economically significant infection of swine caused by the classical swine fever virus (CSFV). CSFV is known to cause hemorrhagic syndrome and immunosuppression in infected swine. CSFV is an enveloped, 12.5 kb positive-sense single strand RNA virus belonging to the genus *Pestivirus* of the *Flaviviridae* family (Figure 4.4-1).[1] The genome of the CSFV possesses a single long open reading frame, flanked by 5' and 3' non-coding regions without a poly A tail. The single reading frame encodes a polyprotein (~3898 amino acids), which is both co- and post-translationally processed into viral proteins by viral and cellular enzymes. From the N- to the C- terminal, the translated viral proteins are: N[pro], capsid protein (C), E[RNS], E1, E2, P7, NS2, NS3, NS4A, NS4B, NS5A and NS5B. C and three envelope glycoproteins Erns, E1 and E2 represent the structural proteins, while the remaining are nonstructural proteins.[2]

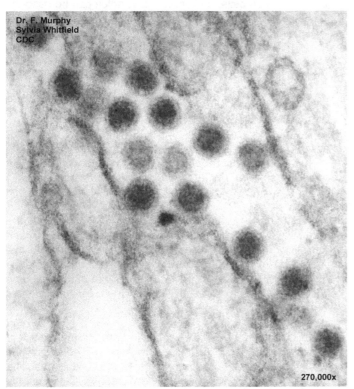

Dr. F. Murphy
Sylvia Whitfield
CDC

270,000x

Figure 4.4-1: Negatively-stained transmission electron micrograph (TEM) showing the presence of numerous virions, that belong to the family Flaviviridae

Glycoprotein E2, presented on the surface of CSFV, possesses a conservative spatial structure. It has been proposed that E2 interacts with surface receptor integrin β3 to gain entry into the host cell. However, the exact manner that the virus obtains entry remains to be elucidated.[3] Using the E2 glycoprotein gene for genotyping and classification, as well as phylogenic analysis, demonstrates a link between genotype and geographical region from where the CSFV isolates originated. CSFV is divided into three main groups and several subgroups. For example, groups 1.1 to 1.3 are found in South America and Russia, groups 2.1 to 2.3 are isolated from Western Europe and group 3.1 to 3.4 are from Asia.[4, 5, 6, 7]

Regardless of the group and/or subgroup, CSFV has the ability to survive for prolonged periods on formites. It has been reported

that this virus can survive up to three months in refrigerated meats, up to 4.5 years in frozen meats, two weeks at 20°C in liquid manure and more than six weeks at 4° C. Treatments such as curing and smoking of meat have very little effect on the survivability of the virus. It has been reported that the virus can survive 17 to 180 days dispite the treatment.[8, 9, 10]

Infected swine are the only reservoir of the virus, where CSFV can be found in blood, tissue, oronasal and lacrimal secretions, urine, feces, and semen. Viral shedding has been reported to begin before the onset of any clinical signs and occurs throughout acute infections. In chronic infections, infected pigs can shed viral particles continuously or intermittently for months.[10]

Transmission of the virus occurs mainly through oral or oronasal routes, either through direct or indirect contact. Pigs can also be infected by CSFV through the conjunctiva, mucus membranes, skin abrasions, sexual contact and artificial insemination.[10, 11] This virus may also be spread on formites or transmitted via insects, birds and other wild or domesticated animals. Airborne transmission does occur, however, the maximum distance that the virus can travel is presently unknown. CSFV can also be spread through the feeding of untreated contaminated garbage to animals. Reports has indicated that infected sows may give birth to persistently infected pigs, indicating transplacental infections.[10]

After the virus gains entry to the host, the first site of CSFV replication is the tonsils. Subsequently, the virus spreads to the regional lymph nodes before proceeding to the bone marrow, visceral lymph nodes and lymphoid structures associated with the small intestines and spleen. The spread of CSFV through the entire body is generally completed in less than six days.[9] A significant reduction of lymphocytes, as well as, an increase of apoptotic lymphocytes can be found in CSFV-infected swine as early as 24 hours post-infection. During this time the infection is asymptomatic and the only location where virally infected cells can be identified is in the tonsils. This result indicates that the depletion of lymphocytes is not the result of direct viral infection, but indirectly by means of virally induced apoptosis. It is speculated that the increased expression of FasL (a member of the tumor necrosis factor family) and decreased expression of Bcl-2 on the lymphocytes indicates an increased susceptibility to apoptosis mediated by Fas-FasL interactions (e.g. Fas-mediated activation-induced cell death). The physiological role of the Fas-FasL system is believed to be involved in the prevention of overstimulation of T lymphocytes during down regulation of the immune response, as well as, being involved in the maintenance of lymphocyte homeostasis. Furthermore, the indirect role of CSFV in the depletion of lymphocytes is supported by the observation that this virus has no cytopathic effect on lymphocyte *in vitro*.[12, 13, 14, 15]

Monocytes and macrophages are targets for CSFV. Once infected, the cells increase production of prostaglandin E_2 (PGE_2), as well as, interleukin-1 (IL-1). It was noted in the report by Knöetig *et al.* (1999), the increase in PGE_2 did not inhibit, but inhanced lymphocyte proliferation, where IL-1 was related to increased lymphocyte activation. It is believed that CSFV infection of monocytes and macrophages in the pig does not contribute to leucopenia, but is involved in the onset of fever and coagulation disorders (e.g. hemorrhagic disturbances such as petechia and infarction) observed in CSF.[16]

Within the bone marrow, the virus targets the bone marrow hematopoietic cells (BMHC) mainly from the myeloid lineages, but the monocytic lineage was most susceptible. CSFV is known to infect the immature, less differentiated cells, such as myeloid progenitors, although their different-iation along the granulocyte lineage was not impaired by infection. It was through this early infection that the more mature, viral positive, granulocytic cells were observed in the peripheral blood of infected pigs. It has also been reported that CSFV do not directly infect the more mature granulocytic cells.[17]

The CSFV infection causes apoptotic cell death in some of infected BMHC. Several key features were identified, most notably an increase in caspase activity. The strong increase in the activity of caspase 3 and 9 indicates the possibility of a mitochondria initiated pathway of apoptosis.[18, 19] Nonetheless, the apoptotic activit-ies were not restricted to infected cells, but also to uninfected cells. It has been reported that the majority of the apoptotic cells were viral negative. Interestingly, this influence of CSFV on uninfected BMHC is not the direct consequence of viral infection and replication. Summerfield et al. (2000) stated that the increased rate of apoptosis of uninfected cells was observed when infected BMHC were in direct contact with them, therefore the apoptotic effect was speculated to be directly related to cell-to-cell contact. This apoptosis of mostly uninfected immature granulocytes is likely the result of the loss of mature granulocytes being replaced by viral positive immature granulocytes in swine blood during a CSFV infection, contributing to leucopenia and atrophy of primary lymphoid tissue.[20, 21, 22, 23]

CSFV is known to cause different levels of infection, depending upon the virulence of the CSFV strains. In highly virulent isolates, acute infections can occur and result in high mortality. In less virulent strains, subacute, chronic, as well as, prenatal forms of infection can occur. In chronic infections, the clinical signs are difficult to recognize; the infection can appear to be mild and resemble septicemias caused by other agents. Furthermore, chronically infected pigs may only appear to have poor reproductive performance or simply fail to thrive.[9, 10]

In domestic pigs, piglets develop more evident clinical signs in comparison with adults. The symptoms of acute infections include high fever (<40° C or 104° F in piglets, and 39.5° C or 103° F in adults), huddling, weakness, drowsiness, lethargy, anorexia, conjunctivitis, respiratory signs and constipation followed by diarrhea. Pigs suffering from acute infections generally display an uncoordinated or unsteady, weaving gait, which progresses to posterior paresis. These infected pigs may vomit yellow bile-containing fluids, while along the abdomen, inner thigh, ears and tail a purple cyanotic discoloration may develop. Hemorrhages may also develop in the skin, as well as, in many internal organs. The mortality associated with this form of disease is extremely high.[9, 10, 24]

Animals suffering from subacute CSFV infections generally demonstrate similar signs as acute infections, but they are less severe. None-theless, fever associated with this form of disease may persist for 2 to 3 weeks. Some pigs suffering from subacute infections may survive, while others may die within a month.[9, 10, 24] In chronic infections, the signs are similar to acute infections, but the course of the disease is less severe. Typical signs include fever (which may last several weeks), depression, periods of constipation and diarrhea, wasting and anorexia. Affected pigs generally improve after several weeks; however, in a short period of time, they will develop recurrent symptoms. These recurrent signs include intermittent fever, anorexia, periods of constipation and diarrhea, wasting or stunned growth, alopecia and skin lesions. These signs may appear and disappear for several months before the animal finally succumbs to the disease.[9, 10]

CSFV is capable of cross placental infection of the fetus in pregnant sows. Depending on the group and/or subgroup of the virus, along with the period of gestation, the virus can induce abortion and stillbirths in early pregnancy or lead to the birth of a persistently viraemic piglet (if the infection takes place at day 50-70 of gestation). These piglets appear to be normal at birth, but quickly demonstrate signs of wasting, as well as, congenital tremors. These piglets shed viruses for several months and are a dangerous reservoir for CSFV.[8, 25]

Since the CSF clinical signs are variable and may be confused with other infections, definitive diagnosis has to be based on laboratory tests. For example, CSFV isolation is based upon the incubation of sample materials (e.g. leukocytes, plasma, whole blood, tissue samples from the tonsils, kidneys, spleen, ileum and the lymph nodes) from infected animals with susceptible porcine cell cultures. Subsequently, after the virus has replicated within the cultured cells, conjugated antibodies can be used via immunohistochemistry to identify the virus.[8, 25, 26, 26] Presently, reverse transcription-polymerase chain reaction (RT-PCR) or real-time RT-PCR are the most sensitive methods for detecting CSFV. For example, small fragments of CSFV RNA are reverse transcribed into DNA fragments, which are later amplified by PCR. The PCR then uses either SYBR green or a fluorogenic-probe hydrolysis (TaqMan) to detect the amplicons.[28, 29, 30, 31, 32] Commercially available enzyme-linked immunosorbant assays (ELISA), such as CIVTEST™ and IDEXX™, are available for detecting CSFV-specific antibodies. These tests are easy to use, inexpensive and do not require complex laboratory facilities.[33, 34] Recently, a new loop-mediated isothermal amplification (LAMP) assay coupled with lateral flow dipstick (LFD) for the detection of CSFV has been developed. This assay, developed for 7 genotypes (1.1, 1.2, 1.3, 2.1, 2.2, 2.3 and 3.1), combines the efficient one-step isothermal amplification of CSF viral RNA and the simplicity of the LFD to read the results within two to five minutes. Chowdry et al. (2014) reported that the performance of this RT-LAMP-LFD assay was similar to that of the real-time RT-PCR with no cross-reactivity to non-CSFV pestiviruses observed.[35]

Although culling the herd and disinfection are the most efficient manner of eliminating CSFV, there are two types of CSFV vaccines available commercially: ① live attenuated/modified live vaccine (MLV) and ② an E2 subunit vaccine (E2subV). Classical live vaccines are used on different attenuated virus strains. The most common used vaccine strain is the Chinese (C) strain, which has been attenuated by hundreds of serial passages in rabbits. Other attenuated virus strains used are Japanese guinea-pig exaltation (GPE)-negative strain, the Thiverval strain and the Mexican PAV strain. It has been reported that MLVs are highly efficacious after a single oral vaccine application, where the onset of protection is initiated within a few days after administration. However, the MLVs do not allow for the discrimination of infected versus vaccinated animals when examined via serology.[9, 36, 37] E2subV uses the E2 glycoprotein of CSFV to induce protective immunity through the formation of anti-E2 antibodies. Non-vaccinated pigs also develop antibodies, but towards a combination of other viral proteins such as E2, E^{RNS} and NS3. This different pathway of immunization allows the distinction via ELISA between vaccinated pigs and non-vaccinated pigs. It has been reported that E2subV are most efficacious after booster injection, while the protective immunity does not start until several weeks after immunization.[9, 38, 39, 40, 41, 42]

References

1. Becher P., Orlich M., Kosmidou A., Konig M., Baroth M., Thiel H.J. Genetic Diversity of Pestiviruses: Identification of Novel Groups and Implications for Classification. Virology, 1999. 262: pp. 64-71
2. Sun S.Q., Yin S.H., Guo H.C., Jin Y., Shang Y.J., Liu X.T. Genetic Typing of Classical Swine Fever Virus Isolates from China. Transboundary and Emerging Diseases, 2013. 60: pp. 370–375
3. Li W., Wang G., Liang W., Kang K., Guo K., Zhang Y. Integrin β3 Is Required in Infection and Proliferation of Classical Swine Fever Virus. Public Library of Science (PLoS) One, 2014. 9: pp. e110911
4. Paton D.J., McGoldrick A., Greiser-Wilke I., Parchariyanon S., Song J.Y., Liou P.P., Stadejek T., Lowings J.P., Bjorklund H., Belak S. Genetic Typing of Classical Swine Fever Virus. Veterinary Microbiology, 2000. 73: pp. 137-157
5. Stadejek T., Vilcek S., Lowings J.P., Ballagi-Pordany A., Paton D.J., Belak S. Genetic Heterogeneity of Classical Swine Fever Virus in Central Europe. Virus Research, 1997. 52: pp. 195-204
6. Bartak P., Greiserwilke I. Genetic Typing of Classical Swine Fever Virus Isolates from the Territory of Czech Republic. Veterinary Microbiology, 2000. 77: pp. 59-70
7. Pereda A.J., Greiser-Wilke I., Schmitt B., Rincon M.A., Mogollon J.D., Sabogal Z.Y., Lora A.M., Sanguinetti H., Piccone M.E. Phylogenic Analysis of Classical Swine Fever Virus (CSFV) Field Isolates from Outbreaks in South and Central America. Virus Research, 2005. 110: pp. 111-118
8. Edwards S. Survival and Inactivation of Classical Swine Fever Virus. Veterinary Microbiology, 2000. 73: pp. 175-181
9. Osterhaus A., Bøtner A. Algers B., Müller-Graf C., Guemene D., Morton D.B., Pfeiffer D.U., Broom D.M., Koenen F., Blokhuis H.J., Sharp J.M., Hartung J., Domingo M., Weirup M., Greiner M., Salman M., Sanaa M., Costa P., Vannier P., Roberts R. Scientific Report. Control and Eradication of Classic Swine Fever in Wild Boar and Animal Health Safety of Fresh Meat Derived from Pigs Vaccinated Against Classic Swine Fever. Scientific Opinions of the Panel on Animal Health and Welfare. European Food Safety Authority, 2007. pp. 1-140
10. The Center for Food Security & Public Health. Iowa State University. Classical Swine Fever. Revised September 16, 2009. Retrieved December 26, 2009. Website: http://www.cfsph.iastate.edu/factsheets/pdfs/classicalswine_fever.pdf
11. Choi C., Chae C. Detection of classical swine fever virus in boar semen by reverse transcription-polymerase chain reaction. The Journal of Veterinary Diagnostic Investigation, 2003. 15: pp. 35–41
12. Summerfield A., Knötig S.M., McCullough K.C. Lymphocyte Apoptosis During Classical Swine Fever: Implication of Activation-Induced Cell Death. Journal of Virology, 1998. 72: pp. 1853-1861
13. Akbar A.N., Berthwick N., Salmon M., Gombert W., Bofill M., Shamsadeen N., Pilling D., Pett S., Grundy E., Janossy G. The Significance of Low bcl-2 expression by CD45RO T Cells in Normal Individuals and Patients with Acute Viral Infections. The Role of Apoptosis in T cell Memory. The Journal of Experimental Medicine, 1993. 178: pp. 427-238
14. Akbar A.N., Salmon M. Cellular Environments and Apoptosis: Tissue Microenvironments Control Activated Cell Death. Immunology Today, 1997. 72: pp. 72-76
15. Lynch D.H., Ramsdell F., Alderson M.R. Fas and FasL in the Homeostatic Regulation of Immune Response. Immunology Today, 16: pp. 569-574
16. Knötig S.M., Summerfield A., Spangnuolo-Weaver M., McCullough K.C. Immunopathogenesis of Classical Swine Fever: Role of Monocytic Cells. Immunology, 1999. 97: pp. 359-366
17. Summerfield A., Hofmann M.A., McCullough K.C. Low Density Blood Granulocytic Cells Induced during Classical Swine Fever are Targets for Virus Infection. Veterinary Immunology and Immunopathology, 1998. 63: pp. 289-301
18. Budihardjo I., Oliver H., Lutter M., Lou X., Wang X. Biochemical Pathways of Caspase Activation during Apoptosis. Review of Cell and Developmental Biology, 1999. 15: pp. 269-290
19. Rathmell J.C., Thompson C.B. The Central Effector of Cell Death in the Immune System. Annual Review of Immunology, 1999. 17: pp. 781-828
20. Summerfield A., Knötig S.M., Tschudin R., McCullough K.C. Pathogenesis of Granulocytopenia and Bone Marrow Atrophy During Classical Swine Fever Involves Apoptosis and Necrosis of Uninfected Cells. Virology, 2000. 272: pp. 50-60
21. Summerfield A., Zingle K., Inumaru S., McCullough K.C. Induction of Apoptosis in Bone Marrow Neutrophil-Lineage Cells by Classical Swine Fever Virus. Journal of General Virology, 2001. 82: pp. 1309-1318
22. Trautwein G. Pathology and Pathogenesis of Disease. Classical Swine Fever and Related Infections. Boston: Matinus Nijhoff. pp. 27-54
23. Thiel H-J., Plagemann P.G.W., Moennig V. Pestiviruses. Field Virology. Third Edition. Philadelphia: Lippincott-Raven. pp. 1059-1073
24. Gregg D. Update on Classical Swine Fever (Hog Cholera). Journal of Swine Health and Production, 2002. 10: pp. 33-37
25. Congenital Tremor in Pigs Farrowed from Sows given Hog Cholera Virus during Pregnancy. American Journal of Veterinary Research, 1981. 42: pp. 135-137
26. Sánchez-Cordón P.J., Romanini S., Salguero F.J., Ruiz-Villamor E., Carrasco L., Gómez-Villamandos J.C. A Histopathologic, Immunohistochemical, and Ultra-structural Study of the Intestine in Pigs Inoculated with Classical Swine Fever Virus. Veterinary Pathology, 2003. 40: pp. 254-262
27. Choi C., Chae C. Localization of Classical Swine Fever Virus from Chronically Infected Pigs by In Situ Hybridization and Immunohistochemistry. Veterinary Pathology, 2003. 40: pp. 107-113
28. Thür B., Hofmann M.A. Comparative Detection of Classical Swine Fever Virus in Striated Muscle from Experimentally Infected Pigs by Reverse Transcription Polymerase Chain Reaction, Cell Culture Isolation and Immunohistochemistry. Journal of Virological Methods, 1998. 74: pp. 47-56
29. Liu S.T., Li S.N., Wang D.C., Chang S.F., Chiang S.C., Ho W.C., Chang Y.S., Lai S.S. Rapid Detection of Hog Cholera Virus in Tissues by Polymerase Chain Reaction. Journal of Virological Methods, 1991. 35: pp. 227-236
30. Roehe P.M., Woodward M.J. Polymerase Chain Reaction Amplification of Segments of Pestivirus Genome. Archives of Virology (Supplemental), 3: pp. 231-238
31. Liu L., Hoffmann B., Baule C., Beer M., Belák S., Widén F. Two Real-Time RT-PCR Assays of Classical Swine Fever Virus, Developed for the Genetic Differentiation of Naturally Infected from Vaccinated Wild boars. Journal of Virological Methods, 2009. 159: pp. 131-133
32. Risatti G.R., Callahan J.D., Nelson W.M., Borca M.V. Rapid Detection of Classical Swine Fever Virus by a Portable Real-Time Reverse Transcriptase PCR Assay. Journal of Clinical Microbiology, 2003. 41: pp. 500-505
33. Moser C., Ruggli N., Tratschin J.D., Hofmann M.A. Detection of Antibodies against Classical Swine Fever in Swine Sera by Indirect ELISA Using Recombinant Envelope Glycoprotein E2. Veterinary Microbiology, 1996. 51: pp., 41-53
34. Colijn E.O., Bloemraad M., Wensvoort G. Improved ELISA for the Detection of Serum Antibodies Directed Against Classical Swine Fever Virus. Veterinary Microbiology, 1997. 59: pp. 15-25
35. Chowdry V.K., Luo Y., Widén F., Qiu H.J., Shan H., Belák S., Liu L. Development of a loop-mediated isothermal amplification assay combined with a lateral flow dipstick for rapid and simple detection of classical swine fever virus in the field. The Journal of Virological Methods, 2014. 197: pp. 14-18
36. Aynaud J.M. Principle of Vaccination. Classical Swine Fever and Related Viral Infections. Dordrecht: Matinus Nijhoff. 1988. pp. 165-180
37. Blome S., Meindl- Böhmer A., Loeffen W., Thuer B., Moennig V. Assessment of Classical Swine Fever Diagnostics and Vaccine Performance. Revue Science et Technique (International Office of Epizootics), 2006. 25: pp. 1025-1038
38. Rumenapf T., Stark R., Meyers G., Thiel H.J. Structural Proteins of Hog Cholera Virus Expressed by Vaccina Virus – Further Characterization and Induction of Protective Immunity. The Journal of Virology, 1991. 65: pp. 589-597
39. König M., Lengsfeld T., Pauly T., Stark R., Thiel H.J. Classical Swine Fever Virus – Independent Induction of Protective Immunity by 2 Structure Glycoproteins. The Journal of Virology, 1995. 69: pp. 6479-6486
40. van Rijn P.A., van Gennip H.G.P., Moormann R.J.M. An Experimental Marker Vaccine and Accomanying Serological Diagnostic Test Both Based on Envelope Glycoprotein E2 of Classical Swine Fever Virus (CSFV). Vaccine 1999. 17: pp. 433-440
41. Moormann R.J.M., Bouma A., Kramps J.A., Terpstra C., De Smit H.J. Development of a Classical Swine Fever Subunit Marker Vaccine and Companion Diagnostic Test. Veterinary Microbiology, 2000. 73: pp. 209-219
42. Prodanov-Radulovic J., Došen R., Polacek V., Stojanov I., Ratajac R., Valcic M. Classical swine fever: active immunisation of piglets with subunit (E2) vaccine in the presence of different levels of colostral immunity (China strain). Acta Veterinaria-Beograd, 2014. 64: pp. 493-509

Photo Bibliography

Figure 4.4-1: A negatively-stained transmission electron micrograph (TEM) revealing the presence of numerous virions belonging to the family Flaviviridae. This electron photomicrograph was taken by Dr. Fred Murphy and Sylvia Whitfield and released by the CDC. Public domain photo

Foot and Mouth Disease (FMD) is a highly contagious, acute systemic, severe, viral disease affecting cloven-hoofed mammals (e.g. cattle, swine, sheep, goats, etc.) and has great potential for causing grave impacts on food production and incurring large economic loss. FMD is caused by foot and mouth disease virus (FMDV), which is the sole member of the genius *Aphthovirus* of the family *Picornaviridae* (Figure 4.5-1). Presently, there are seven known serotypes of the FMDV – A, O, C, Asia-1, South African Territories (SAT) – 1, SAT-2, SAT-3 and more than 60 strains have been identified. FMDV serotypes and strains vary within each geographic region, although serotype O is the most common worldwide.[1, 2, 3]

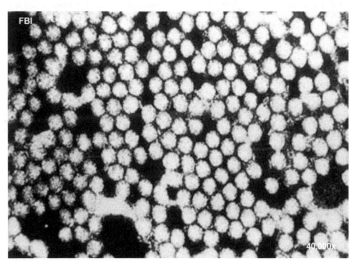

Figure 4.5-1: A transmission electron photomicrograph (TEM) of Foot and Mouth Disease virus

The virus contains a positive-sense, single-stranded RNA genome (~8500 nucleotides) that functions as an mRNA. The viral RNA is linked covalently at its 5' terminus to a small protein, VPg, while the viral genome contains a unique open reading frame flanked by 2 non-coding regions. The initiation of FMDV RNA translation is directed by a large (~440 nucleotides) RNA *cis*-acting element, also known as the internal ribosome entry site (IRES) element. Researchers proposed that the IRES adopt a secondary structure that mediates RNA–protein interactions essential for ribosome recognition.[4, 5, 6] The translation of the genome yields a single viral polyprotein (L-P1-P2-P3), that is subsequently cleaved mainly by virus-encoded proteases (from the P1 region) to form viral structural proteins (VP1-VP4), as well as, non-structural viral proteins such as viral-specific protease 3C and viral specific RNA polymerase 3D.[7, 8]

The viral capsid is non-enveloped, showing icosahedral symmetry with a diameter of approximately 300 Å. The capsid is composed of 60 copies of VP1-VP4 structural proteins with VP1-VP3 (~24 kDa) possessing surface components, while VP4 (~8.5 kDa) is the internal component.[7, 8]

The viral RNA genome also acts as the template for RNA replication.[9] It has been reported that due to the lack of proofreading mechanism, the viral genome undergoes rapid mutation at average rates of 10^{-3} to 10^{-5} substitution per nucleotide copied. Therefore, the population of FMDV possesses various mutants or viral quasispecies.[10] It is believed that this high rate of mutation influences FMDV's evolution, in addition to causing the ever-changing targets for antiviral strategies, including

vaccination.[11]

Due to the seriousness of the disease, FMD prompted the World Organization for Animal Health (OIE) to establish an official list of countries and zones with or without vaccination programs.[12] Recognizing that FMDV is a potential anti-livestock weapon, the Soviet Union established the Main Directorate for Scientific and Production Enterprises (Biokombinat) and the project code named Ecology that developed FMD as an agricultural biological weapon. According to Alibek (1999), FMDV was engineered to be spread from Ilyushin bombers and flown over a target area in a straight line (a line source pattern) to ensure an extended coverage area. Even if only a few animals are infected, the contagious nature of the pathogen would ensure that it would spread and potentially wipe out livestock activities in that region for a long period of time.[13]

FMDV is relatively stable and can persist for extended periods of time in favorable conditions. For example, the virus can remain viable up to a year in cell culture medium, meat, bone marrow and in wool, chilled at 4° C (39° F). Additionally, it can survive for more than three months on bran and hay in laboratory conditions, as well as, two to three months in bovine feces. FMDVs survival is enhanced when it is protected from sunlight and prevented from drying. This virus is inactivated when pH levels fall below 6.5 or rise above 11.[3, 14, 15]

In acutely infected animals, FMDV can be found in all secretions and excretions, such as expired air, saliva, milk, urine, feces and semen. It is known that animals can shed viruses for up to four days before the onset of the first symptoms. Transmission can occur via direct or indirect contact with infected animals or contaminated formites. The main route of transmission of FMDV is through the inhalation of aerosolized virus, but this disease may also spread through the alimentary tract and skin lesions.[1, 3, 16, 17]

The main attachment site on the cell, as well as, the immunodominant region for FMDV, is located on the trypsin-sensitive areas of VP1 within a highly conserved region with Arg-Gly-Asp (RGD) motif. Within this region, there are several overlapping B lymphocyte epitopes (140S particle of VP1) which are able to induce both neutralizing and non-neutralizing antibody responses. However, the high sequence variability seen in this region across the various strains of FMDV accounts for the low cross-reactivity of antibodies between serotypes.[18, 19, 20, 21, 22, 23, 24] The RGD motif, which comprises the main attachment site, targets the host cell surface protein, integrin $\alpha_v\beta_3$, the vitronectin receptor.[25, 26, 27, 28, 29] It is believed that in addition to the main attachment site, there are at least two more mechanisms in which the virus enters the host cell. For example, certain isolates of FMDV use heparin sulfate (HS) as a predominant host cell surface ligand to gain entry. In addition, it has been reported that FMDV may use the antibody-dependent enhancement pathway, where FMDV binds to virus-specific antibodies, gaining entry to the host cell via Fc receptors.[17, 30, 31, 32, 33]

Initially, the virus replicates in the epithelial cells of the pharynx, nasal mucosa and the trachea and subsequently enters the blood stream. Following a three to five day period of febrile viraemia, it spreads throughout the organs and tissues, causing areas of secondary infection. The clinical signs of this disease include fever and vesicles (blisters) on the feet, around the mouth (e.g.

tongue, dental pad, gums, soft palate, nostrils and/or muzzle) and the mammary glands. On occasion these blisters may appear on other locations such as vulva, prepuce or pressure points on the infected animals' legs. These vesicles often rupture rapidly and become erosions (lesions), which are highly painful (Figure 4.5-2). Lesions located on the coronary band (the upper circular limit of the hoof capsule) may cause growth arrest lines on the hoof where, in severe cases, the hoof may slough off (Figure 4.5-3). The discomfort from these lesions leads to a variety of other signs such as anorexia, depression, lameness, excessive salivation, profuse nasal discharge and reluctance to move or rise. Although FMDV does not cross the placenta and infect the fetus, this infection does cause spontaneous abortion in pregnant animals. FMD rarely causes deaths in adult animals, but it does produce high mortality rates in young animals, where it can cause severe lesions of the myocardium.[1, 3, 16, 17]

An asymptomatic persistent infection can be established in ruminants for weeks to years (< 3.5 years), as a consequence of acute infection or due to the vaccination with live-attenuated virus. Animals suffering from a persistent infection are also known as carriers, where they become a reservoir for FMDV.[3, 34, 35, 36]

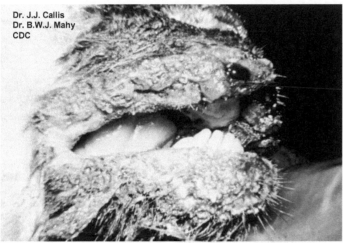

Figure 4.5-2: From the "Illustrated Manual for the Recognition and Diagnosis of Certain Animal Diseases", published in 1982, by the Mexico-United States Commission for the Prevention of Foot and Mouth Disease, this image depicts a close view of proliferative lesions around the mouth of a goat with accompanying detachment of the epithelial lining of the animal's lips, all due to contagious ecthyma

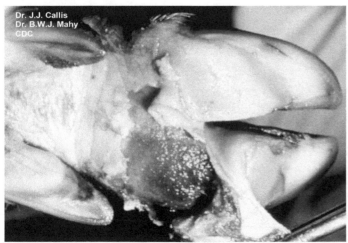

Figure 4.5-3: From the "Illustrated Manual for the Recognition and Diagnosis of Certain Animal Diseases", published in 1982, by the Mexico-United States Commission for the Prevention of Foot and Mouth Disease, this photograph depicts a close-up, ventral view of a pig's foot, displaying a large region of epithelial detachment, due to a foot-and-mouth disease infection

Identification of the foot-and-mouth disease varies with the stage of the disease. For example, in acutely infected animals, FMDV, along with the viral antigens or nucleic acids, can be found in vesicular fluid, epithelial tissue, nasal and oral secretions, esophageal-pharyngeal fluids, blood, milk and in tissue samples (e.g myocardium collected at necropsy, primary bovine thyroid cells or primary pig, calf or lamb kidney cells). Carriers can only be identified through virus isolation and/or the detection of nucleic acids via esophageal-pharyngeal fluids.[3, 37, 38]

Baby hamster kidney (BHK)-21 cell line or porcine kidney cell line, IB-RS-2 cells, can also be used to isolate the viruses via cell culture, but are less sensitive than primary cell cultures.[3, 37, 38] FMDV can be identified from cell cultures by using enzyme-linked immunosorbent assay (ELISA), as well as, compliment fixation (CF), however, it has been reported that ELISAs are superior to CF. ELISA uses monoclonal antibodies designed to detect specific epitopes on the capsid of the FMDV (e.g. 12S protein subunit).[39]

Reverse transcription polymerase chain reaction (RT-PCR) tests can also be used to identify FMDV from cell culture, or real-time reverse transcriptase-PCR (rRT-PCR) may be used to directly detect viral RNA from the blood of the infected animal. However, by using rRT-PCR the virus may be undetectable, until three to five days after the onset of clinical signs of the disease.[40, 41] Serological tests (ELISA) can be used to detect antibodies to viral non-structural proteins (NSP) and diagnose previous or current infections in unvaccinated animals. For example, FMVD diagnostic kits, such as Ceditest ®, UBI ® and a FMDV 3ABC-I-ELISA kits developed at the Lanzhou Veterinary Research Institute are commercially available. The sensitivity and specificity of both Ceditest ® and FMDV 3ABC-I-ELISA kit was 100% sensitive, however, the sensitivity of the UBI ® kit was only 81.8%. Nonetheless, with sera from naive or vaccinated non-infected animals, the specificity of all tests exceeded 90%.[42]

Vaccination has been one of the most efficient manners by which FMDV infections are controlled and eradicated. The first vaccine, a whole-virus live attenuated vaccine, was developed in 1925 by Vallee and collegues, using formaldehyde inactivation of tongue tissue from infected cattle.[43] This manner of vaccine production has been essentially unaltered, with the exception that other tissues, such as fragments of tongue epithelium, BHK-21 cell line, IB-RS-2 cell lines, pig or calf kidney cell monolayer can be used. Following incubation *in vitro*, the virus is inactivated with ethyleneimine (aziridine), absorbed onto aluminum hydroxide and mixed with saponin prior to inoculation. However, this conventional vaccine has its draw- backs. First, the vaccine must be kept at low temperatures in order to preserve its immunogenicity, but this is problematic in certain areas of the world with difficult terrain and warm climate conditions. Secondly, there is the potential that FMDV may escape deactivation and cause a new outbreak, establishing a reservoir of the virus in ruminants. Lastly, the draw-back of conventional vaccines comes from the high antigenic diversity of the FMDV. As indicated previously, FMDVs have seven serotypes and 60 different strains and are constantly mutating to form viral quasispecies. The vaccine must match a particular strain of the virus to immunize the animal from of the disease. Nonetheless, the development of the conventional vaccine did make possible for the comprehensive vaccination programs which resulted in the elimination of the disease by 1989 from Western Europe.[2, 17, 44, 45, 46] Presently, there is ongoing research and development for a synthetic, molecularly engineered vaccine. Some of these experimental vaccines are designed to target the FMDV B-cell epitope located within the protein VPI, however, despite impressive progress, a peptide vaccine that can match the classical vaccine with respect to efficacy has not yet materialized.[47, 48]

References

1. Woodbury R.L. A Review of the Possible Mechanisms for the Persistence of Foot–and-Mouth Disease Virus. Epidemiology and Infection, 1995. 114: pp. 1-13
2. Kitching R.P. A Recent History of Foot-and-Mouth Disease. Journal of Comparative Pathology, 1998. 118: pp. 89-108
3. The Center for Food Security & Public Health. Iowa State University. Classical Swine Fever. Revised April 2014. Retrieved January 10, 2015. Website: http://www.cfsph.iastate.edu/Fact sheets/pdfs/foot_and_mouth_disease.pdf
4. Belsham G.J., Brangwyn J.K. A region of the 5' non-coding region of foot-and-mouth disease virus RNA directs efficient internal initiation of protein synthesis within cells; interaction with the role of the L protease in translational control. The Journal of Virology, 1990. 64: pp. 5389–5395
5. Kuhn R., Luz N., Beck E. Functional analysis of the internal translation initiation site of foot-and-mouth disease virus. The Journal of Virology, 1990. 64: pp. 4625–4631
6. Belsham G.J., Martinez-Salas E. Genome Organization, Translation and Replication of Foot-and-Mouth Disease Virus RNA. Foot-and-Mouth Disease Current Perspectives. London: Horizon Scientific Press. 2004. pp 19–52
7. Domingo E., Escarmís C., Martínez M.A., Martínez-Salas E., Mateu M.G. Foot-and-Mouth Disease Virus Populations are Quasispecies. Current Topics in Microbiology and Immunology, 1992. 176: pp. 33-47
8. Acharya R., Fry E., Stuart D., Fox G., Rowlands D., Brown F. The Three-dimensional Structure of Foot-and-Mouth Disease Virus at 2.9 Å Resolution. Nature, 1989.337: pp. 709-716
9. Belsham G.J. Translation and replication of FMDV RNA. Current Topics in Microbiology and Immunology, 2005. 288: pp. 43–70
10. Domingo E, Pariente N, Airaksinen A, Gonzalez-Lopez C, Sierra S, Herrera M, Grande-Perez A, Lowenstein PR, Manrubia SC, Lazaro E, Escarmis C: Foot-and-mouth disease virus evolution: exploring pathways towards virus extinction. populations are quasispecies. Current Topics in Microbiology and Immunology, 2005. 288: pp. 149-173
11. Domingo E, Escarmis C, Baranowski E, Ruiz-Jarabo CM, Carrillo E, Nunez JI, Sobrino F: Evolution of foot-and-mouth disease virus. Virus Research, 2003. 91: pp. 47–63
12. World Organization for Animal Health. Foot-and-Mouth Disease. Revised April 22, 2002. Retrieved December 29, 2009. Website: http://www.oie.int/Eng/maladies/fiches/a_A010.htm
13. Alibek K. Biohazard. New York: Dell Publishing. 1999. pp. 37-38
14. Bartley L.M., Donnelly C.A., Anderson R.M. Review of Foot-and-Mouth Disease Virus Survival in Animal Excretions and on Formites. The Veterinary Record, 2002. 151: pp. 667-669
15. Tomasula P.M., Konstance R.P. The Survival of Foot-and-Mouth Disease Virus in Raw and Pasteurized Milk and Milk Products. Journal of Dairy Science, 2004. 87: pp. 1115-1121
16. Domingo E., Mateu M.G., Martínez M.A., Dopazo J., Moya A., Sobrino F. Genetic Variability and Antigenic Diversity of Foot-and-Mouth Disease Virus. Applied Virology Research. Volume 2. New York: Plenum Publishing Company. 1990. pp. 233-266
17. Doel T.R. Natural and Vaccine-induced Immunity to Foot-and-Mouth Disease: The Prospects for Improved Vaccines. Revue Science et Technique (International Office of Epizootics), 1996. 15: pp. 883-911
18. Laporte J., Lenoir G. Structural Proteins of Foot-and-Mouth Disease Virus. Journal of General Virology, 1973. 20: pp. 161-168
19. Cavanagh D., Sangar D.V., Rowlands D.J., Brown F. Immunogenic and Cell Attachmnet Sites of Foot-andMouth Disease Virus: Further Evidence for Their Location in a Single Capsid Polypeptide. Journal of General Virology, 1977. 35: pp. 149-158
20. Strohaier K., Franze R., Adam K.H. Location and Characterization of the Antigenic Portion of the Foot-and-Mouth Disease Virus Immunizing Protein. Journal of General Virology, 1982. 59: pp. 295-306
21. Cheung A., DeLamarter J., Weiss S., Küpper H. Comparison of the Major Antigenic Determinants of Different Serotypes of Foot-and-Mouth Disease Virus. The Journal of Virology, 1983. 48: pp. 451-459
22. Beck E., Feil G., Strohmaier K. The Molecular Basis of the Antigenic Variation of Foot-and-Mouth Disease Virus. European Molecular Biology Organization (EMBO) Journal, 1983. 2: pp. 555-559
23. Oulridge E.J., Barnett P.V., Parry N.R., Syred A., Head M., Rweyemamu M.M. Demonstration of Neutralizing and Non-Neutralizing Epitopes on the Trypsin-Sensitive Site of Foot-and-Mouth Disease Virus. Journal of General Virology, 1984. 65: pp. 203-207
24. Grubman M.J., Zellner M., Wagner J. Antigenic Comparison of the Polypeptides of Foot-and-Mouth Disease Virus Serotypes and Other Picornaviruses. Birology, 1987. 158: pp. 133-140
25. Fox G., Parry N.R., Barnett P.V., McGinn B., Rowlands D.J., Brown F. The Cell Attachment Site on Foot-and-Mouth Disease Virus includes the Amino Acid Sequence RGD (Arginine-Glycine-Aspartic Acid). Journal of General Virology, 1989. 70: pp. 625-637
26. Verdaguer N., Mateu M.G., Andreu D., Giralt E., Domingo E., Fita I. Structure of the Major Antigenic Loop of Foot-and-Mouth Disease Virus Complexed with a Neutralizing Antibody: Direct Involvement of Arg-Gly-Asp Motif in the Interaction. European Molecular Biology Organization (EMBO) Journal, 1995. 14: pp. 1690-1696
27. Verdaguer N., Mateu M.G., Bravo J., Domingo E., Fita I. Induced Pocket to Accommodate the Cell Attachment Site Arg-Gly-Asp Motif in a Neutralizing Antibody Against Foot-and-Mouth Disease Virus. Journal of Molecular Biology, 1996. 256: pp. 364-376
28. Berinstein A., Rovivain M., Hovi T., Mason P.W., Baxt B. Antibodies to the Vitronectin Receptor (Integrin $\alpha_v\beta_3$) Inhibits Binding and Infection of Foot-and-Mouth Disease Virus to Cultured Cells. The Journal of Virology, 1995. 69: pp. 2664-2666
29. Jackson T., Ellard F.M., Abu-Ghazaleh R., Brookes S.M., Blakemore W.E., Corteyn A.H., Stuart D.I., Newman J.W.I., King A.M.Q. Efficient Infection of Cells in Culture by Type O Foot-and-Mouth Disease Virus Requires Binding to Cell Surface Heparan Sulfate. The Journal of Virology, 1996. 70: pp. 5282-5287
30. Sá-Carvalho D., Rieder E., Baxt B., Rodarte R., Tanuri A., Mason P.W. Tissue Culture Adaptation of Foot-and-Mouth Disease Virus Selects Viruses that Binds to Heparin and are Attenuated in Cattle. The Journal of Virology, 1997. 71: pp. 5115-5123
31. Mason P.W., Baxt B., Brown F., Harber J., Murdin A., Wimmer E. Antibody-complexed Foot-and-Mouth Disease Virus, but Not Poliovirus, can Infect Normally Insusceptible Cells via the Fc Receptor. Virology, 1993. 192: pp. 568-577
32. Jackson T., Sharma A., Abu-Ghazaleh R., Blakemore W.E., Ellard F.M., Simmins D.L., Newman J.W.I., Stuart D.I., King A.M.Q. Arginine-Glycine-Aspartic Acid-specific Binding by Foot-and-mouth Disease Viruses to the Purified Integrin $\alpha_v\beta_3$ in vitro. The Journal of Virology, 1997. 71: pp. 8357-8361
33. Ruiz-Jarabo C.M., Sevilla N., Dávila M., Gómez-Mariano G., Baranowski E., Doningo E. Antigenic Properties and Population Stability of a Foot-and-Mouth Disease Virus with an Altered Arg-Gly-Asp Receptor Recongnition Motif. Journal of General Virology, 1999. 80: pp. 1899-1909
34. Gebauer F., de la Torre J.C., Gomes I., Mateu M.G., Barahona H., Tiraboschi B., Bergmann I., Augé de Mello P., Domingo E. Rapid Selection of Genetic and Antigenic Variants of Foot-and-Mouth Disease Virus During Persistence in Cattle. The Journal of Virology, 1988. 62: pp. 2041-2049
35. Hernández A.M.M., Carrilo E.C., Servilla N., Doningo E. Rapid Cell Variation can Determine the Establishment of a Persistent Viral Infection. Proceedings of the National Academy of Science United States of America, 1994. 91: pp. 3705-3709
36. Alexanderson S., Zhang Z., Donaldson A.I., Garland A.J.M. The Pathogenesis and Diagnosis of Foot-and-Mouth disease. Journal of Comparative Pathology, 2003. 129: pp. 1-36
37. Chapman W.G., Ramshaw I.A. Growth of the IB-RS-2 Pig Kidney Cell Line in Suspension Culture and Its Susceptibility to Foot-and-Mouth Disease Virus. Applied Microbiology, 1971. 22: pp. 1–5
38. Herrera M., Grande-Pérez A., Perales C., Domingo E. Persistence of Foot-and-Mouth Disease Virus in Cell Culture Revisited: Implications for Contingency in Evolution. Journal of General Virology, 2008. 89: pp. 232-244
39. Smitsaart E., Saiz J.C., Yedloutschnig R.J., Morgan D.O. Detection of Foot-and-Mouth Disease Virus by Competitive ELISA using a Monoclonal Antibody Specific for the 12S Protein Subunit from Six of the Seven Serotypes. Veterinary Immunology and Immunopathology, 1990. 26: pp. 251-265
40. Goris N., Vandenbussche F., Herr C., Villers J., van der Stede Y., de Clercq K. Validation of Two Real-Time RT-PCR Methods for Foot-and-Mouth Disease Diagnosis: RNA-Extraction, Matrix Effect, Uncertainty of Measurement and Precision. Jorunal of Virological Methods, 2009. 160: pp. 157-162
41. Juleff N., Widsor M., Reid E., Seago J., Zhang Z., Monaghan P., Morrison I.W., Charleston B. Foot-and-Mouth Disease Virus Persists in the Light Zone of Germinal Certres. Public Library of Science (PLoS) One, 2008. 3: pp. 1-9
42. Cao Y-M., Lu Z-J., Liu Z-X., Xie Q-G. Comparison of three ELISA Kits for the Differentiation of Foot-and-Mouth Disease Virus-Infected From Vaccinated Animals. Virologica Sinica, 2007. 22: pp. 74-79
43. Lombard M., Pastoret P.P., Moulin A.M. A brief history of vaccines and vaccination. Scientific and Technical Review of the Office International des Epizooties, 2007. 26: pp. 29-48
44. Mason P.W., Piccone M.E., McKenna T. St.C., Chinsangaram J., Grubman M.J. Evaluation of a Live-attenuated Foot-and-Mouth Disease Virus as a Vaccine Candidate. Virology, 1997. 227: pp. 96-102
45. Doel T.R. Optimization of the Immune Response to Foot-and-Mouth Disease Vaccine. Vaccinie, 1999. 17: pp. 1767-1771
46. Brown F. Foot-and-Mouth Disease and Beyond: Vaccine Design, Past, Present and Future. Archives of Virology, 1999. 15: pp. 179-188
47. Meloen R.H., Langeveld J.P.M., Schaaper W.M.M., Slootstra J.W. Synthetic Peptide Vaccines: Unexpected Fulfillment of Discarded Hope? Biologicals, 2001. 29: pp. 233-236
48. Zhang Z., Pan L., DingY., Zhou P., Lv J., Chen H., Fang Y., Liu X., Chang H., Zhang J., Shao J., Lin T., Zhao F., Zhang Y., Wang Y. Efficacy of synthetic peptide candidate vaccines against serotype-A foot-and-mouth disease virus in cattle. Applied Microbiology and Biotechnology, 2014. 10: pp. 1007

Photo Bibliography

Figure 4.5-1: A transmission electron photomicrograph (TEM) of Foot and Mouth Disease Virus. This photograph was taken and released by the Federal Bureau of Investigations (FBI). Public domain photo

Figure 4.5-2: From the "Illustrated Manual for the Recognition and Diagnosis of Certain Animal Diseases", published in 1982, by the Mexico-United States Commission for the Prevention of Foot and Mouth Disease, this image depicts a close view of proliferative lesions around the mouth of a goat with accompanying detachment of the epithelial lining of the animal's lips, all due to contagious ecthyma. The photograph was taken by Dr. Jerry J. Callis and Dr. Brian W.J. Mahy and released by the CDC. Public domain photo

Figure 4.5-3: From the "Illustrated Manual for the Recognition and Diagnosis of Certain Animal Diseases", published in 1982, by the Mexico-United States Commission for the Prevention of Foot and Mouth Disease, this photograph depicts a close-up, ventral view of a pig's foot, displaying a large region of epithelial detachment, due to a foot-and-mouth disease infection. The photograph was taken by Dr. Jerry J. Callis and Dr. Brian W.J. Mahy and released by the CDC. Public domain photo

Newcastle disease (ND), also known as fowl pest, is an acute viral disease of domestic poultry and many other bird species (~250 species in 27 orders), with a wide range of clinical signs extending from mild to severe, depending on the pathotype of the virus and the susceptibility of the host.[1] The first documented cases of ND simultaneously occurred in Java, Indonesia and Newcastle-upon-Tyne, England in 1926; the latter is where the disease obtained it name.[2] Presently, ND is still endemic in many countries in Asia, Africa, and the Americas, where it causes considerable economic losses, high flock mortality rates, as well as, subsequent trade restrictions for that nation following an outbreak.[3]

ND is caused by viruses in the serotype avian paramyxovirus type 1 (APMV-1), which are members of the newly formed genus *Avulavirus* (previously classified as genus *Rubulavirus*), belonging to the family Paramyxoviridae. APMV-1 has also been referred to as the Newcastle disease virus (NDV), or at times referred to pigeon paramyxovirus type 1 (PPMV-1), due to the various strains that have been maintained in pigeon populations, and posseses some antigenic differences. APMV-1 isolates are divided into two classes (class I and class II) based on the genetic relationship among the isolates.[4, 5] For example, the vast majority of the strains belong to class II, divided into nine genotypes (I-IX), while class I isolates are found mainly in wild waterfowl and are usually low in pathogenicity (Figure 4.6-1).[4, 5, 6, 7, 8, 9]

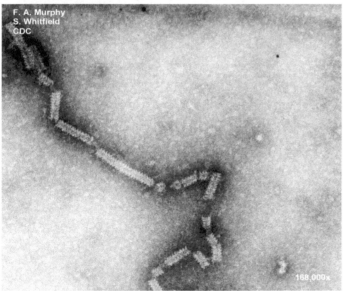

F. A. Murphy
S. Whitfield
CDC

168,000x

Figure 4.6-1: A transmission electron photomicrograph (TEM) of *Paramyxoviridae*

APMV-1 strains are classified into three pathotypes, based on their virulence in chickens. Velogenic strains, also known as exotic Newcastle Disease (END), are the most virulent and cause acute fatal infections in chickens of all age groups, with clinical findings of neurological signs and extensive hemorrhagic lesions of the gastrointestinal tract. Velogenic strains are further subdivided into two forms: the neurotropic form, which is generally associated with respiratory and neurological symptoms, and viscerotropic form which is associated with hemorrhagic intestinal lesions.[4, 10, 11, 12, 13] Mesogenic strains, are moderately virulent with occasional nervous and respiratory signs, while lentogenic strains are of low virulence and are commonly used as live vaccines in healthy chickens.[4, 12, 14]

The genome of the APMV-1 is a single stranded, enveloped, ~15,186 nucleotide, negative-sense RNA that contains six genes that encode for at least eight proteins.[15, 16, 17] For example, the nucleoprotein (NP), phosphoprotein (P), and large polymerase protein (L) form the nucelocapsid while the hemagglutinin-neuraminidase (HN) and the fusion protein (F) constitute the external envelope. [1, 13, 16, 17, 18, 19, 20, 21] The APMV-1 genes are tandemly linked in the order of 3'-NP-P-M-F-HN-L-5' and are separated by junction sequences consisting of gene-end (GE), intergenic (IG) and gene-start (GS). The replication of the viral genome is dependent upon encapsidation of the RNA by the NP, which acts as a template for a polymerase complex composed of L and P cofactors. It is believed that the viral RNA-polymerase complex enters the genomic RNA at a single 3' entry site and transcribes the genome by a sequential start to stop mechanism.[13, 22, 23, 24]

It has been reported that the F protein cleavage site is the major determinant of APMV-1 virulence. It is known that the precursor, F_0 glycoprotein must be cleaved into F_1 and F_2 for the progeny virus to be infectious. The matrix (M) protein forms the inner layer of the virion while the alternative mRNA that are generated by RNA editing process during P gene transcription yield two more non-structural proteins: V and W.[1, 16, 17, 18, 19, 20, 21, 24] Huang *et al.* (2003), have reported that V proteins are zinc-binding interferon-α (IFN-α) antagonists by selectively targeting the STAT1 protein for degradation while the function of the W protein remains to be elucidated.[25]

APMV-1 are transmitted either through the inhalation of aerosolized viruses and/or through the fecal-oral route (e.g. ingestion of contaminated food or water). It is known that infected birds shed virus in exhaled air, respiratory discharges, eggs laid during an infection and feces. In addition, APMV-1 are found in all parts of the infected bird and the ingestion of contaminated meat could result in the transmission of the virus. Furthermore, insect vectors may also be involved in the transmission of the disease.[25] APMV-1 are relatively hardy and have been reported to remain viable for up to 255 days in a henhouse (-11° C/12° F to 36° C/97° F), survive in contaminated litter for 10 to 14 days at 23-29° C (73-84° F), and in the soil for 22 days at 20° C (68° F).[4]

APMV-1 HN binds to host epithelial cells via sialic acid-containing host cell receptors. Subsequent to the binding the F protein mediates the fusion of viral and host cellular membrane. The RNA genome of the virus is then released into the cytoplasm and undergoes replication and transcription. It has been reported that HN can induce caspase-dependent (e.g. caspase-8 and -9) intrinsic and extrinsic apoptotic pathways in chicken embryo fibroblast cells; and it is suggested that it may have a similar effect on avian lymphoid cells, leading to lymphoid depletion in APMV-1-infected birds.[18] It is believed that the assembly of the viral component takes place at the host cell membrane while the mature virus is release via budding.[23, 27]

During an infection caused by velogenic strains, the onset of clinical signs is rapid both in individual and at the level of the flock, within 2 to 12 days after aerosol exposure. The spread is slower if the disease is transmitted via fecal-oral route. The signs observed are dependent on the strain of virus and its predilection for the respiratory, digestive or nervous system. Nonetheless, sudden death, with few or no signs may also occur.[4] Initial signs of lethargy, lack of appetite, conjunctival reddening, edema and ruffled feathers are common signs of velogenic infections (Figure 4.6-2). Birds may develop watery, greenish-white diarrhea, coupled with respiratory signs of depression, gasping, coughing and sneezing are commonly observed. In addition, the infected birds will also develop cyanosis (bluish coloration of the skin), as well as, swelling of tissues in the head and neck. Occurring concurrently, or most often seen in the later stages of the infection, are neurological signs which include tremors, paralyzed wings and/or legs, torticllis (twisted necks), circling, clonic spasms or complete paralysis. Egg production will decline dramatically during the course of the disease. Eggs that are laid during the course of the infection may be abnormal in color, rough or thinned shelled, irregular in shape with watery albumen. Mortality is variable, but can be as high as 100%.[4, 28, 29, 30]

ND can be diagnosed by isolating APMV-1 from infected birds. The virus can be insolated by inoculating samples into 9 to 11 days old chicken embryos. Subsequently, chorioallantoic fluids from the eggs are examined for hemagglutination. Any agents that cause hemagglutination are examined for hemmagglutination inhibition (HI) with a monospecific antiserum to APMV-1. The pathogenicity of the virus can be calculated by the mean death time (MDT) of the chicken embryo (e.g. MDT for velogenic is >60 hours, 60-90 hours for mesogenic, and lentogenic <90 hours), intracerebral pathogenicity index (ICPI) in one day old chicks and intravenous pathogenicity (IVPI) index in 6 week old chickens.[4, 31, 32]

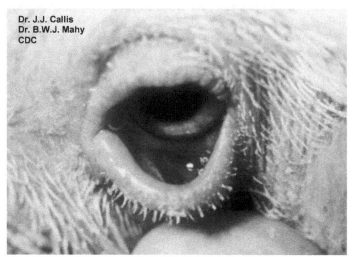

Dr. J.J. Callis
Dr. B.W.J. Mahy
CDC

Figure 4.6-2: This image shows a close lateral view of chicken's eye, demonstrating conjunctivitis and edema of the eyelids, resulting from New Castle disease

Reverse transcription polymerase chain reaction (RT-PCR), nucleotide sequencing, restriction endonuclease analysis are all capable of identifying APMV-1 in the eggs of clinical specimens and their pathotype. Most highly virulent forms of APMV-1 have a particular amino acid sequence, 112R/K-R-Q-K/R-R116, at the C-terminus of the F2 protein and phenylalanine at residue 117 of the F1 protein.[4, 32, 33, 34, 35, 36] Serological examinations, such as enzyme linked immunosorbent assays (ELISA), can also be used to identify ND infections.[37]

Live lentogenic vaccines (e.g. B1 and LaSota strains) are widely used and are administered to poultry through drinking water, spray or individual administration via the nares or conjunctival sac. Administering live-attenuated vaccines has shown to produce protective mucosal immunity mediated by immunoglobulin A (IgA) antibodies.[38, 39] Vaccination should be completed between days one to four after hatching although delaying vaccination until the second or third week avoids maternal antibody interference

with an active immune response. Oil-adjuvanted inactivated vaccines could be used alone or administered following live vaccine administration. The combinations of live attenuated and inactivated vaccines are generally applied in countries where virulent NDV is endemic. Administration of inactivated vaccines produces high levels of serum antibodies which produce humoral immunity; however the lack of local immunity has been reported.[40, 41]

References

1. Alexander D.J. Newcastle Disease and Other Paramyxoviridae Infections. Diseases of Poultry. Tenth Edition. Ames: Iowa State University Press. 1997. pp. 541-569
2. Lancaster J.E. A History of Newcastle Disease with Comments on its Economic Effects. World's Poultry Science Journal, 1976. 32: pp. 167-175
3. Leslie J. Newcastle Disease: Outbreak Losses and Control Policy Costs. The Veterinary Record, 2000. 146: pp. 603-606
4. The Center for Food Security & Public Health. Iowa State University. Newcastle Disease. Revised July 14, 2008. Retrieved December 29, 2009. Website: http://www.cfsph.iastate.edu/Facts heets/pdfs/Newcastle disease.pdf
5. van Regenmortel M.H.V., Ranquet C.M., Bishop D.H.L., Carstens E.B., Estes M.K., Lemon S.M., Maniloff J., Mayo M.A., McGeoch D.J., Pringle C.R., Wickner R.B. Virus Taxonomy. 7th Report of International Committee on Taxonomy of Virus. San Diego: Academic Press. 2000. pp. 1024
6. Seal B.S., King D.J. Characterization of Newcastle Disease Virus Isolates by Reverse Transcription PCR coupled to Direct Nucleotide Sequencing and Development of Sequence Database for Pathotype Prediction and Molecular Epidemiological Analysis. Journal of Clinical Microbiology, 1995. 33: pp. 2624-2630
7. Czegledi A., Ujvari D., Somogyi E., Wehmann E., Werner O., Lomniczi B. Third Genome Size Category of Avian Paramyxovirus Serotype I (Newcastle Disease Virus) and Evolutionary Implications. Virus Research, 2006. 120: pp. 36-48
8. Kim L.M., King D.J., Curry P.E., Suarez D.L., Swayne D.E., Stallknecht D.E., Slemons R.D., Pedersen J.C., Senne D.A., Winker K., Afonso C.L. Phylogenetic Diversity Among Low-virulence Newcastle Disease Virus from Waterfowl and Shorebirds and Comparison of Genotype Distribution to Those of Poultry-Origin Isolates. The Journal of Virology, 2007. 81: pp. 12641-12653
9. Liu X.F., Wan H.Q., Ni X.X., Wu Y.T., Liu W.B. Pathotypical and Genotypical Characterization of Strains of Newcastle Disease Virus Isolated from Outbreaks in Chicken and Goose Flocks in Some Regions of China during 1985-2001. Archives of Virology, 2003. 148: pp. 1387-1403
10. Seal B.S., King D.J., Locke D.P., Senne D.A., Jackwood M.W. Phylogenetic Relationship among Highly Virulent Newcatle Disease Virus Isolates Obtained from Exotic Birds and Poultry from 1989-1996. Journal of Clinical Microbiology, 1998. 36: pp. 1141-1145
11. Pedersen J.C., Seene D.A., Woolcock P.R., Kinde H., King D.J., Wise M.G., Panigrahy B., Seal B.S. Phylogenetic Relationships among Virulent Newcastle Disease Virus Isolates from the 2002-2003 Outbreak in California and Other Recent Outbreaks in North America. Journal of Clinical Microbiology, 2004. 42: pp. 2329-2334
12. Jindal N., Chander Y., Chockalingam A.K., de Abin M., Redig P.T., Goyal S.M. Phylogenetic Analysis of Newcastle Disease Virus Isolated from Waterfowl in the Upper Midwest Region of the United States. Virology Journal, 2009. 6: pp. 1-9
13. Absalón A.E., Mariano-Matías A., García L.J., Morales-Garzón A., Toscano-Contreras A., Lucio-Decanini E., Cortés-Espinosa D.V. Complete genome analysis of velogenic Newcastle disease virus reference strain "Chimalhuacan": evolution of viral lineages in Mexico. Virus Genes, 2014. 49: pp. 233-236
14. Chellappa M.M., Dey S., Gaikwad S., Kataria J.M., Vakharia V.N. Complete Genome Sequence of Newcastle Disease Virus Mesogenic Vaccine Strain R2B from India. The Journal of Virology, 2012. 86: pp. 13814–13815
15. Krishnamurthy S., Samal S.K. Nucelotide Sequence of Trailer Nucleocapsid Protein Gene and Intergenic Region of Newcastle Disease Virus Strain Beaudette, C, and Completion of the Entire Genome Sequence. Journal of General Virology, 1998. 79: pp. 2419-2424
16. de Leeuw O.S., Peeters B. Complete Nucleotide Sequence of Newcastle Disease Virus: Evidence for the Existence of a New Genus within the Subfamily Paramyxocivinae. Journal of General Virology, 1999. 80: pp. 131-136
17. Steward M., Vipond I.B., Millar N.S., Emmerson P.T. RNA Editing in Newcastle Disease Virus. Journal of General Virology, 1993. 74: pp. 2539-2547
18. Ravindra P.V., Tiwari A.K., Sharma B., Rajawat Y.S., Ratta B., Palia S., Sundaresan N.R., Chaturvedi U., Kumar G.B.A., Chindera K., Saxena M., Subudhi P.K., Rai A., Chauhan R.S. HN Protein of Newcastle Disease Virus Causes Apoptosis in Chicken Embryo Fibroblast Cells. Archives of Virology, 2008. 153: pp. 749-754
19. Peeters B.P.H., de Leeuw O.S., Koch G., Gielkens A.L. Rescue of Newcastle Disease Virus from Cloned cDNA: Evidence that Cleavability of the Fusion Protein is a Major Determinant for Virulence. The Journal of Virology, 1999. 73: pp. 5001-5009
20. McGinnes L., McQuain C., Morrison T. The P protein and the Nonstructural 38K and 29K proteins of Newcastle Disease Virus are Derived from the Same Open Reading Frame. Virology, 1988. 164: pp. 256-264
21. Jordan I.K. Sutter IV B.A., McClure M.A. Molecular Evolution of the Paramyxoviridae and Rhabdoviridae Multiple-protein-encoding P Gene. Molecular Biology and Evolution, 2000. 17: pp. 75-86
22. Hamaguchi M., Yoshida T., Nishikawa K., Naruse H., Nagai Y. Transcriptive Complex of Newcastle Disease Virus. I. Both P and L proteins are required to Constitute and Active Complex. Virology, 1983. 128: pp. 105-117
23. Lamb R.A., Kolakofsky D. Paramyxoviridae: the Viruses and Their Replication. Fields Vriology. Third Edition. Philadelphia: Lippincott-Raven. Pp. 1177-1204
24. Zhao H., Peeters B.P.H. Recombinant Newcastle Disease Virus as a Viral Vector: Effect of Genomic Location of Foreign Gene on Gene Expression and Virus Replication. Journal of General Virology, 2003. 84: pp. 781-788
25. Huang Z., Krishnamurthy S., Panda A., Samal S.K. Newcastle Disease Virus V Protein is Associated with Viral Pathogenesis and Functions as an Alpha Interferon Antagonist. The Journal of Virology, 2003. 77: pp. 8676-8685
26. Chakrabarti S., King D.J., Afonso C., Swayne D., Cardona C.J., Kuney D.R., Gerry A.C. Detection and Isolation of Exotic Newcastle Disease Virus from Field-collected Flies. Journal of Medical Entomology, 2007. 44: pp. 840-844
27. Simons K., Garoff H. The Budding Mechanisms of Enveloped Animal Viruses. Journal of General Virology, 1980. 50: pp. 1-20
28. National Agriculture Biosecurity Center, Kansas State University. Revised: 2009. Retrieved: December 31, 2009. Website: http://nabc.ksu.edu/content/factsheets/category/

Exotic%20Newcastle%20Disease

29. Friend M., Franson J.C. Biological Resources Division. Field Manual of Wildlife Diseases General Field Procedures and Diseases of Birds. Washington D.C.: United States Department of Interior. United States Geological Survey. 1999. pp. 175-180

30. Samour J. Newcastle Disease in Captive Falcons in the Middle East: A Review of Clinical and Pathologic Findings. Journal of Avian Medicine and Surgery, 2014. 28: pp. 1–5

31. Alexander D.J. Newcastle Disease. A Laboratory Manual for the Isolation and Identification of Avian Pathogens. Jacksonville: American Association of Avian Pathologists. 1989. pp. 110-112

32. Chang P.C., Hsieh M.L., Shien J.H., Grahm D.A., Lee M.S., Shieh H.K. Complete Nucleotide Sequence of Avian Paramyxovirus Type 6 Isolated from Ducks. Journal of General Virology, 2001. 82: pp. 2157-2168

33. Creelan J.L., Graham D.A., McCullough S.J. Detection and Differentiation of Pathogenicity of Avian Paramyxovirus Serotype 1 from Field Cases Using one-step Reverse Transcriptase-Polymerase Chain Reaction. Avian Pathology, 2002. 31: pp. 493-499

34. Zou J., Shan S., Yao N., Gong Z. Complete Genome Sequence and Biological Characterizations of a Novel Goose Paramyxovirus-SF02 Isolated in China. Virus Genes, 2005. 30: pp. 13-21

35. Mohan C.M., Dey S., Kumanan K. Restriction Enzyme Analysis of Tissue Culture-adapted Velogenic Newcastle Disease Virus. Veterinary Research Communications, 2006. 30: pp. 455-466

36. Al-Habeeb M.A., Mohamed M.H.A., Sharawi S. Detection and characterization of Newcastle disease virus in clinical samples using real time RT-PCR and melting curve analysis based on matrix and fusion genes amplification. Veterinary World, 2013. pp. 239-243

37. Stanislawek W.L., Wilks C.R., Meers J., Horner G.W., Alexander D.J., Manvell R.J., Kattenbelt J.A., Gould A.R. Avian Paramyxoviruses and Influenza Viruses Isolated from Mallard Ducks (Anas platyrhynchos) in New Zealand. Archives of Virology, 2002. 147: pp. 1287-1302

38. Parry S.H., Aitken I.D. Immunoglobulin A in the Respiratory Tract of Chicken Following Exposure to Newcastle Disease Virus. The Veterinary Records, 1973. 42: pp. 258-260

39. Jayawardane G.W.L., Spardbrow P.B. Mucosal Immunity in Chickens Vaccinated with the V4 Strain of Newcastle Disease Virus. Veterinary Microbiology, 1995. 46: pp. 69-77

40. van Eck J.H.H. Immunity to Newcastle Disease in Fowl of Different Breeds Primarily Vaccinated with Commercial Inactivated Oil-emulsion Vaccines: a Laboratory Experiment. Veterinary Quarterly, 1987. 9: pp. 296-303

41. Folitse R., Halvorson D.A., Sivanandan V. Efficacy of Combined Killed-in-oil Emulsion and Live Newcastle Disease Vaccines in Chickens. Avian Diseases, 1998. 42: pp. 173-178

Photo Bibliography

Figure 4.6-1: A transmission electron photomicrograph (TEM) of *Paramyxoviridae*. The electron photomicrograph was taken by S. Whitfield and F. A. Murphy and released by the CDC. Public domain photo

Figure 4.6-2: This photograph is from the "Illustrated Manual for the Recognition and Diagnosis of Certain Animal Diseases", published in 1982, by the Mexico-United States Commission for the Prevention of Foot and Mouth Disease. This image shows a close lateral view of chicken's eye, demonstrating conjunctivitis and edema of the eyelids, resulting from to New Castle disease. This photograph was taken by Dr. Jerry J. Callis and Dr. Brian W.J. Mahy in 1982 and released by the CDC. Public domain photo

Rinderpest, also known as cattle plague or Steppe murrain, is caused by the rinderpest virus (RPV). RPV is a non-segmented, single stranded, enveloped negative-sense RNA virus and is the only serotype belonging to the genus *Morbillivirus* of the family *Paramyxoviridae*. There are three distinct lineages of rinderpest virus that have been identified (lineage 1 to 3) from different geographical areas around the world (Figure 4.7-1).[1, 2]

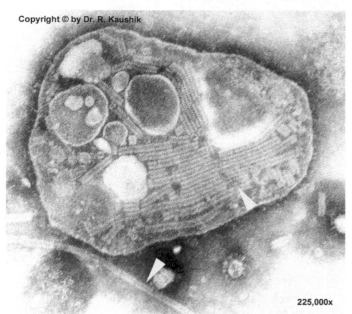

225,000x

Figure 4.7-1: A transmission electron micrograph (TEM) revealed the ultrastructural appearance of rinderpest viruses (arrows), a member of the genus *Morbillivirus* of the family Paramyxoviridae

Rinderpest is an acute, highly infectious and deadly disease of domestic cattle and other hoofed animals (e.g. sheep, goats, pigs, buffalo, giraffe, wildebeest, etc.). In the past, epidemics of rinderpest appeared regularly in Eurasia, but in 1887 a cattle shipment from India to Africa (Eritrea) spread the disease to that continent. This initial epidemic killed approximately 90% of the cattle in sub-Saharan Africa, as well as, great numbers of sheep and goats. Wildlife, such as buffalos, giraffes and wildebeasts, were also greatly affected and their populations were decimated. The loss of livestock and wildlife caused mass starvation in the human population and one-third of Ethiopia's population perished.[3, 4, 5, 6, 7, 8]

By the early 20th century, rinderpest had been eradicated from Europe, and in the 1960s an international project to eradicate the virus globally through a vaccination program began. This program was initiated by the Organization of African Unity in 1962, which included 22 countries, with the launch of the Joint Project 15. Initially, the project was a success, as cattle in African countries were vaccinated. However, gradually many countries begin to lapse in the vaccination program due to the expenses involved. Finally, the project was terminated after non-compliance. This ill timed termination allowed the disease to reemerge from remaining pockets of infection (the Mali-Mauritiana border and Southern Sudan) and re-colonize larger areas of the African continent during the 1980's.[9] This rinderpest epizootic resulted in the initiation of the Pan African Rinderpest Campaign (PARC). Later, in 1992, the United Nations Food and Agriculture Organization (FAO) initiated the Global Rinderpest Eradication Programme (GREP) with the goal of completely eradicating the virus by the year 2010. By utilizing zoosanitary measures with vaccination, lineage 3 was last seen in 2000, while in 2001, lineage 1 was last observed. Lineage 2 has been eradicated from most of Africa, however, a pocket may still exist in the Somali pastoral ecosystem (southern Somalia, northeast Kenya and southeastern Ethiopia).[1, 3, 8] In response to this potential pocket of RPV lineage 2 in Somali pastoral ecosystem, the Somali Ecosystem Rinderpest Eradication Coordination Unit (SEREGU) was developed in 2006 to monitor and eradicate this disease. Finally, in 2011, the 79th General Session of the World Assembly of the World Organisation for Animal Health (OIE) and the 37th Food and Agriculture Organization of the United Nations (FAO) adopted a resolution declaring the world free from rinderpest.[10] However, the stocks of RPV still exist and there remains a risk of reintroduction. Pathways leading to the reappearance of RPV include deliberate or accidental use of virus in laboratories, deliberate or accidental use of vaccines, host exposure to an environmental source of virus, and use of virus for anti-animal biological warfare.[11]

Transmission of RPV is usually through direct or indirect contact with infected animals. The incubation period for RPV ranges from 3 to 15 days. Prior to the onset of clinical signs (one to two days), RPV can be isolated in small amounts from nasal and ocular secretions, saliva, milk, blood, urine, fecal matter and tissues. After the onset of clinical signs, during first week of infection, large numbers of virus particles can be found in all the infected animals' secretions and excretions such as nasal and ocular secretions, saliva, milk, blood, semen, vaginal discharges, urine, fecal matter and also in tissues. It has been reported that even the expired air of infected animals contains RPV. Certain species of pigs can become infected with rinderpest if they ingest contaminated tissues and can subsequently transmit the virus to other hoofed animals.[1, 2, 12, 13]

RPV can remain viable for at least a week in meat kept at 4° C (39° F), however, it can be easily deactivated by exposure to sunlight or drying. RPV are known to remain viable on un-shaded pastures for approximately six hours, while it remains viable for approximately 18 to 48 hours in shaded pastures. Within bare enclosures, RPV can remain infective for approximately 48 hours and remain viable in an enclosed building for a minimum of 96 hours.[1]

Rinderpest may appear in subacute or acute (classical) forms depending on the virulence of the viral strain involved and the innate resistance of various breeds of cattle and other hoofed animals. For example, Saudi/81 RPV strain is generally involved with the severe acute (classical) form of the disease, while the mild or subclinical form is generally caused by Kenya/Kudu/96 and Egypt/84 strains. However, the genetic determinants that lead to the variation of pathogenesis are presently unknown.[14, 15]

The preacute form of the disease is characterized by high fever, depression, deep congestion of visible mucosae, severe panting, racing pulse and sudden death of the animal. This form of the disease is common among young and newborn animals.[13] The acute form of the disease is divided into five phases: incubation, prodromal fever, erosive mucosa, diarrhea and convalescence. The incubation period ranges from 2 to 15 days with little or no overt signs, followed by the sudden onset of the prodromal phase. The prodromal phase begins with high fever, which may lasts six to nine days, depression, decreased appetite, reduction in milk production, congestion of the mucous membranes and serous ocular and nasal discharges are commonly observed. Within two to five days, the development of necrotic oral lesions (erosive mucosa phase) will appear on the lips, tongue, gums, buccal mucosa and both the soft and hard palates of the animal. Initially, these lesions will appear as pinpoints but will enlarge rapidly into gray plaques or form thick yellowish-pseudomembrane, after which they will slough to form shallow, non-hemorrhagic erosions. Severe salivation, turning purulent, will appear along with the lesions (Figure 4.5-2). The muzzle of the animal will eventually become dry and cracked; the animal will become anorexic and develop mucopurulent ocular and nasal discharges. Subsequently, necrotic lesions may also be found on the nares, vulva, vagina and preputial sheath. Within a few days after the development of the oral necrosis, the diarrhea phase will begin. At first the diarrhea will be profuse and watery, but will develop into a form that is mucus filled, bloody and may contain shreds of the animals' epithelium. During this time the animal will demonstrate severe abdominal pain, thirst and tenesmus. Affected animals generally arch their back due to the strain and expose their congested and eroded rectal mucosae. Respiration of the animal will become labored and painful, characterized by a noticeable grunt when exhaling. Dyspea may be observed, as well as, maculopapular rash that forms in the areas such as the groin and axillae. Death usually occurs six to nine days after the appearance of the signs and generally results from severe dehydration. If the animal manages to survive (~25 days), the convalescence can be prolonged and may be accompanied by secondary infections.[1, 3, 12, 13, 15]

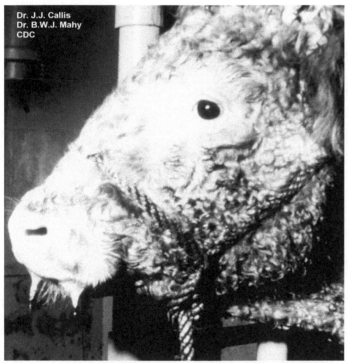

Figure 4.7-2: From the "Illustrated Manual for the Recognition and Diagnosis of Certain Animal Diseases", published in 1982, by the Mexico-United States Commission for the Prevention of Foot and Mouth Disease, this photograph depicts a bovine showing signs of a Rinderpest infection, also known as cattle plague, which can be seen as excessive salivation. This sign follows the appearance of oral lesions in this disease

Acute rinderpest infections in goats and sheep is similar with the respect to the signs to those described for cattle, with the exception that the course of the disease is shorter and displays more prominent pneumonic signs. Animals display high fever concurrently with mucosal erosions, although at times the signs of erosive stomatitis are absent. Soon after the onset of initial signs, the animals will show depression, and inappetence soon follows. Animals frequently stand "hair-on-end" with their heads thrust forwards and downwards with their backs arched. Panting, sneezing and coughing are frequent occurrences. Serious nasal and lacrimal secretions are common with the secretions turning mucopurulent during the later stages of infection. Many animals will succumb to the disease within six to seven days.[13, 15]

Acute rinderpest infections have only been observed in Asiatic sway-back pigs and the preacute disease is marked by sudden onset of fevers and death before other signs develop. The onset of the acute form of the infection is also abrupt with signs such as fever, depression and inappetence. Within 48 hours, the pigs are shivering, vomiting and bleeding from the nose, while shallow erosions appear in the oral mucosa and vesicles erupt in the perineal skin. Diarrhea soon appears after the previous described signs. At first it is watery becoming streaked with blood during the later stages. The loss of fluids will cause the animals to become dehydrated and emaciated. Many animals will succumb to the disease within 5 to 9 days.[13, 15]

RPV has a high affinity for lymphoid tissues and the alimentary mucosa, where it replicates and produces a focal necrotic stomatitis and enteritis. During the course of the infection, a transient leukocytosis appears prior to the onset of fever and immediately afterwards a dramatic decrease in the white blood cell counts (leucopenia) develops during the erosive mucosa phase.[13, 16] RPV uses CD150 (SLAM) receptors, found only on certain type of leukocytes. Therefore, this virus selectively grows and destroys CD4+, CD8+ alpha/beta T-lymphocytes, gamma/delta T-lymphocytes and B-lymphocytes, but not the memory cells.[17, 18] In addition, the numbers of basophils are severely reduced and disappear at the onset of fever, while the number of eosinophils falls with the lymphocytes and completely disappears during the erosive mucosa phase of the disease.[13]

RPV can readily replicate in B95a, an Epstein-Barr virus-transformed marmoset B lymphoblastoid cell line. This is the required method of RPV identification during any outbreak of the disease as dictated by the Global Rinderpest Eradication Programme (GREP). Direct isolation of RPV is essential for subsequent virus characterization and molecular epidemiological studies.[1, 13, 19] RPV can also be identified via viral antigen with agar gel immunodiffusion (AGID) tests, counter-immunoelectrophoresis, reverse phase passive hemagglutination (RPHA) tests or immuno-capture enzyme-linked immunosorbent assay (ELISA). AGID is a serological examination where soluble antigens in agar are precipitated by the addition of a specific antibody. The AGID test is useful under field conditions, however, it does not differentiate between RPV and other members of Paramixoviridae family (e.g. pest-des-pestits-ruminants virus).[1, 13, 20] Counter-immunoelectrophoresis is a technique that combines AGID and electrophoresis. This technique uses the electrophoretic flow of the antigen preparations through a gel towards the anode (+) and the couterelectroendosmotic flow of antibody towards the cathode (-). Comparatively, counter-immunoelectrophoresis detection of rinderpest antigens is between four and 16 times more sensitive than AGID and takes less time to complete. Nonetheless, this method runs into the same problem as AGID, where it cannot differentiate between RPV and other members of Paramixoviridae family.[1, 13, 21] RPHA is a classical immunological diagnostic tool that uses a preserved red blood cell-linked antigen or antibody within a simple agglutination test. This technique has been reported to be more sensitive and rapid than precipitation tests.[1, 13, 22] Immunocapture ELISA, are monoclonal antibody-based indirect sandwich ELISA. This method is more rapid, sensitive, virus specific and can be useful in a definitive diagnosis between RPV and pest-des-pestits-ruminants virus.[1, 13, 23]

Other diagnostic methodologies have been devised to detect RPV. For example, a pen-side monoclonal antibody-based, latex particle agglutination test has been developed for rapid, and reportedly accurate field diagnosis.[1, 24] Direct immunofluorescence and immunoperoxidase with monoclonal and polyclonal antibodies have also been developed to identify RPV.[1, 13, 25, 26] In addition, a reverse-transcription polymerase chain reaction (RT-PCR) assay has been used to specifically identify RPV. This diagnostic tool first uses reverse transcription to convert RPV RNA genome into DNA. Subsequently, a defined segment of the target DNA is copied repeatedly by using specific genome- and anti-genome-sense primers, which are usually separated by 200-400 nucleotides on the genome. This methodology allows the researchers to accurately identify RPV and distinguish the various lineages.[1, 13, 27]

A tissue-cultured rinderpest vaccine was developed from one immunogenic type of RPV that produces a mild infection, but it induces the development of host antibodies that will protect the animal from all other known strains of RPV. Currently, the vaccine used is called Plowright's tissue culture rinderpest vaccine (RBOK strain), and gives both full protection and lifelong immunity, however, this vaccine is highly thermolabile and requires a cold chain from vaccine production until delivery. The requirement of constant refrigeration makes it difficult to deliver the vaccine to remote areas where refrigeration may not be available. Therefore, much research has gone into finding a thermostabile vaccine.[28, 29] In 2005, CIRAD, a French agricultural research organization identified and produced three synthetic interfering RNAs that can inhibit peste-des-petits from ruminants and RPV replication by over 80% in vitro. This therapeutic vaccine targets the messenger RNA of the nucleoprotein gene of the causal viruses, thus blocking the virus propagation process.[30]

References

1. The Center for Food Security & Public Health. Iowa State University. Rinderpest. Revised August 8, 2008. Retrieved December 29, 2009. Website: http://www. cfsph.iastate.edu/ Factsheets/pdfs/rinderpest.pdf
2. Wagner E.K., Hewlett M.J. Basic Virology. Malden. Blackwell Publishing Company, 2004. pp. 264-265
3. Pereira N. Cattle Plague Wiped Away. Current Science, 2008. 94: pp. 1355-1356
4. Barrett T., Rossiter P.B. Rinderpest: the Disease and its Impact on Human and Animals. Advances in Virus Research, 1999. 53: pp. 89-110
5. Scott G.R. Rinderpest. Advances in Veterinary Science, 1964. 9: pp. 113-224
6. Rossiter P.B., Hussain M., Raja R.H., Moghul W., Khan Z., Broadbent D.W. Cattle Plague in Shangri-La: Observations on a Severe Outbreak of Rhiderpest in Northern Pakistan 1994-1995. Veterinary Record, 1998. 143: pp. 39-42
7. Barrett T., Rossiter P. Rinderpest: the Disease and its Impact on Humans and Animals. Advances in Veterinary Science, 1999. 53: pp. 89-110
8. Barrett T., Pastoret P-P., Taylor W.P. Rinderpest and Peste des Petits Ruminants. Virus Plagues of Large and Small Ruminants. London: Academic Press. 2006. pp. 86-130
9. Lepissier H.E. Joint campaign against Rinderpest in Central and West Africa. General technical report on OAU/STRC Joint Campaign against Rinderpest in Central and West Africa (1961-69). Lagos: Scientific, Technical and Research Commission of the Organization of African Unity. 1971. pp. 1-201
10. Njeumi F., Taylor W., Dialloi A., Miyagishima K., Pastoret P.P., Vallatw B., Traore M. The long journey: a brief review of the eradication of rinderpest. Revue Scientifique et Technique De L'Office International des Epizooties, 2012. 31: pp. 729-746
11. Fournié G., Jones B.A., Beauvais W., Lubroth J., Njeumi F., Cameron A., Pfeiffer D.U. The risk of rinderpest re-introduction in post-eradication era. Preventive Veterinary Medicine, 2014. 113: pp. 175-184
12. Matin M.A., Rafi M.A. Present Status of Rinderpest Disease in Pakistan. Journal of Veterinary Medicine B, 2006. 53: pp. 26-28
13. Anderson J., Barrett T., Scott G.R. Manual on the Diagnosis of Rinderpest. Second Edition. Rome: Food and Agriculture Organization of the United Nations. 1996. pp. 1-7; 9-10; 13-14; 40-80
14. Barrett T., Rossiter P.B. Rinderpest: the Disease and its Impact on Humans and Animals. Advances in Virus Reseach, 1999. 53: pp. 89-110
15. Taylor W.P. Epidemiology and Control of Rinderpest. Revue Scientifique Et Technique, 1986. 5: pp. 407-410
16. Ogilvie T.H. Large Animal Internal Medicine. Oxford: Blackwell Publishing Company. 2005. pp. 60-61
17. Rossiter P.B., Herniman K.A., Gumm I.D., Morrison W.I. The Growth of Cell Culture-attenuated Rinderpest Virus in Bovine Lymphoblasts with B cells, CD4+ and CD8+ Alpha/Beta T cell and Gamma/Delta T cell Phenotypes. The Journal of General Virology, 1993. 74: pp. 305-309
18. Baron M.D. Wild-type Rinderpest Virus Uses SLAM (CD150) as its Receptor. Journal of General Virology, 2005. 86: pp. 1753-1757
19. Kobune F., Sakata H., Sugiyama M., Sugiura A. B95a, a Marmoset Lymphoblastoid Cell Line, as a Sensitive Host for Rinderpest Virus. Journal of General Virology, 1991. 72: pp. 687-692
20. White G. A Specific Diffusable Antigen of Rinderpest Virus Demonstrated by the Agar Double-Diffusion Precipitation Reaction. Nature, 1958. 181: pp. 1409
21. Rossiter P.B., Mushi E.Z. Rapid Detection of Rinderpest Virus Antigens by Counter-immunoelectrophoresis. Tropical Animal Health and Production, 1980. 12: pp. 209-216
22. Bansal R.P., Joshi R.C., Sharma B., Chandra U. Reverse Phase Passive Haemagglutination Test for the Detection of Rinderpest Antigen. Tropical Animal Health and Production, 1987. 19: pp. 53-55
23. Abraham G., Berhan A. The Use of Antigen-capture Enzyme-linked Immunosorbent Assay (ELISA) for the Diagnosis of Rinderpest and Peste des Petits Ruminants in Ethiopia. Tropical Animal Health and Production, 2004. 33: pp. 423-430
24. Brüning A., Bellamy K., Talbot D., Anderson J. A Rapid Chromatographic Strip Test for the Pen-side Diagnosis of Rinderpest Virus. Journal of Virological Methods, 1999. 81: pp. 143-154
25. Rossiter P.B., Jessett D.M. Detection of rinderpest virus Antigen in vitro and in vivo by Direct Immunofluorescence. Research in Veterinary Science, 1982. 33: pp. 198-204
26. Wamwayi H.M., Rossiter P.B., Wafula J.S. Confirmation of Rinderpest in Experimentally and Naturally Infected Cattle using Microtitre Yechniques. Tropical Animal Health and Production, 1991. 23: pp. 17-21
27. Couacy-Hymann E., Bodjo S.C., Koffi M.Y., Danho T. Observations on Rinderpest and Rinderpest-like Diseases Throughout West and Central African Countries During Rinderpest Eradication Projects. Research in Veterinary Science, 2007. 83: pp. 282-285
28. House J.A., Mariner J.C. Stabilization of Rinderpest Vaccine by Modification of the Lyophilization Process. Developments in Biological Standardizations, 1996. 87: pp. 235-44
29. Raut A., Singh R.K., Malik M., Joseph M.C., Bakshi C.S., Suryanarayana V.V., Butchaiah G. Development of a Thermoresistant Tissue Culture Rinderpest Vaccine Virus. Acta Virologica, 2001. 45: pp. 235-241
30. de Almeida R.S., Keita D., ve Libeau G., Albina E. Control of Ruminant Morbillivirus Replication by Small Interfering RNA. Journal of General Virology, 2007. 88: pp. 2307-2311

Photo Bibliography

Figure 4.7-1: A transmission electron micrograph (TEM) revealed the ultrastructural appearance of numerous virions of rinderpest virus (yellow arrow), a member of the genus Morbillivirus of the family Paramyxoviridae. The transmission electron photomicrograph was taken by Dr. Rajnish Kaushik, (with special thanks to Professor M. S. Shaila) of the Department of Microbiology and Cell Biology Indian Institute of Science, Bangalore, India. The electron photomicrograph is copyrighted © by Dr. Rajnish Kaushik and permission granted for reprint through Creative Commons Attribution-Share Alike 2.5 Generic license.

Figure 4.7-2: From the "Illustrated Manual for the Recognition and Diagnosis of Certain Animal Diseases", published in 1982, by the Mexico-United States Commission for the Prevention of Foot and Mouth Disease, this photograph depicts a bovine showing signs of a Rinderpest infection, also known as cattle plague, which can be seen as excessive salivation. This sign follows the appearance of oral lesions in this disease. The photograph was taken by Dr. Jerry J. Callis, and Dr. Brian W.J. Mahy in 1982 and released by the CDC. Public domain photo

Magnaporthe grisea is the sexually reproductive phase (teleomorph) of the organism known as *Pyricularia grisea* (syn. *P. oryzae*). This organism is a haploid, filamentous, ascomycete fungus that is heterothallic, with mating controlled by the alternative mating loci: Mat1-1 and Mat1-2. Mating of this fungus occurs readily when opposite mating types are mixed on oatmeal agar. *M. grisea* is an efficient and devastating organism and its various strains can cause blast disease on a variety of grasses, including rice, wheat, pearl millet, and barley (e.g. rice blast, wheat blast, finger millet blast, barley blast etc.). The most serious of these infections is the rice blast, which causes losses of between 10 to 30% of the rice harvest annually and poses the most serious disease to the world's most important food security crop. It has been stated that few plant pathogens have this kind of impact on a global scale with regards to nutrition, livelihoods and economic well-being. Therefore, *M. grisea* has been recognized as a potential biological weapon and a worldwide pathogenic threat (Figure 4.8-1).[1, 2, 3, 4]

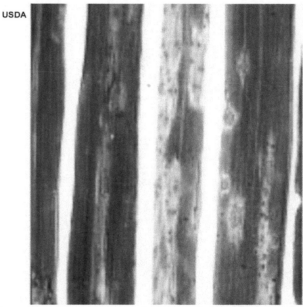

USDA

Figure 4.8-1: A photograph of lesions caused by the rice blast fungus, *Magnaporthe grisea*, on rice plant leaves

During World War II, plans were developed by the U.S. military to decimate Japan's rice crops. Although the biological attack on Japan was never implemented, the research on *M. grisea*'s potential as a biological weapon continued. For example, between the years of 1961 and 1962, the U.S. Army tested the potential of *M. grisea* as a biological weapon at least a dozen times in Okinawa, Japan during the post-war occupation.[5, 6]

Rice blast infection is initiated when an asexual non-motile spore (conidiospore) lands on the surface of a rice leaf and attaches itself to the cuticle through the release of an adhesive via a large periplasmic deposit at the apical compartment of the spore.[7] Conidiospore germination begins approximately two hours after attachment, where a polarized germ tube is formed from one of the apical cells of the conidium and extends for ~15-30 μm before changing direction. It becomes flattened against the leaf surface through a process known as "hooking." The process of "hooking" is believed to constitute the recognition phase of development, before committing to appressorium morpho-genesis.[8] The development of the appressorium requires the

presence of a hard, hydrophobic surface and the absence of exogenous nutrients. Nonetheless, the availability of cutin monomers, such as cis-9, 10-epoxy-18-hydroxyoctadecanoic acid or lipid monomers, like 1, 16-hexa-decanediol, can also trigger appressorium formation even on non-inductive surfaces.[9, 10]

The appressorium of *M. grisea* is a dome shaped structure with a highly differentiated cell wall structure, rich in chitin and containing a layer of melanin on its interior surface. The melanin is believed to aid the fungus by providing an impermeable layer to prevent leakage of an osmotically active metabolite, responsible for tugor pressure generation (~8.0 MPa). The high tugor pressure is essential for providing the physical force needed to insert the penetration peg (composed of numerous microfilaments, filasomes and microtubules) through the cuticle of the plant.[8, 11] Once the penetration of the plant is completed, the penetration peg differentiates into a series of bulbous, branched, infectious, hyphae which fills the initial plant epidermal cells. Subsequently, longer and more conventional, cylindrical hyphae ram out into the adjacent tissue and proceed with colonization. *M. grisea* also generates toxins, such as tenuazoinic acid, pyricularin, pyrichalasin, *etc.* during tissue invasion, however, the exact mechanisms of the toxin function remains to be elucidated.[2, 12]

M. grisea may infect most above ground parts of a plant, which includes leaves, leaf collars, nodes, panicles and the grains. In addition, this fungus may infect rice at different stages of growth and has adapted to both upland and lowland rice ecosystems.[13, 14] Infections that occur in the leaves typically consist of elongated diamond-shaped lesions with gray or white centers and brown and reddish margins. Leaf collar infections produce a brown or reddish-brown necrotic area at the junction of the leaf blade which may kill the entire attached leaf. Stem node infections may result in a blackened node and the death of the tiller above the infection. Infections just below the panicle will result in a brown or black lesion, encircling the entire node. This form of infection may result in the blanketing of the panicle or incomplete grain filling. Additionally, panicle branches and spiklets may also be infected, which may result in reduced yield and poor milling quality. Once established on a rice plant, the fungus rapidly produces thousands of spores, which are readily carried through the air via wind or rain, infecting neighboring plants.[15, 16, 17, 18]

Continuous efforts are being made to control blast disease. Fungicides, pesticides and other chemical compounds are presently being used, however, the long term effects of these chemicals may include damage to soil fertility for future crops and potentially pose an environmental hazard. Chemicals such as blasticidin S, kasugamycin, iprobenphos (IBP), edifenphos (EDDP), isoprothiolane, ferimzone and metominostrobin have demonstrated excellent results in controlling this pathogen. These chemicals generally act on the growth of *M. grisea* (e.g. act upon the primary metabolism of the pathogen such as protein and phospholipid biosynthesis) by exhibiting specific fungicidal effects. However, the long term use of these chemicals may cause the development of resistance in the pathogen. Non-fungicidal agents are also being used that pose no threat in developing resistance in the pathogen. Non-fungicidal agents, including melanin biosynthesis inhibitors (MBIs) such as fthalide, tricyclazol, pyroquilon, carpropamid, diclocymet and fenoxanil have been shown to be effective in controlling the fungus. In addition, plant defense activators, such as probenazole,

273

acibenzolar-S-methyl and tiadinil have shown to increase host resistance against pathogen attack.[19, 20, 21]

In 2014, Li *et al.* explored the possibilities of using citral as an alternative to the synthetic fungicides currently used against *M. grisea*. Their study revealed that citral caused a series of marked hyphal morphological and structural alterations, as well as, inhibited hyphal growth of *M. grisea in vitro*. Citral demonstrated the ability to significantly inhibit colony development and mycelial growth. Additionally, citral was shown to reduced spore germination and germ tube length in a concentration-dependent manner.[22]

References

1. Correll J.C., Harp T.L., Guerber J.C., Zeigles R., Liu B., Cartwright R.D., Lee F.N. Characterization of *Pyricularia grisea* In the United States using Independent Genetic and Molecular Markers. Phytopathology, 2000. 90: pp. 1396-1404
2. Talbot N.J. On the Trail of a Cereal Killer: Exploring the Biology of *Magnaprthe grisea*. Annual Review of Microbiology, 2003. 57: pp. 177-202
3. Anderson P.K., Cunningham A.A., Patel N.G., Morales F.J., Epstein P.R., Daszak P. Emerging Infectious Diseases of Plants: Pathogen Pollution, Climate Change and Agrotechnology Drivers. Trends in Ecology and Evolution, 2004. 19: pp. 535-544
4. Mitchell T.K., Thon M.R., Jeong J-S., Brown D., Deng J., Dean R.A. The Rice Blast Pathosystem as a Case Study for the Development of New Tools and Raw Materials for Genome Analysis of Fungal Plant Pathogens. New Phytologist, 2003. 159: pp. 53-61
5. Martin J.W., Christopher G.W., Eitzen E.M. History of Biological Weapons: From Poisoned Darts to Intentional Epidemics. Aspects of Biological Warfare. Chapter 1. Washington D.C.: The Surgeon General United States Army Medical Department Medical Center and School Borden Institute. 2007. pp. 1-20
6. U.S. conducted bioweapon tests in Japan in early 1960s. Homeland Security News Wire. Revised January 17, 2014. Retrieved January 11, 2015. Website: http://www.homelandsecuritynewswire.com/dr20140117-u-s-conducted-bioweapon-tests-in-japan-in-early-1960s
7. Hamer J.E., Howard R.J., Chumley F.G. Valent B. A Mechanism for Surface Attachment in Spores of a Plant Pathogenic Fungus. Science, 1988. 239: pp. 288-290
8. Bourett T.M., Howard R.J. *In Vitro* Development of Penetration Structures in the Rice Blast Fungus *Magnaporthe grisea*. Canadian Journal of Botany, 1990. 68: pp. 329-342
9. Gilbert R.D., Johnson A.M., Dean R.A. Chemical Signals Responsible for Appressorium Formation in Rice Blast Fungus. Physiological and Molecular Plant Pathology, 1996. 48: pp. 335-346
10. Dean R.A. Signal Pathways and Appressorium Morphogenesis. Annual Review of Phytopathology, 1997. 35: pp. 211-234
11. Howard R.J., Ferrari M.A., Roach D.H., Money N.P. Penetration of Hard Substrate by a Fungus Employing Enormous Tugor Pressure. Proceedings of the National Academy of Science United States of America, 1991. 88: pp. 11281-11284
12. Valent B., Chumley F.G. Molecular Genetic Analysis of Rice Blast Fungus *Magnaprthe grisea*. Annual Review of Phytopathology, 1991. 29: pp. 443-467
13. Bonman J.M., Khush G.S., Nelson R.J. Breeding Rice for Resistance to Pests. Annual Review of Phytopathology, 1992. 30: pp. 507-528
14. Teng P.S. The Epidemiological Basis for Blast Management. Rice Blast Disease. Wallingford: International Rice Research Institute and Commonwealth Agricultural Bureaux International. 1994. pp. 409-433
15. Pinnschmidt H.O., Teng P.S., Luo Y. Methodology for Quantifying Rice Yield Effects of Blast. Rice Blast Disease. Wallingford: International Rice Research Institute and Commonwealth Agricultural Bureaux International. 1994. pp. 381-408
16. Hashimoto A. Water Droplets on Rice Leaves in Relation to the Incidence of Leaf Blast. Use of the Dew Balance for Forecasting the Disease. Review of Plant Protection Research, 1981. 14: pp. 112-126
17. Sanyal P., Patel S.C. Pattern Recognition Method to Detect Two Diseases in Rice Plants. The Imaging Science Journal, 2008. 56: pp. 319-325
18. Zhu Y.Y., Fang H., Wang Y.Y., Fan J.X., Yang S.S., Mew T.W., Mundt C.C. Panicle Blast and Canopy Moisture in Rice Cultivar Mixtures. Phytopathology, 2005. 95: pp. 433-438
19. Yamaguchi I. Fungicides for Control of Rice Blast Disease. Journal of Pesticide Science, 1982. 7: pp. 307-316
20. Yamaguchi I. Overview on the Chemical Control of Rice Blast Disease. Rice Blast Interaction with Rice and Control. Dordrecht: Kluwer Academic Publishers. 2004. pp. 1-13
21. Gouramanis G.D. Biological and Chemical Control of Rice Blast Disease (*Pyricularia oryzae*) in Northern Greece. Cahiers Options Méditerranéennes, 1988. 15: pp. 61-68
22. Li R-Y., Wu X-M., Yin X-H., Liang J-N., Li M. The Natural Product Citral Can Cause Significant Damage to the Hyphal Cell Walls of *Magnaporthe grisea*. Molecules, 2014. 19: pp. 10279-10290;

Photo Bibliography

Figure 4.8-1: A photograph of lesions caused by the rice blast fungus, *Magnaporthe grisea*, on rice plant leaves. Photograph was taken and released by United States Department of Agriculture. Public domain photo

Black stem rust is a serious disease that affects wheat, barley, oat and rye crops, as well as, many other economically important grasses. This disease is caused by *Puccinia graminis*, an obligated biotroph, belonging to the family *Pucciniaceae* which contains 17 genera and approximately 4121 species. *P. graminis* is a typical heteroecious rust fungus with five distinct spore stages, which occur during asexual reproduction on its gramineous host, as well as, sexual reproduction that begins in the resting spore stage and finishes on alternative hosts (*Berberis* spp. or *Mahonia* spp.).[1,2] The host range of *P. graminis* is extremely broad, affecting approximately 365 species of cereals and grasses in 54 genera. For example, in one species of wheat stem rust, *P. graminis* f.sp. *tritici* has been shown to be capable of infecting 74 species in 34 genera during artificial inoculations of seedlings. Nonetheless, out of the species infected during laboratory conditions, only 28 species, belonging to eight genera are known to be natural hosts for the fungus (Figure 4.9-1).[3]

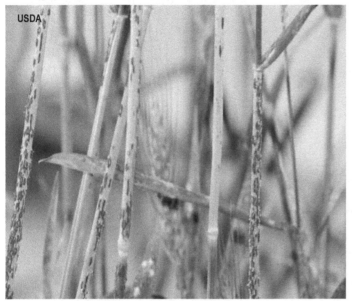

Figure 4.9-1: A photograph of black stem rust on wheat

Stem rust is primarily a warm and/or temperate climate disease although, it is able to infect susceptible crops over broad geographical regions. *P. graminis* generally produces a black, thick-walled, two celled teliospore, which is also known as the resting spore stage or over-winter stage, towards the end of the growing season of the host.

When first formed, each of the teliospore cells is dikaryotic although karyogamy occurs early in teliospore maturation. Meiosis begins shortly after karyogamy, however, it is suspended at diplonema of the first meiotic division during the resting spore stage (e.g. period of telisopore dormancy).[2,4] During the resting spore stage, the teliospore stalks remain intact, while the spores are not dispersed from the telial pustule. Alternatively, both teliospore stalks and spores remain dormant in the infected straws, until spring when they germinate in synchrony with the bud break and new leaf growth in the alternative host (*Berberis* spp. or *Mahonia* spp.).[2,5,6]

During the spring, one or both of the cells of the teliospore produces a promycelium (also known as a basidium), which is a hyphal protrusion. Upon the completion of meiosis, the 4 haploid nuclei are separated in the promycelium by three transverse septa. Subsequently, a projecting sterigma form on each of the promycelium cells, where on its tip, the sterigma expands as it forms thin-walled, colorless basidiospores. The newly formed haploid nuclei then migrate through the sterigma and into the basidiospores. There they proceed thru mitosis, and two identical haploid nuclei are formed.[2,5]

Since *P. graminis* is heteroecious, once mitosis is completed, the mature basidiospores are ejected from the sterigma and carried by wind to infect the alternative hosts such as the common barberry (e.g. *Berberis vulgaris*). Basidiospores germinate and produce a haploid mycelium, which colonizes the leaf tissue. Older barberry leaves are resistant to *P. graminis*, mainly because their thick cuticles prevent the basidiospore germ tube from penetrating. Therefore, the infection of the fungi is limited to the production of flask-shaped pycnia (also referred to as spermagonia) on the surface of the barberry leaves. Pycnia produce receptive hyphae and small thin-walled pycniospores (also referred to as spermatia, male gametes consisting of single haploid nuclei). They are formed within the pycnium and exude from its tip in drops of pycnial nectar. The pycnial nectar is sticky honeydew, highly attractive to insects, which serve to disseminate pycniospores. In addition, droplets of rain can also serve to aid in the cross-fertilization. For example, the insect will disseminate the pycniospores to flexuous (receptive) hypha, extending out of the top of the pycnia, which serve as the female gametes.[2,6]

P. graminis possesses two mating types, which are designated as + and − strains. Only the pycnial nectar of one mating type is known to induce cap formation on pycniospores of opposite mating type.[7,8,9] When a pycniospore of one mating type comes into contact with the flexuous hypha of the opposite mating type, plasmogamy will occur through the formation of a fusion tube. The formation of the fusion tube allows the haploid nucleus from the pycniospore to migrate from the pycniospore into flexuous hypha. Then it proceed through the monokaryotic hyphae until reaching the cells of the proto-aecium at the base of the pycnium.[2,10] Over a period of days, after nuclear division and paired association of the + and − nuclei, a dikaryotic state (e.g. dikaryotic mycelium) is reached. Continuation of growth of the fungi produces a cup-shaped dikaryotic aecium, below the pycnium, which eventually ruptures the lower epidermis of the barberry leaf. During this time of growth, chains of single celled dikaryotic aeciospores are produced which are designed to only infect the targeted gramineous hosts (e.g. wheat and other grasses).[2,5,6]

After the aeciospores settle and infect the targeted gramineous host, the *P. graminis* produces a dense mat of hyphae or dikaryotic mycelium beneath the host epidermis. Within one to two weeks, the sporophores grow from the mat and initate the production of masses of brick-red, spiny, single-celled dikartyotic urediniospores which also ruptures the host leaf or stem epidermis and produces a pustule, known as the uredinium. The uredium is an elongated mass, measuring approximately 2x5 mm. It is cinnamon brown in color and turns almost black as it develops. The germination of the uredospore and the growth of the germ tube are oriented perpendicular to the ventilation of the leaf which makes the ability of the germ tube in locating a stomatal pore more efficient. Urediniospores are wind dispersed and can re-infect the gramineous host. Under favorable environmental conditions, multiple, repeated infections of the same wheat plant and neighboring wheat plants can result in explosive epidemics.[2, 6, 11, 12, 13, 14] In North America, stem rust can still occur in temperate regions even if the alternative host, such as the barberry, are not present. For example, during cases of natural infection in the absence of barberry, the windborne urediniospores can reach wheat in the spring via southerly winds. These urediniospores are produced on winter wheat crops in the mild climate of the south.[2, 6, 15, 16, 17]

The infection of cereals or grasses occurs mainly on stems and leaf sheaths, although occasionally the infection can spread to the blades of the leaves, as well as, glumes. Initially, small chlorotic flecks appear after a few days post infection. Approximately eight to ten days afterwards, a pustule several millimeters (mm) long and wide form from the rupture of the host epidermis due to the pressure of a mass of brick-red urediniospores. These uredinial pustules are generally linear or diamond shaped and may enlarge to approximately 10 mm long. In time, the infection ceases production of brick-red urediniospores and begins producing a layer of black teliospores, which causes the heavily infected gramineous host to appear blackened late in the growing season. Severe infection by the disease interrupts nutrient flow to the developing heads of the crops resulting in shriveled grain. In addition, stems heavily infected by the fungus are prone to lodging, thereby resulting in the further loss of grain. Gramineous host which appear to be healthy three weeks before harvest, can be devastated by stem rust if adequate numbers of pathogens arrive from infected crops from adjacent regions.[2, 6]

One of the manners by which black stem rust is being combated is through breeding resistant gramineous varieties. However, due to mutations and parasexual processes resulting in somatic recombination in *P. graminis,* new infective strains are constantly being produced, making any advantages of the newly bred varieties of gramineous varieties short-lived.[6] As of 2006, there were approximately 53 distinct and officially designated genes for resistance to various races of wheat stem rust. There are an additional 24, presumably distinct, resistance genes that have received provisional designations. Each of these genes requires a matching avirulence gene in the *P. graminis* that is required for recognition and initiation of the resistance response. Out of the 53 known resistance genes, 23 were found originally in hexaploid bread wheat (*Titicum aestvum*), nine were transferred to bread wheat from wild of cultivated durum wheat (tetraploid *T. turgicum*), 3 were tranbsferred from *T. monococcum*, four from cultivated rye (*Secale cereale*) and the remaining were transferred from various wild wheat relatives such as *T. comosum*, *T. speltoides*, *T. tauschii*, *T. timopheevii*, *T. ventricosum* and *Thinopyrum ponticum*. Fungicides such as pyraclostrobin (Headline), azoxystrobin (Quadris Flowable Fungicide), propiconazole (Bumper 41.8 EC), metconazole (Caramba), tebuconazole (Folicur 3.6F, Muscle 3.6F, Orius 3.6F, propiconazole (proline 480 SC, PropiMax 3.6 EC, Tilt), propiconazole + tebuconazole (Prosaro 421 SC), tebuconazole (Tebuzol 3.6F, Tegrol 3.6F, Toledo Agricultural Fungicide), azoxystrobin + propiconazole (Quilt), propiconazole + trifloxystrobin (Stratego Fungicide) and pyraclostrobin + metconazole (TwinLine) can also be used to control black stem rust. However, the use of these chemicals is generally cost prohibitive.[2, 18, 19]

References

1. Kirk P.M., Cannon P.F., David J.V., Stalpers J.A. Ainsworth and Bisby's Dictionary of the Fungi. Ninth Edition. Wallingford: Commonwealth Agricultural Bureaux International. 2001. pp. 569, 610, 624
2. Leonard K.J., Szabo L.J. Stem Rust of Small Grains and Grasses Caused by *Puccinia graminis*. Molecular Plant Pathology, 2005. 6: pp. 99-111
3. Anikster Y. The Formae Speciales. Cereal Rusts. Volume one. Orlando: Academic Press. 1984. pp. 115-130
4. Boehm E.W.A., Wesnstrom J.C., McLaughlin D.J., Szabo L.J., Roelfs A.P., Bushnell W.R. An Ultrastructural Pachytene Karyotype for *Puccinia graminis* f.sp.*tritici*. Canadian Journal of Botany, 1992. 70: pp. 410-413
5. Roelfs A.P. Wheat and Rye Stem Rust. The Cereal Rust. Volume Two. Orlando: Academic Press. 1985. pp. 3-37
6. Raven P.H., Evert R.F., Eichhorn S.E. Biology of Plants. New York: W.H. Freeman and Company Publishers. 2005. pp. 278-279
7. Roelfs A.P., Groth J.V. *Puccinia graminis* f.sp.*tritici*, Black Stem Rust of Triticum spp. Genetics of Plant Pathogenic Fungi, Advances in Plant Pathology. Volume Six. London: Academic Press. 1988. pp. 345-361
8. Anikster Y., Eilam T., Mittelman L., Szabo L.J., Bushnell W.R. Pycnial Nectar of Rust Fungi induces Cap Formation on Pycniospore of Opposite Mating Type. Mycologia, 1999. 91: pp. 858-870
9. Anikster Y., Eilam T., Bushnell W.R. Interspecific Transfer of Pycnial Nectar Induces Pycniospore Caps in Rust Fungi in a Manner Related to Mating Type within Species. Mycological research, 2000. 104: pp. 311-316
10. Johnson T., Newton M. Specialization, Hybridization, and Mutation in the Cereal Rusts. The Botanical Review, 1946. 12: pp. 337-392
11. Staples R.C., Macko V. Germination of Urediospores and Differentiation of Infection Structures. The Cereal Rust. Volume one. Orlando: Academic Press. 1984. Pp. 255-289
12. Lewis B.G., Day J.R. Behaviour of Uredospore Germ-tubes of *Puccinia graminis tritici* in Relation to the Fine Structure of Wheat Leaf Surfaces. Transactions of the British Mycological Society, 1972. 58: pp. 139-145
13. Staples R.C., Hoch H.C., Epstein L., Laccetti L., Hassouna S. Recognition of Host Morphology by Rust Fungi: Responses and Mechanisms. Canadian Journal of Plant Pathology, 1985. 7: pp. 314-322
14. Parry D.W. Plant Pathology in Agriculture. New York: Cambridge University Press. 1990. pp. 192-193
15. Browder L.E., Johnston C.O., Pady S.M. Cereal Rust Epidemiology in Kansas in 1959. Plant Disease Reporter, 1961. 5: pp. 894-898
16. Browder L.E., Young Jr H.C. Further Development of an Infection Type Coding System for the Cereal Rust. Plant Disease Reporter, 1975. 59: pp. 964-965
17. Eversmeyer M.G., Kramer C.L. Epidemiology of Wheat Leaf and Stem Rust in the Central Great Plains of the USA. Annual Review of Phytopathology, 2000. 38: pp. 491-513
18. McLintosh R.A., Wellings C.R., Park R.F. Wheat Rusts: An Atlas of Resistance Genes. Boston: Kluwer Academic Publishers. 1995. pp. 1-200
19. Singh R.P., Hodson D.P., Jin Y., Huerta-Espino J., Kinyua M., Wanyera R., Njau P., Ward R.W. Current Status, Likely Migration and Strategies to Mitigate the Threat to Wheat Production from Race Ug99 (TTKS) of Stem Rust Pathogen. Commonwealth Agricultural Bureaux (CAB) Reviews: Perspectives in Agriculture, Veterinary Science, Nutrition and Natural Resources, 2006. 1: pp. 1-13

Photo Bibliography

Figure 4.9-1: A photograph of black stem rust on wheat. The photograph was taken and released by the United States Department of Agriculture. Public Domian Photo

Unlike an attack with explosives or chemical weapons, nearly all of the effects of biological agents are delayed for hours, days or even weeks due to their incubation period. This lull poses an additional threat with certain contagious biological agents, since these asymptomatic individuals have the potential to infect others. For example, biological incapacitating agents often possess relatively extended incubation periods, whereby allowing the agent to spread into an unsuspecting population before they are ever diagnosed or detected by laboratory tests.[1, 2] During the incubation period, it is impossible for any clinicians to diagnose the disease without advance notices and warnings from federal agencies. If the warnings are not forthcoming, the first indications of an attack may be a large number of symptomatically similar individuals appearing at a hospital or clinic within a short period of time. Unfortunately, many of the biological agents may not be endemic to the location where they are released and most likely will cause confusion due to differential diagnoses. Therefore, an efficient surveillance system, with trained individuals to perform in depth epidemiological investigations will be needed to analyze the distribution patterns of patients and demonstrate possible clustering to help determine the specific biological agent involved in the event and in turn, save lives.[1, 3]

Prior to September 11, 2001, the Center for Disease Control and Prevention (CDC) oversaw various passive infectious disease surveillance systems. The best known of these surveillance systems is the National Notifiable Disease Surveillance System (NNDSS), which relied on voluntary collaborations with clinicians and health laboratories to initiate reports of specific diseases, which are then passed to local or state health departments, before finally being conveyed to the NNDSS. Clinicians, hospitals and laboratories in each of the 50 states, along with the District of Columbia, and the territories are required by regulations to report cases of approximately 50 diseases, caused by known biological agents, such as, anthrax, botulism, brucellosis, and plague.[1] Unfortunately, the reliability of passive surveillance is low, and the timeliness of the voluntary reporting of suspicious cases is inefficient at best. Even with the potential legal ramifications faced by clinicians, hospitals or laboratories for failing to file a report in a timely manner, such punishments are rarely imposed, thereby providing little incentive for compliance. These inadequacies were highlighted in a 1996 report, which stated that there was little or no federal funding provided to local health departments to support disease surveillance. Because of inadequate funding, 12 states have no professional position dedicated to diseases surveillance.[1, 4]

However, since the terrorist attacks on September 11, 2001, financial shortfalls have been addressed though bioterrorism preparedness funding via The Bioterrorism Act of 2002, also known as the Public Health Security and Bioterrorism Preparedness and Response Act – H.R. 3448. The increased funding to local and state health agencies is managed through the Department of Health and Human Services (HHS) and its divisions, such as the Centers for Disease Control and Prevention (CDC), as well as, Health Resources and Services Administration (HRSA). For example, after 2001, federal funding for state public health preparedness programs increased from 67 million in fiscal year (FY) 2001 to approximately 1 billion in FY 2002. Included in the awards, is targeted funding to expand the Cities Readiness Initiative (CRI) in all 50 states. The goal of CRI is to ensure that the hospitals in selected cities are prepared to provide oral medications to 100% of their populations during a public health emergency (Figure 5.1-1). In 2006, the CRI was expanded to include to other public health emergencies. The Pandemic and All-Hazards Preparedness Act of 2006 (P.L. 109-417) emphasizes an all-hazards approach to public health preparedness planning. In 2013, President Obama signed the Pandemic and All Hazards Preparedness Reauthorization Act into law. This reauthorization of PAHPA build on the work the U.S. Department of Health and Human Services on national health security, which included authorizing funding for public health and medical preparedness programs, such as the Hospital Preparedness Program and the Public Health Emergency Preparedness Cooperative Agreement. Based on information provided by HHS and U.S. Department of Veterans Affairs, Congressional Budget Office estimates that implementing the act would cost ~11 billion dollars over the 2014-2018 period.[5, 6, 7]

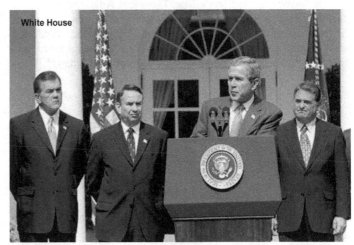

White House

Figure 5.1-1: President George W. Bush at the signing of H.R. 3448, the Public Health Security and Bioterrorism Response Act of 2002 in The Rose Garden on Wednesday, June 12

Additional funding has also been appropriated for the Early Warning Infectious Disease Surveillance program specifically for states bordering Canada and Mexico. Furthermore, HHS and HRSA have also provided funds for states to develop medical surge capacity and the capability to deal with mass casualty events. These targeted improvements of hospitals includes increased numbers of hospital beds, improvements to isolation capacity, establishing pharmaceutical caches, providing mental health services, improving trauma and burn care, communications, personal protective equipment and hiring new health care personnel. Between the years of 2001 to 2004, approximately 14.5 billion dollars were allocated by the federal government towards funding civilian bioterrorism-preparedness measures.[8, 9, 10, 11, 12]

In addition to the increased funding to the local and state health agencies, The Bioterrorism Act of 2002 also provided legal authority in a bureaucratic effort to increase the effectiveness of local, state and federal surveillance and response to a potential biological terrorist act. For example, the act allows for the establishment of the Assistant Secretary for Public Health Emergency Preparedness within the HHS, allocated hundred of millions of dollars to bolster the national stockpile of vaccines, antibiotics and antitoxins, created regulations to bolstered the safety of laboratory and individuals in handling biological hazardous agents, and instituted measures to strengthen the protection of the nation's food, drug and water supplies.[12] In

2004, Section 564 of the Federal Food, Drug and Cosmetic Act (21 U.S.C 360bbb-3) was amended by the Project Bioshield Act of 2004 (Public Law 108-276). The Project Bioshield Act 2004 permits the Food and Drug Administration (FDA) Commissioner to authorize the use of unapproved medical products or unapproved use of approved medical products during a declared emergency.[13] Additionally, the United States government has also established the National Pharmaceutical Stockpile Program (NPS), under the supervision of the CDC. NPS is designed to insure the availability of essential antidotes, pharmaceuticals and other medical supplies and equipment necessary during a biological terrorism attack. Presently, the caches of medical supplies are strategically placed at multiple sites around the United States in environmentally controlled warehouses stored in shipping containers referred to as "push packages." Each of the "push packages" contains 50 tons of materials that are designed to meet the needs of mass casualty events and are capable of being deployed promptly (within 12 to 24 hours) in the case of an incident (Figure 5.1-2). Furthermore, a team of CDC advisors, designated as Technical Advisory Response Unit (TARU), will accompany each of the "push packages" for the purpose of advising local health officials on receiving, distributing, dispensing, and replenishing the package, as well as, recovering unused assets when the event subsides.[14, 15]

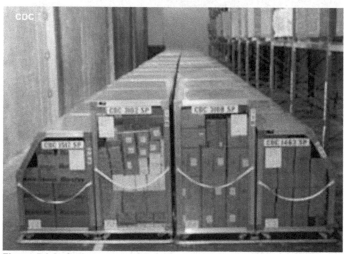

Figure 5.1-2: A photograph of "push packages" stockpiled for a declared emergency

In the United States, the state government has the constitutional authority to mandate healthcare providers (e.g. clinicians, hospitals, laboratories etc.) to report specific diseases and other specific health conditions. It is important to note that the United States Supreme Court has upheld public health reporting requirements in rulings on cases alleging that such requirements violate individual privacy. Therefore, clinicians (also hospitals and clinics) should be aware that the Health Insurance Portability and Accountability Act (HIPAA) Privacy Rule afford them the right to report conditions of public health importance to public health officials.[10, 16] In addition, HIPAA also authorizes private health insurers, managed care organizations, Medicaid, Medicare, The Veterans Health Administration, as well as, healthcare clearinghouses (e.g. billing services, repricing companies and community health information systems) to disclose protected health information to public health officials, if the individual has been exposed to a communicable disease or may be at risk in contracting or spreading a disease or condition.[10]

Presently the reporting of specific diseases and health conditions to a national surveillance system is voluntary and passive, where the flow of information begins with the local health care providers to

their local or state health departments and laboratories. The state and local public health agencies and laboratories then report any information to the HHS office of the Assistant Secretary for Public Health Emergency Preparedness for coordination and response, as well as, the CDC's Epidemic Intelligence Services for testing and advice. The CDC established the Epidemic Information Exchange (Epi-X), a secure, web-based communications network that serves as a powerful communication exchange between the CDC, state and local health departments, poison control centers, and public health professionals. The system has promised rapid reporting, immediate notification, editorial support, and coordination of health investigations for public health professionals.[17] Subsequently, the information will be shared with the Department of Homeland Security offices of Emergency Responses (e.g. Disaster Medical Assistant Teams, Disaster Mortuary Operational Response Teams and National Medical Response Teams), Federal Emergency Management Agency, Department of Justice Federal Bureau of Investigations (FBI) and the Department of Defense (US Army Medical Research Institute of Infectious Diseases) (Figure 5.1-3)[9, 10]

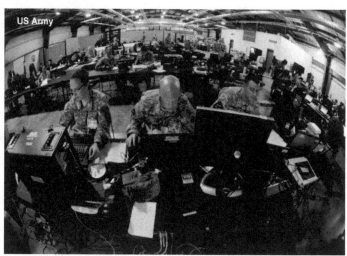

Figure 5.1-3: A photograph of the military's Defense Chemical, Biological, Radiological and Nuclear Response Force conducting field training exercise

With the additional funding, state and local health departments have made improvements to their response capacities to small- to large-scale emergencies. However, since 2004, federal funding to support all-hazards preparedness has declined steadily. The funds granted to the states, territories, and large cities were cut by $20 million in Fiscal Year 2004 (August 31, 2004 to August 30, 2005) and by an additional $97 million in Fiscal Year 2006 (August 31, 2006 to August 30, 2007). Presently, concerns put forth by local health officials with regards to the impact that these repeated cuts will have on the sustainability of their relatively new preparedness programs have not been heeded.[8, 9, 18, 19] In addition to federal and local financial issues, other gaps still remain in state and local disease surveillance systems. For example, it is known that there are still significant workforce shortages in state and local health departments, consequently a large opening remains within the communication systems, necessary for the regional coordination of the response to outbreaks or bioterrorist events. In addition, some of the regional laboratory facilities are outdated and do not possess the necessary equipment for accurate and timely analysis. Finally, there is still a general consensus that America's hospitals are still the weakest link in the preparedness for a biological terrorist attack.[1, 18, 19, 20]

The preparedness issue on both state and federal level finally came to light during 2014 Ebola cases on American soil. The confusion over treatment protocols, shortages in trained medical professionals, and a lack of specialized medical facilities showed that the U.S. is far from ready to deal with and manage a biological attack.[21]

No matter if a disease outbreak occurs naturally or due to the intentional release of a biological agent, the initial response would occur at the local level, particularly in hospitals and their emergency departments. Therefore, it would be the hospital personnel that first identify an infectious disease outbreak or a bioterrorist event. Even though most hospitals have trained their staff with respect to biological agents and planning coordination efforts with public health entities, preparedness limitations may impact the hospitals' ability to conduct disease surveillance. Furthermore, many hospitals still lack the capacity to respond to large-scale infectious disease outbreaks. Presently, most emergency departments across the country are regularly experiencing some degree of overcrowding. These crowded conditions may be exacerbated during a disease outbreak or bioterrorist attack, where considerable numbers of infected individuals with similar symptoms may appear at once at the emergency department for treatment.[1, 18, 19, 20]

References

1. Committee on R&D Needs for Improving Civilian Medical Response to Chemical and Biological Terrorism Incidents Health Science Policy Program Institute of Medicine and Board of Environmental Studies and Toxicology commission on Life Sciences National Research Council. Chemical and Biological Terrorism. Research and Development to Improve Civilian Medical Response. Washington D.C.: National Academy Press. 1999. pp. 65-71
2. Nicolson G.L., Nicolson N.L. New Emerging Infections: Their Development, Testing and Resulting Diseases. Journal of Degenerative Diseases, 2008. 9: pp. 50-53
3. Lewis M.D., Pavlin J.A., Mansfield J.L., O'Brian S., Boomsma L.G., Elbert Y.E., Kelley P.W. Disease Outbreak Detection System Using Syndromic Data in the Greater Washington SC Area. American Journal of Preventive Medicine, 2002. 23: pp. 180-186
4. Osterholm M.T., Birkhead S., Meriwether R.A. Impediments to Public Health Surveillance in the 1990s: The Lack of Resources and the Need for Priorities. Journal of Public Health Management and Practice, 1996. 22: pp. 11-15
5. Cities Readiness initiative. Center for Disease Control and Prevention. September 11, 2013. Retrieved January 11, 2015. Website: http://www.cdc.gov/phpr/stockpile/cri/
6. Assistant Secretary Nicole Lurie statement on the Pandemic and All Hazards Preparedness Reauthorization Act. U.S. Department of Health and Human Services. Released March 13, 2013. Retrieved January 11, 2015. Website: http://www.hhs.gov/news/press /2013pres/03/20130313a.html
7. H.R. 307, the Pandemic and All-Hazards Preparedness Reauthorization Act of 2013. Congressional Budget Office. Released February 21, 2013. Retrieved January 12, 2015. Website: http://www.cbo.gov/publication/43948
8. HHS Announces $1.2 Billion In Funding To States For Bioterrorism Preparedness. News release. United States Department Health and Human Services. Revised June 7 2006. Retrieved January 10, 2009. Website: http://www.hhs.gov/news/press/2006pres/20060607.html
9. Heinrich J. Testimony before the Subcommittee on Emergency Preparedness and Response, Select Committee on Homeland Security, House of Representatives. Infectious Diseases Gaps Remain in Surveillance Capabilities of State and Local Agencies. Wednesday, September 24, 2003. Government Accountability Office. GAO-03-1176T
10. Melnick A.L. Biological, Chemical and Radiological Terrorism. Emergency Preparedness and Response for the Primary Care Physician. New York: Springer. 2008. pp. 221-236
11. Public Health Security and Bioterrorism Preparedness and Response Act. Public Law, 2002. 107th Congress. pp. 107-188
12. Shuler A. Billions for Biodefense: Federal Agency Biodefense Funding, FY2001 – FY2005. Biosecurity Bioterrorism, 2004. 2: pp. 86-96
13. The Project Bioshield Act. Public Law, 2004. 108th Congress. Public Law pp. 108-276
14. National Pharmaceutical Stockpile Aids Homeland Health Security. American Journal of Health-System Pharmacy, 2001. 58: pp. 2112-2115
15. Summary of the Second Executive Session on Emergency Preparedness and the Pharmaceutical Supply Chain. American Journal of Health-System Pharmacy, 2002. 59: pp. 1057-1065
16. Gostin L.O. Public Health Law: Power, Duty and Restraint. Turning Point. Collaborating for a New Century in Public Health. University of Washington, Turning Point National Program Office, December 1999. pp. 1-55
17. The Epidemic Information Exchange (Epi-X). Center for Disease Control and Prevention. Retrieve January 10, 2009. Website: http://www.cdc.gov/mmwr/epix/epix.html
18. Brief Report: Terrorism and Emergency Preparedness in State and Territorial Public Health Departments --- United States, 2004. Morbidity and Mortality Weekly Report (MMWR), 2005. 54: pp. 459-460
19. Johnson V., Bachir Z., Leep C., Troutman N., Brown D., Briggs E. Federal Funding for Public Health Emergency Preparedness: Implications and Ongoing Issues for Local Health Departments. Washington D.C.: National Association of County and City Health Officials. 2007. pp. 1-16
20. Krenzelok E.P. Biological and Chemical Terrorism: A Pharmacy Preparedness Guide. Bethesda: American Society of Health-System Pharmacists. 2003. pp. 135-144
21. Could US handle biologic attack? The Hill. Released October 21, 2014. Retrieved January 12, 2015. Website: http://thehill.com/policy/defense/221329-after-ebola-experts-fear-nation-isnt-ready-for-a-biological-attack

Photo Bibliography

Figure 5.1-1: President George W. Bush at the signing of H.R. 3448, the Public Health Security and Bioterrorism Response Act of 2002 in The Rose Garden on Wednesday, June 12. The photo was taken and released by the White House. Public domain photo

Figure 5.1-2: A photograph of "push packages" stockpiled for a declared emergency. The photo was taken in 2011 by the Office of Public Health Preparedness and Response and released by the CDC. Public domain photo

Figure 5.1-3: A photograph of the military's Defense Chemical, Biological, Radiological and Nuclear Response Force conducting field training exercise. The photo was taken in August 2011 and released by the United States Army. Public domain photo

Due to the highly mobile population of the United States and the inconsistencies of the health regulations from state to state, there is a necessity for the federal government to address both foreign and interstate threats posed by communicable diseases. The Federal Public Health Service Act gives the Secretary of the HHS the authority to create and enforce regulations needed to prevent the "introduction, transmission or spread of communicable diseases from foreign countries into the states or possessions, or from one state or possession into any other state or possessions."[1] Federal quarantine laws and regulations give authority to HHS to apprehend and examine "any individual reasonably believed to be infected with a communicable disease in a qualifying stage and ① to be moving or about to move from a State to another State; or ② to be a probable source of infection to individuals who, while infected with such disease in a qualifying stage, will be moving from a State to another State."[2] The language "qualifying stage" allows the Federal government preemptive authority to intervene if a person is suspected of being infected with a disease that is likely to cause a public health emergency (Figure 5.2-1 and 5.2-2).[2, 3]

"insufficient to prevent the spread of any of the communicable diseases from such State or possession to any other State or possession."[2, 3] Presently, the list of communicable diseases for which the CDC may institute a quarantine that may supersede local and state authority are cholera, diphtheria, infectious tuberculosis, plague, smallpox, yellow fever, viral hemorrhagic fevers (e.g. Lassa, Marburg, Ebola etc.), severe acute respiratory syndrome (SARS), and avian influenza.[4]

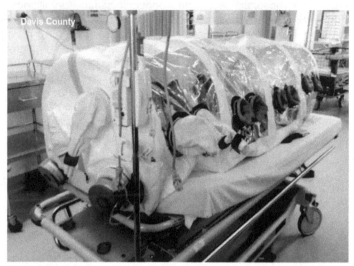

Figure 5.2-2: An ISO-POD isolation unit for transporting infectious patients

In an effort to protect the military personnel and individuals associated with the United States military during the times of war, the Secretary of the HHS, in consultation with the Surgeon General, is authorized to apprehend and examine "any individual reasonably believed ① to be infected with such disease and ② to be a probable source of infection to members of the armed forces of the United States or to individuals engaged in the production or transportation of arms, munitions, ships, food, clothing, or other supplies for the armed forces."[8]

References

1. United States Code - Title 42: The Public Health and Welfare - 42 USC § 264 - Sec. 264. Regulations to Control Communicable Diseases. January 2003. Website: http:// www.bt.cdc.gov/legal/42USC264.pdf
2. Khardori N. Bioterrorism Preparedness. Medicine – Public Health – Policy. Weinheim: Wiley-VCH. 2006. pp. 243-244
3. United States Code - Title 42 (e): The Public Health and Welfare - 42 USC § 264 (e) - Sec. 264. Regulations to Control Communicable Diseases. January 2003. Website: http://vlex.com
4. /vid/regulationscontrolcommunicablediseases9250396
5. Code of Federal Regulations - Title 42: Public Health – 42 CFR § 70.2. Measures in the event of inadequate local control. December 2005. Website: http://cfr.vlex.com/vid/70-measures-event-inadequate-local-19796469
6. Executive Order 13295: Revised List of Quarantinable Communicable Diseases. April 4, 2003. Website: http://www.cdc.gov/ncidod/sars/pdf/executiveorder040403.pdf
7. Executive Order: Amendment to E.O. 13295 Relating to Certain Influenza Viruses and Quarantinable Communicable Diseases. April 1, 2005. Website: http://edocket.access.gpo.gov/cfr_2006/janq tr/pdf/3CFR13375.pdf
8. United States Code - Title 42: The Public Health and Welfare - 42 USC § 266, Special Quarantine Powers in Time of War. January 2003. Website: http://vlex.com /vid/special-quarantine-powers-time-war-19250368

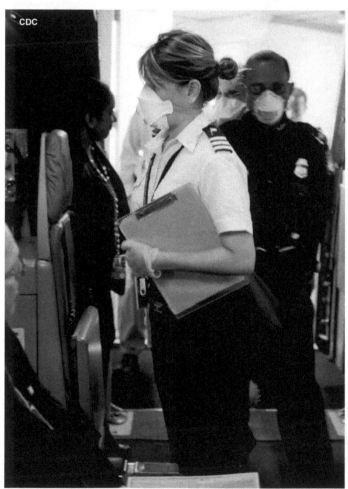

Figure 5.2-1: CDC quarantine officer Danitza Tomianovic, as she was entering a plane in order to assess the status of an ill traveler at the Miami International Airport

Although state laws take precedence in most circumstances involving quarantine and isolation, the Director of the CDC has the authority to take "measures to prevent such spread of the diseases as he/she deems reasonably necessary"[2] when the measures taken by the local and state health authorities are

In order to develop an effective defense against biological weapons, accurate and timely intelligence is essential. Unfortunately, at present, there are no available technologies that are capable of attaining an acceptable timeframe between the release and the detection of the biological weapon. This timeframe, also known as 'detect to warn', is essential in issuing a timely warning to don masks and other protective equipment. Additionally, most of the treatment of weaponized microbes and viruses must begin prior to the appearance of initial symptoms; any delay will result in the death of the individual. Figure 5.3-1 shows a graph plotting the concentration of various biowarfare agents needed for an unprotected person with normal respiration rate to get an infectious dose against time. For example, at a concentration of 100 particles/liter of *Bacillus anthracis,* an individual would become infected within 10 minutes, while at a concentration of only 10 particles/liter, a person would become infected with *Francisella tularensis* in less than a minute (Figure 5.3-1).[1]

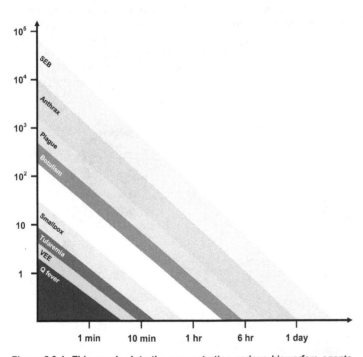

Figure 5.3-1: This graph plots the concentration various biowarfare agents concentration needed for an unprotected person with normal respiration rate to get an infectious dose against the estimated amount of time it takes for the infection to take place. Please note that staphylococcal enterotoxin B is abbreviated SEB and Venezuelan equine encephalitis is abbreviated VEE

Interim systems for detecting dispersed biological agents are only available in limited numbers, although they have yet to achieve the accuracy and reliability necessary to adequately guard against biological attacks. Presently, the only indication that a biological attack has occurred will most likely be the large numbers of affected individuals appearing at the local emergency facilities. Therefore, the development of real-time detection method of biological weapon agents has become one of the most challenging, as well as, high-priority areas of research by both the Department of Defense (DOD) and civilian sectors.[2]

The classic approach to microbial detection has been outlined under each of the biological agent sections within this text under the heading "Detection." Most of these identification methods involve the use of differential assays, such as immunohistochemistry, enzyme-linked immuno-sorbent assay (ELISA), and polymerase chain reaction (PCR) tests. to determine the particular species in the case of most bacteria or the use of cell culture and serodiagnostic methods in detecting specific antibodies found within human sera through immunohistochemical techniques, ELISA, haemaglutination inhibition or neutral-ization techniques and reverse transcription polymerase chain reactions (RT-PCR), etc. Unfortunately, most of these methodologies require adequately equipped laboratories, as well as, time for accurate diagnosis. In times of potential biological attack or epidemics, these requirements may prove to be the limiting factor in the identifying pathogen(s) in a timely manner (Figure 5.3-2). Therefore, new methodologies are currently being researched in order to provide accurate and rapid biodetection.[3]

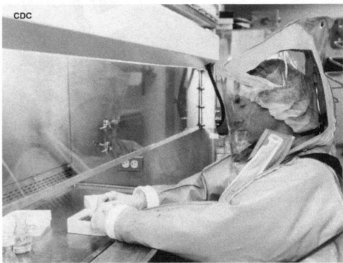

Figure 5.3-2: A CDC scientist conducts laboratory research in the Biosafety Level 4 laboratory, Atlanta, GA

One of these novel avenues is referred to as probe technology, based on nucleic acids, antibody/antigen binding and ligand/receptor interactions. Nucleic acid based probes use the extreme selectivity of DNA and RNA recognition. Probes are engineered single DNA or RNA strands that are highly sensitive and specific to the complimentary strands located within the pathogen. Subsequently, these probes can be directly detected by tagging with a signal molecule, such as a molecular fluorescent tag. The disadvantages that need to be overcome with this technology are the difficulties in the isolation of DNA samples from pathogens, degradation of the probes and interference from related sequences that may provide false positives.[3]

GeneChip™ developed by Affymetrix®, uses ~100 thousand fluorescence-tagged hybridization probes and scanning confocal optical readouts to detect various specific human disease such as HIV, SARS, as well as, H1N1.[4, 5, 6] Diagnostic tests that combine Affymetrix' GeneChip® DNA probe array technology with RMS' PCR gene amplification technology are being tested for applications in HIV drug resistance to help in disease management of HIV infected individuals and AIDS patients, as well as, the p53 gene for cancer staging. In addition, the Roche AmpliChip Cytochrome P450 Genotyping test uses the Affymetrix® GeneChip™ Microarray Instrument-ation System to detect certain common genetic mutations that alter the body's ability to break down (metabolize) specific types of drugs from a patient's blood (Figure 5.3-3).[4, 7] The United States Army Medical Research Institute for Infectious Diseases (USAMRIID) has attempted to adapt GeneChip™ technology to develop a real-time detection device for the identification of biological weapons, as their characterized sequences are recognized. For example, the Zebra (Z) chip project, represents an attempt to develop a comprehensive surveillance network to detect biological threats by using Z-chip (GeneChip™). The Z-chip consists of an array of DNA probes designed to detect various gene sequences. The resulting DNA pattern should reveal the identity of the infectious organism (Figures 5.3-3 and 5.3-4).[2, 8]

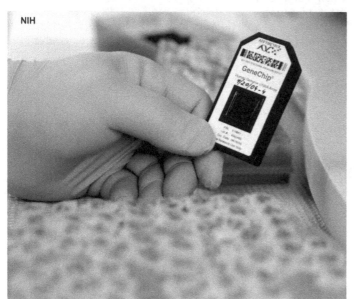

Figure 5.3-3: An Affymetrix® GeneChip™ microarray loaded with RNA extracted from a single patient

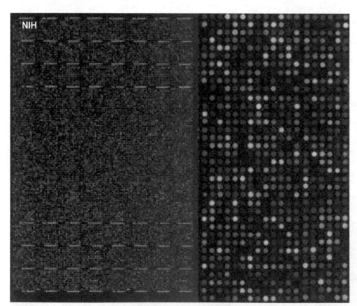

Figure 5.3-4: This photograph shows an array of colored dots indicating the results of a GeneChip™ experiment that compares the gene-expression patterns of the DNA probes and unknown DNA sample

In 2005, a joint research project funded by the Office of Naval Research and Tuffs University developed and tested a fiber-optic, microsphere-based, multiplexed array that is capable of rapidly screening and simultaneously identifying multiple biological weapon agents. This system is designed with DNA probe-functionalized micro-spheres that are randomly distributed into microwells generated on the end of an etched coherent optical fiber bundle that contains 6K to 50K individual fibers. A multiplexed array was created by distributing up to 18 different microsphere sensors into the optical fiber array with species-specific 50-mer DNA probes. These probes are designed to multiply targeting six biological agents (e.g. *B. anthracis, Y. pestis, F. tularensis, B. melitensis, C. botulinum*, vaccinia virus and *B. thuringiensis kurstaki*, a simulant), which reduce the potential of false-negatives and -positives. The researchers reported that the microsensors enabled a detection limit as low as 10 fmol/L (in 50 μL volumes) with 30 minutes of hybridization time. This multiplex array is designed to be expandable as new probes are created when the genome sequences of other biological agents becomes available.[9, 10, 11]

Genetic analysis of samples that have been collected could also be tested through the Joint Biological Agent Identification and Diagnostic System (JBAIDS®). JBAIDS®, produced by Idaho Technology™, is similar in design as the ruggedized, advanced pathogen identification device (RAPID®) and light-cycler®. JBAIDS® is portable, reusable thermocycler that is capable of reliable, quick and specific identification of biological agents from various clinical specimens and environmental samples by employ real time RT-PCR technology (Figure 5.3-5).[2, 12] Since 2009, JBAID® has been approved by the Food and Drug Administration and is presently deployed by the U.S. Army to identify potential biological warfare agents in battle-field conditions. In Iraq, this system demonstrated 100% specificity (95% CI 63-100%) in identifying *Coxiella burnetii*, the causative agent of Q fever. Similarly, JBAIDS was used in Afghanistan to identify *Bacillus anthracis* with 98% (95%, CI, 98-100%) specificity.[13, 14]

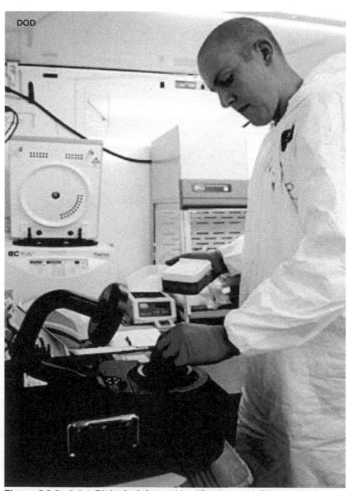

Figure 5.3-5: Joint Biological Agent Identification and Diagnostic System analyzer is loaded with biological samples

Immunosensors or antibody-based probes are another avenue

explored in the real-time detection of biological agents. Immunosensors are designed to recognize specific sites or cellular components (epitopes) of a bacterium or the envelope of a virus. The binding of an antibody to the epitope can be monitored directly with a transduction method such as luminescence, electrochemical signal or sandwich assay in which a second antibody labeled with fluorescent dye is used to bind to the probe antibody. Indirect monitoring may be accomplished through the competition between the bound epitope with a standard epitope labeled with a fluorescent dye. Fluorescence-based fiber optic immunosensors have demonstrated the detection of 10^4 microbial cell/mL and immunochemical sensors have demonstrated the detection at 10^3 cells/mL.[3, 15, 16] The problem associated with this detection system is the degradation of the antibodies, reproducibility of the antibodies, the ability to produce the monoclonal or polyclonal antibodies towards a specific pathogen and/or cross-reactivity of the antibodies. In addition, some viruses possess hypervariable coat proteins, therefore, one antibody targeting a virus may be completely useless in detecting another virus of the same species after it has propagated for several generations. Nonetheless, some of the most sensitive sensors that are presently available are based on antibody probe technology. For example, immunoPCR, is a variation of the existing system by combining antigen-antibody complex with a short strand of DNA which takes advantage of PCR amplification. It has been reported that E.I. DuPont Company and USAMRIID are attempting to adapt this technology to simultaneously identify multiple biological agent threats.[3, 17]

USAMRIID has adapted immunosensor technology to various interim systems available to the military. For example, hand-held assays (HHA) are simple one-time-use immuno-chromatography devices that are used on non-porous surfaces (metal, plastic and glass) which can provide a presumptive yes-no response to the presence of 10 biological agents (4 stimulant agents), within 15 minutes. The presence of a biological agent is indicated by the degree of color change (Figure 5.3-6). HHAs are currently employed in virtually all field military biological detection systems and are also present in developmental systems, such as Biological Integrated Detection System (BIDS), Portal Shield, Joint Biological Point Detection System (JBPDS) and Dry Filter Units (DFU).[2, 18, 19, 20]

US Army

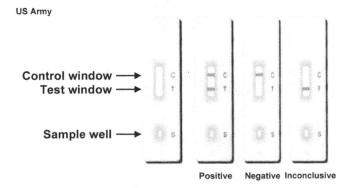

Figure 5.3-6: Graphics showing hand-held assays (HHA). HHAs are one-time-use immune-chromatography devices that can provide a presumptive yes-no response to the presence of biological agents within 15 minutes

BIDS is a remote manned point detection system designed with a shelter (S-788 Lightweight Multipurpose Shelter) mounted on a high mobility multi-purpose wheeled vehicle (M1097 HMMWV). This system includes a trailer-mounted 15-kilowatt PU-801 generator to provide electrical power to ensure uninterrupted operation for at least three days. The complete BIDS system also includes a second HMMWV that is used to carry two out

of four BIDS crew and as a support vehicle to carry additional spares and repairs, and transport suspect samples to a collection point. BIDS is capable of concentrating aerosol particles (2-10 μm) from environmental air for counting, sizing, analyzing for biological activity (presence of ATP), as well as, subsequently subjecting the particle sample to immunosensors for selected agents. The first version of BIDS (without immunosensors) was fielded by the U.S. Army's 310th Chemical Company (Reserve) in 1996 and the second version equipped with immunosensors (BIDS P3I) was fielded to the 7th Chemical Company in October, 1999. BIDS has been reported to be capable of detecting eight biological warfare agents within 45 minutes (Figure 5.3-7).[2, 3, 19, 20]

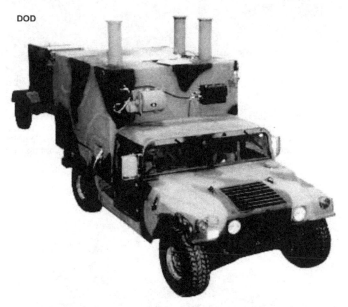

DOD

Figure 5.3-7: A photograph of biological integrated detection system (BIDS)

The Interim Biological Agent Detection System (IBADS) is a shipboard semi-automatic point detector system, a marine version of the BIDS, was first deployed in 1994 aboard the ship USS LaSalle (Figure 5.3-8). This system utilizes a combined particle counter/sizer, wetted-wall cyclone mounted on the forecastle of the ship, and a HHA that are employed manually inside the ship. The particle counter continuously monitors the ambient air for a significant rise in particulate concentration. If a significant rise of particulate concentration is detected, the instrument will automatically collect a sample and alert the ship's damage control center for the need to screen it using the HHA for identification. It has been reported that IBADS is capable of detecting the same eight BW agents as the BIDS but in a shorter amount of time (~25 minutes).[2, 19, 20]

Portal Shield ACTD, is a portable fully automated independent aerosol collector, which also uses a wetted-wall cyclone to collect particles into an aqueous sample. In addition, this system is composed of 12 to 20 or more sensory systems that can be interfaced and networked to a central command post computer that monitors the sensors operational status controls the networked sensors, evaluates network data to determine if a biological attack has occurred and alerts the operator to biological agent detection. The central command post also comes complete with decision-aid algorithms to assist in protective posture decisions, and can interface with the Joint Service Warning and Reporting Network (JWARN). This system is capable of detecting up to eight biological warfare agents within 25 minutes, using antibody-based detection. Although portable, this system is designed for fixed installations and in January 1999, the Portal Shield went into production and was the initial attempt to fulfill the requirement of providing biological protection for Ports and Airfields (Figure 5.3-9).[2, 19, 20]

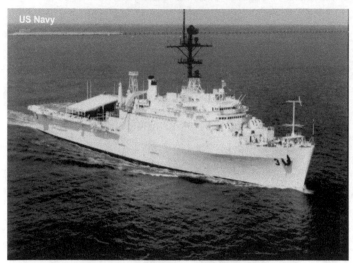

Figure 5.3-8: A photograph of USS La Salle (AGF-3) which the Interim Biological Agent Detection System (IBADS) a shipboard semi-automatic point detector system was first deployed in 1994. USS La Salle was decommission in 2005 and sunk as target in 2007

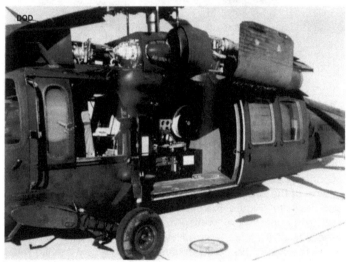

Figure 5.3-9: This photograph shows the fully portable, automated aerosol collector called Portal Shield. Please note that the biological detection system is installed within a Black Hawk helicopter

The JBPDS is an automated point detection system that is designed for multiple platforms. Similar to Portal Shield, it can be interfaced and networked with chemical warfare sensors. This system is designed to detect 10 biological warfare agents and is designed to a have a process time of less than 18 minutes and is presently being integrated onto HMMWVs and ships. Unfortunately, due to its size and power requirements, JBPDS is limited as to where it can be deployed (Figure 5.3-10).[3, 20]

Dry Filter Units (DFU) is a standardized point detection system that is designed to collect aerosolized bio-particulates from ambient air and then subjected for analysis by several complementary technologies (Figure 5.3-11). These complimentary technologies includes HHAs and real-time polymerase chain reaction assays (RT-PCR) etc.[2]

The Long-Range Biological Standoff Detection System (LR-BSDS) is designed to provide a first-line biological standoff detection ability with a "detect to warn" capability. The LR-BSDS is designed to be flown as close to the forward-line troops as

possible by UH-60 helicopter to allow detection of biological agents before they reach the military forces, thereby allowing time to adopt protective measures. This system utilizes an infrared laser to detect aerosol clouds at a standoff distance of up to 30 kilometers and is designed to accommodate fixed-site applications and/or be deployable aboard aircrafts. The LR-BSDS NDI was fielded to the 310th Chemical Company along with the BIDS systems.[2, 19, 20]

Presently under development is the Short-Range Biological Standoff Detection System (SR-BSDS), which will employ ultraviolet and laser-induced fluorescence to detect biological aerosol clouds at distances of up to five kilometers. SR-BSDS like the LR-BSDS is designed to provide early warning to a potential biological attack, thereby enhancing contamination avoidance efforts. However, these systems do not have the capabilities to identify the specific agent. Confirmation of the biological agent or toxin could be accomplished subsequent to detection via BIDS, DFU, etc.[2, 20]

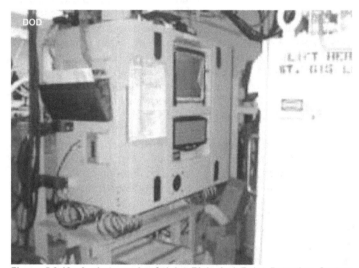

Figure 5.3-10: A photograph of Joint Biological Point Detection System (JBPDS)

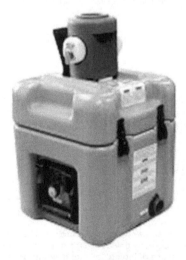

Figure 5.3-11: A photograph of Dry Filter Unit (DFU) 1000

References

1.   Primmerman C.A. Detection of Biological Agents. Lincoln Laboratory Journal, 2000. 12: pp. 3-32
2.   Darling R.G., Woods, J.B. USAMRIID's Medical Management of Biological Casualties Handbook. Fifth Edition. Fort Detrick: US Army Medical Research Institute of Infectious Diseases, 2004. pp. 109-111
3.   Committee on R&D Needs for Improving Civilian Medical Response to Chemical and Biological Terrorism Incidents Health Science Policy Program Institute of Medicine and

Board of Environmental Studies and Toxicology commission on Life Sciences National Research Council. Chemical and Biological Terrorism. Research and Development to Improve Civilian Medical Response. Washington D.C.: National Academy Press. 1999. pp. 78-96

4. Vahey M., Nau M.E., Barrick S., Cooley J.D., Sawyer R., Sleeker A.A., Vickerman P., Bloor S., Larder B., Michael N.L., Wegner S.A. Performance of the Affymetrix GeneChip HIV PRT 440 Platform for Antiretroviral Drug Resistance Genotyping of Human Immunodeficiency Virus Type 1 Clades and Viral Isolates with Length Polymorphisms. Journal of Clinical Microbiology, 1999. 37: pp. 2533–2537

5. Lorence M., O'Kelly J. FDA Grants Emergency Use Authorization for TessArae(R) 2009 H1N1 Influenza A Virus Assay Based on the Affymetrix(R) GeneChip(R) Platform. Revised December 21, 2010. Retrieved January 11, 2009. Website: http://phx.corporateir.net/preview/phoenix.zhtml?c=116408&p=irolnews-Article&ID=13683 08

6. Roche Molecular Systems and Affymetrix combine Genechip® Technology and PCR for New Diagnostic Products. Revised April 27, 1998. Retrieved December 19, 2010. Website: http://www. roche.com/home/media/med_div/med_dia/med_dia_1998/med_dia_1998-04-27.htm

7. Roche AmpliChip Cytochrome P450 Genotyping test and Affymetrix GeneChip Microarray Instrumentation System - K042259. Revised December 23, 2004. Retrieved January 19, 2010. Website: http://www.accessdata. fda.gov/cdrhdocs/ pdf4/k042259.pdf

8. Casman E.A. The Potential of Next-Generation Microbiological Diagnostics to Improve Bioterrorism Detection Speed. Risk Analysis, 2004. 24: pp. 521-536

9. Walt D.R. Bead-based Fiber-optic Arrays. Science, 2000. 287: pp. 451-452

10. Ferguson J.A., Steemer F.J., Walt D.R. High-density Fiber-optic DNA Random Microsphere Array. Analytical Chemistry, 2000. 72: pp. 5618-5624

11. Song L., Ahn S., Walt D.R. Detecting Biological Warfare Agents. Emerging Infectious Diseases, 2005. 11: pp. 1629-1632

12. Joint Biological Agent Identification and Diagnostic System (JBAIDS) UA 9409. U.S. Army Medical Material Agency LIN J00447 6545-01-537-1100. Support and Consumables Handbook. Revised October 2008. Retrieved January 20, 2009. Website: http://www. usamma.army.mil/assets/docs/Handbooks/UA9409_Joint%20Biological%20Agent%20Identification%20and%20Diagnostic%20System%20(JBAIDS)_112409.pdf

13. Hamilton L.R., George D.L., Scoville S.L., Hospenthal D.R., Griffith M.E. PCR for rapid diagnosis of acute Q fever at a combat support hospital in Iraq. Military Medicine, 2011. 176: pp. 103-105

14. Pace S., Steigelman D., Norton S.A., Krivda S. Field-Based PCR for Rapid Diagnosis of Cutaneous Anthrax in the Deployed Setting Using the Joint Biological Agent Identification and Diagnostic System. Military Medicine, 2013. 178: pp. e944-e947

15. Thompson V.S., Maragos C.M. Fiber-Optic Immunosensor for the Detection of Fumonisin B_1. Journal of Agriculture and Food Chemistry, 1996. 44: pp. 1041-1046

16. Taniguchi M., Akai E., Koshida T., Hibi K., Kudo H., Otsuka K., Saito H., Yano K., Endo H., Mitsubayashi K. 3rd Kuala Lumpur International Conference on Biomedical Engineering, 2007. 15: pp. 308-311

17. Joerger R.D., Truby T.M., Hendrickson E.R., Young R.M., Ebersole R.C. Anylate Detection with DNA-labeled Antibodies and Polymerase Chain Reaction. Clinical Chemistry, 1995. 41: pp. 1371-1377

18. Emanuel P.A., Dang J., Gebhardt J.S., Aldrich J., Garber E.A.E., Kulaga H., Stopa P., Valdes J.J., Dion-Schultz A., Recombinant Antibodies: a New Reagent for Biological Agent Detection. Biosensors and Bioelectronics, 2000. 14: pp. 751-759

19. Fatah A.A., Barrett J.A., Arcilesi R.D., Ewing K.J., Lattin C.H., Moshier T.F. An Introduction to Biological Agent Detection Equipment for Emergency First Responders. NIJ Guide 101-00. U.S. Department of Justice. Office of Justice Programs. National Institute of Justice. 2001. pp. 1-53

20. Clark D., Cypret G., Gonsalves C., Hoesly N., Moore A., Saulnier N., Scales-Brown P., Slack M., White R., Buley D., Boulet C., Ellis R., Famini G., Foster R., Long S.R., Phelps K., Wall R., Wong N. Biological Detection System Technologies. Technology and Industrial Base Study. A Primer on Biological Detection Technologies. Final Report. North American Technology and Industrial Base Organization (NATIBO). 2001. pp. 5-5 - 5-9

Photo Bibliography

Figure 5.3-2: A CDC scientist conducts laboratory research in the Biosafety Level 4 laboratory, Atlanta, GA. The photograph was taken and released by CDC. Public domain photo

Figure 5.3-3: An Affymetrix® GeneChip™ microarray loaded with RNA extracted from a single patient. The photograph was taken and released by the National Institutes of Health (NIH). Public domain photo

Figure 5.3-4: This photograph shows an array of colored dots indicating the results of a GeneChip™ experiment that compares the gene-expression patterns of the DNA probes and unknown DNA sample. The photograph was taken by Brian Oliver of the National Institute of General Medical Sciences of the National Institute of Health. Public domain photo

Figure 5.3-5: Joint Biological Agent Identification and Diagnostic System analyzer (JBAIDS ®) is loaded with biological samples. This photograph shows U.S. Army Spc. Paul Miller, from the 9th Area Medical Laboratory at Aberdeen Proving Ground, Md. Utilizing JBAIDS®. The analyzing time of JBAIDS® generally takes 40 minutes per sample once the extraction process of a suspect biological warfare agent specimen is complete. The photograph was taken by Jerry Stillwagon and released by the Department of Defense. Public domain photo

Figure 5.3-6: Graphics showing hand-held assays (HHA). HHAs are one-time-use immune-chromatography devices that can provide a presumptive yes-no response to the presence of biological agents within 15 minutes. The graphic was developed and released by Dugway Proving Ground, United States Army. Public domain photo

Figure 5.3-7: A photograph of biological integrated detection system (BIDS). The photograph was taken and released by Department of Defense. Public domain photo

Figure 5.3-8: A photograph of USS La Salle (AGF-3) which the Interim Biological Agent Detection System (IBADS) a shipboard semi-automatic point detector system was first deployed in 1994. USS La Salle was decommission in 2005 and sunk as target in 2007. The photograph was taken and released by the United States Navy. Public domain photo

Figure 5.3-9: This photograph shows the fully portable, automated aerosol collector called Portal Shield. Please note that the biological detection system is installed within a Black Hawk helicopter. The photograph was taken and released by the Department of Defense. Public domain photo

Figure 5.3-10: A photograph of joint biological point detection system (JBPDS). The photograph was taken and released by the Department of Defense. Public domain photo

Figure 5.3-11: A photograph of dry filter units (DFU) 1000. Photograph was taken and released by the Federal Emergency Response Agency (FEMA). Public domain photo

Decontamination is the process by which hazards are removed from the environment, property and/or life forms in an effort to prevent further contamination and optimize the chance for full recovery after proper treatment. First responders, such as the fire department and hazardous material (Hazmat) teams are the ones that are faced with this daunting task and have classified the decontamination process into two subcategories: Ⓐ technical decon and Ⓑ patient decon. Technical decon is the process used to clean vehicles and protective equipments (PPE), while patient decon is the process by which contaminated individuals are cleansed to eliminate any hazardous agents.[1]

Technical decontamination is most commonly performed by first responders and generally consists of sequential nine steps process. In the Hot Zone where dangerous concentrations of hazardous agents are likely present, the first responders perform the following: ① place the contaminated tools and equipment onto a plastic sheet. ② Place the plastic sheet containing tools and equipment into a trash drop and proceed into the Warm Zone. The Warm Zone, is defined as a location where the concentration of hazardous agents is reduced or not present (Figure 5.4-1).[1]

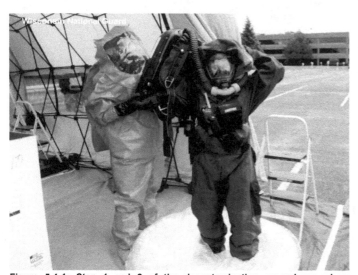

Figure 5.4-1: Step 1 and 2 of the decontamination procedures where contaminated tools and equipment are removed

Once inside the Warm Zone, first responders should proceed to carry out ③ a primary garment wash, which includes cleaning of their boots, outer gloves, suit, SCBA and mask followed by ④ the removal of garments (Figure 5.4-2). The first responders should then proceed to perform step, ⑤ secondary garment wash, where the inner protective garments and gloves are cleansed. This is followed by ⑥ face piece and ⑦ boots removal and drop and finally, ⑧ where the individual should remove their inner gloves which is followed by ⑨ a shower and change of clothing (Figure 5.4-3).[1]

The cleaning solutions used in technical decontamination involve water and one or more of the 4 cleaning solutions (solutions A, B, C, D), depending upon the type of contaminant. For example, solution A contains 5% sodium bicarbonate and 5% trisodium phosphate, and is used to clean materials contaminated by biological pollutants, organic compounds, inorganic acids, acid caustic wastes, solvents, plastic wastes and polychlorinated biphenyls (PCBs). Solution B contains a concentrated solution of sodium hypochlorite, where a 10% solution is used for biological contaminations, organic wastes, pesticides, radioactive materials, chlorinated phenols, dioxin, PCB, cyanide, ammonia and inorganic wastes. Solution C contains 5% trisodium phosphate and it is used for organic compounds, solvents, PCB and polybrominated biphenyls. Solution D contains diluted hydrochloric acid and is used to decontaminate inorganic bases, alkalis and alkali caustic wastes. Once the technical decontamination process is completed, the equipment is most often return to service.[1]

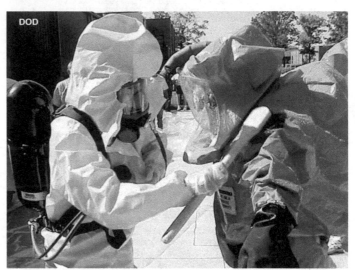

Figure 5.4-2: Step 3 and 4 of the decontaminated procedures. N.D. Air national guardsman go through decontamination procedure during Emergency Management Training hosted at the 119th Wing

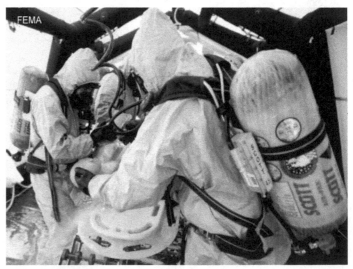

Figure 5.4-3: Steps 5-9 of the decontaminated procedures

Patient decontamination generally involves three stages: gross, secondary and definitive decon-tamination. Gross decon involves ① evacuating the individual from the high risk area (<300 feet), ② removal of the patient's clothing and performance of a one-minute head-to-toe rinse with soap and water or a fresh solution of 0.5% sodium hypochlorite. It has been reported that the removal of the patient's clothing will eliminate approximately 70-80% of the contaminates.[1, 2, 3] The secondary decon can be performed in the field or at a hospital where the patient receives ① a full body rinse, ② a wash from head-to-toe with water or decontamination solution and ③ receives an additional full body rinse. The definitive decon should be performed at the hospital where the patient is ① washed from head-to-toe once again, until clean, ② rinsed thoroughly and ③ dried and given clean clothes prior to examination and treatment (Figure 5.4-4).[1]

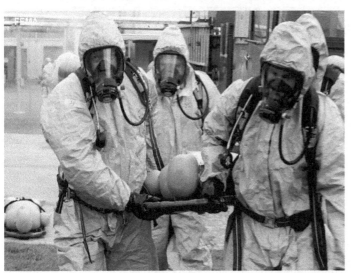

Figure 5.4-4: This photograph shows the removal of the individual from the high risk area (<300 feet) and the removal of the patient's clothing which may be contaminated

Emergency shower systems are commercially available, generally equipped with provisions for capturing contaminated runoff. However, in the event where emergency shower systems are not available, a fire hose (operating at a reduced pressure) can be used for gross decon. Although hospitals are required by the Joint Commission on Accreditation of Healthcare Organizations (JCAHO) to be prepared for Hazmat emergencies, most hospitals do not see the need to invest in a once in a life time event. Therefore, most hospitals at this time do not have decontamination facilities and even fewer have outdoor facilities or an easy way of expanding their decontamination facilities as could be required. In an event of a terrorism act, most hospitals would be overrun with walk in patients and unannounced ambulances delivering the infected which would place hospital staff and patients at great risk (Figure 5.4-5).[1]

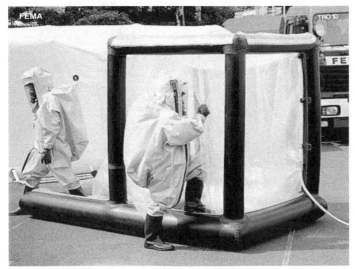

Figure 5.4-5: Emergency shower system is shown to decontaminated potentially contaminated health workers

References

1. Committee on R&D Needs for Improving Civilian Medical Response to Chemical and Biological Terrorism Incidents Health Science Policy Program Institute of Medicine and Board of Environmental Studies and Toxicology commission on Life Sciences National Research Council. Chemical and Biological Terrorism. Research and Development to Improve Civilian Medical Response. Washington D.C.: National Academy Press. 1999. pp. 78-96
2. Emergency Response Guidebook for Weapons of Mass Destruction Incidents. U.S. Department of Justice. Office of Justice Programs. Office for State and Local Domestic Preparedness Support. Louisiana State University, Academy of Counter-Terrorist Education. 2001. pp. 37
3. Cox R.D. Decontamination and Management of Hazardous Materials Exposure Victims in the Emergency Department. Annals of Emergency Medicine, 1994. 23: pp. 761-770

Photo Bibliography

Figure 5.4-1: Steps 1 and 2 decontamination procedure where contaminated tools and equipment are removed. Photograph was taken and released by the Wisconsin National Guard. Public domain photo

Figure 5.4-2: Air national guardsman go through decontamination procedure during Emergency Management Training hosted at the 119th Wing, North Dakota. Photograph taken and released by the Department of Defense. Public domain photo

Figure 5.4-3: Steps 5-9 of the decontaminated procedures at the decontamination corridor at the Pentagon. Photo taken and released by the Federal Emergency Management Agency. Public domain photo

Figure 5.4-4: This photograph shows the removal of the individual from the high risk area (<300 feet) and the removal of the patient's clothing which may be contaminated. The photograph was taken and released by Federal Emergency Management Agency. Public domain photo

Figure 5.4-5: Emergency shower system to decontaminate potentially contaminated health workers. Photo taken and released by the Federal Emergency Management Agency. Public domain photo

Personal protection equipment (PPE) varies significantly depending upon the type of hazard. For chemical material protection, the PPE required is typically designed to afford respiratory, as well as, whole-body protection since most of the agents can be absorbed through the skin or inhaled. PPE for radiological material protection should be designed to prevent radiological materials, such as alpha and beta particles, neutrons, and gamma rays, from being inhaled or penetrating the skin. However, most available PPE do not provide radiation shielding. PPE for biological protection, on the other hand, concentrates on preventing the biological materials from being inhaled, coming into contact with the mucous membrane of the eyes and/or nasal passage, and come into contact with lesions in the skin.

The PPE designed for biological protection depend upon the Biosafety Level that is required when experimenting or transporting specific biological agents. Biosafety Levels (BSLs) are based upon the danger posed by the pathogen. For example, BSL-1 labs can be found in all college campuses, where faculty and students alike, can work on microorganisms or viruses that do not pose a health hazard. Organisms and viruses that are allowed in BSL-1 consist of those that belong to Risk Group 1 (Tables 1 and 2). BSL-2 is used when working with pathogens that can cause disease, but are generally treatable and will not spread from one individual to another through aerosolized transmission. Organisms and viruses that are allowed in BSL-2 consist of those that belong to Risk Group 2 (Table 1 and 2). In BSL-2, any work that may involve splashes or aerosols should be completed in glove boxes. The PPE required for BSL-2 consist of splash protective clothing (e.g. a lab coat), gloves and face protection. BSL-3 is used when working with pathogens that may have serious health consequences and can be transmitted via aerosol. Organisms and viruses that are allowed in BSL-3 consist of those that belong to Risk Group 3 (Table 1 and 2). In BSL-3, any work that may involve splashes or aerosols should be completed in glove boxes. PPE for BSL-3 includes splash protection, gloves, goggles and a respirator. BSL-4 is required for work with high-risk pathogens that can produce extremely serious human or animal disease. Pathogens that are grouped in BSL-4 are those that belong to Risk Group 4. These pathogens are often untreatable and can be easily spread. Personnel that handle these pathogens must wear one-piece positive pressure suits and all work must be conducted in a sealed environment (Table 1 and 2).

Potentially dangerous pathogens are assigned Risk Groups 1-4; where Risk Group 1 pathogens are not known to consistently cause disease in healthy adults, while Risk Group 4 consist of serious pathogens that are highly likely to cause serious or fatal disease and are able to be transmitted as aerosols (Table 2).

Table 1: The Biosafety Levels and laboratory equipment and laboratory types. Please note that BSC stands for biological safety cabinets

Biosafety	Lab Type	Equipment needed
Level 1	Open bench	Basic teaching and research
Level 2	Open bench plus biological safety cabinets	Primary health services, diagnostic and research
Level 3	BSC and other primary devices for all activities	Special diagnostic and research
Level 4	Class III BSC, positive pressure suits with Class II BSC, filtered air, double ended autoclave	Dangerous pathogen Units

Table 2: Risk Groups 1 to 4 as listed by the World Health Organization

Risk Group	Organism Types
1	Pathogen that are unlikely to cause disease in either animals or humans
2	Pathogen that can cause human of animal disease but is unlikely to be a serious hazard to laboratory workers, the community, livestock or the environment
3	Pathogen that can cause serious diseases in humans and animals but does not ordinarily spread from one individual to another. Effective treatment and preventive measures are available
4	Pathogen that can cause serious diseases in humans and animals that can readily spread (directly or indirectly) from one individual to another. Effective treatment and preventive measures are not usually available

RESPIRATORS

Respirators are designed to supply clean, breathable air to their users. Respirators are categorized into two groups: atmospheric-supplying and air purifying respirators.

Atmospheric-Supplying Respirators

Atmospheric-supplying respirators are high-level respirators that supply air from a source independent of the surrounding atmosphere. These respirators include open-circuit self-containing breathing (SCBA) apparatus, closed-circuit supplied-air respirators and supplied-air respirators. For example, the open-circuit self-containing breathing apparatus is designed to supply air to the user from a high-pressure compressed air tank and expels its exhaust to the surrounding atmosphere. These units are commonly used by first responders and depending upon the tank size, the amount of air contained could last anywhere from 30 to 60 minutes. This apparatus weighs approximately 25 to 30 pounds and could be used for Biosafety Levels 3 for pathogens in the Risk Group 3 (Figure 5.5-1).

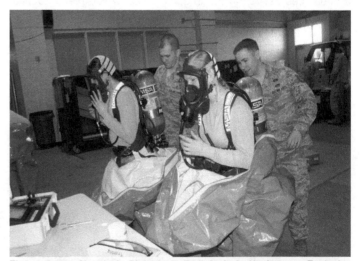

Figure 5.5-1: Chemical, Biological, Radiological, Nuclear or Explosive Emergency Response Force (CERF) from Malmstrom Air Force Base, Montana removes their Level A suits and their self-contained breathing apparatus after simulating entry and detection hazardous materials

The closed-circuit self-contained breathing apparatus is designed to recycle usable air by circulating the exhaled air through a scrubber to remove carbon dioxide and replenish the consumed oxygen through a stored container. The closed-circuit system is designed to provide the wearer up to 4 hours of air supply. The closed-circuit self-contained breathing apparatus weighs approximately 35 to 40 pounds and could be used for Biosafety Levels 3 for pathogens in the Risk Group 3 (Figure 5.5-2).

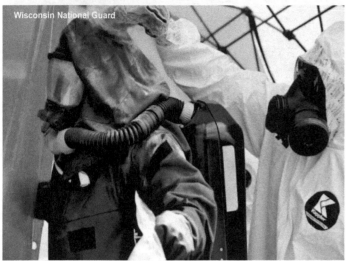
Figure 5.5-2: The closed-circuit self-contained breathing apparatus is designed to recycle usable air by removing carbon dioxide and replenish the consumed oxygen

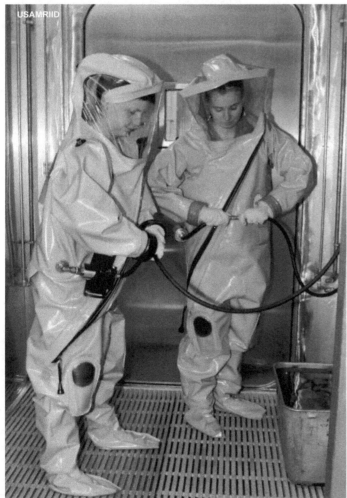
Figure 5.5-3: supplied-air respirator system is designed to supply compressed air from a stationary source that is located outside of the hazardous area

The supplied-air respirator system is designed to supply compressed air from a stationary source such as an air tank or a compressor that is located outside of the hazardous area. The

cleaned air is supplied to the wearer through a hose, which will provide the necessary protection from biological agents, as well as, increasing the wearer's air supply from hours (depending on the side of the air tank) to unlimited air supply if a compressor is used. However, the mobility of the wearer is limited by the length of the hose. This respirator system is generally found on positive pressure suits and could be used for Biosafety Levels 3 and 4, for pathogens in the Risk Groups 3 and 4 (Figure 5.5-3).

Air-Purifying Respirators

The air-purifying respirators are subdivided into three groups: ① particulate-removing respirators, ② vapor- and gas-removing respirators and ③ combination respirators.

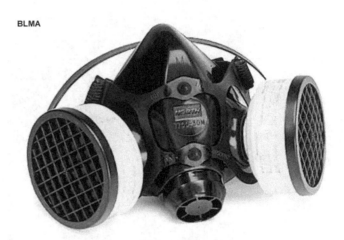
Figure 5.5-4: A particulate-removing respirator with disposable cartridges is designed to mechanically filter the inlet air and reduce the amount of potentially hazardous particulates that the user inhales

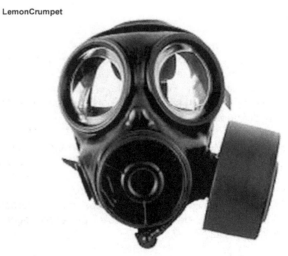
Figure 5.5-5: An example of vapor- and gas-removing respirators. This respirator is designed to have canisters or cartridges that contain sorbent bed to remove of chemically neutralize vapor or gases in the air

The particulate-removing respirators are designed to mechanically filter the inlet air and reduce the amount of potentially hazardous particulates that the user inhales. The mask could be made out of the filter material in a disposable mask or could also be designed with disposable filter cartridges. Both types of particulate-removing respirators are designed to have a maximum acceptable exposure limits not less than 0.05 milligram per cubic meter (mg/m^3) of air (Figure 5.5-4).

The vapor- and gas-removing respirators are designed to have canisters or cartridges that contain sorbent bed to remove of chemically neutralize vapor or gases in the air. The type of cartridge utilized will determine the type of vapors and/or gases that the wearer is protected from. Nonetheless, a general sorbent is activated carbon which will remove many vapors (Figure 5.5-5).

The combination respirators use cartridges that contain filters and sorbent beds to remove particulates, vapors and gases. These filters are designed to direct inhaled air first through a particulate filter and then through a sorbent bed. Nonetheless, this type of filtering unit tends to offer more resistance to breathing. To compensate, some combination respirators possess battery powered blowers to draw air into the filter, as well as, provide additional pressure to push the air to the wearer (Figure 5.5-6).

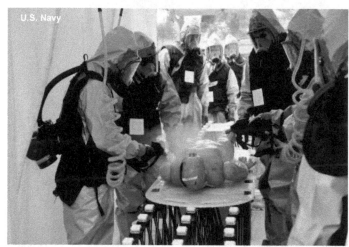

Figure 5.5-6: The decontamination team at U.S. Naval Hospital Yokosuka decontaminates a simulated patient during a training session. Please note that the combination respirator is used by the decontamination team

CLOTHING

Protective clothing is necessary to prevent exposure of the skin with any hazardous chemicals, liquids, vapors and infectious pathogens. As with the case in respirators, protective clothing differs in different situations. For example, clothing that provides adequate protection against biological agents may be ineffective against chemical agents and vice versa.

There are various materials that are employed in protecting the wearer against chemical and biological attacks. The first material used is called Tyvek®. Tyvek® is a light weight, durable, high-density polyethylene material that is commonly employed as a single-use suit to provide splash protection from hazardous materials, as well as, an effective means of protection against biological agents (Figure 5.5-7).

The second material used is called Texshield. This is a fabric system that activated carbon beads are placed between the outer shell fabric and a lightweight nonwoven fabric. Texshield is used in the Joint Services Lightweight Integrated Suit Technology (JSLIST) over-garments (Figure 5.5-9). The third fabric is a selectively-permeable polytetrafluoroethylene membrane laminated between a tightly woven nylon outer shell and tricot inner shell. This relatively new technology is presently being considered for an advanced protective ensemble for the United States military. The fourth fabric is composed of polymerically encapsulated carbon topstitched with elasticized threads and is presently being used as protective undergarments by the United States military. Finally, the fifth fabric is carbon-impregnated foam with tricot laminate. Presently, this material is being used as the

inner layer of the United States Army Battle Dress Over-garment.

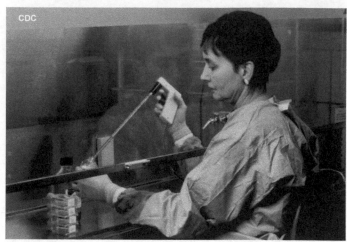

Figure 5.5-7: A photo of a CDC laboratory technician wearing single use Tyvek® protective suit

GLOVES

Like protective clothing, the types of gloves used are selected based upon the hazard that the wearer will be facing. There are several tradeoffs influencing the selection. For example, heavy gloves are more resistant to physical hazards, while lightweight gloves offer better dexterity. Nitrile gloves are highly resistant to hydrocarbons and oils and offer protection form may types of chemicals, while Vitron® gloves are resistant to chlorinated aromatic solvents. Norfoil® gloves, made out of laminated plastic, are highly resistant to various chemical corrosives. For biological pathogens, double latex gloves provide adequate protection and dexterity for field work. Ordinary latex gloves are generally adequate for laboratory conditions (Figure 5.5-8).

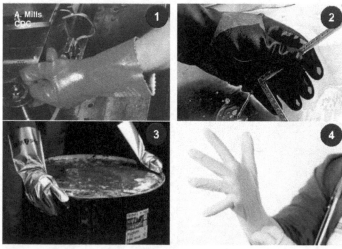

Figure 5.5-8: Examples of gloves used during exposure to chemical and biological hazards. ① Nitrile gloves ② Viton® gloves ③ Norfoil® gloves and ④ typical laboratory latex gloves

MILITARY PROTECTIVE EQUIPMENT

At present, the field military chemical and biological protective equipment includes the M40 protective mask, Joint Services Lightweight Integrated Suit Technology (JSLIST), a replacement for the battle dress over-garment, protective gloves, and multi-purpose over-boots (MULO) (Figure 5.5-9).

The M40 full face-piece respirator is a United States military standard issue mask available in three sizes. With two styles of optical inserts for individuals requiring optical correction, M40 is designed to protect the face, eyes, and respiratory tract. The mask is complete with a drinking tube that allows the wearer to rehydrate while in a contaminated environment. It is important to note that the wearer should disinfect the canteen and tube by wiping with a 5% hypochlorite solution before use. M40 employs a single, standard screw-on C2A1 filter element. The C2A1 filter element, developed by 3M™, contains both a carbon bed and particulate filter. The particulate filter is at least 99.97% efficient in a 0.3 mm MMAD (Mass Median Aerodynamic Diameter) aerosol challenge at 85 L/min. The carbon bed filter has been created to United States military specifications and has been effective in protecting soldiers from hydrogen cyanide, cyanogen chloride, phosgene and the nerve agent simulant dimethyl methylphosphonate (Figure 5.5-10).[1]

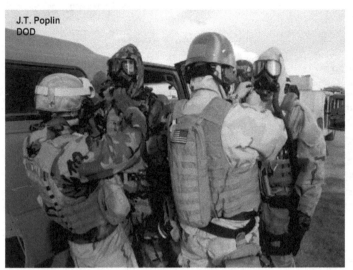

Figure 5.5-9: U.S. Sailors assigned to Explosive Ordnance Disposal Mobile Unit 8 help each other don M45 gas masks and joint service lightweight integrated suit technology suits during a training exercise at Naval Air Station Sigonella, Italy

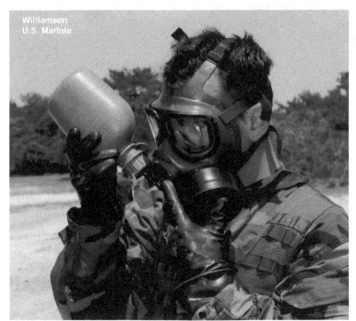

Figure 5.5-10: A soldier from the 31st Marine Expeditionary Unit drinks water through the drinking system in his M40 Field Protective Mask during Nuclear, Biological and Chemical training in Okinawa, Japan

JSLIST is available in seven sizes, with woodland and desert camouflage patterns. This protective suit can be used continuously for 45 days in an uncontaminated environment. In a contaminated environment the suit can be laundered up to 6 times and may be worn continuously for 24 hours. Once the suit reached its life expectancy, it should be either incinerated or buried.[1]

Chemical and biological protective gloves, as well as, over-boots are made from butyl rubber and come in various sizes. This equipment is durable and may be decontaminated and reissued, although they must be visually inspected and decontaminated as needed after every 12 hours of exposure, in a contaminated environment.[1]

Non-military personal protective equipment standards are established by the Occupational Safety and Health Administration (OSH), the Occupational Safety and Health Administration (OSHA) and the Environmental Protection Agency (EPA). This standard for protective equipment is based upon the type of hazards and duration of exposure anticipated; therefore an assessment of any potential hazardous environment must be carefully made. For example, Level A protective equipment provides maximal protection against vapors and liquids and consists of a fully encapsulating, chemical resistant suit, outer and inner gloves and steel toed boots. In addition, this level demands either a self-contained breathing apparatus (SCBA) or a pressure-demand (positive pressure) supplied air respirator with an escape SCBA. Level A is designed to protect workers in an environment that may be immediately dangerous to health and life (Figure 5.5-3).[2, 3, 4]

Level B protective equipment is used when full reparatory protection is needed, while the danger to the skin is less severe. This level incorporates a hooded, non-encapsulating, splash-protective, chemical resistant suit (slash suit) that is not air tight, chemical resistant outer and inner gloves, chemical resistant steel toe boots and a SCBA or positive pressure supplied air respirator with escape. Level B is designed for the minimum protection for workers in danger of unknown chemicals or biological hazards (Figure 5.5-6).[2, 3, 4] Level C protective equipment uses a hooded splash suit, chemical resistant outer and inner gloves, and chemical resistant steel toe boots along with a full-covering positive or negative pressure respirator (e.g. gas mask) rather than a SCBA.[2, 3, 4] Level D allows for the least amount of protection where it is limited to coveralls, steel toe boots, safety glasses or goggles, hard hat, escape mask, face shield and chemical resistant gloves.[2, 3, 4]

The isolation procedures for patient care are dependent upon the specific type of biological agents. USAMRIID guide-lines have been prepared to determine the level of containment should be utilized for each individual patient (see Table 3).[5]

At USAMRIID, located at Fort Detrick, MD, patients can be brought into the BSL-4 suite directly from the outside through specialized ports with unique patient-isolation equipment. In addition, USAMRIID maintains unique teams (each team lead by a specially trained physician, a registered nurse and eight volunteers), known as Aeromedical Isolation Team (AIT). These teams are specially trained to provide evacuation capability for casualties suspected of being infected with highly transmittable and infectious diseases. AIT are specially equipped with special adult size Vickers isolation units (e.g. Vickers Medical Containment Stretcher Transit Isolator®), which are designed to completely isolate a patient from the external environment. The Vickers isolation units are aircraft transportable and are enveloped by a transparent plastic that maintains negative air pressure through an air supply system in order to avoid the exit

Table 3: Isolation Procedures for Patients and Care Providers at USAMRIID[5]

Biological Agents	Biosafety Level
Ebola Virus	BSL-4 isolation suite admission for patients and care providers in positive-pressure protective suits
Marburg Virus	BSL-4 isolation suite admission for patients and care providers in positive-pressure protective suits
Crimean-Congo Hemorrhagic Fever Virus	BSL-4 isolation suite admission for patients and care providers in positive-pressure protective suits
Smallpox (Variola) Virus	BSL-4 isolation suite admission for patients and care providers in positive-pressure protective suits
Monkeypox Virus	BSL-4 isolation suite admission for patients and care providers in positive-pressure protective suits
Yersinia pestis (pneumonic)	BSL-4 isolation suite admission for patients and barrier nursing procedures
Lassa Fever Virus	BSL-4 isolation suite admission for patients and barrier nursing procedures
Junin Virus	BSL-4 isolation suite admission for patients and barrier nursing procedures
Machupo Virus	BSL-4 isolation suite admission for patients and barrier nursing procedures
Venezuelan Equine Encephalitis Virus	Normal hospital room for patients and depending on the agent barrier nursing procedures or secretion precautions
Rift Valley Fever Virus	Normal hospital room for patients and depending on the agent barrier nursing procedures for secretion precautions
Chikungunya Virus	Normal hospital room for patients and depending on the agent barrier nursing procedures or secretion precautions
Dengue Virus	Normal hospital room for patients and depending on the agent barrier nursing procedures or secretion precautions
Brucella species	Normal hospital room for patients and depending on the agent barrier nursing procedures or secretion precautions
Bacillus anthracis (pulmonary or cutaneous forms)	Normal hospital room for patients and depending on the agent barrier nursing procedures or secretion precautions
Francisella tularensis (pulmonary form)	Normal hospital room for patients and depending on the agent barrier nursing procedures or secretion precautions
Yersinia pestis (bubonic or septicemic)	Normal hospital room for patients and depending on the agent barrier nursing procedures or secretion precautions
Coxiella burnetii (Q fever)	Normal hospital room for patients with no special precautions
Botulinum Toxin	Normal hospital room for patients with no special precautions
Staphylococcal Enterotoxin B	Normal hospital room for patients with no special precautions
Ricin Toxin	Normal hospital room for patients with no special precautions
Trichothecene Mycotoxins	Normal hospital room for patients with no special precautions

of potentially contaminated air.[5, 6]

References

1. Woods, J.B. USAMRIID's Medical Management of Biological Casualties Handbook. Sixth Edition. Fort Detrick: US Army Medical Research Institute of Infectious Diseases, 2005. pp. 117-119
2. Committee on R&D Needs for Improving Civilian Medical Response to Chemical and Biological Terrorism Incidents Health Science Policy Program Institute of Medicine and Board of Environmental Studies and Toxicology commission on Life Sciences National Research Council. Chemical and Biological Terrorism. Research and Development to Improve Civilian Medical Response. Washington D.C.: National Academy Press. 1999. pp. 78-96
3. Melnick A.L. Biological, Chemical and Radiological Terrorism. Emergency Preparedness and Response for the Primary Care Physician. New York: Springer. 2008. pp. 113-118
4. Guidance on Emergency Responder Personal Protective Equipment (PPE) for Response to CBRN Terrorism Incidents. Department of Health and Human Services. Centers for Disease Control and Prevention National Institute for Occupational Safety and Health (NIOSH). 2008. pp. 1-8
5. Franz D.R., Parrott C.D., Takafuji E.T. The U.S. Biological Warfare and Biological Defense Programs. Medical Aspects of Chemical and Biological Warfare. Washington D.D.: Office of the Surgeon General Department of the Army, United States of America. 1997. pp. 425-436
6. Ippolito G., Nicastri E., Capobianchi M., Do Caro A., Petrosillo N., Puro V. Hospital Preparedness and Management of Patients Affected by Viral Haemorrhagic Fever or Smallpox at the Lazzaro Spallanzani Institute, Italy. Eurosurveillance, 2005. 10: pp. 36-38

Photo Bibliography

Figure 5.5-1: Chemical, Biological, Radiological, Nuclear or Explosive Emergency Response Force (CERF) from Malmstrom Air Force Base, Montana removes their Level A suits and their self-contained breathing apparatus after simulating entry and detection hazardous materials. Photograph was taken and released by Airman 1st Class Kristina Overton, U.S. Airforce. Public domain photo

Figure 5.5-2: The closed-circuit self-contained breathing apparatus is designed to recycle usable air by removing carbon dioxide and replenish the consumed oxygen. Photograph was taken and released by the Wisconsin National Guard. Public domain photo

Figure 5.5-3: supplied-air respirator system is designed to supply compressed air from a stationary source that is located outside of the hazardous area. This photograph was released by U.S. Army Medical Research Institute of Infectious Diseases. Public domain photo

Figure 5.5-4: A particulate-removing respirator with disposable cartridges is designed to mechanically filter the inlet air and reduce the amount of potentially hazardous particulates that the user inhales. This photograph was released by LemonCrumpet via Wikicommons. Public domain photo

Figure 5.5-5: An example of vapor- and gas-removing respirators. This respirator is designed to have canisters or cartridges that contain sorbent bed to remove of chemically neutralize vapor or gases in the air. This photograph was released by the DCI Counterterrorist Center, Central Intelligence Agency in May 2003. Public domain photo

Figure 5.5-6: The decontamination team at U.S. Naval Hospital Yokosuka decontaminates a simulated patient during a training session. Please note that the combination respirator is used by the decontamination team. The photo was taken by Richard McManus on September 16, 2010 and released by the United States Navy. Public domain photo

Figure 5.5-7: A photo of a CDC laboratory technician wearing single use Tyvek ® protective suit. The photo was taken by Jim Gathany and released in 2005 by the CDC. Public domain photo

Figure 5.5-8: Examples of gloves used during exposure to chemical and biological hazards. ① Nitrile gloves ② Viton® gloves ③ Norfoil® gloves and ④ typical laboratory latex gloves. Photographs taken by Amanda Mills in 2011 and released by the CDC. Public domain photo

Figure 5.5-9: U.S. Sailors assigned to Explosive Ordnance Disposal Mobile Unit 8 help each other don M45 gas masks and joint service lightweight integrated suit technology suits during a chemical warfare training exercise at Naval Air Station Sigonella, Italy. The photograph taken by Communication Specialist 2nd Class Jason T. Poplin on Jan. 27, 2009 and released by the Department of Defense. Public domain photo

Figure 5.5-10: U.S. sailor wearing a M45 gas mask and joint service lightweight integrated suit technology suits during a mass casualty field training exercise. The photograph taken by Lance Cpl. Craig Williamson and released by U.S. Marine Corps. Public domain photo

Figure 5.5-11: CDC scientist in her level A protection suit. Photo taken by James Gathany in 2007 and released by the CDC. Public domain photo

Figure 5.5-12: CDC scientist working in his level B protection suit. Photo taken by James Gathany in 2005 and released by the CDC. Public domain photo

Many terrorist groups have the technical capability to produce biological agents using improvised laboratory equipment from common objects. Biological pathogen production generally involves acquiring an infectious bacterial or viral strain, which is then grown and isolated. It is possible that the infectious cell strains can be stolen or obtained from medical or research facilities, or obtained from natural sources, such as soil, plants, animals or animal products.

The culturing method used by terrorist groups may be as simple as a cell culture growth method, which includes growing bacteria on a petri dish containing nutrient or growth media or multiplying viruses in cell cultures contained within flat-bottom flasks. If larger quantities are desired, a secondary growth method may be employed. The secondary method involves large containers, such as bacterial fermenters, embryonated chicken eggs for viruses (Figure 5.6-1), or even living creatures.

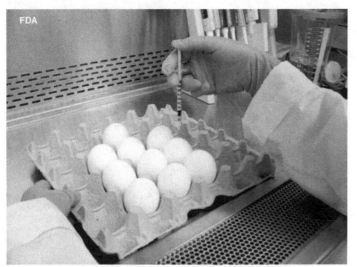

Figure 5.6-1: A technician in the process of injecting an embryonated egg with the influenza virus. Historically, eggs have been used for viral cultures

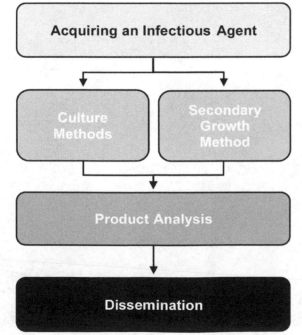

Acquiring an Infectious Agent

Culture Methods

Secondary Growth Method

Product Analysis

Dissemination

Figure 5.6-2: Stepwise process of biological agent production

After the infectious bacteria or viruses have been produced or the desired toxins manufactured, they are separated from the growth media and wastes. In more sophisticated laboratories, product analysis may be used to determine the virulence of the pathogen or the toxicity of the toxin; however, in smaller laboratories, this step may not be possible (Figure 5.6-2).

PRODUCTION

The first step in pathogen production that a would-be terrorist or terrorist group would do is the acquisition of a pure strain of the bacteria or virus to be used as a starting material. Infectious pathogens can be purchased or stolen from biological supply houses, universities, health care facilities and/or research laboratories. Nonetheless, highly infectious agents are tightly controlled and are difficult to acquire. It is known that some pathogenic materials can be extracted from natural sources. Anthrax, for example, can be extracted from soil, usually from animal pastures. Other pathogens could be isolated from the blood of an infected animal, spoiled meat or tainted canned goods. However, samples obtained from natural sources will contain microorganisms other than the pathogen of interest and have to be further processed and purified to achieve the desired results.

Growing cultures is the second step in producing pathogens. For example, bacteria will thrive in culture media and divide through bacterial fission until the desired concentration of bacterial pathogen is reached. Bacterial cultures are typically grown in Petri dishes containing the necessary agar and nutrients (Figure 5.6-3). Viruses, in contrast, will require a host cell to replicate. As mentioned previously, embryonated eggs may be used for virus replication or the host cells grown in flat bottom flaks, also known as, culture flask (Figure 5.6-1 and 5.6-4).

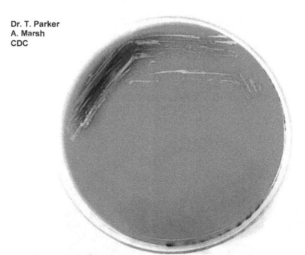

Dr. T. Parker
A. Marsh
CDC

Figure 5.6-3: This photograph depicts the colonial morphology displayed by Gram-negative *Brucella abortus* bacteria, which was grown on a medium of sheep blood agar (SBA), for a 48 hour time period, at a temperature of 37°C

In order to achieve optimal pathogen growing conditions, the environment must be controlled. For example, if a sterile environment is not maintained, undesirable microorganisms may invade the culture, start to grow, and may out-compete the desired pathogen. Therefore, special clothing must be worn to prevent contamination. Substances, such as alcohol and bleach, are commonly used to clean the laboratory area, while high pressure steam from equipment, such as a commercially available pressure cooker (Figure 5.6-5), or an autoclave may be used to sterilize equipment (Figure 5.6-6).

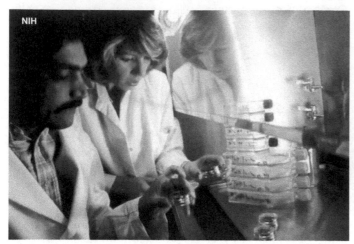
Figure 5.6-4: Scientists examining culture flasks under a laminar flow hood

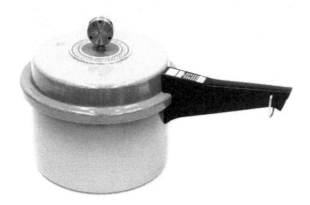
Figure 5.6-5: A commercial available pressure cooker that can be used to sterilize equipment

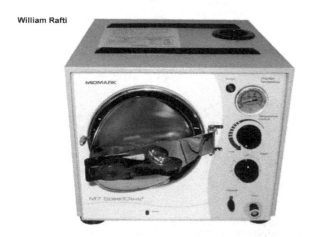
Figure 5.6-6: A commercial available autoclave that can be used to sterilize equipment

Once the desired bacteria or viruses are isolated, they are typically cultured in Petri dishes or flat bottom flasks and stored within a controlled environment provided by incubators. However, if an incubator is not available, a would-be terrorist could use a household oven or even modify a large cooler to provide the pathogen with an optimal environment for growth (Figure 5.6-7).

Depending on the type of pathogen, gases such as carbon dioxide (CO_2) or oxygen (O_2) may be used to enhance cell growth. For example, both CO_2 and O_2 are commercially available gases readily available for purchase from retailers. Makeshift equipment can be rigged so that the gases are pumped into the growing area. Evidence of tampering or modification of an incubator or a household oven may be an indication of pathogen production.

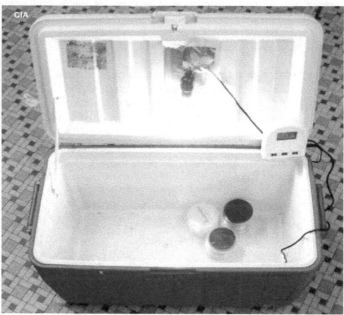
Figure 5.6-7: A photograph of a makeshift incubator made from a commercially available cooler

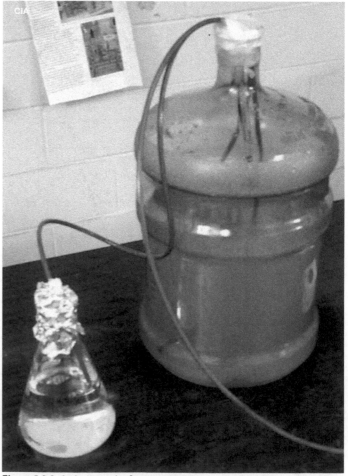
Figure 5.6-8: A photograph of a converted water container into an improvised fermenter

Certain pathogens require constant monitoring of the pH levels or their growth will be reduced or even completely halted. Both pH meters and paper are commercially available. For example, a pH meter designed for a saltwater aquarium could easily be used in illegal pathogen production. After the bacteria have been given enough time to multiply, they could be transferred to a fermenter for mass production. Fermenters are large, close containers that hold growth media for bacterial propagation. Resourceful terrorists could use simple converted plastic jars (Figure 5.6-8), yogurt makers, jugs used in home-made beer kits, to industrial-scale vats, to accomplish their tasks. The size of the fermenter will determine the amount of bacteria that can be produced.

Virus production, on the other hand, generally involves introducing the virus into embryonated eggs (Figure 5.6-1) or host animals and allowing these obligated intracellular parasite to continue their replication within the host cells. If the virus is introduced into a host animal, the virus should cause the animal to die in several days. Subsequently, the viruses are extracted. The extraction process is difficult and generally only a small amount of viral agent is recovered.

ISOLATION

Filtration is generally the method of choice for separating biological agents from their amalgam. For example, if a fermenter is used to grow bacteria cultures, the pathogen must be separated from the growth media or nutrient broth. Filtration methods vary in sophistication and the one used depends on the desired purity of the product. A filtration system may be as simple as a coffee filter, cheesecloth, laboratory filter paper, to a vacuum or industrial filtration system (Figure 5.6-9). Additionally, centrifugation techniques may also be used to isolate the bacteria.

After the pathogens are successfully separated from the growth media or nutrient broth, they will exist in a slurry, or "wet" phase. Additional steps must be taken to dry and mill the pathogen, thereby allowing for aerosol dissemination. The drying and milling process is highly dangerous, as well as, technically challenging. Equipment used in the process includes drum pelletizers, pan dryers, spray or freeze drying equipment, or even rock tumblers.

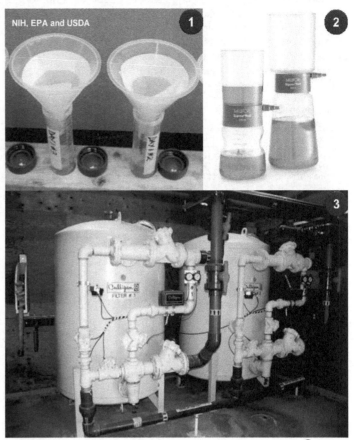

Figure 5.6-9: Composite photographs of various filtration systems. ① Simple filtration, ② vacuum filtration and ③ industrial filtration system

PRODUCTION DIFFICULTIES

Although it is possible for a terrorist or terrorist group to produce any and all biological agents for targeted or mass dissemination as described within this book, there are certain inherent challenges with production. The following charts list

Table 1: High impact diseases. Highly contagious diseases and with high degree of difficulties to obtain and handle

Agent	Mode of Deployment	Comments
Variola Virus (smallpox)	Aerosol dispersal or person to person contact	Highly contagious
Ebola Virus	Aerosol dispersal or person to person contact	Highly contagious & lethal
Marburg Virus	Aerosol dispersal or person to person contact	Highly contagious & lethal
Congo Crimean Hemorrhagic Fever Virus	Aerosol dispersal or person to person contact	Moderately contagious

Table 2: Moderate impact diseases. Highly to rarely contagious and with moderate degree of difficulties to obtain and handle

Agent	Mode of Deployment	Comments
Venezuelan Equine Encephalitis Virus	Aerosol dispersal or through infected mosquitoes	Moderately contagious
Coxiella burnetii (Q-Fever)	Aerosol dispersal	Low-level contagion
Yersinia pestis (Pneumonic Plague)	Aerosol dispersal or through infected fleas	Highly contagious & lethal
Burkholderia mallei (Glanders)	Aerosol dispersal	Highly contagious & lethal

Table 3: Low impact diseases or toxin. Highly to rarely contagious and with low degree of difficulties in obtain and handle

Agent	Mode of Deployment	Comments
Shigella spp. (Shigellosis)	Aerosol dispersal of food/water contamination	Rarely contagious
Salmonella typhi (Typhoid Fever)	Food/water contamination	Rarely contagious
Rhinderpest Virus	Aerosol dispersal and infections of animals	Highly contagious
Newcastle Disease Virus	Aerosol dispersal and infections of animals	Highly contagious
Foot and Mouth Disease	Aerosol dispersal and infection of animals	Highly contagious
Botulinum Toxin	Aerosol dispersal or food/water contamination	Not contagious
Ricin	Aerosol dispersal or food/water contamination	Not contagious

the various biological warfare agents in descending order of relative difficulties. The following lists are based on a number of factors, including acquisition of agent or supplies, relative ease of production and dissemination, and agent stability. As a rule of thumb, toxins are the easiest to produce, while bacteria are more challenging, and viruses, the most difficult. The various agents or toxins are ranked based on their impact and their degree of difficulty in obtaining and handling (Tables 1, 2 and 3).

Photo Bibliography

Figure 5.6-1: A technician in the process of injecting and egg with the influenza virus. Historically, eggs have been used for replicating viruses. The picture was taken and released by the Food and Drug Administration. Public domain photo

Figure 5.6-3: This photograph depicts the colonial morphology displayed by Gram-negative *Brucella abortus* bacteria, which was grown on a medium of sheep blood agar (SBA), for a 48 hour time period, at a temperature of 37˚C. This Petri dish and its contents were incubated in a CO_2 incubator. *B. abortus* bacteria are known to cause the disease brucellosis. This photograph was taken by Dr. T. Parker and A. Marsh in 2010 and released by the CDC. Public domain photo

Figure 5.6-4: Scientists examining culture flasks under a laminar flow hood. Picture was taken by the Nation Cancer Institute, under the direction of National Institute of Health. Public domain photo

Figure 5.6-5: A commercial available pressure cooker that can be used to sterilize equipment. This photograph was released by the DCI Counterterrorist Center, Central Intelligence Agency in May 2003. Public domain photo

Figure 5.6-6: A commercial available autoclave that can be used to sterilize equipment. This photograph was released by the DCI Counterterrorist Center, Central Intelligence Agency in May 2003. Public domain photo

Figure 5.6-7: A photograph of a makeshift incubator made from a commercially available cooler. This photograph was released by the DCI Counterterrorist Center, Central Intelligence Agency in May 2003. Public domain photo

Figure 5.6-8: This photograph depicts a converted water container into an improvised fermenter. This photograph was released by the DCI Counterterrorist Center, Central Intelligence Agency in May 2003. Public domain photo

Figure 5.6-9: Composite photographs of various filtration systems. ① Simple filtration, ② vacuum filtration and ③ industrial filtration system. These photographs were acquired from NIH, EPA and USDA. Public domain photo

About the Authors

William E. Houston (ret. Colonel U.S. Army) received his doctorate in Molecular Microbiology from Vanderbilt University in 1971. Colonel Houston served as the Director, U.S. Army Medical Chemical Defense Research Program, Office of the Surgeon General, Washington D.C. from 1982-1985. Presently, he is a consultant and lecturer for the National Center for Biomedical Research and Training for Louisiana State University, a program sponsored by the Department of Homeland Security.

Phillip Yuan Pei Jen received his doctorate in Human Anatomy and Physiology from The Chinese University of Hong Kong in 1995. Presently, Dr. Jen is an Associate Professor of Biology at Gordon State College located in Georgia.

Amanda Duffus received her doctorate in Biological Sciences from Queen Mary University of London in 2010. Presently, Dr. Duffus is an Assistant Professor of Biology at Gordon State College located in Georgia.

Mustapha Durojaiye received his doctorate in Biological Sciences from Clark Atlanta University in 1981. Presently Dr. Durojaiye is Interim Department Head of Biology and Professor of Biology at Gordon State College located in Georgia.

CPSIA information can be obtained
at www.ICGtesting.com
Printed in the USA
LVHW061813111120
671417LV00009B/531